BIOMEDICAL ENGINEERING, TRENDS, RESEARCH AND TECHNOLOGIES

Edited by **Małgorzata Anna Komorowska**
and **Sylwia Olsztyńska-Janus**

INTECHOPEN.COM

Biomedical Engineering, Trends, Research and Technologies
Edited by Małgorzata Anna Komorowska and Sylwia Olsztyńska-Janus

Published by InTech
Janeza Trdine 9, 51000 Rijeka, Croatia

Edition 2014

Publishing Process Manager Ana Nikolic

Technical Editor Teodora Smiljanic

Cover Designer InTech Design Team

Image Copyright Olivier Le Queinec, 2010. Used under license from Shutterstock.com

Additional hard copies can be obtained from orders@intechopen.com

Biomedical Engineering, Trends, Research and Technologies,
Edited by Małgorzata Anna Komorowska and Sylwia Olsztyńska-Janus
p. cm.
ISBN 978-953-307-514-3

INTECH
open science | open minds

Contents

Preface

"Biomedical Engineering encompasses fundamental concepts in engineering, biology and medicine to develop innovative approaches and new devices, materials, implants, algorithms, processes and systems for the medical industry. These could be used for the assessment and evaluation of technology; for prevention, diagnosis, and treatment of diseases; for patient care and rehabilitation, and for improving medical practice and health care delivery". This remarkable citation after Wikipedia provides the very essence of the scientific and technical fields known as biomedical engineering. Parallel to the technical achievements widely introduced into medicine, scientists are looking for even more efficient examination methods for complex biological systems and phenomena at the molecular level. Physicochemical methods combined with numerous interdisciplinary techniques have been accepted as powerful tools leading to better understanding of biological processes and diseases.

This book has been organized in 8 sections corresponding to sub-disciplines within the biomedical engineering. First chapter in section 1 introduces the ethical and legal contexts of medical sciences. The next one contains an analysis of the style of writing the biomedical papers. Section 2 focuses on methods for the chemical and structural characterization of biomolecules. Four chapters in this section demonstrate how the molecular spectroscopy can be applied for the structural resolution of biological systems at the molecular level within cells, organelles and large molecular complexes. The next two sections deal with novel developments in creation of nanotechnological devices and introduction of cell therapies. Section 5 contains 6 chapters concentrating on different types of natural medicines, dietary supplements and also on the study of biomaterials such as hydroxyapatite. Closing sections 6 and 7 are devoted to the remarkably increasing subdiscipline – bioinformatics. Applications in medical diagnosis are presented in section 6, achievements in organization, education and information retrieval supported by informatical tools are described in section 7. Final section is devoted to the technological and instrumental aids; very interesting discussion is presented focusing on the question: how far can we expand the application of single use medical devices?

This book is addressed to scientists and professionals working in the wide area of biomedical studies from biochemistry, pharmacy to medicine and clinical engineering. The panorama of problems presented in this volume may be of special interest for the young, looking for new, original technologies and new trends in biomedical engineering.

December 2010

Prof. Małgorzata Komorowska and Ph.D. Eng. Sylwia Olsztyńska-Janus
Wrocław, Poland

Part 1

The Ethical and Legal Contests

1

Conceptual Models of the Human Organism: Towards a New Biomedical Understanding of the Individual

Stephen Lewis
University of Chester
United Kingdom

1. Introduction

Central to the conduct of ethical medical practice is the need to have some conception of what disease and health might be. It is the concept of disease which prompts medical intervention and that of health which either prevents unwarranted intervention in the first place or informs its cessation when the patient is deemed to be well again. As highlighted by Reznek (1987), it is not only those directly involved in clinical activities who are affected by these concepts. The work of scientists in medically-related fields can also be directed by how these concepts are understood. What is and what is not an appropriate project may be affected by how disease and health are understood with the granting of funds and other resources similarly affected.

An individual's legal status and the responsibilities expected of them may also be affected by how they are classified medically. Somebody with a psychiatric disturbance may be excused for an act which, in others, might be deemed wilfully criminal by virtue of their condition. Alternatively, somebody with what is classed as a disability may be provided with financial assistance and/or specialised equipment at public expense. They may even be excused the expectation of work altogether.

How individuals are labelled medically - how their 'condition' is classified - is important. However, defining the terms 'disease' and 'health', upon which much of this has rested, has proven to be extremely difficult and it may well be that an alternative approach is long overdue.

2. The current biomedical model

The prevailing model upon which much of modern Western medicine relies is the so-called 'biomedical model' (Davey & Seale, 1996). Sometimes this may be shortened to simply 'medical model'. Indeed, the terms tend to be used somewhat interchangeably to refer to the same way of thinking about the well-being and ailments of individuals. There is certainly no appreciable difference in the way the terms 'biomedical model' and medical model' are used. In addition, the title 'disease model' may also be sometimes used. This title is perhaps more telling. One of the central characteristics of Western medical thinking is its emphasis on disease and with anything else which might be deemed to be 'wrong' with the patient.

As the term implies, the biomedical model is an attempt at combining biological and medical thinking in the clinical setting. There are two inter-linked ways in which the biomedical model can be seen working in practice.

Firstly, scientific knowledge gained from non-clinical research is often used to inform patient treatment. Secondly, clinical practice itself is undertaken in a scientific way by adopting the same methodology and intellectual rigour as found in pure scientific research. This approach became typical of the style of medicine practised in the West particularly during the twentieth century and it has become for us that century's medical legacy. Indeed, it is still the prevailing model by which the medical profession operates and, as a result, it is also the way in which people's ailments are understood and treated. Furthermore, this impacts on the attitude shown to the people affected. Once the medical focus is fixed upon what is wrong with the patient, that patient can very easily become a bystander and less of a participant in their own ailments as their bodies are probed and exposed to various treatments.

Seedhouse (2001) identified in this model the following characteristics:

1. That health is the absence of disease.
2. That health is a commodity with a wide-ranging commercial/business-like dimension.
3. That medical science has produced an accumulation of knowledge which can be applied to bodies as physical objects rather than to bodies as people.
4. That the best way to cure disease is to reduce bodies to their smallest constituent parts.
5. That health can be quantified in relation to norms for populations, particular groups of individuals, and individuals.
6. That medicine is and should be a form of engineering.

In essence, the biomedical model explains a patient's ailments as being the result of some anatomical or physiological cause which, in turn, is deemed to be a fault with the patient's body. Understanding the causal processes leads directly - or so it is assumed - to appropriate treatments: remove the cause and one removes the source of suffering and, subsequently, the suffering itself with the result that the patient is restored to health. The logic seems reasonable enough and, to an extent, this approach seems to have been successful. Arguably, the biomedical model has provided clinicians with exactly what they have needed to do their job: a clear and direct way of approaching the identification and remedying of their patients' problems. However, this apparent success may be somewhat illusory.

The emphasis of the biomedical model is on the patient's body. The psychological, behavioural, social and wider environmental aspects of their ailments are not integrated into this model – certainly not overtly. Whether or not a particular clinician chooses to include these aspects is another matter. If they do, it will tend to be at their own discretion and in their own particular style and manner. Significantly, the biomedical model does not oblige clinicians to make any such consideration.

Furthermore, the biomedical model fails to recognise and take into account the multi-factorial nature of cause. If the cause of a patient's ailment is multi-factorial, then effecting some form of cure is likely to require a multi-factorial approach too. By following this model, health professionals limit themselves to dealing primarily with the patient's physical state when other aspects of their lives might need particular attention for complete well-being to be achieved. For example, a patient may be unwell because of a lifestyle choice such as over-eating, smoking or excessive alcohol consumption. The simplistic biomedical remedy is to prescribe a change in diet, a cessation of smoking and a limitation of alcohol consumption to safe levels, respectively. While these recommendations, if adopted, may well bring about beneficial physical effects in the patient's body, this approach completely overlooks what might be described as the 'cause of the cause'. The patient's eating, smoking and drinking habits may stem from some non-physical problem or set of problems to do with the wider aspects of their life. Factors which may have led to these habits in the first place are largely ignored. A patient who adopts the recommendation to change their lifestyle habits in the way described may be physically improved but still have what might be described as 'quality of life' problems. These, because they fall outside the biomedical model, are not usually seen as specifically clinical problems and have not become an integral part of medical thinking. Yet they can impact directly on an individual's overall well-being.

In the biomedical model, there is also a tacit separation between the mind and the body. Indeed, a mind-body dualism is arguably central to this model. Exactly why this should be is unclear. As will be noted below, the biomedical model does not seem to have appeared as the result of a specific formulation but seems instead to have evolved over a period of time and while there is a historical and philosophical precedent for a separation of mind and body in the work of René Descartes (1596-1650), the biomedical separation may have a much more prosaic explanation. There is a sense in which each individual feels as if they are a person with or within a body. It is not uncommon for people to use expressions such as 'my hand' or 'my heart' as if they were objects which belonged to them rather than being integral parts of them. The linguistic environment within which people operate is not one conducive to an integration of mind and body but rather one of separation. Thus, to the average individual, mind and body are not continuous; they are not a unity and it is, therefore, very easy for people - including clinicians - to make such a separation.

Consequently, the extent to which a patient's experience of pain and suffering are part of the biomedical model is also a moot point. There is no mention of these in Seedhouse's characterisation above. That a patient is in some form of distress is only implicit in the biomedical model in that it is taken for granted that this is what causes people to seek medical help in the first place. Thereafter, however, once medical help has been procured, attention is focussed primarily on the cause of the ailment and upon its removal or, failing this, on the treatment of symptoms until the individual gets well of their own accord. Pain gets treated quite separately via the provision of analgesia. It does not get considered from a psychological perspective. The prevailing notion is that pain is experienced because of some physical cause within the body. Analgesia is given to take away that experience while the task of removing the physical cause is undertaken. In effect, there is no fully developed theory of suffering in its wider sense within the biomedical model.

Another effect of the mind-body dualism is an assumption that mind and body can be treated separately. The body, it is further assumed, can be treated as a machine and a mechanical metaphor for how it operates can be adopted. Accordingly, the biomedical model assumes that diseases can be characterised as resulting from identifiable physical causes - that is, there must be a mechanical element to disease. As a corollary to this, it is assumed that applying ever more sophisticated technological investigations in determining the mechanical nature of the disease can only be to the increasing benefit of the patient. However, this may not necessarily be the case. Tinetti and Fried (2004) have noted that "(a) primary focus on disease ... inadvertently leads to undertreatment, overtreatment, or mistreatment". Confronted with this, it may well be the clinician who, in fact, benefits most from these technological advances - or at least some of them. Being better informed does not necessarily lead to better treatment. What an extensive battery of diagnostic tests certainly can do is allow clinicians to guard themselves against liability for misdiagnosis and inappropriate choice of treatment.

Historically, the biomedical model never had a single definitive founding moment. Instead, a series of events in the history of biology and medicine appear to have contributed to its gradual emergence. These include the work of Giovanni Battista Morgagni (1682-1771) in founding the field of pathology in the eighteenth century, the general progress made in establishing physiology as a science in the nineteenth century (with the work of Claude Bernard (1813-1878) occupying a significant and enduring position as a forerunner to the notion of homeostasis developed by Walter Cannon (1871-1945) in the 1920s) and the specific proposals about the nature of medical training made early in the twentieth century in the Flexner Report (1910). However, as Keating and Cambrosio (2003) have noted "... the object of medicine is not the body per se but, rather, models of the body". The emphasis that the biomedical model places on the body is, in fact, an emphasis on a model of the body: an abstraction.

The models we use influence and may even drive our understanding of the object to which those models apply. Here, our models of the human body influence the practice of medicine itself. Until the nineteenth century, the prevailing model of the body in Western medicine was based upon the ancient notion of humoralism. How well or unwell one felt was thought to be the product of the way in which four supposed bodily humors - black bile, yellow bile, phlegm and blood - were in proportion to each other. Therapies and treatments were delivered not in accordance with physical observations about the nature of the body alone but in terms of how these observations were interpreted in terms of humoral theory. For example, if a patient's ailment was deemed to be related to an excess of the humor blood, this excess was alleviated by subjecting them to the process of blood-letting. Any anaemia that may have resulted from this process seems to have gone unnoticed. While we have moved on since then to become more accurately informed about the true physical nature of the body, we still adhere to conceptual models via which to operate, as the example of the biomedical model illustrates. Any model by which we operate is an abstraction from what is currently known. As a result, such models are always in need of refinement as knowledge and understanding develop.

Given this historical background, one might reasonably expect the biomedical model to be something which continues to evolve and to be refined as new knowledge and understanding emerge. While research does produce new findings from which new treatments and therapeutic techniques are developed within the context of the current model, the conceptual basis upon which the biomedical model is founded appears to be somewhat more static. Arguably, the biomedical model has not, strictly speaking, kept pace with wider intellectual developments. In practice, it is now quite clear that the cause-effect relationship does not hold. Frequently, clinicians are confronted with patients whose ailments are without apparent physical cause. Similarly, routine screening can bring to light potentially life-threatening lesions for which there is an absence of any experienced symptoms. Those conditions which cannot be accommodated by the biomedical model often cause clinicians considerable problems in terms of decision making (Marinker, 1975). Yet, the central cause-effect assumption remains. This reflects, in part at least, a too rigid application of the wider scientific expectation that all observable phenomena within the physical universe are explicable in physical terms. It is questionable whether the body, even if seen merely as a set of physical processes, really operates in quite that way.

One is compelled to ask not only to what extent the prevailing biomedical model is useful in contributing to clinical practice but also to what extent this model truly represents the biology of the individuals concerned. Ailing, in the absence of apparent physical cause, and the absence of symptoms, in the presence of life threatening lesions, seem to refute the viability of the biomedical model as currently formulated. Indeed, the conceptual bases upon which much of Western medicine is founded may not be as sound as might be expected.

One of the core problems with the prevailing biomedical model is its focus on disease. Health, it tends to be assumed, is merely the absence of disease. In effect, something that exists because of the absence of something else - some sort of default status. This is in contrast to the constitutional statement of the World Health Organization which holds that '(h)ealth is a state of complete physical, mental and social well-being and not merely the absence of disease or infirmity' (WHO, 1948). While the first part of this statement has its critics, the latter clause tends to receive little criticism. Those whom one might have expected to be most exercised by the problem of defining the notions of health and disease - because they are core to their professional practice - are those who seem least interested in their conceptual foundations. When posing the question 'What is health?' Richard Smith, editor of the British Medical Journal (BMJ) stated that '(f)or most doctors that's an uninteresting question. Doctors are interested in disease, not health. Medical textbooks are a massive catalogue of diseases.' However, when it comes to diseases, defining what these are seems to be equally difficult as surveys published in the BMJ have discovered (Campbell et al., 1979; Smith, 2002). Offered a list of named conditions with which clinicians frequently deal, different groups of people - including medical academics and general practitioners - were asked to say which they thought were diseases and which they thought were not. Noticeably, there was not complete agreement. There were differences of opinion within and between the groups surveyed. Clearly, deciding whether something merits being called a disease is not a simple proposition.

One finds there to be in the philosophy of medicine, however, much more debate about how to define the terms 'disease' and 'health' with two different schools of thought having emerged (Nordenfelt, 1986; 2007a,b). One school of thought, sometimes called 'descriptivism' or 'naturism' because it holds that disease and health can be understood in physical terms, is represented by the work of Christopher Boorse (1975; 1977; 1997). His work has been particularly prominent within this debate and is in some respects a formulation of the biomedical model. There is certainly a pathological and physiological emphasis within Boorse's description of what constitutes disease The other school, sometimes called 'normativism' because it sees the ascription of the terms 'disease' and 'health' as labels expressing a value-judgement, has come to be associated with the work of Lennart Nordenfelt (Khushf, 2007). While not overlooking the pathological and physiological, Nordenfelt takes a different approach. His emphasis is on health and, using action theory, the individual's ability to achieve various 'vital goals' associated with daily living.

A simple dichotomy between health and disease - or of being well and unwell - seems to pervade biomedical thinking which has become somewhat linear in nature. In various pictorial descriptions, a simple line is used to represent the health-disease (well-unwell) dichotomy (Seedhouse, 2001; Downie et al 1996). This is also, arguably, a tacit assumption within the philosophical debate about the definition of disease and health. Health and disease are largely seen as dichotomous categories into which patients may be placed. By portraying 'disease' and 'health' in this way, as if at opposite ends of a single axis, the biomedical model has not contributed to the resolution of the philosophical debate and finding philosophically rigorous definitions of these terms remains elusive. Indeed, it may be argued that the biomedical model, at least as currently formulated, has contributed to the apparent obfuscation. At best, the biomedical model can only be said to provide a heuristic by which clinicians work.

Sadegh-Zedah (2000) has strongly criticised this bipartite 'either-or' aspect of thinking about disease and health. This he attributed to an uncritical adherence to another aspect of scientific thinking, Aristotelian logic with its law of the excluded middle. Instead, he suggested, it might be more appropriate to apply Fuzzy Logic recognising a continuity between the two extremes. Adhering to the dichotomy - and even allowing for this continuity - means that those scenarios described above, which cannot be accommodated by the biomedical model, are still simply left in abeyance.

The healthy or 'well' state is also assumed to be the 'normal' state; the diseased or 'unwell' is assumed to be the 'abnormal' state. This attitude, deemed to be currently prevailing in medical schools and textbooks, has been labelled 'Naïve Normalism' (Sadegh-Zedah, 2000). The prescription of normal and abnormal states is typically undertaken by comparison to population means for given anatomical or physiological parameters. Deviations outside prescribed limits either side of these statistical means forms a basis for clinical concern. The individual is constantly compared to others in order to determine what is and what is not 'normal' for them. However, as Sadegh-Zedah (2000) has also pointed out, what 'normal' really is - apart its numerical interpretation - remains unclear.

3. The biopsychosocial model – an attempt at improvement

One of the most prominent critics of the biomedical model and advocate for change was the American psychiatrist, George Engel (1913-1999). Having identified the need for a new model (Engel, 1977), he proposed an alternative: the biopsychosocial model (Engel, 1981; 1997). Engel intended this model to be a "conceptual framework to guide clinicians in their everyday work with patients" (Engel, 1997) as well as a framework for a wider more scientific understanding of what he called the "human domain". That is, a model to act as a general framework to guide theoretical and empirical exploration, not only of processes or states that are called illnesses or diseases but something more inclusive when trying to understand the human condition as a whole. Importantly, Engel's work highlighted how easy it is to forget that it is a person who is central to any understanding of suffering and its causes. It is not only the physical processes involved when an individual is feeling unwell that should command centre stage but a whole range of features at a number of different hierarchical levels of interaction (Figure 1). It is the individual as a whole - as a physical organism and as a person interacting with the world around - that is essential to any understanding of the notions of disease and health.

Despite initial optimism when first proposed, the biopsychosocial model failed to find the key role in clinical medicine for which it was intended. While Engel's ideas still attract followers (see, White, 2005), his proposals have met with limited success and have not fully entered mainstream medical thought. The main legacy of that model appears to be that the term 'biopsychosocial model' has come to be used to mean something akin to 'holistic'. When the term 'biopsychosocial' is used, it is more likely to be as a form of shorthand implying 'widely-inclusive' or 'all-encompassing' rather than offering a way of detailing what is going on at the different levels Engel had envisaged.

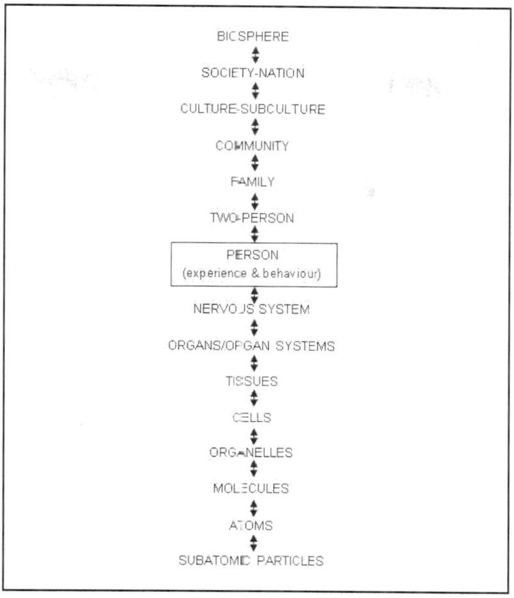

Fig. 1. The Systems Hierarchy (Levels of Organisation) of the Biopsychosocial Model (after Engel, 1981)

The biopsychosocial model does improve upon the standard biomedical model in that it recognises a link between mind and body. The two influence each other but exactly how is unclear. The biopsychosocial model does not set out to explain what the mechanisms involved might be. This is, perhaps, a good thing. To have speculated was not strictly necessary and to have speculated and found to be wrong would have cast a shadow over the rest of his ideas. Instead, the biopsychosocial model recognises there to be a link between mind and body in a somewhat more empirical way.

The biopsychosocial model is not without its critics. It has been criticised for not explaining how the levels Engel highlights interact (Malmgren, 2005). It is true that the biopsychosocial model does lack what might be called a theory of the organism. The list of different levels at which different effects may be observed is left without a detailed explanation of the way in which these levels influence each other being given. The biopsychosocial model is able to accommodate a good deal of information about what occurs at each level as was demonstrated using the clinical example of a myocardial infarction (Engel, 1981). However, its explanatory and predictive capabilities are quite limited. Indeed, Engel's model begs the question of how much detail is necessary in order to understand the organism as a whole.

Instead of a series of hierarchical levels, an alternative is to conceive of a series of nested (or Chinese) boxes (Grobstein, 1965). Where Engel encounters a problem is that his readers require of him an explanation of how the different levels - or nested boxes - influence each other (Malmgren, 2005). It may not be strictly necessary for all the minutiae to be explained before an acceptable picture of the organism emerges. Might one reasonably choose instead to put a lid on one or other of the boxes and to view the operation of each box separately without going into the finer detail of the workings within? Indeed, the biopsychosocial model owes much to Ludwig von Bertalanffy's (1901-1972) 'General Systems Theory' (Malmgren, 2005). In such an approach, it is usually more informative to explain the behaviour of a system as a whole. Such behaviour is not merely the summation of the behaviour of the parts. Emergent properties may only manifest themselves at certain levels of organisation and might be missed by looking too deeply at fine detail.

In engineering, a black box is a something which can be viewed purely in terms of its input, output and the transfer function that gives the relationship between the two rather than in terms of the details of internal operation. There need be no knowledge of the processes occurring within the black box for it to be understandable in some way (Figure 2). Instead of requiring increasingly precise amounts of information about different levels of organisation, it may be more desirable, in order to understand a system as a whole more clearly, to put a lid on one of the conceptual boxes and deliberately ignore what lies within. This produces a form of black box. More appropriately, perhaps, one might refer to this as a 'closed box'. 'Closed', that is, in the sense that the contents and their various processes are hidden from view and 'closed' in the sense that the lid has been deliberately put on. This is a somewhat counter-reductionist approach. While Engel attempts to look at all levels associated with the individual simultaneously, a way of understanding just the individual as a single whole may prove to be a better starting point.

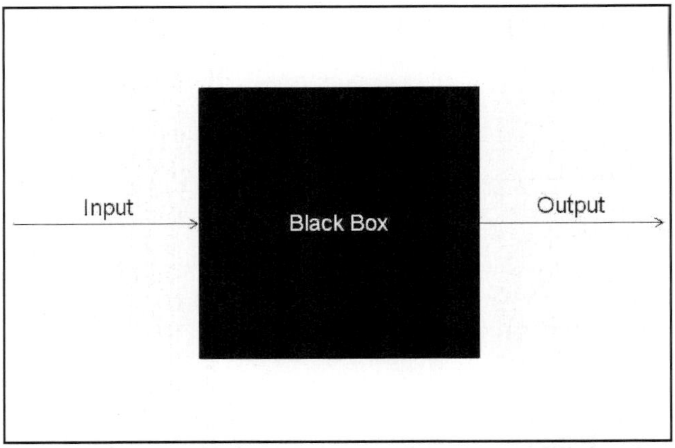

Fig. 2. A Black Box. Only the input and output are known and, as a result, the transformation that has taken place within the black box.

4. Another way ahead

Despite various criticisms, the biomedical model still occupies a prominent place in Western medicine. Indeed, it has proved useful despite its flaws and its complete removal or replacement is likely to prove virtually impossible as Engel's attempts with the biopsychosocial model have demonstrated. The persistence of the biomedical model is, perhaps, not surprising. It has, in many respects, withstood the test of time, having been very successful in acting as a useful - if imperfect - heuristic. However, that is not to say that the biomedical model cannot be improved. Instead of attempting a complete replacement, a more productive approach might be to build upon its useful features, correct its flaws and expand it as necessary. A revision of the existing biomedical model is needed. Such a revision would need to ensure that there was a firm foundation in biological science such that a range of biomedical and biomechanical disciplines could operate in a more informed manner when dealing with individual patients.

Although the name biomedical model suggests that there is already a strong biological component, not every aspect of biology pertinent to medicine can be said to have been utilised by this model. For example, it is only in recent years that the need for a place for evolutionary biology in medicine has been highlighted with the emergence of the field of evolutionary (Darwinian) medicine - and that well over one hundred years after the publication of Darwin's 'On The Origin of Species' (see, for example, Williams & Nesse 1991; Nesse & Williams, 1995, 1999; Nesse, 2001a,b; Nesse et al., 2006).

Out of a consideration of the range of ideas that evolutionary biology can bring to medicine comes the question of the relationship between the notion of individual 'survival' and a patient's overall state as an integrated physical, experiential and interactive system. 'Survival' should not be seen as simply a matter of whether or not one can stay alive. There is a 'quality of life' element as well which influences whether one merely survives in the sense of just barely staying alive or whether one survives well and flourishes. It is in the latter context that the biological imperative of reproduction can be best performed. For example, those female animals which are required to invest much of themselves in producing and raising offspring would, if experiencing a low quality of life, be less likely to succeed in bringing many to full reproductive maturity. In seeking medical help, an individual is, in effect, seeking help with their quality of life - although not, of course, necessarily with the aim of enhancing reproductive success in mind. Somebody who visits their doctor with an ailment is, in effect, acknowledging a diminution of some perceived aspect of their quality of life. Thus, what biology has to say about this in relation to notions of survival and quality of life is relevant to medical practice.

As a result, one may reasonably propose that one should first seek to understand, in biological terms, what contributes to the individual's quality of life via an examination of the notion of individual survival before going on to try to define the notions of 'disease' and 'health' *per se*.

4.1 On modelling

The need to explain complex systems such as the human body in disease and in health leads to the development of models which in themselves are interpretations of reality. All models are, by their very nature, abstractions. A drawing of a bird that is intended to help bird-watchers identify different species is, in effect, a model, an abstraction. Such a drawing is not an exact likeness of any particular bird that one is likely to see. Rather it is a representation of a whole species. There is, in that drawing, a certain generality.

Similarly, in medicine, it is necessary to identify different types of people. Firstly, there are those who should and those who should not be classified as 'patients'. Secondly, of those who should be classified as patients, it is necessary to differentiate between different types of patient. That is, those who are in need of different kinds of medical attention. A way of distinguishing between these different categories is needed. However, the distinction between 'patient' and 'non-patient' need not mirror the dichotomy between 'disease' and 'health' - which seems to be what the biomedical model seeks to do. Help with enhancing one's quality of life is broader than this.

One must be clear about the purpose of making models. Two major types of model may be identified. These may be described as 'Models of' and 'Models for'. 'Models of' are those models which simply describe an object or process in simplified (although not necessarily simplistic) terms. 'Models for' are those models which have been constructed with a particular purpose in mind. 'Models for' may also share some of the characteristics of 'models of' type models. They may include some form of description of an object or process which then provides something with a practical use. Astrophysical models of star or black hole formation, for example, are models of how something happens but these models may have no immediate practical usefulness on Earth. Models of physiological processes can be models of what occurs within a body and can be of purely theoretical interest - especially if that process occurs in a species quite unlike our own. However, when they are applicable clinically, some physiological models allow for understanding a patient's pathophysiological processes better and may help in remedying their ailments more effectively. It follows that it is of paramount importance in the medically-related fields that the best possible models are devised in order to provide the best possible patient care.

5. Understanding the individual in two biomedical dimensions

In organismal terms, human individuals are not simply physical objects or even sets of physical processes; they are persons - minds as well as bodies. In particular, an individual can be considered as having two concurrent and interwoven characteristics. Firstly, the individual is a materially self-referential system in that there are numerous physiological processes that are monitored and regulated at a physical level via different forms of feedback. Secondly, the individual is experientially self-aware in that conscious and also sub-conscious monitoring and regulation are also being affected at a higher level. If, for example, the body becomes dehydrated, this is not merely a physical change accompanied by concomitant physiological responses. There is also a higher level experience of 'thirst'. Biologically, being 'known' to oneself in these various ways allows the individual to respond accordingly so as to ensure continued survival - in this example, by drinking.

5.1 The physical dimension

At the non-conscious physical level, biochemical and physiological pathways and their regulatory mechanisms are involved. It is with these that the current biomedical model is largely concerned - with much of the emphasis being confined to biochemical and physiological detail. However, if considered from an organismal perspective, these processes have a much greater significance. They can operate in such a way as to ensure organismal survival or they can operate in a way that endangers the survival of the whole organism - or any gradation in between. If these processes work *en masse* so as to ensure survival, we may consider this form of operation to be 'ordered' or 'orderly'. If these processes do not work *en masse* to ensure survival, we may consider this form of operation to be 'disordered' or 'disorderly'. The criteria for conferring these appellations are quite simple, being based on the overall effect on the survival of the individual as an organism. By concentrating on biochemical or physiological detail alone, it is easy to overlook the organism-level role played by the numerous physiological processes occurring within the human body simultaneously. Here one seeks to avoid this by using the black box approach described above. One is looking primarily at how the whole organism operates, not the sum of its parts. One has closed the box at organism level.

5.2 The experiential dimension

Human beings also have a capacity for self-awareness. They are conscious of how they feel. In particular, the ability to feel unwell or otherwise distressed seems to be especially significant as these experiences are often indicative of some physical disorder. Raised to the conscious attention of the individual, remedial action is possible. While consciousness may be something that concerns the psychologist or the philosopher, the notion of self-awareness is something that has been rather under-represented in biology - especially in relation to the experience of illness (Lewis, 2007a,b) - and, unsurprisingly, is missing from the biomedical model. This is unfortunate as this is an important capacity for an organism to possess. Without the capacity for self-awareness - at conscious and/or sub-conscious levels - one would lack the ability to be aware of any need to respond to disadvantageous changes in one's internal environment. Should this capacity become disturbed, it would impact negatively on individual survival.

Although akin to the separation of mind and body, this division into physical and experiential is subtly different. The notion of 'mind' usually implies consciousness and cognitive self-awareness. Within the experiential dimension as envisaged here, all organismal feedback mechanisms are included whether or not one is aware of them.

5.3 A two-dimensional (biomedical) model

The two dimensions described above may be represented graphically as a plane as depicted in Figure 3 (Lewis, 2009). Importantly, the axes are arranged so that as one moves along

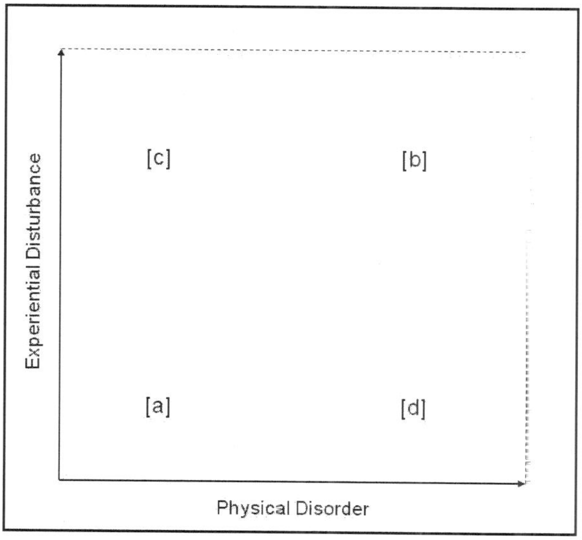

Fig. 3. A new two-dimensional biomedical model

them, there is an increase in physical disorder and experiential disturbance the further one travels away from the origin. With these increasing levels of disorder and disturbance come increasing levels of threat to individual survival. As one moves from left to right along the horizontal axis, the level of physiological disorder increases such that life is increasingly less viable and a point ultimately reached when the individual dies. As one moves up the vertical axis, the level of experiential disturbance increases to a point where the effectiveness of its contribution to survival declines and ultimately ceases.

The intention here is to depict something of the overall state of the individual. They are not being fitted into one or other of the dichotomous states of 'disease' or 'health' at either end of a line, as occurs in the current biomedical model. Instead, they are being given a position on a plane, the different points upon which represent different overall states of the individual and different abilities to survive. Positions on the plane are not static. The position that an individual occupies can vary as their physical and experiential states change. This may occur during the progress of a pathological or psychiatric condition or due to the changes concomitant with the normal course of life.

5.4 Representing clinical cases

An individual who feels well and whose physical processes are operating in an orderly way may be represented somewhere to the lower left of the plane [a]. Likewise, an individual who feels unwell and whose physical processes are not operating in an orderly way may be represented somewhere to the upper right of the plane [b]. Exactly where on the plane one might choose to place a particular individual is a matter of clinical judgement rather than mere physiological measurement. However, in a clinical consultation, what may be more important is using this model as a tool for assessing the patient more informatively. It is not simply a case of the individual being fitted into a category. Rather, it is a matter of assessing the individual and developing a better mental picture of their own particular overall state. By separating out these two dimensions of the individual so that they become available during clinical consultation, the examining clinician is more readily alerted to the need to take not only the physical but the experiential into account.

As noted earlier, not all cases presenting to the clinician can be accommodated by the old biomedical model and these caused clinicians serious problems (Marinker, 1975). These were cases where an individual felt unwell but for which there was no obvious physical cause and cases where the individual felt well yet had a lesion of some sort. While these cannot be fitted into the current biomedical model, they can now be represented by this two-dimensional model quite readily. Position [c] represents the situation when the individual feels unwell but for which there is no obvious physical cause. Here, there is an experience of disturbance but no obvious physical disorder. Position [d] represents the situation where the individual feels well but has a lesion of some sort. Here, there is no feeling of being unwell but there is a degree of physical disorder. Thus, lesion-less symptoms and symptom-less lesions can now be represented alongside the more easily accommodated states.

In a clinical consultation, this would again act as a useful tool. In both cases, there is now a way of characterizing and understanding the patient better. Furthermore, this model also allows phenomena such as the placebo and nocebo effects to be represented. When somebody takes a dummy pill or undergoes a sham operation, they may feel better (placebo effect) or worse (nocebo effect) afterwards. This may be represented by a downward shift from one's previous position on the plane or by an upward shift respectively.

6. Understanding the individual further - a third dimension

While physical and experiential aspects of an individual can be represented using a two-dimensional model, there still remain other aspects which both contribute to individual survival and are potentially of clinical relevance. These concern the behaviours expressed by an individual. It is through behaviour that the individual interacts with the wider world - drawing upon what can prove beneficial or trying to counter that which is disadvantageous, as appropriate. Each can have the express aim of contributing to individual survival. Although humans display a diverse range of behaviours, those primarily directed at survival through such activities as eating, drinking, finding safety, maintaining general hygiene etc. are those that are of particular importance here. Any one or more of these needs (see, for example, Maslow, 1943), if left unattended would impinge negatively upon the survival of the individual.

Thus, to the two axes already considered, a third - behavioural - axis may be added (Figure 4). This is an axis of behaviour in terms of an individual's ability to perform actions conducive to their individual survival; an axis concerned with interaction with the world. In particular, this is an axis which describes the extent to which those abilities are constrained. In keeping with the approach adopted for the first two axes, the further one moves away from the origin, the greater the constraint there is upon those abilities. That is, as one moves away from the origin, the greater the deleterious effects on survival become.

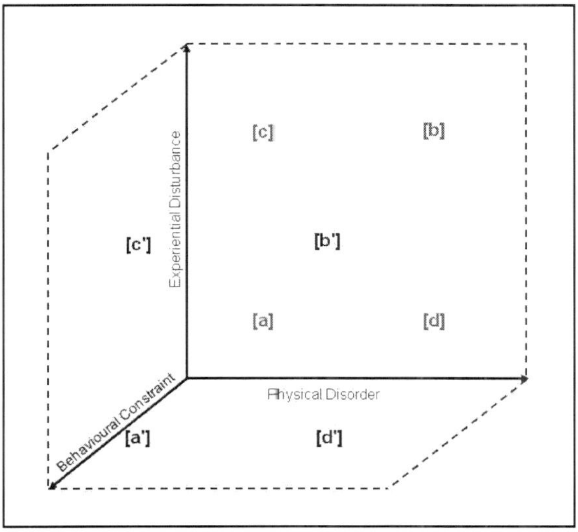

Fig. 4. A new three-dimensional biomedical model

Although it is possible, for clinical purposes, to assess a patient in terms of just the first two dimensions described above, the third is not without clinical relevance. When a patient is discharged from hospital, their ability to look after themselves, or be looked after, is often assessed. Those patients who cannot adequately look after themselves are often discharged into the care of someone who can support them. This assessment is, in effect, an assessment of the patient's ability to behave in a way conducive to their individual survival. Adding this axis formalises the process.

Taking the four previously considered areas ([a]-[d] on Figure 3) and relating each to what the third axis depicts, position [a'] depicts an individual who feels well and has no physical lesions yet for some reason is constrained in the performance of those tasks conducive to individual survival. Position [b'] depicts an individual who feels unwell and has a lesion and for this, or some other reason, is constrained in performing the necessary survival tasks. Position [c'] depicts an individual who feels unwell but has no physical lesion and because they feel unwell, or some other reason, is constrained in performing the necessary survival tasks while position [d'] depicts an individual who feels well but has a physical lesion and for this, or some other reason, is similarly constrained.

When the constraints on an individual's ability to perform tasks conducive to their survival arise from some internal, physical cause, then there are likely to be medical connotations that need to be considered. When constraints result from some external source - for example, a constraint due to some aspect of the lived environment or habitat in which the individual lives - the issue is more likely to be one needing the auspices of some other agency such as social services. Both, however, may be interpreted as modern out-workings of the notion of biological survival.

6.1 Disability (vs inability)

The addition of a third axis has the effect of separating out the issue of physical disability - formerly known as 'physical handicap' - as a distinct issue for consideration. The question of how people with a physical disability should be considered within the biomedical model is often queried; should they be treated from a medical perspective or in some other way? Based on the current biomedical model, it is sometimes hard for clinicians to afford disabled people the status of being fully healthy. At the same time, neither do they fit neatly into a category equivalent to 'diseased'. Separating out the idea of the ability to behave in ways conducive to individual survival from the dimensions depicted on the first two axes frees disabled people from this dilemma. This model does not necessarily prescribe how behaviours conducive to individual survival ought to be performed or by whom. The precise way one actually ensures one's survival is not dependent on whether or not one has a full range of physical or mental abilities or whether one requires the help of others. This is an axis representing increasing levels of constraint encountered by the individual when interacting with the wider world. An individual without the benefit of modern technological aids would be more constrained in this respect than they would be had they the benefit of them. Using the model described here, it is feasible to envisage a scenario in which a so-called 'disabled person' may be just as successful at ensuring their daily survival as a so-called 'able-bodied' person. Prosthetic devices such as artificial limbs can help reduce the constraints experienced by those individuals who use them and, in some cases, could even allow the so-called 'disabled' person a level of performance which exceeds that of an 'able-bodied' person – as the evidence of the Paralympics is beginning to demonstrate. This model allows for such a distinction whereas the current biomedical model does not.

Instead of being concerned primarily with the physical state of the body, the model presented here provides scope for the individual's experience of their own body and the extent to which the individual is able to interact with the world to be considered. Indeed, for an individual to be located on either of these models, two or three dimensions need to be taken into account simultaneously. It is not enough to assume that a physical change is all that is needed to effect an improvement in an individual's life. A fuller consideration of their overall state needs to be made.

7. A mental image of biomedical states

The intention of the model described above is to provide a mental image or impression of the overall state of the patient in two or three dimensions as fits the needs of a particular clinical consultation. It is not intended that any clinician should try to draw or plot an exact point representing a patient. The current biomedical model shepherds clinical assessment into thinking in dichotomous terms. The aim of the model described here is to help move thinking on from this single, linear perspective and bring other aspects of a patient's life more fully into consideration. Engel (1981; 1997) was right to want to include the social and psychological factors pertinent to a patient's condition. However, he did not provide a simple way of making an assessment of these factors. Instead, there were numerous potentially interacting levels that needed to be considered simultaneously. The model described here gives a way of assessing the individual as a whole. That does not mean that there should not be detailed and thorough investigation of what makes up that whole where appropriate. The causes and mechanisms involved in any physical disorder, experiential disturbance or behavioural constraint should be explored and the appropriate, specifically directed treatment given. However, that treatment should not be considered in isolation from the effects it may have on the other dimensions considered here. This model is not just for use at the first clinical consultation. It is a tool for continued patient assessment. Having some notion of how a patient's overall state changes, in two or three dimensions, between consultations is important. Furthermore, some treatments aimed at effecting a physical benefit have psychological side-effects which may have, in turn, disadvantageous effects on an individual's ability to look after themselves. In order to bring about the desired overall effect of improving a patient's well-being, some treatments need to be accompanied by assistance in over-coming the effects that may be produced and manifest in the other non-physical dimensions.

7.1 Relevance to other clinical practice – some examples

Not every procedure performed under the auspices of the medical profession is concerned with the cure of ailments. Significant among these is pregnancy. This is a natural phenomenon for which clinical support is typically offered in Western medical settings. However, it is not a medical problem *per se* and the potential medicalisation of this most fundamental of human biological phenomena causes some disquiet. The model described above can be used to represent an individual woman's particular state at any stage during pregnancy without overt medicalisation since it seeks primarily to characterise the individual's overall state.

Physically, the pregnant woman's body undergoes a series of natural changes which have the potential to be hazardous but which may equally be undergone without undue harm. Her conscious self-experience may be, at times, a little more volatile than usual but this is not necessarily to her detriment. Because of her physical changes, the ways in which she is able to interact with the world will change as the pregnancy progresses but again, this is not necessarily to her detriment. Where a particular woman will be represented within the two- or three-dimensional model at any particular stage during pregnancy depends on her particular state. For the uneventful pregnancy, that state will tend to be represented consistently close to the origin. In a condition such as pre-eclampsia, however, her physical state may become more disorderly and one may imagine a horizontal shift to the right in the representation of her overall state. With increasing severity, a vertical shift may ensue leading, in turn, to a shift in the third dimension if the woman becomes disorientated or loses consciousness.

The model presented here helps visualise what may occur – how a clinical condition may progress – while at the same time also helping one to remember that a pregnant woman can occupy much the same location as a non-pregnant person. Although she is seen in a clinical setting, upon assessment, her closeness to the origin of the plane/space can help all concerned remember that she is not an object for medical concern but a person in need of simple humane assistance. Should her condition prove problematic for her (and her baby) in any way, she would become localised in a different part of the model where medical attention might be deemed necessary.

It does not follow that just because somebody has lived for a long time that they are necessarily diminished in some way by the aging process. It does not follow that the representation of the overall state of an elderly person is necessarily further from the origin of the model than was the case when they were younger or that the older person cannot be represented closer to the origin than a younger person. This model helps prevent jumping to simplistic conclusions based on outward appearances by requiring considered assessment in two or three dimensions, as appropriate.

However, as individuals age, this natural process is often associated with increased medical involvement. Yet, like pregnancy, we choose not to label aging as a disease. However, what the model described here does reveal is the potential for the same location on the two- or three-dimensional model to be occupied by one individual due to the effects of age and by another due to a quite different pathological process. This model helps reveal something that the biomedical model was unable to envisage. This is a particularly interesting scenario for the debate about the definitions of disease and health to consider: a state that can be labelled disease and not disease at the same time, the label being ascribed largely because of the way in which the state came about.

Cosmetic procedures, where an individual's appearance is altered, may be performed for medical or purely aesthetic purposes. For medical reasons, cosmetic surgery may be performed to benefit an individual psychologically. For example, some procedures are performed to relieve the effects of distress due to some facial disfigurement. For aesthetic purposes, some individuals simply want to change their appearance to suit some perceived notion of beauty. Such procedures cannot be accommodated easily by the current biomedical model; the decision whether to perform such procedures is not usually based on a straightforward 'well'-'unwell' assessment. However, the new model presented here does allow such cases to be accommodated.

A disfigured individual may not be physically disordered in that their disfigurement may not threaten their physical survival and their ability to interact with the world may not be constrained but their self-esteem may be so damaged as to cause them significant distress. Some individuals might become deeply depressed, despondent or even suicidal, because of their perception of their appearance. In extreme cases, that individual's survival may even be compromised by the threat of self-harm. Such conscious self experiences are represented on the vertical axes of Figures 3 and 4. One might locate such an individual higher on the vertical axis than might otherwise be the case because their experiential distress is potentially injurious.

An individual who wants cosmetic surgery purely for reasons of vanity is by definition somebody whose survival is not adversely affected in any of the dimensions of the new model described above. In such cases, it may be possible for the individual to live perfectly well without undergoing the requested procedure. One might locate such an individual near the origin of Figures 3 and 4. The question for the clinician when confronted by either patient is whether to perform the procedure simply as requested or to address what is essentially an issue relating to each individual's experiential state (i.e. their self-perception) via psychological counselling instead of surgery. It is for the clinician, armed with the model described here and their knowledge of the patient, to make that assessment.

It may be argued that some of the assessments that the model described here seeks to foster are already part of clinical practice. This is not disputed. However, these assessments are not necessarily formalised into a discrete model that can be taught or practised consistently. They are not a formal part of the prevailing biomedical model. At the heart of the model described here is the aim of formally representing the individual as a biological whole.

8. A survival triad

Although the emphasis has been on the improvement of the biomedical model and on its clinical use, the model described here may be seen to be much more than this. The three axes, taken together, provide a model of the individual's ability to survive in a wider biological sense. The individual must remain as close as possible to the origin for all three parameters in order to continue to survive in the world. Too great a deviation from the origin in any one or more of the parameters can compromise the individual's survival chances. The three parameters constitute therefore a 'survival triad'. The three-dimensional model considers the individual very much in their lived context being concerned as it is with ability to interact with the world. Should that world - the environment within which the individual lives - change, there will be an effect on the individual the model represents. Thus, the three-dimensional model provides a way of envisaging how external changes have an effect on the well-being of individuals.

It is important to stress here that this relates to individual survival. Much of modern biology tends to focus on population level effects. Indeed, it is in the population related sense and not in an individual sense that fitness is usually understood with that of the individual organism largely ignored. In a clinical setting, it is the other way around; it is the individual and not the population that matters most. In setting out to improve upon the biomedical model, a contribution to biology may also be made: that of bringing together into a triad those features which are crucial to understanding an individual organism's survival.

9. Conclusion

For a long time, the biomedical model has prevailed even though it has been known to be flawed. Yet, at the same time, it has been able to perform its basic task in such a way that its complete abandonment has proved impossible. Indeed, the approach adopted here has assumed that attempts at its abandonment may be unfruitful - even undesirable - and suggestions have been given instead with a view to its improvement. To that end, axes in addition to the purely physical have been added and the notion of an individual's overall biological state developed.

The prevailing biomedical model tries to match the individual to labels such as 'healthy' or 'diseased', 'well' or 'unwell'. The aim of this work has not been to produce a model of labels but a model of that to which those labels are applied: the individual. The model described here seeks to first describe the individual and then, where necessary, allows a label to be ascribed at the discretion of the clinician. As was noted above (Campbell et al., 1979; Smith, 2002), classifying a particular condition as a disease can vary even between health professionals. Here, need for assistance in personal survival and quality of life has taken precedence over any argument about what is and what is not a disease. Whether a clinician chooses to ascribe a particular disease label to a patient or not is of secondary importance so long as the desired outcome of improving that patient's well-being is attained. Indeed, medically, giving the wrong label but bringing about the desired outcome is preferable to giving the correct label and not bringing about that outcome. In this respect, the model presented here is not prescriptive. Other than those points near the origin where it might be reasonable to suggest that a state of health may be ascribed, no other point on the two- or three-dimensional diagrams has a prescribed label. Indeed, it is possible that under different circumstances, a given state may warrant different labels.

Expressed in two- and three-dimensional forms, the model described here incorporates physiological, experiential and behavioural aspects of the individual into an integrated system which directly relates to an individual's ability to survive in a biological sense. In its two-dimensional form, it extends and improves upon the current biomedical model by integrating the physical and experiential aspects of the individual patient. Instead of a linear 'well'-'unwell' dichotomy, the physical and experiential states of the individual are represented as moveable points upon a plane. This version of the model has particular application to clinical situations. In its three-dimensional form, a third axis is added to allow an individual's ability to interact with the world to be considered. In particular, this allows the question of disability to be accommodated. Disability is not something that has been successfully integrated into the prevailing biomedical model. Indeed, it has largely been ignored. This version of the model particularly suits those dealing with disability issues, for example, those engaged in various branches of bioengineering.

Furthermore, although separate axes have been used, the intention has been to model the individual as a single, integrated biological entity in all lived states and not simply as a 'patient'. Hence, a point combining two- or three-dimensions in a phase space has been used to represent that individual. It has certainly not been the intention to model the individual as a set of distinct physiological processes. As a biological organism, the individual is a single systemic whole: something that has to survive as a unified, albeit changeable, entity within the world in which it finds itself; it does not survive as a series of separate parts or part-functions.

Since the model offers a fuller biological description of the individual, it is conceptually applicable in a wide range of clinical and clinically-related settings. A wider range of states than those traditionally labelled as simply 'diseased' or healthy', 'well' or 'unwell' are discernible and states previously outside the scope of the prevailing biomedical model are now accommodated. The model informs the clinical view of the individual and it informs the application of other technologies in their pursuits of the maintenance and enhancement of well-being and the remedy of ailments and disabilities.

It should not be assumed that all of the criticisms that have been levelled at the biomedical model have been addressed here. Only problems with a biological perspective, in particular those relating to individual survival, have been considered. Shortcomings highlighted by commentators from other fields relevant to human well-being, for example, criticisms by those in the social sciences, have only been touched upon. However, despite the present biological emphasis, it is hoped that commentators from other fields might find the ideas presented to be potentially useful and that they can be built upon within their own particular disciplines.

Originally, these models were developed as part of an exploration into the philosophical problem of defining 'disease' and 'health' and are still intended to contribute to that debate which, after many years, still shows no sign of resolution having been also described as having "ended up in a blind alley" (Sadegh-Zadeh, 2000) and *cul-de-sac* (Khushf, 2007). Care has been taken to avoid entering that debate here but modelling the changeable states of the individual as presented above, if valid, should lead inevitably to new ways of approaching the notions of 'disease' and 'health' (see, for example, Lewis 2007c). Furthermore, a closer conceptual association between the 'biological' and the 'medical' perspectives should also be possible and a more thorough 'bio-medical' understanding be possible by the introduction of the notion of an individual's overall state via a 'biomedical (state) model'. Given the ways in which biology and medicine intersect, it may be timely to reconsider not only the nature of the biomedical model and how its improvement might help the patient but also the place of the individual in biology. While, as already noted, the biomedical model needs a fuller inclusion of biological ideas, biology itself needs a greater appreciation of the individual. This may be especially important if ideas of disease and health - which only properly relate to individuals - are to be understood from both a biological and a medical perspective.

10. Acknowledgements

I would like to thank the trustees and fellows of the Konrad Lorenz Institute, Altenberg, Austria, where, as a Visiting Fellow, I was able to develop many of the ideas outlined here. I would also like to thank Annette Lewis for her help in the preparation of the manuscript of this chapter.

11. References

Boorse, C. (1975). On the distinction between disease and illness. *Philosophy and Public Affairs*, 5, 49-68, ISSN 0048-3915

Boorse, C. (1977). Health as a theoretical concept. *Philosophy of Science*, 44, 542-573, ISSN 0031-8248

Boorse, C. (1997). A Rebuttal on Health. In J. Humber & K. Almeder (Eds.), *What is Disease?* 3-134, Humana Press, ISBN 089603352X, Totowa, New Jersey

Davey, B & Seale, C. (1996). *Experiencing and explaining disease*, (2nd edn.) Open University Press, ISBN 0335192084, Buckingham

Downie, R., Tannahill, C., & Tannhill, A. (1996). *Health Promotion: Models and Values* (2nd ed.). Oxford University Press, ISBN 0192625918, Oxford

Campbell, E., Scadding, J., & Roberts, R. (1979). The concept of disease. *BMJ*, 2, 757-762, ISSN 1759-2151

Engel, G. (1977). The need for a new medical model: a challenge for biomedicine. *Science*, 196, 129-136, ISSN 0036-8075

Engel, G. (1981). The clinical application of the biopsychosocial model. *Journal of Medicine and Philosophy*, 6, 101-123, ISSN 0360-5310

Engel, G. (1997). From Biomedical to Biopsychosocial - being scientific in the human domain. *Psychosomatics*, 38, 521-528, ISSN 0033-3182

Grobstein, C. (1965) *The Strategy of Life*. W H. Freeman and Co., ISBN 0716706350, San Francisco & London

Keating, P., & Cambrosio, A. (2003). *Biomedical Platforms - Realigning the Normal and the Pathological in Late-Twentieth-Century Medicine*. MIT Press, ISBN 0262112760, Cambridge, Mass.

Lewis, S. (2007). Illness - An Under-Rated Biological Phenomenon. Retrieved 5th September, 2010, from https://sites.google.com/site/sjlewis55/presentations/sshb2007. (Abstract: Annals of Human Biology 34, 688, ISSN 0301-4460)

Lewis, S. (2007b). Putting Illness In Its Place. Retrieved 5th September, 2010, from https://sites.google.com/site/sjlewis55/presentations/temah1

Lewis, S. (2009). Seeking a new biomedical model. How evolutionary biology may contribute. *Journal of Evaluation in Clinical Practice*, 15, 745-748, ISSN 1356-1294

Malmgren, H. (2005). The theoretical basis of the biopsychosocial model, In: *Biopsychosocial Medicine - An integrated approach to understanding illness*, White, P. (Ed.), 21-38, Oxford University Press, ISBN 0198530331, Oxford

Marinker, M. (1975). Why make people patients? *Journal of Medical Ethics*, 1, 81-84, ISSN 0306-6800

Maslow, A. (1943). A Theory of Human Motivation. *Psychological Review*, 50, 370-396, ISSN 0033-295X

Nesse, R. (2001). How is Darwinian medicine useful? *Western Journal of Medicine*, 174, 358-360, ISSN 0093-0415

Nesse, R. (2001). Medicine's missing basic science. *The New Physician* (December 2001), 8-10, ISSN 0028-6451

Nesse, R., Stearns, S., & Omenn, G. (2006). Medicine Needs Evolution. *Science*, 311, 1071-1073, ISSN 0036-8075

Nesse, R., & Williams, G. (1995). *Evolution and Healing - The new science of Darwinian medicine*, Weidenfeld and Nicolson, ISBN 0460861409, London

Nesse, R., & Williams, G. (1999). On Darwinian medicine. *Life Science Research*, 3, 1-17, ISSN 1007-7847

Nordenfelt, L. (1986). Health and disease: two philosophical perspectives. *Journal of Epidemiology and Community Health*, 40, 281-284, ISSN 0141-7681

Nordenfelt, L. (2007). The concepts of health and illness revisited. *Medicine, Health Care and Philosophy*, 10, 5-10, ISSN 1386-7423

Nordenfelt, L. (2007). Establishing a middle-range position in the theory of health: A reply to my critics. *Medicine, Health Care and Philosophy*, 10, 29-32, ISSN 1386-7423

Reznek, L. (1987). *The Nature of Disease*, Routledge and Kegan Paul, ISBN 0710210825, London

Sadegh-Zadeh, K. (2000). Fuzzy health, illness, and disease. *Journal of Medicine and Philosophy*, 25, 605-638, ISSN 0360-5310

Seedhouse, D. (2001). *Health - The Foundations for Achievement* (2nd edn.), John Wiley and Sons, Ltd., ISBN 0471490113, Chichester

Smith, R. (2002). In search of "non-disease". *BMJ*, 324, 883-885, ISSN 1759-2151

Smith, R. (2008). The end of disease and the beginning of health. Retrieved 5th September, 2010, from http://blogs.bmj.com/bmj/2008/07/08/richard-smith-the-end-of-disease-and-the-beginning-of-health/

Tinetti, M.E., & Fried, T. (2004) The end of the disease era. *American Journal of Medicine*, 116, 179-85, ISSN 0002-9343

White, P. (Ed.). (2005). *Biopsychosocial Medicine - An integrated approach to understanding illness*, Oxford University Press, ISBN 0198530331, Oxford

World Health Organization. (1948). WHO Constitution. Retrieved 5th September, 2010, from http://apps.who.int/gb/bd/PDF/bd47/EN/constitution-en.pdf

Williams, G., & Nesse, R. (1991). The dawn of Darwinian medicine. *The Quarterly Review of Biology*, 66, 1-22, ISSN 0033-5770

2

Factors Affecting Discourse Structure and Style in Biomedical Discussion Sections

Ian A. Williams
University of Cantabria
Spain

1. Introduction

Over the last three decades or so, increasing interest has been paid to scientific discourse, and in particular to the research article, from a variety of perspectives. Sociological studies (Gilbert & Mulkay, 1984; Latour & Woolgar, 1979) established that the research article is not an objective representation of scientific enterprise as it is performed, but a rhetorical artefact that seeks to construct knowledge and persuade readers to accept the validity of the claims made by writers, and thus to promote the personal and professional interests of the researchers and research groups (Hyland, 1998). Gilbert & Mulkay (1984) showed that scientists have two ways of representing science: a formal "empiricist repertoire" expressed through impersonal public statements of evidence and procedures, and an informal "contingent repertoire" that stresses personal and social factors and which they use to discuss their discipline and practices among themselves in less restricted and private settings. Myers (1994) refers to the *narrative of science*, which researchers use when writing up their research for publications in journals for their peers: "they follow the argument of the scientist, arrange time into a parallel series of simultaneous events all supporting their claim, and emphasize in their syntax and vocabulary the conceptual structure of the discipline" (Myers, 1994). In contrast, Myers found that the same scientists used the *narrative of nature* to popularise their research for a less specialised audience; in this sequential narrative "the plant or the animal, not the scientific activity, is the subject, the narrative is chronological, and the syntax and vocabulary emphasize the externality of nature to scientific practices" (Myers, 1994).

Other studies (Knorr-Cetina 1981; Myers 1985) have investigated the changing shape of research articles and their discourse as they passed through the peer review system. Myers (1985) found that while the biologists he studied always sought to achieve the highest level claim they could, they inevitably had to lower their aims and accept a lower level. Knorr-Cetina (1981) performed a textual study tracing writing of a paper from laboratory notes to the final draft, and found that the Introduction and Discussion sections were those that underwent the greatest transformation. Again the language had to be carefully modified by eliminating "dangerous" claims and excessive speculation. These case studies, therefore, show how the discourse is reconstructed in the negotiation process and support the artefactual nature of the scientific article.

It is pertinent here to return to Latour and Woolgar's 1979 study since in their analysis of statements in scientific discourse, they sought to establish a hierarchical taxonomy of knowledge claims, distinguishing five statement types according to the degree of certainty conveyed. Knowledge represented by type 5 is not actually stated but presupposed and refers to that wealth of knowledge that is shared by experts and is so obvious that in the context does not require expression. Type 4 statements are explicit assertions on uncontroversial subject matter that are more typical of textbooks than research articles: "Two anatomicoclinical variants of pemphigus have been recognized according to the suprabasal or superficial site of the blister: pemphigus vulgaris and its rare vegetating form, pemphigus vegetans, on the one hand, pemphigus foliaceus on the other". Type 3 statements express uncertainty through signals that indicate that the information they convey cannot be taken for granted. This may be achieved by simple attribution to the source through the citation system: "In fact, lesional OCP [ocular cicatricial pemphigoid] tissue is characterized by a marked infiltration of T cells (including interleukin 2 receptor-positive activated T cells), Langerhan's cells, and macrophages,[44-46] similar to those of lichen planus.[47]" Removal of the citation sources transforms type 3 into type 4. Type 2 statements are far more tentative, and contain a wide range of linguistic devices denoting the uncertainty of the status of the claim: "The significantly increased frequency of IgA deposits in this subset as well as the antigenic specificity of the IgA autoantibodies to BP Ag in these patients,[21] suggest that the occurrence of mucosal lesions in anti-BP Ag mucosal pemphigoid may be related to the development of IgA autoantibodies." Type 1 statements are even more speculative in nature: "One could speculate that this difference in apneic pause frequency is related to the fact that approximately 50% of these black children, who were healthy siblings of children with sickle cell anemia, can be expected to have sickle trait (Hb AS)." Hyland (1998), while accepting the validity of this transformation of speculation and knowledge claim from the research article to textbook knowledge and beyond, criticises the scale in that it does not offer a systematic framework for analysis, nor do the authors provide sufficient authentic examples, or support their classification empirically.

Parallel to these sociological developments, linguistic analysis of scientific discourse and the research article has also progressed over this period. From the early attempts at classifying linguistic components of scientific discourse, such as verb forms and tense, *that* nominals, and use of the passive voice (Barber, 1962; Tarone et al., 1981; West, 1980; Wingard, 1981), there came a major shift in orientation with the pioneering work of Swales (1981). In this work, the author took the concept of Move, hitherto used to analyse oral discourse (Sinclair & Coulthard, 1975), and applied it to written text, the Introduction section of research articles across several disciplines. Move analysis essentially assigns a function to a stretch of text, and identifies its typical exponents or manifestations. If a pattern emerges, it is tested on further texts. Swales initially identified four moves that appeared in the Introduction section in a generally regular way. The author later revised the 4-move model, replacing it with a modified 3-move system called the Create a Research Space (CARS) model (Swales, 1990), and based on an ecological metaphor: establish the field, create a niche and occupy the niche. Swales' models, whether the 4-move or 3-move version, have been verified as valid, albeit with certain variations, for a number of disciplines (Cooper, 1985; Crookes, 1986; Peng, 1987). Move analysis has also been applied to other sections such as Results (Brett, 1994; Williams, 1999) and Discussion (Dudley-Evans, 1994; Hopkins & Dudley-Evans, 1988; Williams, 2009), or to the whole research article (Nwogu, 1997; Skelton, 1994; Swales, 2004). Together with this increasing interest in the macrostructure of the research article and the rhetoric of the individual sections, other researchers have examined specific aspects of this discourse, such as reporting verbs (Thomas & Hawes, 1994; Thompson & Ye, 1991);

citation (Thomas, 1991); evaluation (Hunston, 1994), and hedging (Salager-Meyer, 1994; Hyland, 1998). As a result, there is now a rich reservoir of linguistic data on which to base empirical research of large quantities of text using electronic corpora and computer-based methods and tools.

With regard to the Discussion section, Move analysis was first applied by Belanger (1982) and McKinlay (1982). McKinlay studied Discussions in medical articles and identified a 4-move structure consisting of background information, statement of result, interpretation of result, and conclusion. This system was validated for Spanish by Vásquez (1987). While other systems, generally with few Moves, have emerged (Kanoksilapatham, 2003; Lewin *et al.*, 2001; Nwogu, 1997), the most elaborate model is that of Hopkins and Dudley-Evans (1988), an 11-move system identified in the Discussions of biology Master's dissertations. Dudley-Evans (1994) revised this model, reducing it to a 9-move model, which is valid for both theses and research article Discussions. In previous studies on the Discussion section (Williams, 2005; Williams, 2009), we have validated the system for both English and Spanish biomedical articles.

Using the system, Dudley-Evans (1994) states that the moves are combined in different ways according to the writers' communicative needs and that cycles usually have a result or finding as head, followed by reference to previous research, or a claim also followed by a reference to previous research. However, the order of pairs of moves can also be reversed. Mauranen (1993) used a simpler model and compared the discourse style of Finnish authors writing in their native language and writers publishing their work in English-language journals. She identified two contrasting styles referred to as "progressive" and "retrogressive", depending on whether the writer placed the main point of the Discussion towards the end or at the start of the section. Finnish writers preferred the progressive style whereas the English-language authors preferred the retrogressive style. In our previous study (Williams, 2009) using Dudley-Evans model, we were able to show this same trend on comparing English-language and Spanish publications. Some 70% of Spanish authors preferred the progressive style and about 58% of the writers in English-language journals used the retrogressive style. However, in that study, the main criterion for classification was the presence of background information, which is not always a reliable guide for the discourse style. In addition, owing to the selection of the English-language subcorpus, this includes both native and non-native writers of English, which was not taken into account. Thirdly, the only criterion for the selection of studies was that they conform to the Introduction-Methods-Results-and-Discussion (IMRAD) format, which covers many different study designs so that this factor may also have an influence on choice of discourse style.

The aim of the present study is to re-examine the discourse style in the English-language and Spanish research articles by applying strict criteria for the identification of the styles, to compare the non-native writers of English with the native authors, and to investigate the influence of study type on the choice of style.

2. Move analysis in the discussion section

The Move analysis for this study was based on the categories established by Dudley-Evans (1994: 225), the descriptions of which have been slightly modified to take into account differences between the progressive and retrogressive discourse styles. The denominations of the nine moves and their subdivisions or "steps" together with the descriptors are shown in table 1.

Background information (Move 1) is a free-floating move that can be found anywhere in the Discussion, but is generally placed at the start of the whole section, subsection or paragraph especially in the progressive discourse style. When background information combines with other moves and is placed after them, it is interpreted as supporting or justifying the statements made in them. Therefore, when a reference to previous research appears in initial position (Move 5a), it is interpreted as providing background information based on one or more studies, a type 3 statement in Latour and Woolgar's typology (1979) but more limited in scope and truth value than contextual information presented as a consensus view, that is their type 4 statement. In contrast, reference to previous research placed after other moves will perform one of the other two functions of this category: comparison of results or findings (Move 5b) and support for claims, explanations and recommendations (Move 5c).

No.	Move and Step	Description
1.	**Information move: BI**	- Introduces background information (BI) about theory, aim of the research, methodology used, or previous research (see Move 5a) that is necessary for interpreting the results and findings of the current study.
2.	**Statement of results: SOR**	- Often the first move of a cycle: presents a numerical /statistical result from the previous Results section for comment.
3.	**Statement of findings: SOF**	- Presents a finding or observation from the Results section for further comment or elaboration: findings are expressed in more general terms than SORs.
4.	**(Un)expected outcome:**	- A special kind of SOR or SOF indicated by comment on the fact that the result is expected or, more usually, unexpected or surprising. Unexpected findings usually require an explanation.
5.	**Reference to previous research: RPR** a) BI b) comparison c) support	- a) Provides the basis for BI, or may constitute the BI itself - b) Combines with SORs/SOFs for comparison (similarity or contrast) - c) Provides support for claims, explanations, and recommendations.
6.	**Explanation**	- Gives a reason for an unexpected outcome or a result/finding that differs from those previously reported, but they may follow other categories (claim or limitation).
7.	**Claim** a) deduction b) hypothesis	- The more general statements arising from the results, and representing the contribution of the article to the research field; a) deductions are more strongly expressed than b) hypotheses.
8.	**Limitation**	- Indicates that aspects of the research (methodology, findings or claims) should be treated with caution: i.e. they restrict the application or interpretation in the more general setting.
9.	**Recommendation**	- Suggestions for future research, for improvements in methodology, for application of the results.

Table 1. Rhetorical Moves in the Discussion section modified from Dudley-Evans (1994)

Statements of findings (Move 3) are expressed in more general terms than numerical statements of results (Move 2). The type of finding is influenced by the kind of study, but there will not be a strict correlation between study type and finding (see Williams, 1999). Comparisons are common in many discussions, but especially in case-control studies and those examining two types of intervention. Findings expressing relationships between different variables are also common to several study designs, but are particularly characteristic of parametric and epidemiological studies that seek to determine effects between factors and a predetermined outcome or invariable factor such as mortality. Time-related findings are typical of longitudinal studies and those comparing pre-treatment and post-treatment levels. In descriptive studies such as those investigating histopathological characteristics, the finding may simply describe what was observed.

The appearance of certain moves in the Discussion often predicts the subsequent presence of another (Tadros, 1994). Thus, references to previous research that conflict with the data of the new study (Move 5b) and unexpected outcomes (Move 4) require subsequent explanation (Move 6) on the part of the authors. Similarly, a limitation (Move 8) on an aspect of the study design, methodology or results is almost always followed by a reply, or counter claim (Move 7), that justifies or attenuates to some degree the impact of the limitation. In both situations the authors by introducing the first Move of the pair into the discourse are seen to acquire a commitment to their readers to provide the second explanatory or damage-limiting Move.

According to Dudley-Evans (1994), the moves are selected and combined in different ways into cycles depending on whether the focus is placed on a result, a finding or a claim. Despite the varying combinations, he did not identify the overall progressive and retrogressive patterns, which Mauranen (1993) discovered in her comparison of native Finnish writers and authors publishing in English-language journals. In a previous study (Williams, 2009), we were able to confirm these different discourse styles in a contrastive study of native Spanish writers and authors publishing in eight English-language journals. The advantage of our study was the size of the corpus (64 research articles per subcorpus) and that the samples were randomly selected to avoid bias. The two discourse styles and the possible combination patterns are represented in figures 1 and 2.

The progressive style (figure 1) typically opens with background information at a general level, followed by details of more specific aspects of previous research and sometimes those relating to the design and methods of the current study. Individual results or findings are then presented and compared to previous research with evaluative comments following. If a result is unexpected, and when there is a discrepancy between current and previously reported findings, an explanation will almost invariably follow. Comparisons and explanations lead on to the main interpretative category of the claim. Explanations and claims, especially the more tentative hypotheses, may be supported by data drawn from external sources. Recommendations, when present, generally appear at the end of the discussion or of an intermediate cycle. Thus, the progressive pattern is iconic and displays a linear chronological sequence.

The retrogressive style (figure 2) places the major claim or claims at the opening of the Discussion, although these may be preceded by some background information. The claims are then explained or justified in relation to evidence available in the current results and findings and in previous research. Discrepancies will again be accounted for, and the significance of the study will be established in the wider context of the field of interest through the formulation of new hypotheses, again supported by data from outside or within the study, and by means of suggestions for practical applications or recommendations for future lines of research.

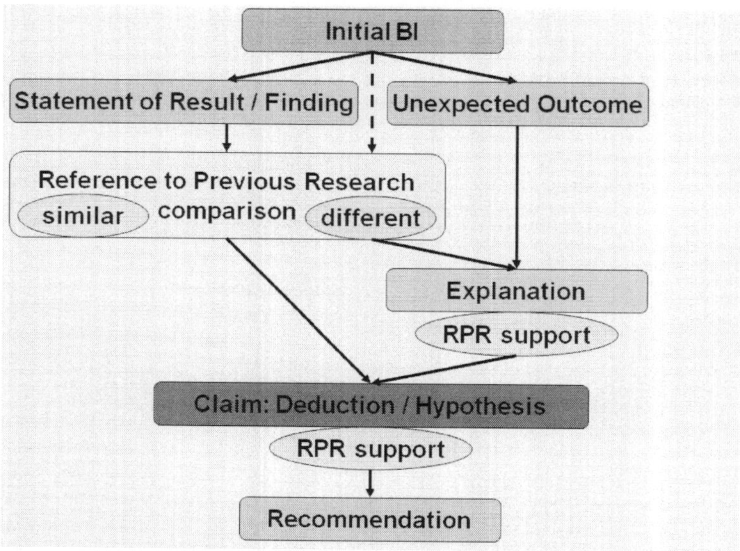

Fig. 1. Pattern of the progressive discourse style in the Discussion section of biomedical research articles

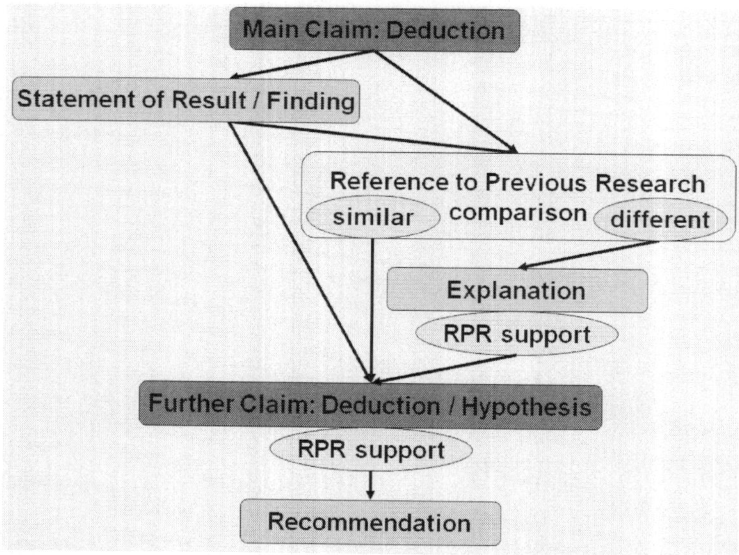

Fig. 2. Pattern of the retrogressive discourse style in the Discussion section of biomedical research articles

For a better understanding of how the Move system works, we provide a worked example of a complete Discussion taken from the English language subcorpus. This discussion section has been chosen as an illustration since it includes a wide range, if not all, of the Moves shown in table 1. The discussion consists of ten paragraphs (marked by the # symbol).

# S1	M7 Claim	# This study demonstrated that oral prednisone was efficacious in reducing the need for hospitalization among a subset of children treated in the ED [emergency department] for acute asthma.
S2	M3 SOF	This benefit was achieved within 4 hours of prednisone's administration and was seen among patients treated frequently with β_2-agonist aerosols.
S3	M5 RPR comparison M6 Explan	There have been several recent studies showing corticosteroids to be efficacious in the management of acute asthma, but none demonstrated the efficacy of oral therapy in the ED and none showed a corticosteroid benefit in the setting of frequent β_2-agonist therapy.
S4-S5	M5 RPR comparison	Storr *et al.*[16] randomly assigned 140 children hospitalized with acute asthma to receive oral prednisolone or placebo soon after admission. At a median time for reexamination of 5 hours, 30% of patients in the prednisolone group were discharged to home compared with 3% in the placebo group (P <.0001).
S6	M6 Explan	However, since these patients were relatively undertreated with β_2-agonists, a steroid benefit in addition to that achieved with frequent β_2-agonist therapy alone was not demonstrated.
S7-S8	M5 RPR comparison	Tal *et al.*[12] randomly assigned 74 children between 6 and 60 months of age in the ED with acute wheezing to receive either 4 mg/kg of intramuscular methylprednisolone or placebo. After 3 hours, 20% of steroid-treated patients required hospitalization compared with 43% in the control group (P <.05).
S9-S10	M6 Explan	However, these patients were also relatively undertreated with β_2-agonists, perhaps making it possible to discern a steroid benefit. Also, it is feasible that some of the younger infants were wheezing secondary to bronchiolitis and that such patients may respond differently to corticosteroid therapy than do older children with asthma.
S11-S12	M5 RPR comparison	Littenberg and Gluck[13] randomly assigned 97 adults in the ED with acute asthma to receive either 125 mg of intravenous methylprednisolone or placebo. Only 19% of steroid-treated patients required hospitalization, compared with 47% in the control group (P <.003).
S13-S14	M6 Explan	However, an early clinical benefit after steroid

		administration was not shown since patients were treated for up to 12 hours in the ED. Also, patients only received β_2-agonist aerosols every 2 hours.[17]
S15-S16	M5 RPR comparison	In contrast, Stein and Cole[15] treated adults with acute asthma with 125 mg of intravenous methylprednisolone or placebo, followed by frequent β_2-agonist aerosols. They found no difference in hospitalization rates between the two groups.
S17	M6 Explan	However, the failure to detect a steroid benefit was most likely the result of the administration of methylprednisolone to some patients in the placebo group, rather than the use of aggressive β_2-agonist therapy.[17]
#S18	M1/5 BI	# A recent meta-analysis of steroid therapy concluded that the oral and intravenous routes are equally efficacious in the initial hours of treatment of acute asthma.[18]
S19	M1/5 BI	In fact, Ratto *et al.*[19] found no significant differences in pulmonary function tests 6 hours after steroid dosing among hospitalized adults treated with oral and intravenous steroids.
S20-S21	M1/5 BI	Engel *et al.*[20] randomly assigned hospitalized adults to receive either intravenous methylprednisolone or oral prednisone. There were no significant differences between the two groups as assessed by hourly measurements of peak expiratory flow during the first 24 hours after admission.
#S22	M1/5 BI	# In a recent review of a 1-year experience at a children's hospital, it was found that only 4% of 3358 children with acute asthma received systemic steroids in the ED, yet 26% were ill enough to require hospitalization.[21]
S23	M1 BI	Establishing intravenous access in a child is often labor-intensive, time-consuming, and painful and may be a primary reason for the underutilization of corticosteroids in the ED.
S24	M7 Claim	The principal benefit of oral prednisone, then, may be that moderately ill patients will receive corticosteroid therapy more consistently and more promptly.
#S25	M1 BI	# There are several aspects of the present study that deserve further comment.
S26	M8 Limit	This study did not attempt to find the time needed for prednisone's peak clinical effect.
S27	M1/5 BI	Recent National Institutes of Health guidelines state that a patient's ED disposition should be decided 2 hours after steroid administration.[22]
S28	M7 Claim	In our study, a similar percentage of patients in each group would have been hospitalized had therapy been restricted to 2 hours.

S29-S30	M2 SOR	However, more than half of those prednisone-treated patients who would have been hospitalized after 2 hours were able to be discharged to home within the next 2 hours; yet hospitalization was prevented in only 17% in the placebo group.
S31	M1 BI	Both groups continued to be treated with frequent β_2-agonists after the 2-hour preliminary disposition was rendered.
S32	M6 Explan (M5 RPR support)	Presumably, then, the lower hospitalization rate for prednisone-treated patients reflected the onset of action of prednisone after the initial delay known to occur with corticosteroid therapy.[23-25]
S33	M7 Claim	It is possible that with a longer period of treatment the prednisone group would have had an even lower hospitalization rate.
S34	M1 BI	However, 4 hours was considered to be a reasonable duration to treat sick asthmatic patients within the constraints of most busy EDs.
S35	M1 BI M3 SOF	# It was decided to stop the study earlier than originally planned when, after an interim review by the study investigators, it was found that three of four study outcomes achieved statistical significance in favor of the use of prednisone.
S36	M7 Claim M1/5 BI + RPR	Based on our data and that of others,[12-14,16] it seemed unethical to fail to treat moderately ill asthmatic patients with corticosteroids, even though this represented the standard of care at this and other centers at the time.[18]
S37	M4 UnexpO	As a result of stopping the study prematurely, the overall hospitalization rate between the two groups did not achieve statistical significance ($P = .10$).
S38	M6 Explan	This failure to achieve statistical significance reflects the observation that many patients experienced a prompt clinical benefit from β_2-agonist aerosols only and were able to be sent home without the need for corticosteroid therapy.
S39	M1 BI M3 SOF	When we considered only those patients with an initial suboptimal response to β_2-agonist therapy, there was a significantly lower hospitalization rate for the prednisone group.
S40	M1 BI M9 Rec	Since it is not possible to preselect those patients who will respond promptly to β_2-agonists, we would advocate treating all moderately ill asthmatic children with prednisone.
#S41-S42	M1/5 BI	# The PI [pulmonary index] is a clinical asthma score that has been shown to correlate significantly with objective pulmonary function studies and hospitalization rates in children older than the age of 6 treated for acute asthma.[26]

		Subsequently, it has been used in the assessment of younger children.[12]
S43	M1 BI	Since our patient population had a wide age range, we modified this PI by adding a second respiratory rate scale.
S44-S45	M1/5 BI M1 BI	Also, since others have shown that oxygen saturation correlates with clinical scores, pulmonary function tests, and the need for hospitalization in children with acute asthma,[27-29] we included oxygen saturation as an additional piece of objective data. It was felt that the modified index, while closely approximating that which has been validated, would better serve as a tool to identify moderately ill children in our patient population.
S46	M3 SOF	In fact, it was found that patients requiring hospitalization had a significantly higher median PI than those who were able to be sent home.
S47	M2 SOR	Also, there was 83% interobserver agreement among the four study investigators assigning PI scores to patients (κ statistic).
#S48	M3 SOF	# There was some overlap among patients with an initial PI greater than 10 and those given a preliminary disposition of "admit".
S49	M2 SOR	However, although there were 24 patients who met both of these criteria, an additional 30 patients met one, but not both, of these criteria.
#S50-S52	M1 BI	# The need for hospitalization was based on the physical examination conducted by the blinded investigators. Guidelines used for admission decisions included an oxygen requirement, continued significant retractions, or continued poor aeration. More explicit criteria for admission were purposely avoided in order to simulate the decision-making as it is carried out in most EDs: that is, reliance on clinical judgment.
S53	M1/5 BI	Also, the lack of explicit admission criteria is consistent with other studies assessing the efficacy of corticosteroids for the ED treatment of asthma.[12,13,15]
S54	M7 Claim M2 SOR	It is not likely that patients who should have been hospitalized were sent home, since none of the 45 patients discharged from the ED relapsed within the first 48 hours.
#S55	M3 SOF M2 SOR	# The capsules used in this study were relatively well tolerated and in no case was a patient too ill to accept oral medication.
S56-S57	M2 SOR	Six (15%) of 39 patients vomited prednisone, and 3 of these patients also vomited the subsequent dose. One placebo-treated patient vomited both the initial and subsequent doses of drug.
S58	M2 SOR	These four patients were excluded from analysis because

	M6 Explan	they, in effect did not receive the study medication.
#S59	M7 Claim	# In summary, this study demonstrated that oral prednisone was efficacious in reducing the need for hospitalization among a subset of children treated in the ED for acute asthma.
S60-S61	M3 SOF	Benefiting most from prednisone therapy were the sickest cohort of patients and those who had suboptimal responses to initial β_2-agonist therapy. These benefits were achieved within 4 hours and were obtained in patients treated frequently with β_2-agonist aerosols.
S62	M9 Rec	Future studies will be needed to substantiate these results, to determine the optimal prednisone dosing, and to compare the oral and intravenous routes of corticosteroid administration in the ED treatment of acute asthma.
S63	M9 Rec	Based on our current knowledge and given the inherent advantages of oral vs parenteral therapy, we recommend that the prompt use of oral prednisone be considered for any moderately ill child with acute asthma.

Sample text 1. Move analysis of a complete Discussion section displaying the retrogressive discourse style

In commenting on this text, we will focus on each of the Move categories in turn and indicate both the features that are typical and those considered to be more personal expression of the repertoire of Moves available. It should be pointed out that this text illustrates the retrogressive style and can be divided into a number of subsections or cycles. The main cycle extends over the first three paragraphs up to sentence 24. A second large cycle covers the next six paragraphs (S25-S58), but as stated in S25 covers several aspects of the study. These subdivisions deal with the questions of the duration (2 hours or 4 hours) of treatment in the emergency department (S26-S34), the influence of stopping the trial prematurely (S35-S40), the relationship between the pulmonary index and hospitalisation (S41-S54), and tolerance of the study drug (S55-S58). In the last paragraph (S59-S63) the authors give their conclusions.

The text includes 12 manifestations of background information (Move 1). Of these, one (S25) is a presentational sentence introducing the four aspects dealt with in the second part of the discussion. Two others provide general contextual knowledge, the first (S23) serving as the basis for a claim and the second (S40) providing the rationale for a recommendation. Both are expressed in the typical present tense. The most frequent function of this move (8 instances) is to present methodological choices and the underlying rationale. While these decisions can be described and justified in the Methods section (Williams, 2010), it is not unusual for authors to delay commenting on them until the discussion section. The selected procedural choices are expressed in the past tense (*continued to be treated, modified, included, was based*), and use of the first person (S43, S44) underlines the fact that the decision deviates from what is considered standard practice. The first person draws attention on to the investigator, leaving readers to judge for themselves the validity of the choice (Hyland, 1998). The underlying rationale, when present, is also expressed in the past but through cognitive verbs (*was considered, was decided, was felt*). The final instance occurs in the conclusion in the last sentence (S63), where general knowledge and the personal experience of the authors are combined to serve as the basis for the final recommendation.

Use of reference to previous research to provide background information (Move 1/5a) is also common in this discussion (11 instances). The typical manifestations of this move are mention of the cited authors (*Ratto et al., Engel et al.*) or an authority (*National Institutes of Health*), general reference to investigators (*other authors*) or institutions (*other centers*), replacement of researchers by the research (*meta-analysis, review, studies*), or use of the impersonal passive (*it has been shown*). When individual studies are cited, the past tense is used (*concluded, found*) whereas citation of an official source can be expressed in the present (*state* S27). When several studies are cited (S44) or when the reference has greater relevance to the current study (S41, S42), the present perfect is the preferred choice (*has been shown, has been used*).

The text includes eight manifestations of numerical statement of results (Move 2). However, none of these open a cycle for discussion; they all follow more general findings (S47, S49, S55-57) or a claim (S29-30) and provide the concrete data that support the validity of those statements. All the results are expressed in the canonical past tense.

More general statements of findings (Move 3) also appear in the text on eight occasions. Unlike the numerical results, these findings could initiate the comment cycle either at the beginning of a paragraph (S48) or after background information (S35, S46, S55), but two findings (S2, S39) validate a claim or an explanation. The findings presented in S60-61 in the conclusion are a restatement of the data given in S2 and also support the main claim of the study. All the findings, like the results, appear in the canonical past tense. The findings include time-related changes (S2, S61), comparisons (S39, S46), relationships (S35, S48), and evaluative observations (S55, S60).

One statement (S37) was classed as an unexpected outcome (Move 4). Although this is not signalled by the authors with any of the typical indicators (*surprising, unexpected, contrary to expectations,* etc.), its status can be deduced from the discourse. Since it refers to the main outcome of the study (hospitalisation rate in the whole study group), it can be assumed that, as with the other three results (S35), the investigators expected to find a statistically significant difference between treatment with the drug and administration of a placebo. However, this did not materialise. The fact that this finding is followed immediately by an explanation is a further indication of its unexpectedness.

References to previous research functioning as comparisons (Move 5b) or support (Move 5c) are also present in the text. The five examples of the former all appear in the long opening paragraph (S3, S4-5, S7-8, S11-12, S15-16). The first provides an overview of relevant previous research (*several recent studies*), and the remainder all cite the authors by name. The opening general reference is in the typical present perfect (*have been*) whereas each specific study is described in the canonical past tense. The single instance of a citation providing support (S32) serves to validate the explanation in which it is embedded.

There are a total of eight explanations (Move 6) in the text. The first five of these (S3, S6, S9-10, S13-14, S17) follow the comparisons with previous research in which differences with the current study are established. All are signalled by a contrastive marker (*but, however*). The repeated pattern - a brief description of a study followed by an evaluation pointing out the differences - appears to be the authors' personal choice. The overall rhetorical effect of this strategy is to boost the claim of originality for the current study. The explanation in S32 is similar but accounts for apparently inconsistent findings within the current study, the hypothetical non-significant 2-hour result compared with the actual statistically significant 4-hour result. Similarly, the explanation in S38 accounts for the unexpected outcome. The final explanation (S58) justifies the decision to exclude six patients from the analysis; these adjustments to the study sample may require explanation because they can introduce bias into the analysis. When the study under consideration, previous or current, is referred to, the past tense is used, but the explanation may be attenuated by hedges such as *perhaps, possible, feasible, may respond, most likely* and *presumably* (S9-10, S17, S32) or strengthened by boosters such as *in effect* (S58). Explanations are also marked by causality, through verbs such as *reflect* (S32, S38) and connectors *since* (S6, S13) and *because* (S58).

Claims (Move 7) are or should be the most important statements in the Discussion since it is through them that authors declare that their research is making a novel contribution to knowledge and assert their right to this intellectual property. Of the seven claims in the discussion under study, only two are strongly asserted, the opening claim (S1) and a verbatim repetition in the conclusion (S59). This claim is presented in an almost prototypical formula - *This study demonstrated that...* - in which the authors are replaced by their research, the strongest possible verb is used (*demonstrate*), and only slight attenuation is evident in that the past tense is used rather than the present. This may be because, as we have seen, the main outcome of the study (hospitalisation rate in the total study population) did not achieve statistical significance. The remaining six claims are expressed more tentatively, and are all modified in some way: *may be* (S24), *would have been* (S28), *it is possible* and *would have had* (S33), *seemed unethical to fail to treat* (S36), and *it is not likely* (S54). It is not our intention to examine hedging in detail (see Hyland, 1998, for an in depth analysis), but these attenuated statements anticipate and avoid criticism from peers, on the one hand, and show respect for others' work, on the other. In this regard, the double negative in S36 stands out since a stronger formulation might have caused offence and drawn criticism from hospitals not applying this treatment.

The only limitation (Move 8) identified in this study (S26) displays a typical form for methodological limitations with the verb expressed in the negative (*did not attempt to find*). There is no explicit counterclaim to this limitation, but the ensuing argument (S27-S34) can be taken to fulfil this role; the 4-hour limit of the study design will have allowed sufficient time for the steroid to have exerted its effect.

Three recommendations appear in this discussion, typically placed at the end of a cycle (S40) or at the very end of the article (S62, S63). The final recommendation (S63) is a repetition of that made earlier in S40. They are personalised recommendations for clinical practice signalled by the verbs *advocate* and *recommend* in the first person, and strongly supported by evidence both from the study data and from consensus opinion. The other recommendation (S62) is for further research but notably suggests filling gaps not covered by the current study. It is indicated by typical markers *future studies* and *need.*

The combinations of the different communicative moves in the discussion analysed corresponds to the retrogressive style overall. The section opens with the strongest claim, which is directly linked to the aim of the study expressed in the Introduction: "Therefore, we designed a randomized, double-blind, placebo-controlled trial to assess the efficacy of oral prednisone combined with frequent β_2-agonist therapy for children treated in the ED for moderate, acute asthma exacerbation." For the other subsections, the presence of initial contextual information does not preclude the retrogressive style. In fact, the subcycles on duration of treatment (S26-S34), on the pulmonary index and hospitalisation rate (S41-S54), and on drug tolerance (S55-S58) also display elements of the retrogressive style since numerical results appear after the more general findings and claims which they support, when iconically the opposite would be true: first the data are produced, then they are compared and interrelated statistically, and finally they are interpreted and evaluated. The only possible exception is the subcycle on the premature stoppage of the trial (S35-S40), where a finding (S35) is placed before a related claim (S36). However, it is unlikely that we will find pure retrogressive or pure progressive discourse styles and what we are concerned with is the style of the major discourse pattern in the Discussion section.

3. Material and methods

3.1 The corpus

The study was carried out on an extensive computerised corpus consisting of 128 research articles with the typical IMRAD format, divided into two subcorpora: a subcorpus of 64 articles (57,650 words) published in eight English-language journals covering the specialities of general medicine (2 journals), cardiology, dermatology, gynaecology and obstetrics, ophthalmology, paediatrics and surgery; and a subcorpus of 64 Spanish research articles (140,250 words) drawn from one or more Spanish journals covering the same specialities as the English-language subcorpus, with eight articles per journal (general medicine) or speciality. The articles were selected in blocks of eight by means of a table of random numbers. The present study used only the Discussion section (English-language texts, 55,360 words; Spanish texts, 59,210 words).

3.2 Analyses

For the analysis of discourse style, the procedure described previously (Williams, 2009) was followed with slight modifications:

Step 1. Each T-unit, defined as a main clause together with all the subordinate clauses dependent on it (Fries, 1994), was assigned one or more of the Move categories defined in table 1.

Step 2. The first statement arising from the current results was identified and the Move category noted for χ^2 analysis. The moves of interest were (1) claim, (2) result, finding or unexpected outcome, (3) reference to previous research for comparison, (4) limitation. Unlike our previous study, we included limitations as a separate category in the quantitative analysis despite the small number of occurrences.

Step 3. The number of T-units preceding the statement identified in step 2 was found and the amount of background information was expressed as a percentage of the whole Discussion section.

Studies with no background information opening with a claim were considered retrogressive, as were those opening with a limitation, followed by a counterclaim with no intervening results or findings, whereas those opening with a result, finding, unexpected outcome or comparison with previous research were classed as progressive. Studies with background information were classified as retrogressive if the background was followed by an early claim (< 25% background information), and where the combination pattern of claim > result or finding > comparison with previous research was clearly evident in the main cycle. When contextual background was followed by a result, finding or comparison, the style was classed as progressive.

In the analysis of native versus non-native writers of English, non-native writers were identified on the basis of the affiliation of first author and co-authors. When all the authors were attached to institutions in countries whose first language is not English, they were classed as non-native writers. For authors whose name suggested they were non-natives (e.g. Chan), their continued affiliation to an institution in an English-speaking country was checked by a computer search.

For the analysis of discourse style in relation to study type, studies were broadly classed using definitions of evidence-based medicine, clinical trial classifications and data for retrospective and prospective studies. On the basis of the data collected, studies were grouped into the following categories: small case series, based on < 30 cases; large retrospective studies, when the studies were defined as such in the Abstract, or in the body of the article; large prospective studies, identified as for retrospective studies; epidemiological studies, when these were population-based, were cohort studies, or were case-control studies defined as epidemiological in the Abstract or body of the text; experimental and investigational studies, which included studies using animal models or in vitro methods and those investigating aspects of medical practice through surveys and questionnaires; and finally clinical trials defined as such in the Abstract or body of the text.

For statistical analysis, categorical variables were compared by χ^2 analysis, with Yates' correction for 2 × 2 tables. With regard to small expected numbers, Everitt (1977) gives the following conservative rule for this type of analysis: the 2 × *c* table can be tested by the conventional χ^2 criterion if all the expectations are 1 or greater, and that it may even be used for tables with expectations in excess of 0.5 in the smallest cell. The amount of background information was compared with the Mann-Whitney test. P values ≤ 0.05 were considered significant.

4. Quantitative analysis

4.1 Background information

Some initial background information was included in 45 of the 64 Spanish language studies but in only 31 of the 64 English language articles (χ^2 = 5.474; 1 df; P = 0.019). However, the presence of initial background information is not sufficient by itself to indicate the type of discourse style; it is also necessary to take into account the category of the Move that opens the discussion of the data emerging from the new study (table 2). There was a significant difference overall (P = 0.002) in the type of Move between the English and Spanish subcorpora. A claim was the preferred choice (35/64; 55%) in the English language texts whereas a statement of results or finding (35/64; 55%) was most often selected in the Spanish texts.

Move	English	Spanish	Total
Claim	35 (24.5)	14 (24.5)	49
SOR	21 (28)	35 (28)	56
RPRcomp	7 (10)	13 (10)	20
Limitation	1 (1.5)	2 (1.5)	3
Total	64	64	128
χ^2 = 14.633; 3 degrees of freedom; P = 0.002			
Numbers in brackets are expected values. SOR: statement of result; RPRcomp: reference to previous research for comparison.			

Table 2. Distribution of Move type in the two subcorpora

When the Move type was analysed according to the presence or not of background information, the level of significance (P = 0.008) was only maintained for texts with no introductory matter (table 3). In the English subcorpus, the selection of an opening claim was made in two thirds of the texts; in contrast, in the Spanish Texts, the choice between a claim, a result or finding and comparison with previous research was found to be fairly evenly distributed.

Move	English	Spanish	Total
Claim	22 (17.8)	6 (10.2)	28
SOR	10 (10.8)	7 (6.2)	17
RPRcomp	0 (3.2)	5 (1.8)	5
Limitation	1 (1.3)	1 (0.7)	2
Total	33	19	52
$\chi^2 = 11.755$; 3 degrees of freedom; $P = 0.008$			
Numbers in brackets are expected values. SOR: statement of result; RPRcomp: reference to previous research for comparison.			

Table 3. Distribution of Move type in Discussions with no initial background information in the two subcorpora

For the discussions that opened with background information (table 4), the significance was lost ($P = 0.062$) although the English language texts again tended to open the commentary with a claim, whereas the Spanish texts showed a strong preference (28/64; 62%) for a statement of result or finding.

Move	English	Spanish	Total
Claim	13 (8.6)	8 (12.4)	21
SOR	11 (15.9)	28 (23.1)	39
RPRcomp	7 (6.1)	8 (8.9)	15
Limitation	0 (0.4)	1 (0.6)	1
Total	31	45	76
$\chi^2 = 7.337$; 3 degrees of freedom; $P = 0.062$			
Numbers in brackets are expected values. SOR: statement of result; RPRcomp: reference to previous research for comparison.			

Table 4. Distribution of Move type in Discussions with initial background information in the two subcorpora

4.2 Discourse style

When the presence and the amount of background information was taken into account together with the Move type to establish the discourse style, a statistically significant difference was found between the English language discussions and the Spanish comparable texts (table 5). Whereas just over half (33/64; 52%) of the former displayed the retrogressive style, the overwhelming preference (54/64; 84%) in the Spanish subcorpus was for the progressive style ($P < 0.001$).

Discourse Style	English	Spanish	Total
Retrogressive	33 (21.5)	10 (21.5)	43
Progressive	31 (42.5)	54 (42.5)	85
Total	64	64	128
$\chi^2 = 16.950$; 1 degree of freedom; $P < 0.001$			
Numbers in brackets are expected values.			

Table 5. Relationship of discourse style with the language used for publication in the two subcorpora

4.3 Non-native writers

The compilation of the original English language subcorpus was based on the random selection of eight research articles with the required IMRAD format for each of the eight journals, and no further selection criteria had to be met. As a result, the authors of the studies included in the corpus could be either native language writers or authors whose mother tongue could well be a language other than English. The application of the identification criteria for the latter yielded a total of 22 authors considered most likely to be non-native writers of English publishing in English language journals. The range of countries of origin was broad: Sweden 5; France 3; Austria, Denmark, Germany and Holland 2 each; Belgium, Israel, Japan, Norway, Spain and Switzerland one each. The number of non-native writers varied per journal. The selection of articles included at least one non-native writer for all the journals, but in the case of the journal *Acta Obstetricia et Gynecologica Scandinavica,* all eight of the selected articles were written by non-native authors.

Comparison of native and non-native writers (table 6) showed no significant difference with regard to the retrogressive and progressive discourse styles (P = 0.657), indicating that non-native writers either share or successfully adopt the appropriate discourse style in these specialised publications.

Style	Native	Non-native	Total
Retrogressive	23 (21.7)	10 (11.3)	33
Progressive	19 (20.3)	12 (10.7)	31
Total	42	22	64
χ^2 = 0.197; 1 degree of freedom; P = 0.657			
Numbers in brackets are expected values			

Table 6. Comparison of native and non-native writers in terms of discourse style

When the non-native writers were compared to the Spanish authors (table 7), a significant difference was observed in the discourse styles used (P = 0.010).

Style	Spanish	Non-native	Total
Retrogressive	10 (14.9)	10 (5.1)	20
Progressive	54 (49.1)	12 (16.9)	66
Total	64	22	86
χ^2 = 6.577; 1 degree of freedom; P = 0.010			

Table 7. Comparison of Spanish authors and non-native writers of English language articles

4.4 Study type

For the analysis of the influence of study type on discourse style in the two subcorpora, studies were divided into six broad groups taking into consideration as far as possible the strength of the evidence afforded by the study design. The groups established were trials, experimental and investigational studies, epidemiological studies, large prospective series, large retrospective series, and small series (< 30 subjects). The distribution of the discourse styles in relation to study type is shown in table 8.

Study Type	English			Spanish		
	Total	Retro	Prog	Total	Retro	Prog
Trials	18 (11)	12	6	4 (11)	2	2
Experimental/investigational	5 (4.5)	2	3	4 (4.5)	2	2
Epidemiological	7 (6.5)	2	5	6 (6.5)	0	6
Large Prospective Series	17 (16.5)	9	8	16 (16.5)	1	15
Large Retrospective Series	9 (14)	4	5	19 (14)	3	16
Small series	8 (11)	4	4	14 (11)	2	13
Total	64	33	31	64	10	54
$\chi^2 = 14.829$; 5 degrees of freedom; $P = 0.011$						
Numbers in brackets are expected values; Retro: retrogressive style; Prog: progressive style						

Table 8. Discourse style in the two subcorpora according to study type

The distribution of study types between the English language and Spanish subcorpora showed a statistically significant difference ($P = 0.011$). In comparison with the English subcorpus, the Spanish studies had a considerable deficit of trials and exhibited smaller excesses of both large retrospective studies and small case series. Owing to the small numbers in many of the individual categories, no formal statistical analysis was performed between styles for the language of publication. Nevertheless, differences are evident from the figures. Two thirds of the trials in the English language subcorpus displayed the retrogressive style whereas only two of the four Spanish studies denominated trials had retrogressive discussions. Although the epidemiological category covers a number of study types with this orientation, it is noteworthy that two English language discussions in this category exhibited a retrogressive style whereas all six Spanish studies displayed the progressive style. In the remaining four study categories, the progressive and retrogressive discourse styles were fairly evenly distributed in the English subcorpus; in contrast, in the Spanish subcorpus, this was true only for the experimental and investigational studies. For small case series and for large series, whether retrospective or prospective in nature, the style of the Spanish discussions was overwhelmingly progressive.

5. Qualitative analysis

5.1 Initial background information

The quantitative analysis showed that significantly more Spanish studies than English language studies opened the discussion section with background information (45 versus 31, respectively). Moreover, our previous study (Williams, 2009) found that overall the Spanish discussions also contained a significantly greater amount of background information (median 14.3% versus 0%); however, when only those texts with background information were considered, the difference was no longer statistically significant (median 24.0% versus 15.8%). This study examined the type of information included as background and again no difference between the subcorpora was found. Of the 45 Spanish discussions with background content, 28 (62%) included only external information, that is, general context and a general or specific review of previous research; 14 (31%) combined external data with details of the current study in the form of a restatement of aims and/or description of selection criteria or methods; and 3 (7%) presented contextual information on the current study only. The corresponding figures for the 31 English language discussions were 18 (58%), 9 (29%), and 4 (13%), respectively.

The following extract (sample text 2) is a typical example taken from the Spanish subcorpus (Note: all English translations from the Spanish subcorpus are mine) of a discussion with only external general content prior to the first statement arising from the current study, which in this case is a numerical result (S7). The background provided consists of three cycles, each in its own paragraph (marked by the symbol #): a definition of granulocyte elastase (S1); its mode of action and the usefulness of Elastase α_1-Proteinase-Inhibitor complex as a biochemical marker (S2-4); and the positive and negative characteristics of the behaviour of free elastase (S5-6). All the background information consists of type 3 and type 4 statements (Latour &Woolgar, 1979).

#S1	# Granulocyte elastase is a glycoprotein with a molecular weight of 30 kD, which is located in the azurophilic granules of polymorphonuclear leukocytes, which contain 3 μg of elastase/10^{-6} cells (11).
#S2	# In the presence of an inflammatory and/or infectious process, the granulocyte elastase released by neutrophils immediately binds to α1-antitrypsin and α2-macroglobulin in a proportion of 90% and 10%, respectively, and they inactivate it in thousandths of a second.
S3	When the local concentration of the elastase exceeds that of α1-antitrypsin and α2-macroglobulin, it acts on a series of biological substrates and increases the inflammatory response.
S4	Therefore, the determination of E-α1-PI complex in blood is a biochemical marker of the inflammatory response in tissues (12).
#S5	# Free elastase performs two types of action: one beneficial by destroying toxins, attacking infectious agents and removing cell debris; and the other harmful by inactivating functional proteins, producing toxic peptides and damaging intact tissues.
S6	Its proteolytic activity also influences different blood systems, such as coagulation, fibrinolysis and the complement cascade (11,12).
#S7	# In this study, the reference values for E-α1-PI complex (median, range) obtained in the plasma of 99 healthy newborns were 189 μg/L (46-196 μg/L).

Sample text 2. External background information in a progressive style Spanish Discussion

An example of a discussion with less background but including not only general contextual information but also details on the current study design is taken from an English cancer trial (sample text 3). Despite the relatively high frequency of pancreatic carcinoma, it presents considerable difficulties for study design and implementation. The authors move rapidly from the general context (S1) through previous studies (S2) to certain aspects of their own design (S3) before stating their first result (S4). The following comparison with previous research (S5), together with the earlier citations, justifies the seemingly low recruitment rate and places the study in a better light. It should be noted that this study was one of the minority of six trials that exhibited the progressive discourse style, and one of the reasons for this choice may have been the poor recruitment rate, which could place the validity of the results in doubt.

As in this example, all the English language discussions which combined general context with specific details on the current study explicitly mentioned at some point the rationale underlying the aim, design, patient selection or a procedure (table 9).

#S1	# Carcinoma of the pancreas is a common condition in the UK (approximately 100 cases per million population annually).
S2	Trials of treatment have often included relatively few patients.[6-8]
S3	This trial was designed to minimize disruption to patient and participating clinician, with the coordinator performing all administrative and clinical duties.
S4	Only 44 patients were randomized during the 2 years of the trial despite 102 patient referrals.
S5	The recruitment rate (43%) was not unusually low for a clinical trial of this type.[16]

Sample text 3. Mixed external and internal background information in a progressive style English language Discussion

1	This study evaluated the relationship between bile duct diameter and the risk of developing an immediate complication of ES [endoscopic sphincterotomy]. Sphincterotomy may be more hazardous in patients with a duct that is not dilated or tapered distally (6), particularly if performed for dysfunction of the sphincter of Oddi (7).
2	In addition, we used Doppler color flow imaging to determine the origin and direction of the mitral regurgitant jet. Use of color jet direction reflects the physiology of the "nozzle" of the regurgitant orifice, which augments anatomic information available from two-dimensional echocardiography alone.
3	Since describing the autologous GvHR [graft versus host reaction] and the ELR [eruption of lymphocyte recovery], we have been interested in the apparent similarities between these entities. […] We were interested to determine whether histologic changes developing in skin affected with autologous GvHR and ELR were consistently different or whether there was sufficient overlap in findings to make distinction difficult or impossible.
4	In the present study, women born 1923, 1929, 1931 or 1933 were chosen since they had previously not been interviewed about their climactic symptoms.
5	Asymmetric patients with primary open angle glaucoma were selected because of the high probability that the perimetrically normal eye would eventually develop a visual field defect, so that temporal relationships between disc and field damage could readily be established.
6	In an attempt to clarify the pathogenesis as well as the definitions used in this report, we elected to exclude cases of pneumonia and suspected pneumonia. The difficulty of diagnosing pneumonia with certainty has been noted by others (18).
7	The goal of this survey was to identify features of staffing patterns, ancillary services, patient follow-up, and clinical issues common to a variety of institutions providing emergency care for children. Through such data collection it is hoped that standards for patient care, teaching, and research can be developed.
8	Complications of noncontact diode cyclophotocoagulation have been few and have included mild uveitis and conjunctival burns that cleared rapidly with topical prednisolone acetate. Several patients have been noted to lose visual acuity, but no other significant complications have been reported (1,6-8). In this study we evaluated patients who underwent noncontact semiconductor diode transscleral cyclophotocoagulation with follow-up for up to 1 year, to evaluate intraocular pressure control, prognostic factors, and complications.

Table 9. Exponents of the expression of the rationale behind study design and methodological choices in the background information of English language Discussions

The variation of expression is great, ranging from the selection of the object of study (1) supported by a hypothesis, and a reasoned choice of procedure (2), through a change of viewpoint in approaching a problem (3), choice of subjects (4 and 5), and justification for patient exclusion (6), to the establishing of aims in the face of novel situations (7 and 8) – namely, development of a new field (paediatric emergency medicine) and application of new technology.

In the 14 Spanish discussions with combined background information, explicit rationale was not always present. In one study, the specific context was limited to a description of the rural location of the hospital. Other studies included repetitions of information provided in other sections: in one case, the justification for the study as in the introduction section but in more detail; in another, the inclusion criteria; and in a third, the description of the age- and sex-matched control group. However, the remaining discussions largely coincided with their English language counterparts. Two studies involving novelty merit special attention since the true comment on the results was delayed almost to the end of the section. The first of these involved the experimental application of a drug by a new route in five patients with Aids-related cytomegalovirus (CMV) retinitis. The authors meticulously examined the problems of treatment with a review of the relevant literature, and proposed four potential advantages of intravitreal foscarnet over the alternative treatment with intravitreal ganciclovir. All of these data (85% of the discussion) motivated the current study (sample text 4)

#S1	# These data led us to carry out intravitreal treatment with 0.1 mL of foscarnet 2,400 microgram solution twice weekly for induction and once a week for maintenance, since the pharmacokinetic data obtained provide a safety margin for these intervals.
#S2	**Conclusion** # The complete response in all patients after intravitreal administration of 0.1 mL of 2.4mg foscarnet opens up a new therapeutic possibility in the treatment of CMV retinitis, and offers a broader therapeutic range so that treatment can be varied according to the response of the disease to the drugs and routes used at any given time.
S3	We recommend the 2.4 mg/0.1 mL dose, which shows no toxicity at the same induction and maintenance frequency as ganciclovir.
S4	Nevertheless, there is a need for a broader clinical study for a comparison with the results obtained by other authors in order to establish the viability of making this treatment a daily reality.

Sample text 4. Late claim in a progressive style Spanish Discussion

The rest of the section consists of a description of the treatment and the underlying rationale (S1), followed by a subsection labelled 'Conclusion' consisting of a claim (S2) for this approach based on the result, which is embedded in the grammatical subject and not expressed in an independent statement, and two recommendations, one for clinical practice (S3) and the other for further research (S4). Although the background information is followed by a claim, the style is progressive, but the authors clearly felt there was no need for further comment on the results.

The studies (4 English and 3 Spanish) in which the background information deals only with the current study are characterised by a very short introduction of two sentences on average (range 1 to 3). In three of the English language discussions, this background was followed by a claim initiating a retrogressive section; the other study had a finding. In contrast, two of the three Spanish studies had statements of results after the background and the other a limitation. Table 10 shows an example of each of the three moves following methodologically oriented contextualisation: 1) numerical result; 2) claim; 3) limitation. In example 1, the choice of the cut-off for definition of adolescent mothers is supported by the rationale, and the ensuing numerical result is compared to previous research. Example 2 restates the aim of the study, which is to compare the argon green laser (AGL) and the krypton red laser (KRL), and this is immediately followed by a claim that answers the study question but the implications of which extend beyond the limits of the current study. In example 3, the theoretical assumptions and precisions of the opening statement require an immediate precautionary statement to avoid the risk of an exaggerated or over-optimistic interpretation of the results, and this is manifested as a limitation. These two sentences form the opening paragraph of the discussion, which is followed by a list of the assumptions that have been made before the results are presented and commented on; this discussion, therefore, displays the progressive discourse style in spite of the claim-like character of the limitation.

1	Our study population included pregnant women 18 years of age or under and although not all authors agree on this age (5,7,8,9), it is based on the fact that in Spain the age of majority is reached at 18 years, a point after which ethical and socioeconomic factors play a significant role. There were 4.08 deliveries in adolescent women with an annual maximum of 4.43% and an annual minimum of 3.55%, figures somewhat higher than those of previous studies (7,9).
2	This clinical trial was designed to determine if either AGL or KRL is superior to the other by one line of visual acuity. This study rejects the hypothesis that KRL is superior by 1 line of acuity (5% probability of error).
3	For calculation of the estimations presented here certain assumptions and precisions have been made concerning the data, methods and objectives used. For this reason, the results presented only claim to be illustrative of the theoretical benefit that could be achieved by preventive intervention.

Table 10. Move types following background information on design and methodological issues

5.2 Studies with no background information

As observed in the quantitative analysis, the English language subcorpus contained many more studies with no background information move than the Spanish comparable subcorpus (33 and 19, respectively). Twenty-two of the English discussions opened with a claim. The main exponents, or phraseological patterns, of these claims are summarised in table 11. The exponents listed in rows 1 to 6 share some features but differ in at least one aspect. They all contain instances of epistemic verbs, which can be roughly graded from strongest to weakest: *demonstrate, show, confirm, provide evidence, indicate,* the choice of which is essentially strategic as writers adjust the strength of their claim to their confidence in its truth value (Hunston, 1994; Hyland, 1998). The variation in choice of tense should also be noted: the present tense expresses the greatest generality and the simple past the greatest specificity, with the perfect tense occupying an intermediate position. The distinctive aspects for each case are that in (1) the presence of the authors through the pronoun *we* indicates that the writers assume responsibility for the claim, freeing the reader to decide whether to accept or challenge it in what Hyland (1998) has identified as a reader-oriented hedge. In (2) and (3) the researchers place the responsibility on the study as a whole or on the data obtained, respectively. In (4) the reported clause is replaced by a noun as the direct object of the verb. This brings the claim closer to a statement of finding; note that the presence of the phrase *for the first time* stakes a claim for originality, and the *different patterns* mentioned in the other instance generalises the individual findings reported in the results section. In (5) the authors have shifted the perspective to have the object of study (*photodynamic therapy*) or an aspect thereof (*benefits of endoscopic surgery*) as the point of departure for the claim, which means use of the agentless passive to maintain "anonymity". In (6) the more usual introductory reporting clause (examples 1-3) is replaced with a subordinate clause, which achieves a similar effect. The remaining instances are of a different character and the last one is a highly personal choice. In (7). the epistemic verb is replaced by *support* and the authors' claim is for the originality of their findings. In (8) it is the presence of the evaluative element *most striking* and *most important* that confers the status of claim on the finding. The same effect is achieved by the evaluative adverb *clearly* in example (9), thus validating the adequacy of the *in vivo* model employed in the study. The final example shows a different writer strategy; the statement displays the form of a counterstatement to anticipated potential criticisms of the study related to selection bias or faulty or irreproducible methodology. Having defended their study with this rather weak claim, the authors proceed to make a stronger claim: "Differences are explained by the different treatments given to the two subgroups of IDA [iron-deficient anaemic] infants".

1	We have shown that ... In this study we provide evidence that ...
2	The current study demonstrates that ... This study demonstrated that ... This study shows that ... This study has shown that ... (2 instances) The present study showed that ... Our trial indicates that ... This trial provides good evidence that ...
3	These results demonstrate that ... The overall results of this trial show that ...
4	This study shows for the first time a reduction ... The study showed different patterns of risk ...
5	In this study, PDT has been shown to be an effective therapeutic modality... The benefits of endoscopic surgery were clearly shown in this study.
6	As confirmed by our study, restenosis after successful coronary angioplasty is not necessarily associated with recurrence of angina ...
7	The data presented support the following three new concepts: ...
8	The most striking finding in this study is the strong relation between ... The most important finding in this study is that ...
9	Interleukin 6 clearly stimulated epithelial wound closure in this simple corneal abrasion model *in vivo*.
10	The randomised blinded design used in this study makes it unlikely that the significant differences between iron and placebo treated infants in changes in mental and motor development scores could depend on errors associated with subject selection or with the administration and nature of the Bayley scales.

Table 11. Exponents of initial claims in the English language Discussion sections

In contrast to this wide range of opening claims, the Spanish subcorpus only contained six instances of initial claims. Of these only one coincided with the formulas observed in the English language discussions by opening with "The results of this study show that". The other five displayed minor variations or were radically different (table 12).

1	The results found in our study population suggest that the activity of itraconazole is similar to that of griseofulvin in the treatment of Tinea manuum and Tinea pedis.
2	According to the results obtained, the three antioxidant agents used in the present study produce a statistically significant reduction in the corneal chemiluminescence values in comparison with the control group both in the study using incubation *in vitro*, with highly significant differences (p <0.001) for all three agents, and after treatment *in vivo*, with significant differences (p <0.05) for the group treated with SOD [superoxide dismutase] and highly significant differences (p <0.001) for the groups treated with DMTU [dimethylthiourea] and bendazac lysine salt.
3	Our results confirm the antiproliferative effectiveness of the different drugs under study although there are differences in the concentrations used.
4	Since the source of the three samples in case 1 is known (amniotic, cystic and ascitic), the values obtained will serve as a reference in the comparison with cases 2 and 3, which although thought to come from the amniotic fluid, must have resulted from the accidental puncture of the hygroma.
5	The absence of Schlemm's canal is thought to be one of the factors that lead to increased intraocular pressure and is considered by some authors to be the main determinant of congenital glaucoma; it cannot, however, be a primary cause, since this structure has been identified in many other cases with high intraocular pressure, as has also been seen in this study.

Table 12. Exponents of initial claims in the Spanish Discussion sections

The variation in (1) lies in the use of *suggest*, which is even weaker than *indicate* on the epistemic scale presented above. Example (2) introduces an alternative to the epistemic verb in the form of the prepositional phrase "According to the results obtained" placed before the claim, which is further supported by the statistical evidence; a more natural translation would use formula 3 of table 10. Example (3) shows that the verb *confirm* can be used for claims in association with evaluative concepts such as efficacy and safety in relation to drug testing. However, the last two complex examples require more detailed explanation. The study from which claim (4) is taken is a series of just five cases and seeks to establish a reliable way of distinguishing between different fluid samples in cases of 45,X monosomy obtained during pregnancy. The opening statement in the discussion contains two claims, both of which are prefaced by background in the form of subordinate clauses. Given the limited evidence, the claims are virtually restricted to the bounds of the study, but the first could establish valid reference values for other cases of the condition. Example (5) has a highly complex structure, and is a non-literal translation of the Spanish sentence that uses a device not available in English. As a result, the English states in two sentences what the Spanish does in one, the first containing background information and the second the claim, but as in the original the claim is stated at the end in the subordinate clause "as has also been seen in this study". It is also the weakest claim of all because of this final position. What the authors are claiming is that "This study has shown that the absence of Schlemm's canal cannot be a primary cause of congenital glaucoma"; however, owing to the state of knowledge at that time and in order to avoid open conflict with other authors, the claim has been so attenuated that it hardly merits the name.

5.3 Studies with background information

In the discussions in which background information was followed by a claim, the formulas used were basically similar, but some differences could be discerned (table 13). In comparison to table 11, there are no instances of a first person epistemic verb, but in (1) the claim is linked to the authors through the possessive *Our study* and is strengthened with the adverb *clearly*. In contrast, in the two claims starting with *results*, the subject is combined with the weaker epistemic verbs *indicate* and *suggest*, the former again boosted by *clearly*, but the use of *suggest* might make readers wonder how confident the authors are about their study; however, it does not stand out so much as the instance in the Spanish discussion. Example 3 combines an epistemic verb with an evaluation *better results* in a study in which the authors were defending the much maligned Angelchik device for treatment of gastric reflux. Example (6) is a good instance of anthropomorphic metonymy (Williams, 2005; Williams, 2008) in which the research replaces the researchers but retains their cognitive abilities to *reject the hypothesis* under consideration. Examples 5 to 7 make claims for originality, interest and merit. The first two are clearly introductory claims that structure the discourse and lead on to a series of aspects for comment and interpretation. The importance of the third claim is justified by the risk of malignancy so that an accurate diagnosis is essential. Examples 8 and 9 are illustrations of weaker or tentative claims that require contextualisation because they could hardly stand at the head of the discussion section. Examples 10 and 11 are late claims preceded by so much general discussion that they constitute conclusions. The study in which the first of these claims appears is a review of six small series on the development of a specific clinical entity, *de novo* detrusor instability, following surgery. The aim is to identify predictive factors. Since the results are mostly negative, no major claim can be made and the progressive style is appropriate. The second study presented a novel surgical technique and is similar to the two Spanish studies described above. The authors discuss the advantages and disadvantages of the alternative approaches and conclude that the new technique is successful in overcoming most, if not all, of them.

All discussions in which the first statement arising from the current results is a result, a finding or an unexpected outcome exhibit the progressive discourse style, whether they include prior background or not. However, analysis of the discussions with and without contextualising background revealed qualitative differences that could be confirmed in a larger corpus. In the English language discussions, eight of the ten texts had one of the more general statements of finding - expressing a comparison, a relationship, or a general observation - and only two opened with a numerical result. In the discussions with initial background information, a trend was evident towards a greater presence of numerical results (5 of 11, 45% of the texts). In the Spanish subcorpus, two of the seven discussions with no background opened with numerical results, and one of them opened with a statement classed as an unexpected outcome. "*Lo primero que nos ha llamado la atención es la baja prevalencia de portadores en nuestra población*"; 'The first thing that has drawn our attention is the low prevalence of carriers in our population'. Although classed as an unexpected outcome, it comes close to the evaluative claim formula of "The most striking result of our study is ..." (table 11). In the discussions with initial contextual background, the numerical results accounted for 18 of the 28 (64%) studies, considerably higher than in the equivalent English language studies.

Similarly, all discussions opening with a comparison with previous research, with or without background information, exhibit the progressive style. However, no English language discussion had this Move as its initial sentence whereas five of the 19 Spanish discussions with no initial background did so (table 14).

1	Our study shows quite clearly that ... This study showed that ...
2	The results of this subgroup analysis clearly indicate that ... The results of this study suggest that midazolam is effective in providing rapid sedation and reduction in anxiety in preschool children during laceration repair.
3	The results of the present trial after 4-6 years of follow-up continue to show marginally better results with the Angelchik device.
4	This study rejects the hypothesis that KRL [krypton red laser] is superior by 1 line of acuity (5% probability of error).
5	Our series of pemphigus foliaceus presents original epidemiologic peculiarities.
6	In our work, the comparison of the two SCC [squamous cell carcinoma] groups revealed some interesting features.
7	Histologically, DPN [deep penetrating nevus] is worth recognition as in approximately 30% of the cases the possibility of malignant melanoma was raised.
8	That thyroid orbitopathy is primarily a disease occurring most often in women is not surprising, as thyroidal Graves' disease also preferentially affects women.
9	For women in Dundee having a termination of pregnancy the non-participation rate of only 3.4% and the exceptionally high proportion (93.2%) opting for an anonymous test might be attributable to the special circumstances of the termination of pregnancy patient compared with the antenatal clinic attender.
10	Only one study has shown that multiple previous operations seems to be a risk factor (9).
11	With our technique, the removal of the posterior lens capsule under positive pressure and in closed-system conditions is highly controlled, and the desired ICCE-like [intracapsular cataract extraction] state is obtained without loss of silicone.

Table 13. Exponents of claims that follow initial background information in the English language Discussion sections

1	Our findings confirm those of previous reports by Sale *et al.* (2), Elliot *et al.* (3), Sviland *et al.* (4) and Lever *et al.* (6) on the presence of necrotic keratinocytes in the normal skin of autologous and allogeneic bone marrow transplant recipients both before and after the conditioning regimen.
2	These results are consistent with those obtained by Diamond and Kaplan (5), who found improvement in visual acuity in 24 of 25 cases of chronic uveitis treated with vitrectomy, with fewer recurrences in the treated group compared with non-treated patients.
3	In our study the survival rate of 98% was slightly higher than that reported in most studies (1-5), even though there were 19 cases of shock (38%), 6 cases of shock with diffuse intravascular coagulopathy (12%) and two cases of acute respiratory failure (4%).
4	The prevalence of iron deficiency of 4.94% found in our study population is higher than that reported in other studies: 3.27% in the group studied by Martin in 1989 in a rural population in Tenerife between four and sixteen years of age (1).
5	The high prevalence of hepatitis B virus infection observed in this study (78%) is not substantially different from that reported in previous studies, in which the prevalence of positive markers in intravenous drug users was between 75% and 85% (7-9), with anti-HBc as the commonest marker.

Table 14. Examples of initial comparisons with previous research in Spanish Discussions

It should be noted that in these section-initial comparisons, two patterns are apparent: the general noun *findings* or *results* refers to the whole of the previous results section (examples 1 and 2), or a numerical result is embedded in a complex expression of the grammatical subject (examples 3-5).

1	The proportion of cases with objective confirmation of the initial diagnosis was not as high in those studies as in our trial.
2	The data obtained in such studies agree well with the 6.5% BZD [benzodiazepine] use found among the 46 controls in this study with a combined review of maternity health records and biochemical screening during early pregnancy.
3	As in other biochemical markers, individual differences were noted in the preoperative serum β-endorphin concentrations as well as the β-endorphin response to the circumcision procedure.
4	Although our patient group was basically similar, our results contradict these findings.
5	Symptoms and clinical findings of our patients are in accordance with reports in the literature.
6	The response rate in the present study, 76%, is well in line with our own study of 60 to 62 year old women (6) and also with other, similarly performed cross-sectional studies (11,12).
7	The rate of rim-area loss of 2.1%/y in eyes with an initial field defect and 1.7%/y in the contralateral eye is comparable with the rate recently shown by Airaksinen *et al* (25).

Table 15. Instances of comparison with previous research in English language discussions with background information

Table 15 shows the instances from the English subcorpus of the comparison with previous research Move that initiates the discussion after the initial contextual information. In these comparisons the movement is both inward from the previous research to the current study (examples 1-3) and outward from the current findings to other researchers' studies (examples 4-7). In tables 14 and 15 taken together, in addition to the characteristic comparative structures *higher than* and *(not) as high as*, other exponents include *in line with, comparable with, in accordance with, consistent with*, and the verbs *confirm* and *contradict*.

A minority choice, both in the English and Spanish discussions with zero background was to open the discussion with a limitation (table 16).

1	The number of foetal heart rate patterns included in this study does not allow analysis of the agreement between the description and evaluation of these patterns and the foetal outcome, as such a correlation would be entirely dependent on the selection of the 11 cases.
2	The data obtained in the present study are not representative of the general reference population taking digoxin, since patients came from a hospital emergency department. They are only representative of a population with heart disease in a phase of decompensation.

Table 16. Instances of limitations that open the Discussion section in the English language and Spanish subcorpora

Although the limitation in (1) is a reflection of the selection of the patterns included in the study and as such a methodological question, it is also a comment on the results obtained for the two aspects, which cannot be correlated and are, therefore, presented separately. In the case of the Spanish discussion (example 2), the limitation of the representativeness of the sample, which is presented as a warning to the reader, is immediately followed by an attenuated claim that the sample does represent the population for which it was intended, that is, patients attended in the emergency department for sudden worsening of their heart condition. This text was finally classified as portraying the retrogressive style.

In the light of the qualitative analysis of the results of the comparison of the English language and Spanish discussions, the following tentative conclusions can be reached. There are clearly differences in the choices made by authors publishing their research in the two languages. The retrogressive discourse style is far more prevalent in English language publications than among Spanish writers publishing their work in their national journals. The number of Spanish studies with background information was higher than in the English subcorpus and the amount included tended to be greater. However, the presence of background information is indicative of, but not exclusive to, the progressive style. In the qualitative assessment, the main difference between the subcorpora was that English language Discussions generally provided the underlying rationale when describing specific points of methodology, both when this information was combined with general contextualisation and when it appeared alone as background. In relation to the retrogressive style, the English language texts displayed a wide range of exponents of the opening claim (Move 7). They varied from standard formulas to individual personalised expressions of this Move, and also showed considerable variation in the strength of the expression, which allows writers to convey the level of commitment to the claim and the degree of certainty. In contrast, the small number of initial claims in the Spanish subcorpus inclined to the lower end of the scale, with weaker lexical verbs and greater uncertainty. Despite a degree of overlap with the English language Discussions, the great majority of the Spanish texts conformed to the progressive style. Whether cultural differences are the only explanation of this will be examined in the following sections.

5.4 Native and non-native writers of English

The quantitative analysis comparing native with non-native writers within the English language subcorpus showed no differences in the choice of the progressive and retrogressive discourse styles ($P = 0.657$). Further analyses of these subsets with regard to use of background information and selection of opening move largely confirmed the overall result. Thus, exactly half (11 of 22 authors) included some initial background compared to 48% (20 of 42) of the native authors. However, native authors were more likely to include background information on the current study, either combined with external context or exclusively (10 of 19 authors, 53%), compared with 3 of 12 non-native writers (25%). As regards the choice of Move to open the commentary, both native and non-native writers predominantly selected a claim (55% in both cases) although two non-native discussions presented late claims and corresponded to the progressive discourse style. However, in the native discussions the statement of result or finding was a clear second choice (16 of 42, 38%), with the comparison with previous research showing only a token presence (3 instances, 7%). In contrast, results/ findings and comparisons were fairly even in the non-native discussions (5 and 4 instances, or 23% and 18%), and there was one opening limitation (see table 16).

These results indicate that non-native writers publishing in the selected journals successfully adapt their discussions to the required discourse style, although from a textual study like this it is not possible to know how the final text was arrived at, what strategies were employed, whether translation or native-speaker editing was used, or what negotiation was required with the referees and editors of the journals.

5.5 Study type and discourse style

For our analysis, the study types were broadly grouped according the strength of the evidence they can be expected to produce according to the design. The studies producing the strongest empirical evidence can be expected to correlate with the retrospective discourse style in which the main claim either opens or is placed fairly close to the start of the Discussion, and alternatively the studies with the weakest design, that is, those most prone to problems such as missing data, selection bias and confounding factors, will probably correlate with the prospective discourse style, since in these circumstances writers will be less likely to be able to make a strong claim for their research and, therefore, will build an argument carefully from initial premises, through relevant data before venturing to make interpretative or speculative statements. The quantitative data largely support this hypothesis, although there are differences between the two subcorpora. In the English language subcorpus, two thirds of the trials have retrogressive discussions, and the studies with weaker designs tend toward equality between the retrogressive and progressive styles. In the Spanish subcorpus, the studies with the strongest design are equally distributed between the discourse styles, but the epidemiological studies and case series strongly favour the progressive style. In what follows, we shall attempt to account for some of the anomalous cases.

Of the six trials in the English language subcorpus that used the progressive style, two were follow-up studies in which *post hoc* subgroup analyses were performed. In these cases, since the object of the new study was not a primary outcome of the original trial, the relevant data may not have been collected with the necessary rigour and will be prone to the problems of bias and confounding factors. Sample text 5 is the opening of the Discussion of one of these trials. It begins with a series of findings (S1-S4), followed by comparison with previous studies (S5) before the authors make their claim for originality (S6-S7).

#S1	# The principal findings of this study are that Holter monitoring detected ST segment depression after acute myocardial infarction in 32% of patients.
S2	This incidence was unrelated to the use of thrombolytic therapy.
S3	Patients with ST depression had more severe stenosis in the infarct-related artery, greater left ventricular dysfunction and a more unfavorable prognosis.
S4	The occurrence of ST depression on Holter monitoring was more closely related to the severity of residual stenosis in the infarct-related artery and to the incidence of cardiac events during follow-up than was the occurrence of ST segment depression during exercise testing.
#S5	# Our findings support the previously reported prognostic significance of ST segment depression after myocardial infarction (1,2,5).
S6	The novel contribution of our study is the identification of a possible pathophysiologic mechanism linking the occurrence of ST depression and unfavorable prognosis.
S7	Our study is the first to establish the association between the occurrence of ST segment depression after myocardial infarction and the severity of lumen narrowing in the infarct-related artery

Sample text 5. Trial with a Discussion displaying the progressive discourse style

In a third trial (see sample text 2) the progressive style was the suitable choice not only because of the small numbers of patients enrolled, but because the overall result was negative. Another trial comparing short-term (4 weeks) and long-term (3 months) anticoagulation for deep vein thrombosis and pulmonary embolism yielded mixed results slightly favouring the long-term treatment overall, but indicating short-term anticoagulation when the thrombosis or embolism developed postoperatively. However, the authors' claim is only tentative and they are careful to warn that this result was based on a *post hoc* analysis: "Our finding of only 1 failure to resolve and 1 recurrence among 60 patients whose DVT or PE developed postoperatively suggests that 4 weeks' treatment may be sufficient for such patients. This conclusion, however, is based on a post-hoc analysis and should be confirmed by a further prospective study solely of postoperative patients." When the claims are only tentative, the progressive style becomes the more likely choice. In a trial of topical anaesthesia with lidocaine cream for the circumcision of newborns, the main claim did not appear until the last sentence of the Discussion: "In summary, under these experimental conditions, this study has demonstrated that a topical 30% lidocaine cream applied prior to circumcision of the term newborn may be a safe and efficacious anesthetic." Despite the strength of the evidential verb *demonstrate*, the authors can only claim that this approach *may be* safe. This uncertainty could well have conditioned their whole discourse strategy in the Discussion and led to the choice of the progressive style. The final trial exhibiting the progressive style is more difficult to account for. The trial was a large multicentre, multinational, double-blind, randomised, placebo-controlled study in acute myocardial infarction with ramipril as the study drug. The Discussion was also one of the longest in the subcorpus. Unlike the previous studies, this trial produced positive results, and yet the authors only went as far as restating the main finding at the head of the section: "Ramipril, administered to patients with clinical evidence of heart failure on the second to ninth day after myocardial infarction for an average of 15 months, caused a highly significant and substantial reduction in all-cause mortality." This is an objective past-tense statement of a time-related change produced by the effect of treatment. There is no boosting (*demonstrate, show*) or attenuation (*suggest*) through evidential verbs, and the strength of the assertion relies wholly on the statistical analysis and the size of the change (Skelton, 1994). It could be that in such a large trial with multiple authorship no agreement could be reached on a stronger claim for the results of the study.

In the Spanish subcorpus, two trials exhibited the retrogressive style although the claim in one was attenuated by the use of *suggest* (see table 12). Of the two trials with the progressive discourse style, one was an open-label trial and the patients were not randomised. This weakening of the study design may have been enough to lead the authors to employ a considerable amount of background, both external and methodological, before making a late claim (after 70% background information) for their study: "The results of our study show that the effectiveness of the two antimicrobial agents is similar with regard to the therapeutic action of eliminating the microorganism, around 92%, and eradication of Chlamydia was maintained until the follow-up visit one month later, a period that is similar to that reported in most studies (17,18)." Note that the claim for effectiveness is supported by a finding and comparison with previous research. In the second case, the Spanish study formed part of a multinational European trial comparing active and passive approaches to the management of labour with the ultimate aim of reducing the caesarean rate. The results were again non-conclusive: "In view of our results and those from the rest of the European

Study, it is difficult to make a definitive pronouncement on one or other of the strategies, since no differences were found for the number of operative deliveries and specifically for caesarean sections."

The experimental and investigational studies covered a variety of designs and were placed together in one category for the convenience of statistical analysis. Nevertheless, the two discourse designs were evenly distributed in the two subcorpora. All the experimental studies with a comparative design with objective quantitative measurement systems showed the retrogressive style, with the exception of a study carried out on the ability of nurses and parents to administer small doses of insulin to paediatric diabetic patients. In this study, the results of the initial measurements were negative in that all the subjects administered doses far in excess of the target dose, and so a second test was performed in which the standard was changed. The Discussion opens by reporting the negative findings of the original design: "Although the administration of low doses of concentrated insulin is common practice in pediatric care facilities, our study revealed a remarkably high error when doses of less than 2.0 U of U100 insulin are dispensed by skilled pediatric nurses. Attempts to deliver doses as low as 0.5 U or 1.0 U resulted in overdosage of 95% and 66%, respectively." Here, after the introductory background in the subclause, the initial finding is presented and this is supported by the numerical result. In this case the finding does not fall far short of classification as a claim. The more general claims for the study were expressed in the conclusion with a strong personal commitment: "We thus believe that the errors reported in this study are a conservative estimate of those that occur in day-to-day administration. We conclude that, until better measuring devices are available, it is impractical to deliver insulin injections of less than 20 μL (2 U of U100)." As seen with the trials, the negative results may be the reason for the choice of the progressive style.

Two Spanish experimental studies had the progressive style. One tested a novel modification to a surgical technique, and as seen in section 5.1, this can lead to choice of the progressive style since writers appear to feel the need for extensive contextual information on alternative procedures before making their claims for the new method. In this case, the authors went through the whole gamut of Moves before concluding with their claims: "From the results obtained, it can be deduced that the omega loop with Braun's anastomosis and an associated antireflux valve is a simple quick and safe technique which presents no risk of torsion or vascular compromise and is effective in preventing entero-hepatic reflux. For these reasons, we believe that this technique should be considered an option in diversion surgery for biliary problems in children." The opening formula (literal translation) for the claim is fairly frequent in Spanish and could be rendered more naturally in English as *The results of this study* + evidential verb; however, which verb to choose is not so clear: *show* – *indicate* – *suggest*. The claim is followed by a recommendation.

The second progressive style Spanish Discussion belonged to a study in which a new evaluation technique for surgical adhesions was applied in a rat model. The method was semi-quantitative and established the degree of severity for six surgical situations, and this may be the reason for the progressive style of the Discussion, which presents the findings in descending order and discusses the characteristics of the adhesions and the implications in each case. The first statement after the background context is: "Our method of adhesion quantification revealed that the aetiological factor resulting in the most postoperative peritoneal adhesions is the presence of a foreign body."

The two studies investigating different aspects of clinical practice by means of questionnaires both displayed the progressive style. One opened with a limitation (see table 16, example 2) but, rather than making a counter claim directly, moved on to provide background information before presenting a finding. The second study aimed at collecting baseline data on the emerging new field of paediatric emergency medicine, mentioned in table 9 (example 7) in relation to background information providing the rationale for the study. Again the first statement arising from the data obtained was a finding. It would seem that this kind of investigation, which produces mainly descriptive quantitative data, lends itself to the progressive discourse style rather than the persuasive character of retrogressive argumentation.

Of the 13 studies classified as epidemiological, only two, both of which were in the English-language subcorpus, displayed the retrogressive style. One was a cohort study; studies of this type are ranked just below randomised clinical trials and higher than case-controlled studies and case series in terms of the quality and reliability of the data obtained, and this could justify a strong initial claim. However, another cohort study opened with the main finding followed by a general reference to previous research before the authors made a claim for the data they have produced which come to fill a gap in current knowledge: "The data presented define the overall and relative risks, although the small numbers of events have resulted in lack of precision with wide confidence intervals." The reason for the modest claim immediately becomes clear from the limitation of the statistical evidence so that the progressive style can be seen as the safer option for this study, in which only 334 patients were analysed in comparison to the 2,846 patients included in the cohort study with the retrogressive style.

The other epidemiological study had a tentative claim that followed some background information (see table 13, example 9). The study used pregnant women as a surrogate group to represent a heterosexual population at risk of contracting the HIV virus. The initial claim is not in fact the main claim for the study, but a claim concerning the quality of the data obtained, the main claim being placed later after more consideration of the study methodology. The authors' claim is that the study establishes baseline data that will serve in the future to measure rates of change in the prevalence of HIV infection. This study is, therefore, something of a hybrid between the two styles.

The main differences in the distribution of the discourse styles between the English language and the Spanish texts was seen in the case series whatever their characteristics, small series of fewer than 30 subjects, retrospective reviews of case notes or prospective studies. Overall, the two styles were evenly distributed in the English language texts but in the Spanish subcorpus there was only one retrogressive style Discussion for every seven progressive sections. To try to account for this discrepancy, we looked at how the research was presented in the Introduction section to see whether this had an influence on the choice of discourse style. In the prospective studies there was a trend for those that explicitly mentioned the testing of hypotheses or asked specific questions in the Introduction to provide answers to these questions in the form of an early claim in the Discussion: only one of six studies addressing this type of specific question had the progressive style. Sample text 6 illustrates this direct relationship in which the opening claims of the Discussion (S1-S3) reflect almost exactly the hypothesis stated in the Introduction (S0) for N-terminal natriuretic peptide (N-ANP).

#S0	# The current study tested the hypothesis that the concentration of N-ANP is raised and serves as a sensitive and specific marker in patients with symptomless left-ventricular dysfunction.
#S1	# The current study demonstrates that patients with proven ventricular dysfunction by radionuclide angiography and without symptoms of heart failure have raised concentration of plasma N-ANP.
S2	Our study also shows that this increased concentration is both sensitive and specific for ventricular dysfunction.
S3	These observations support a role for N-ANP as an important noninvasive marker for symptomless left-ventricular dysfunction.

Sample text 6. Discussion showing strong links between claims and the study aim stated in the Introduction

Other studies which expressed their aims in more general terms such as "to characterize patients with asymptomatic restenosis, and to determine the usefulness of late exercise testing..." or "we wanted to further define the success rate, complications and prognostic factors associated with semiconductor diode transscleral cyclophotocoagulation" could be related to weaker initial claims, or the claims were first motivated by an amount of background information. However, this type of study aim was more likely to lead to a progressive style Discussion, as illustrated by sample text 7.

#S0	# To better classify this heterogeneous group of subepithelial blistering mucous membrane diseases, we conducted a 6-year comprehensive study on all new patients whose diagnoses fit within the spectrum of bullous pemphigoid, benign mucous membrane pemphigoid, and ocular cicatricial pemphigoid.
#S1	# Distinct patterns of immunopathology and antigenic specificity of autoantibodies correlated with distinct subsets of patients with immune-mediated subepithelial blistering diseases of mucous membranes.
S2	Because the patient population was drawn from the departments of dermatology, ophthalmology, and oral pathology and identified through a diagnostic test administered by the pathology department, selection bias toward predominant expression in any one organ system is minimized.
S3	Our data indicate that at least two distinct groups can be clearly defined within this heterogeneous group of patients.

Sample text 7. Discussion with progressive style related to a descriptive aim in the Introduction section

In this example, the Discussion opens with a statement of finding (S1) signalled by the typical past tense. This is supported by a minor claim on the methodology (S2) that validates the finding before the main claim that the authors have clarified the classification of these blistering diseases. The neutral evidential verb *indicate* and the fact that only two groups "can be clearly defined" attenuate the claim and motivate the choice of the progressive discourse style. The Discussion then moves into a descriptive mode characterising in turn the different patient groups analysed. In another study, as we have seen in relation to randomised trials, a negative result correlates with choice of the progressive style.

What we have observed for prospective studies also appears to hold true for large retrospective studies and small case series. Statement of a clear study design in the Introduction will be reflected at the start of the Discussion with a claim if the evidence is strong enough. "In this study, we compared the outcome of aortic valve replacement for aortic stenosis in patients >80 years old with that of patients 65 to 75 years old." This comparative design leads to an evaluative claim at the opening of the Discussion: "The most important finding in this study is that despite their poorer postoperative condition, patients >80 years old who undergo aortic valve replacement for aortic stenosis have a favourable postoperative course that is similar in many respects to that of the younger age group." This is clearly not a plain statement of the finding itself, but is coloured by the authors' subjective evaluation through the adjectives "most important" and "favourable", while use of the present tense generalises the finding in the context of aortic replacement in the elderly. While not as strong as the claims in the prospective studies, the evidence is strong enough for the authors to choose the argumentative retrogressive style without fear of having severe criticism levelled at them for overstating their knowledge claim.

Even in the studies with the weakest design structure, a claim to originality can justify choice of the retrogressive style. In one dermatology study, the case series was presented in purely descriptive terms: "We report 20 cases of pemphigus foliaceus, all of them involving young women seen from November 1985 through January 1987 in Sousse, Tunisia." Nevertheless, the data supported an early claim for originality in the Discussion section: "Our series presents original epidemiologic peculiarities." After this, the Discussion again moves into the descriptive mode.

Thus, there is some evidence in the English language subcorpus that in prospective studies, retrospective studies and small case series, it is the strength of the evidence that determines the choice of discourse style. The strong link between the presentation of the study in the Introduction and the style of the Discussion, especially when the retrogressive style is chosen, lends support Swales' (1984) contention that Introductions are written late, or rewritten, after the other sections have been completed, and are "essentially exercises in public relations". It also confirms that the research article is an artefact that constructs knowledge through persuasive argument rather than narrating scientific research in the chronological order in which it was carried out (Myers, 1994).

In the Spanish subcorpus, the situation is clearer in that, for case series of all types, authors prefer the progressive style, which is suitable both for the largely descriptive series reporting the authors' experience with a particular entity or technique and for other studies where writers prefer to build an argument in an iconic chronological order reflecting how the study developed and the data emerged. A previous contrastive study (Williams, 2005) on the same corpus revealed a different attitude to research and research reporting between English language and Spanish articles. Articles published in English language journals are characterised by a "separatist" view of research that distinguishes between the performing of the study (past tense: *The study showed*) and the act of writing or publication (present tense: *This report describes*). In contrast, Spanish Discussions reveal a "unitary" view of research, as illustrated by the word *trabajo* (literally 'work' but more usually 'study', 'report', 'paper' depending on the context), which covers the whole research process, and through greater use of the present tense, which signals relevance to the ongoing development of the argument in the Discussion. Spanish Discussions, therefore, often return to the start of the process and contextualise and motivate the study, restate aims, and mention methods before coming to the interpretation of the results, which is often assumed to be the function of the Discussion.

Sample text 8 is a complete short Discussion section with this kind of progressive through-argumentation. From the initial report in 1984, the authors give a rapid overview of relevant research (S1), and then state the problem to be addressed, the adequate dose (S2). The text then moves inward to the current study and gives the range of doses used and the overall result (S3). There follows a series of more general findings (S4-S7) on different aspects of the study. It should be noted that S5 also includes a limitation on the data, which weakens the strength of the evidence. The final statement (S8) conflates the main claim (*we believe*) with a recommendation for clinical practice with the conditions for use.

#S1	# Since 1984, when Bunn *et al* (1) reported an objective response rate of 45% with interferon alpha in advanced stages of cutaneous T-cell lymphomas, there have been numerous published studies that in general support the effectiveness of this treatment in cutaneous T-cell lymphoma in different stages both when used alone (2,4-11) and when combined with etretinate (12-14) or PUVA [psoralen + ultraviolet A therapy] (15,16).
S2	The optimum dose has not been established, but it appears that low doses may be less effective than larger doses.
#S3	# In our centre, patients with early and advanced stage T-cell cutaneous lymphoma were treated with doses varying from 3 MU/3 times to 18 MU/day and the mean objective response rate was 86%.
S4	The response was somewhat better in early (100%) than in late stages (70%).
S5	The response was also slightly better in patients who tolerated larger doses of interferon although the number of patients was too small to draw conclusions.
#S6	# Recurrences were frequent with no clear relationship with clinical stage or tolerated dose.
#S7	# In our experience, the treatment is well tolerated and, although the adverse effects required treatment to be suspended in four patients, they were always reversible.
#S8	# Thus, we believe that this treatment should be considered in cutaneous T-cell lymphoma, especially in cases of extensive plaques of fungoid mycosis for which PUVA is not possible, and in advanced stages refractory to other treatments.

Sample text 8. Complete Spanish Discussion exhibiting the progressive discourse style and a unitary view of research

However, there are six exceptions in the Spanish subcorpus where authors have selected to open the Discussion with a claim. Two of these have already been mentioned (see table 12, examples 4 and 5) as examples of weak claims. A third Discussion opened with a limitation (table 12, example 2), which, as is often the case, is followed by a counterclaim or rejoinder that restricts or nullifies the effect of the limitation. In this case, the writer is well aware of the nature of the retrospective data he has drawn on, and warns the reader from the outset.

#S0	# Recently, analysis of the rearrangement of the bcr/abl gene by the Southern blotting technique is being used as a clinical laboratory test for diagnosis and monitoring of therapy in chronic myeloid leukaemia (CML) (8).
S0	This article presents the current authors experience in this respect and also analyses six of the patients with CML in blastic crisis.
#S1	# In this study DNA analysis was performed in all cases with the Bg/II restriction enzyme and the complementary DNA probe TransProbe 1, since the results of our previous unpublished studies with the Bg/II and Bam HI enzymes and the Pr-1 probe showed lower sensitivity in the analysis.
S2	This has been confirmed by other studies (8,14-16).
S3	Nevertheless, the complementary use of the two probes in the DNA study of each patient allows us to delimit the breakpoint cluster region and, thus, to determine whether there is a relationship between this breakpoint and the onset of the blastic crisis or with shorter patient survival time (16-19).
#S4	# The results of this study indicate that use of the Southern blotting technique to analyse the bcr/abl gene rearrangement is a sensitive and specific method for the diagnosis of CML, as has been reported by other authors (8,14,15).

Sample text 9. Spanish Discussion with retrogressive style related to a descriptive aim in the Introduction section

Of the remaining three studies, two were large retrospective series and one a prospective study. In two studies, background context preceded the opening claim and only one retrospective study opened with this Move. As in the English language examples, there was a close link between the presentation of the research in the Introduction and the early claim, even when the study lacked an explicit goal, as in sample text 9. This text also illustrates the Spanish tendency to open the Discussion with contextual background adding more detail to the information provided in the Introduction. The first three statements (S1-S3) justifying the methodology used could well have been adapted and inserted between the last two sentences of the Introduction (S0). The claim (S4) displays one of the characteristic formats, but since the findings of the current study merely confirm those previously reported, the neutral verb *indicate* reduces the force of the assertion.

Much the same can be said for the other retrospective study in which the aim was expressed in broad descriptive terms: "The aim of our retrospective study was to assess the frequency and epidemiological characteristics of invasive Hib infections in Spain." Nevertheless, the opening claim used one of the strongest formulas: "The results of this study show that Hib infections are a common cause of serious illness in the paediatric age." The authors stress the seriousness of the problem, and this allows them to construct a persuasive case for the introduction of a vaccination campaign into the Spanish immunisation programme, as has been recommended in the USA and other European countries.

The final retrogressive style Discussion belongs to a complex cardiology study in which the authors use measurement of peak oxygen consumption (peak VO_2) to relate cardiac output with a number of variables in patients with hypertension. These are clearly stated at the end of the Introduction. The Discussion opens with considerable background information (20% of the section) mainly on the methodology and its underlying rationale. In spite of this, the style from then on is clearly retrogressive and opens with the strongest of the formulas: "Our data demonstrate that hypertensive patients without antecedent angina or infarction who have shown left ventricular failure with preserved systolic function may, after control of pulmonary congestion with a diuretic, present a clinical and physiological profile similar to that of patients with hypertensive disease who never showed symptoms." It should be noted that the strength of the formula is later attenuated with the modalised verb *may present*. After this broad general claim for this patient group, the authors go on to analyse the factors mentioned in the Introduction in cycles that are mainly retrogressive but include progressive elements.

6. Conclusion

This study provides empirical evidence of two clearly differentiated discourse styles that are used in the Discussion sections of medical research articles. The statistical and qualitative analyses comparing the two subcorpora indicate differences between the style of the English language publications in which the retrogressive style predominates and that of the Spanish journals where an even stronger preference is observed for the progressive style. Although cultural factors undoubtedly play a role in the choice of style, it is not a sufficient explanation in itself for the choice of discourse style since both styles were evident in the two subcorpora. The subanalysis performed on the English language articles distinguishing between native authors and non-native writers of English showed that the non-native writers, who came from a wide range of national backgrounds, are successful in adapting to the disciplinary and stylistic requirements demanded by English language journals.

The most important determinant of choice of discourse style to emerge from the analyses is the type of study. Studies with the most rigorous design yield the best empirical evidence and were found to correlate with the retrogressive style since this style enables authors to foreground the strongest knowledge claim which they believe they can persuade their peers to accept. The larger proportion of randomised clinical trials in the English language subcorpus accounted for much of the difference between the English and Spanish texts. However, even among the study types with less rigorous designs, the English language writers sought to take every opportunity to make as strong a knowledge claim as possible right from the outset. Conversely, any weakness in the data produced with the strongest study design could lead to a weakening of the claim, covering the claim with background information, and in the last resort switching to the progressive style.

The scant presence of the retrogressive style among the case series - whether prospective, retrospective, or small case series - suggests that the progressive style is an almost automatic choice for Spanish writers in their native language. If this is the case, they must make a great rhetorical effort in order to have their work published in English language journals and thus emulate the non-native writers included in the sample studied here.

The data and the sample texts presented in this paper can serve as models and guidelines for the structuring of the two discourse styles, and as an indication of how the key moves are expressed. More general recommendations suggested by the data would be to reduce the background information in the Discussion by including it in a more elaborately developed Introduction section, written or reworked even after completion of the other sections. This could be achieved by constructing the Introduction along the lines proposed by Swales (1984) as a promotional exercise so that it ends with a clear statement of the hypothesis to be tested, the question or questions to be addressed, or the primary and secondary aims of the study. Depending on the quality and strength of the data obtained, these hypotheses, questions and aims can be linked to the strongest possible claim either at the head of, or as early as possible, in the Discussion. Claims for originality and evaluative statements may be sufficient justification for choosing the retrogressive discourse style since these make it clear to readers where the argument is going to take them, and this can be followed by a switch to a more descriptive style as an alternative option.

If methodological questions are deemed necessary as background information, they should be motivated by stating the underlying rationale. Negative outcomes and any fundamental weaknesses in the data appear to make the retrogressive discourse style incompatible and require a carefully constructed progressive argument to make a convincing case for publication and acceptance by peer readers.

In conclusion, this study has shown that the choice of the retrogressive or the progressive discourse style for the Discussion section of medical research articles is only partly dependent on cultural differences in the use of rhetoric, and that the type of study undertaken and the quality of the evidence produced exert a complementary and stronger influence on this choice. The finding that non-native writers are successful in adopting the appropriate discourse style is testimony to the great rhetorical effort they may have to make if the discourse style does not conform to their cultural mind set and their professional and disciplinary recognition and advancement depends on publishing their work in leading scientific journals.

7. References

Barber, C. (1962). Some measurable characteristics of modern scientific prose, In: *Episodes in ESP*, J. Swales (Ed.), 3-14, Prentice Hall, ISBN 0-13-283383-2, London

Belanger, M. (1982). A preliminary analysis of the structure of the discussion sections in ten neuroscience journal articles (mimeo)

Brett, P. (1994). A genre analysis of the results sections of sociology articles. *English for Specific Purposes*, 13, 1, 47-59, ISSN 0889-4906

Cooper, C. (1985). Aspects of article introductions in IEEE publications, Unpublished M.Sc. dissertation, University of Aston, UK

Crookes, G. (1986) Towards a validated analysis of scientific text structure. *Applied Linguistics* 7, 1, 57-70, ISSN 0142-6001

Dudley-Evans, T. (1994). Genre analysis: an approach to text analysis for ESP, In: *Advances in Written Text Analysis,* M. Coulthard (Ed.), 219-228, Routledge, ISBN 0-415-09519-0, London & New York

Everitt, B. (1977). *The Analysis of Contingency Tables*, Chapman & Hall, ISBN 0-412-39850-8, London

Fries, P. (1994). On theme, rheme and discourse goals, In: *Advances in Written Text Analysis,* M. Coulthard (Ed.), 229-249, Routledge, ISBN 0-415-09519-0, London & New York

Gilbert, G. & Mulkay, M. (1984). *Opening Pandora's Box: a Sociological Analysis of Scientific Discourse*, Cambridge University Press, ISBN 0-521-27430-3, Cambridge

Hopkins, A. & Dudley-Evans, T. (1988). A genre-based investigation of the discussion sections in articles and dissertations. *English for Specific Purposes*, 7, 1, 113-122, ISSN 0889-4906

Hunston, S. (1994). Evaluation and organisation in a sample of written academic discourse, In: *Advances in Written Text Analysis,* M. Coulthard (Ed.), 191-218, Routledge, ISBN 0-415-09519-0, London & New York

Hyland, K. (1998). *Hedging in Scientific Research Articles*, John Benjamins, ISBN 90-272-5067-7, Amsterdam & Philadelphia

Kanoksilapatham, B. (2003). A corpus-based investigation of scientific research articles: Linking move analysis and multidimensional analysis. Unpublished Ph.D dissertation, Georgetown University

Knorr-Cetina, K. (1981). *The Manufacture of Knowledge*, Pergamon, ISBN 0080257771, Oxford

Latour, B. & Woolgar, S. (1979). *Laboratory Life: The Social Construction of Scientific Facts*, Sage Publications, ISBN 0-691-02832-X, Beverly Hills, Cal.

Lewin, B., Fine, J. & Young, L. (2001). *Expository Discourse: A Genre-based Approach to Social Science Research Texts*, Continuum, ISBN 0826449131, London

Mauranen, A. (1993). *Cultural Differences in Academic Rhetoric: A Textlinguistic Study.* Peter Lang, ISBN 3631464746, Frankfurt

McKinlay, J. (1982). An analysis of discussion sections in medical journal articles, Unpublished M.A. dissertation, University of Birmingham, UK

Myers, G. (1985). Texts as knowledge claims: the social construction of two biology articles. *Social Studies of Science* 15, 4, 593-630. ISSN 0306-3127

Myers, G. (1994). Narratives of science and nature in popularizing molecular genetics, In: *Advances in Written Text Analysis,* M. Coulthard (Ed.), 179-190, Routledge, ISBN 0-415-09519-0, London & New York

Nwogu, K. (1997) The medical research paper: Structure and functions. *English for Specific Purposes,* 16, 1, 119-138, ISSN 0889-4906

Peng, J. (1987). Organizational features in chemical engineering research articles. *ELR Journal* 1, 79-116, ISSN 1746-6830

Sinclair, J. & Coulthard, M. (1975). *Towards an Analysis of Discourse,* Oxford University Press, ISBN 0194360113 , Oxford

Skelton, J. (1994). Analysis of the structure of original research papers: an aid to writing original papers for publication. *British Journal of General Practice* 44, 387, 455-459, ISSN 0960-1643

Swales, J. (1981). *Aspects of Article Introductions,* University of Aston, Birmingham, UK

Swales, J. (1984). Research into the structure of introductions to journal articles and its application to the teaching of academic writing, In: *Common Ground: Shared Interests in ESP and Communication Studies,* R. Williams, J. Swales & J. Kirkman (Eds.), 77-86, Pergamon, ISBN 0-08-031055-9, Oxford

Swales, J. (1990). *Genre Analysis: English in Academic and Research Settings,* Cambridge University Press, ISBN 0-521-32869-1, Cambridge

Swales, J. (2004). *Research Genres. Explorations and Applications.* Cambridge University Press, ISBN 0-521-82594-6, Cambridge

Tadros, A. (1994). Predictive categories in expository text, In: *Advances in Written Text Analysis,* M. Coulthard (Ed.), 69-82, Routledge, ISBN 0-415-09519-0, London & New York

Tarone, E., Dwyer, S, Gillette, S. & Icke, V. (1981). On the use of the passive in two astrophysics journal papers. *The ESP Journal* 1, 2, 123-40, ISSN 0889-4906

Thomas, S. (1991). A merging of voices: An investigation of the way discourse is reported in medical research articles, Unpublished Ph.D. dissertation, University of Birmingham, UK

Thomas, S. & Hawes, T. (1994). Reporting verbs in medical journal articles. *English for Specific Purposes,* 13, 2, 129-148, ISSN 0889-4906

Thompson, G. & Ye, Y. (1991). Evaluation of the reporting verbs used in academic papers. *Applied Linguistics* 12, 4, 365-382, ISSN 0142-6001

Vásquez, F. (1987). A comparative study of the rhetorical structure of the discussion sections in English and Spanish medical articles, Unpublished Master's dissertation, Aston University, Birmingham, UK

West, G. (1980). That-nominal constructions in traditional rhetorical divisions of scientific research papers. *TESOL Quarterly* 14, 4, 483-489 ISSN 0039-8322

Williams, I. (1999). Results sections of medical research articles: Analysis of rhetorical categories for pedagogical purposes. *English for Specific Purposes*, 18, 4, 347-366, ISSN 0889-4906

Williams, I. (2005). Thematic items referring to research and researchers in the discussion section of Spanish biomedical articles and English-Spanish translations. *Babel* 51, 2, 124-160, ISSN 0521-9744

Williams, I. (2008). Semantico-syntactic environments of the verb *show* and *demonstrate* and Spanish *mostrar* and *demostrar* in a bilingual corpus of medical research articles. *International Journal of Corpus Linguistics* 13, 1, 38-74, ISSN 1384-6655

Williams, I. (2009). Discourse style and theme-rheme progression in biomedical research article discussions: a corpus-based contrastive study of translational and non-translational Spanish. *Languages in Contrast* 9, 2, 225-266, ISSN 1387-6759

Williams, I. (2010). Getting the ACCENT right in translation studies, In: D. Gile, G. Hansen & N. Pokorn (Eds.), *Why Translation Studies Matters*, John Benjamins, ISBN 978-90-272-2434-7, Amsterdam & Philadelphia

Wingard, P. (1981). Some verb forms and functions in six medical texts, In: L. Selinker, E. Tarone & V. Hanzelli (Eds.), *English for Academic and Technical Purposes: Studies in honor of Louis Trimble*, 53-65, Newbury House, ISBN 0883771780, Rowley, MA

Part 2

Molecular Methods of Analysis

3

An Overview of Analytical Techniques Employed to Evidence Drug-DNA Interactions. Applications to the Design of Genosensors

Víctor González-Ruiz[1], Ana I. Olives[1], M. Antonia Martín[1]
Pascual Ribelles[2], M. Teresa Ramos[2] and J. Carlos Menéndez[2]
[1]S. D. Química Analítica,
[2]D. Química Orgánica y Farmacéutica,
Facultad de Farmacia, Universidad Complutense, 28040-Madrid,
Spain

1. Introduction

The demonstration of the existence of non-covalent bonding interactions between different biomolecules (DNA, enzymes, proteins) and drugs or potentially mutagenic agents requires sensitive analytical techniques. Technological advances in key techniques, together with the miniaturization in fluorescence or surface plasmons resonance techniques, have allowed obtaining information in real time concerning the nature, the localization and the strength of drug-DNA interactions. The present chapter describes these analytical techniques and their application to achieve two fundamental goals, namely a deeper knowledge of the nature of the interactions and their application to the design of different devices (aptamers, molecular beacons, DNA-arrays, genosensors) consisting of short single stranded oligonucleotides produced *in vitro* by well-established methods (polymerase chain reaction, PCR; systematic evolution of ligands by exponential enrichment, SELEX,...) that are capable to detect genetic peculiarities and diseases, biological entities (micro-organisms, genetically modified seeds...) and also genotoxic agents in the environment and in foodstuffs.

2. Chemical structure of DNA

In order to facilitate the discussion of spectral properties of DNA, we present its structure in Figure 1.A. In the biological field, hydrogen bonding is key for molecular recognition, as exemplified by the way a single strand of DNA (ss-DNA) nucleobases recognizes the complementary sequence with high specificity to produce double strand DNA (ds-DNA), as shown in Figure 1.B.

3. A brief summary of the modes of drug-DNA interaction

Supramolecular chemistry is a fascinating and interdisciplinary field of chemistry that involves different phenomena in the frontiers of chemical, physical and biological sciences. One of the keystones of supramolecular chemistry is molecular recognition, a process in which molecules (small or large) selectively recognize each other through different types of

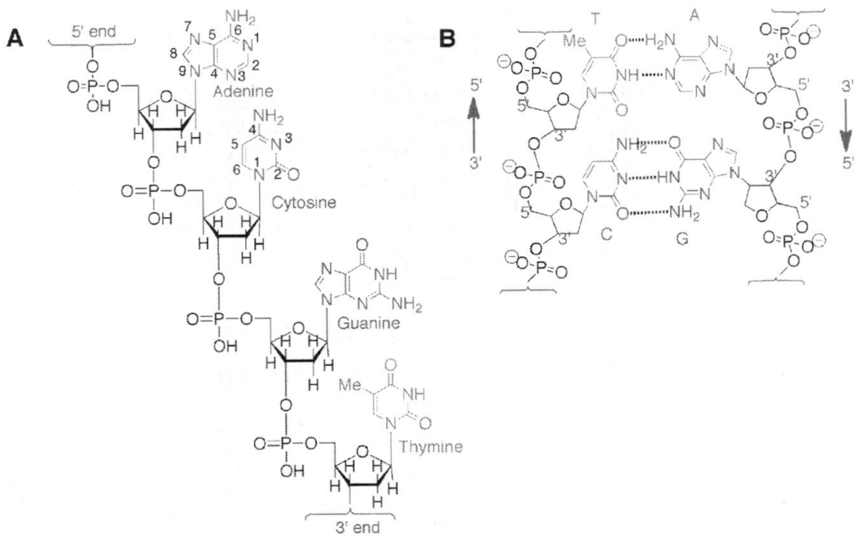

Fig. 1. A. Structure of a DNA single strand. B. Watson-Crick pairing between purine and pyrimidine bases in complementary DNA strands.

molecular interactions, *i.e.*, electrostatic, dipole-dipole, hydrogen bonding, π-π and van der Waals interactions, whose strength determines the stability of the resulting supramolecular complexes (Table 1). The main chemical driving forces for both the stability of ds-DNA and DNA-drug recognition are hydrogen bonding interactions, electrostatic and π-π interactions between the aromatic rings of base pairs.

Type of Interaction	*Strength*	*Distance at which it is effective*
Electrostatic	+++++	+++
Hydrogen bonding	+++++	+++++
π -π stacking	++++	+++
Ion-dipole	++++	++
Dipole-dipole	+++	++
Dipole-induced dipole	++	+
Van der Waals	+	+

Table 1. Types and main characteristics of non-covalent molecular interactions.

The chemical and physicochemical properties of the interacting molecules, as well as their stereochemistry, determine the different modes of interaction, including covalent bonding (in the case of mutagenic and severely genotoxic agents) and non-covalent interactions, which comprise intercalation between bases, binding to the helical minor and major grooves or ionic interactions with the sugar-phosphate backbone (Serganov & Patel, 2006), as schematized in Figure 2. A large number of drugs with anti-tumour activity intercalate into DNA or are selectively recognized by specific regions of DNA, specially the minor groove.

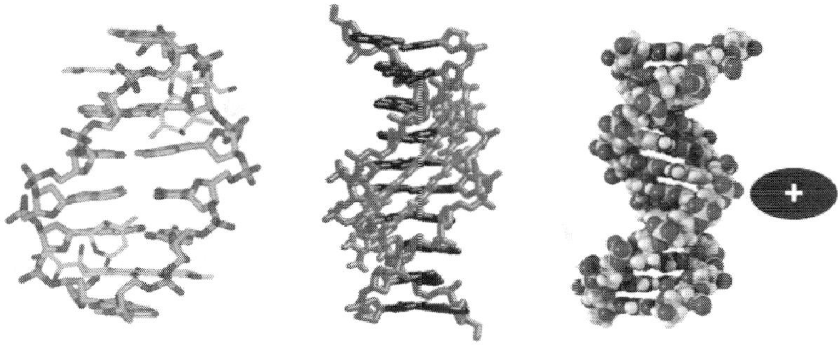

Fig. 2. Modes of non-covalent interaction of small molecules with DNA.

4. Analytical techniques to evidence drug-DNA interactions

The number and variety of techniques devoted to evidence drug-DNA interactions is continuously growing. From the classical UV-vis spectrophotometry or competition dialysis assay to the renewed gel mobility electrophoresis assay or the powerful tandem HPLC-MS or capillary electrophoresis-mass spectrometry, the number of new specific assays and methodologies is overwhelming (Tian et al., 2005). We will describe below some of the most useful techniques, with the exception of separation methods such as chromatography and conventional or capillary electrophoresis, which would require a whole chapter; for further information on this subject, see (Baba, 1999; Krylova et al., 2010; Kral et al., 2010; Koster et al., 2008; Araya et al., 2007; Su et al., 2007a; Su et al., 2007b).

4.1 Vibrational spectroscopy: IR and Raman spectrometries

Infrared spectroscopy (IR) has been widely used for the structural analysis of DNA because it can distinguish among A-, B-, and Z-forms of DNA, triple stranded helices, and other structural motifs. It has also been a useful tool to study interactions of nucleic acids with drugs and the effects of such interactions in the structure of DNA, providing some insights about the mechanism of drug action. A major advantage is that samples can be analyzed in different aggregation states, *i. e.*, as solids or crystals, and also in solution, making it possible to establish a comparison with results from other techniques. In addition, small quantities of sample are needed and collection of spectra is not time consuming.

The region of interest in IR studies dealing with DNA in aqueous solutions is between 1800 and 800 cm^{-1}. Due to interfering absorption bands of water at 1650 cm^{-1} and below 950 cm^{-1}, spectra are generally recorded also in D_2O, where these bands move to 1200 cm^{-1}, and below 750 cm^{-1}. Combination of results from both spectra allows to obtain a complete spectrum. The use of D_2O also causes shifts in nucleic acid absorptions, resulting from deuterium exchange of labile NH protons, and these can be used to monitor H-D exchange processes. A method to remove water signals in the spectra is water substraction, using a NaCl solution as reference. The characteristic IR bands of nucleic acids have been compiled and discussed in a review (Banyay et al., 2003); four regions are considered, each one containing marker bands reflecting either nucleic acid interactions and/or conformations, as shown in Figure 3.

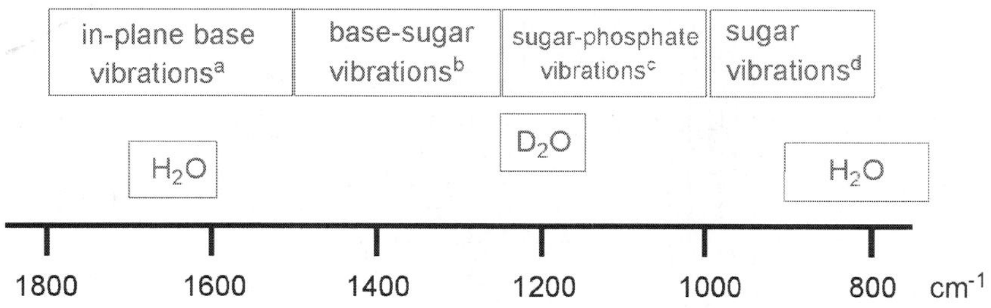

Fig. 3. Approximate position of IR bands of DNA and aqueous solvents. a) 1800-1500 cm^{-1} region, sensitive to effects of base pairing and base stacking. b) 1500-1250 cm^{-1} region, sensitive to glycosidic bond rotation, backbone conformation and sugar pucker. c) 1250-1000 cm^{-1} region, sensitive to backbone conformation. d) 1000-800 cm^{-1} region, sensitive to sugar conformation.

Fourier transform IR (FTIR) has been used alone or supporting other techniques to determine drug binding sites and sequence preference, as well as conformational changes due to drug-DNA interaction (Jangir et al., 2010; Mandeville et al., 2010; Neault & Tajmir-Riahi, 1996). Additional evidence for drug-DNA interaction can be obtained from observed changes (shift or intensity) in the bands of drug spectra upon DNA binding, and even groups involved in the complexation can be inferred.

Raman spectroscopy also depends on the vibrational frequencies of characteristic groups and has been used sometimes in conjunction with infrared spectra to study DNA-drug interactions since it provides complementary information. An advantage of Raman is that water makes an ideal solvent (weak scattering properties and only one broad weak band around 3600 cm^{-1}).

4.2 NMR spectroscopy

Nuclear Magnetic Resonance (NMR) is based on the fact that atomic nuclei endowed with a property called nuclear spin will align with an applied magnetic field. The degree of this alignment depends not only on the strength of the magnetic field, but also on the type of nucleus and its chemical environment. Every nucleus with spin gives rise to a signal or peak which represents a transition between a ground and an excited state. Each magnetically active nucleus is characterized by different parameters such as chemical shift (the position or frequency of the spectral line), multiplicity (the fine structure observed on the spectral lines), *J*-couplings (the separations within a multiplet), relaxation data and Nuclear Overhauser Effect (NOE) connectivities that can be used to obtain detailed structural information about the molecule under study.

Among the atomic nuclei available for the study of DNA (^{1}H, ^{13}C, ^{15}N and ^{31}P), ^{1}H is the most common, but ^{31}P NMR is especially useful for studying the effects of ligand binding on the phosphate groups of DNA. NMR experiments are very versatile and the information can be obtained at different temperatures, solvents, pH values, ionic strengths and dielectric constants.

The typical chemical shift for ^{1}H NMR spectra of nucleic acids at room temperature has previously been reported (Barber et al., 1993), and Table 2 summarizes the most representative values.

Proton type	*Expected chemical shift* [a]
T 5 (CH_3)	1.00 – 2.00 ppm
Sugar 2′ (CH_2)	2.00 – 3.00 ppm
Sugar 5′ terminal (CH_2)	3. 70 ppm
Sugar 5′ (CH_2); 4′(CH)	4.00 – 4.50 ppm
Sugar 3′ (CH)	4.50 – 5.20 ppm
Sugar 1′ (CH)	5.30 – 6.20 ppm
C 5 (CH)	5.30 – 6.20 ppm

Proton type	*Expected chemical shift* [a]
A 2 (CH); A 8 (CH); G 8 (CH); T 6 (CH) C 5 (CH)	6.50 – 8.20 ppm
C 4 (NH_2) (H-1)[b]	6.40 – 6.80 ppm
C 4 (NH_2) (H-2)[b]	8.30 – 8.50 ppm
G 1 (NH)	12.50 – 13.00 ppm
T 3 (NH)	13.50 – 14.00 ppm

Table 2. Typical chemical shift ranges for proton resonances in NMR spectra of nucleic acids. [a] Chemical shifts relative to internal TSP (3-(trimethylsilyl)propionic acid). [b] For Watson-Crick base pairs (CG).

Based on these values, any significant change in the chemical shift will be attributed to a binding between ligand and DNA molecule. Variation of chemical shift is mainly a consequence of neighbouring group effects. For instance, un-stacking of base-pair double-helical DNA by thermal denaturing to form two ss-DNAs is usually accompanied by the downfield shift of ^1H resonances for non-exchangeable protons. A plot of chemical shift change *vs* temperature will yield the melting temperature, T_m, at which half of the ds-DNA has converted to ss-DNA.

The *Nuclear Overhauser Effect* (NOE) is a measure of inter-atomic separation that enables scalar coupling transmitted through space up to a distance of approximately 5 Å. It is usually negative due to the slow tumbling time of the molecule in solution. The combination of substantial signal overlap and poor resolution, especially for ^1H nuclei, imposes major limitations on the assignment of spectra of DNA and ligand-DNA complexes. For this reason, 2D and 3D NMR methods have emerged as the principal sources of both assignments and structural and dynamic information on such materials.

The most useful 2D-NMR experiments are: *Homonuclear Shift Correlated Spectroscopy* (COSY), which provides scalar coupling information which is transmitted over covalent bonds, and *Nuclear Overhauser Enhancement Spectroscopy* (NOESY), which provides information related to the spatial arrangements of atoms relative to one another and can show whether the double-helical is left or right handed. Additional experiments such as *Total Correlation Spectroscopy* (TOCSY), *Rotating Frame NOESY* (ROESY), *Heteronuclear Multiple Quantum Correlation* (HMQC) and *Heteronuclear Multiple Bond Correlation* (HMBC) can also be used. These last 2D experiments can be combined with COSY or NOESY experiments to produce 3D and 4D spectra.

1D ^{31}P-NMR spectroscopy may provide useful information about the binding of intercalators to DNA. Chemical shifts of ^{31}P are sensitive to conformational changes in DNA, and intercalating drugs cause downfield shift in the ^{31}P signal, whereas divalent cations cause upfield shifts.

DNA-binding drugs specific for the minor groove of DNA generally prefer AT-rich, rather than GC-rich regions of DNA. These drugs are usually planar with crescent shapes. and donor/acceptor functionalities. The DNA minor groove possesses an electrostatic potential minimum attractive to many such ligands. The broadening of DNA ^1H NMR resonances upon addition of a suitable minor-groove binding compound has often been taken as primary evidence of complex formation. The broadening is a reflection of the increased rotational correlation time of the DNA with a ligand tightly bound to it. The ^{1}H spectrum of a drug-DNA complex is dependent on its rate of dissociation; free ligands and ligand-bound oligonucleotides have clearly resolved signals when the ligand to oligonucleotide molar ratio is <1:1. Most of the contacts are between imino and adenine C-2 hydrogens and drug aromatic/NH hydrogens.

Many anti-tumour drugs bind to the major groove, and they usually do it covalently through N-7 of guanine but their modes of interaction have been studied with techniques different from NMR.

4.3 UV-VIS absorption spectroscopy

The drug-DNA interaction can be detected by UV-Vis absorption spectroscopy by measuring the changes in the absorption properties of the drug or the DNA molecules. The UV-Vis absorption spectrum of DNA exhibits a broad band (200-350 nm) in the UV region with a maximum placed at 260 nm. This maximum is a consequence of the chromophoric groups in purine and pyrimidine moieties responsible for the electronic transitions. The probability of these transitions is high and thus the molar absorptivity (ε) is of order of 10^4 $M^{-1}cm^{-1}$. The use of this versatile and simple technique allows estimating the molar concentration of DNA on the basis of the measurement of the absorbance value at 260 nm. In practice, the molar concentration of DNA is evaluated in terms of the concentration of pairs of bases. The absorbance ratios (A_{260}/A_{280} and A_{260}/A_{230}) can also characterize the DNA molecules (Paul et al., 2010). Slight changes in the absorption maximum as well as the molar absorptivity can be appreciated with the variations in pH or ionic strength of the media. The ε values (λ_{max}= 260 nm) of free oligonucleotides are higher than the ones corresponding to the same oligonucleotides in single strand DNA (ss-DNA) and double strand DNA (ds-DNA) because base-base stacking results in a *hypochromic effect*. This behaviour can be exploited to verify denaturalization of DNA by measuring its absorbance values before and after denaturing treatment. The *hypochromic effect* can also be employed to verify the existence of drug-DNA interactions, due to the fact that the monitoring of the absorbance values allows studying the melting behaviour of DNA. Melting temperature (T_m) is the temperature value corresponding to the conversion of 50 % of the double strands into single strands, according to the equilibrium shown in Equation (1).

$$\mathrm{ds-DNA} \rightleftarrows \mathrm{ss-DNA} \qquad (1)$$

For native ds-DNA, the separation of the strands starts near to T_1 and ends close to T_2. These temperature values change depending on the origin and nature of DNA (viral, bacterial, duplex, quadruplex...). The temperature value corresponding to one half of DNA existing as ds-DNA and the other half as ss-DNA is named melting temperature. This value corresponds to the inflexion point in the absorbance-temperature plot (Figure 4). An increase in the absorbance value with the increase of temperature is observed because the ε (260 nm) of ss-DNA is higher than the ε (260 nm) of ds-DNA. When a drug–DNA interaction exists, T_m is shifted to values different from native ds-DNA. The magnitude of the shift depends on the type of interaction. Thus, for intercalating agents the increase observed in the T_m value is higher than in the case of agents interacting through the DNA minor or major grooves. The changes in the T_m value can be followed by other techniques such as fluorescence, circular dichroism, NMR or calorimetry, but UV-Vis absorption spectrometry is the most frequently employed method due to its good sensitivity, reproducibility, simplicity and versatility.

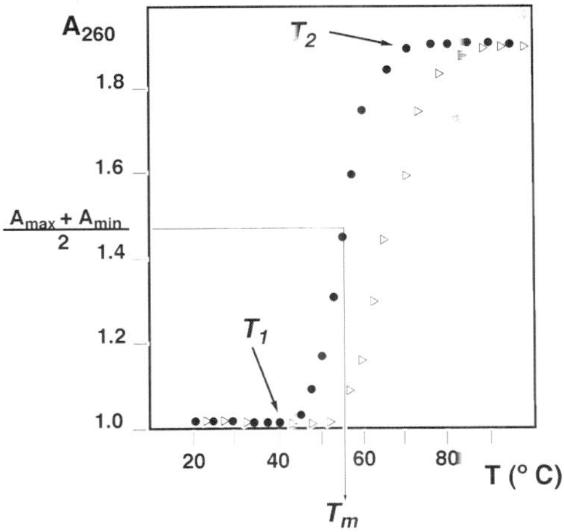

Fig. 4. Absorbance thermal melting profiles of native DNA (●) and the DNA-drug complex (▷). A_{260}: normalized absorbance values at 260 nm, T: temperature (Celsius).

Drug-ds-DNA interactions can be resolved by comparison of UV-Vis absorption spectra of the free drug and drug-DNA complexes, which are usually different. As shown in Figure 5, the maximum absorption can be 20-70 nm shifted towards red wavelengths upon DNA interaction. *Hypochromic* or *hyperchromic* effects usually accompany these shifts, as is the case of ethidium bromide or acridinium salts. In the case of weaker interactions, only *hypochromic* or *hyperchromic effects* are observed without significant changes of shifts in the spectral profiles.

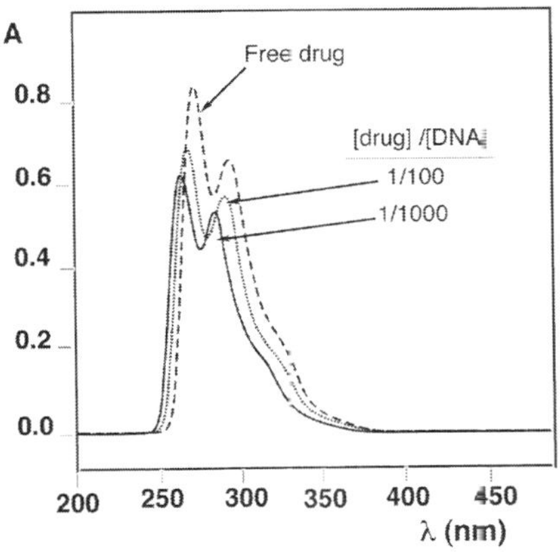

Fig. 5. Effect of the addition of DNA on the UV-Vis absorption spectrum of a drug.

The drug-DNA association constants can be obtained on the basis of the quantitative changes of the drug absorption spectrum in the presence of increasing amounts of DNA. The equilibrium constants can be determined by data fitting to the Scatchard model (Wu et al., 2009). Sometimes Scatchard plots reveal a non-cooperative binding and thus the use of McGhee-von Hippel treatment results more convenient (Islam et al., 2009).

4.4 Circular and linear dichroism

Circular and linear dichroism spectroscopies are useful techniques to probe non-covalent drug-DNA interactions, which affect the electronic structure of the molecules and also alter their electronic spectroscopic behaviour. Polarized light spectroscopy allows to quickly characterize drug-DNA complexes using a small amount of sample. Linear dichroism (LD) provides structural information in terms of the relative orientation between the bound drug molecule and the DNA molecular long axis, and also about the effects of ligand binding on the host. Circular dichroism (CD) provides additional structural details of the complex.

When electromagnetic radiation reaches DNA, the macromolecules present a certain degree of alineation in the direction of the electric field vector, and this molecular alignment is measured by the light polarised absorbance. When a drug binds to DNA, its spectrum will be modified if this binding causes changes in DNA conformation. Circular dichroism is defined as the difference in absorption of left and right circularly polarised light (Equation 2, where ε_l and ε_r are the molar absorptivities for the absorption of left and right circularly polarized light for the selected wavelength).

$$CD = \varepsilon_l - \varepsilon_r \tag{2}$$

When a drug binds to DNA, an induced CD (ICD) spectrum is observed because of the interaction with DNA. This may result from either a geometric change in the drug or from coupling between its electronic transitions and those of the DNA. Similarly, DNA gets an ICD contribution to its CD spectrum from its interaction with the drug. Therefore, what is finally observed is a combination of DNA CD, DNA ICD, drug CD (which is zero for an non-chiral drug and nonzero for a chiral drug), and drug ICD. If an ICD signal is observed in the absorption band of a non-chiral ligand, this is evidence for interaction with DNA.

In contrast to CD, which depends on both electric and magnetic interactions, LD only depends on the electric field vector. LD spectroscopy involves measuring the difference in absorption of two linear polarizations of light, which usually are parallel and perpendicular to a sample orientation direction.

Small molecules that tumble freely in solution are not oriented and in contrast to DNA-bound molecules do not give any LD signal in their absorption region, so the presence of a detectable LD proves that the ligand is bound to the oriented DNA.

Light that is polarised parallel to the transition moment has a high probability of absorption in the region of spectral interest, whereas if light is perpendicularly polarized to the transition moment, no absorption takes place. In practice, this means that intercalating agents that stack closely to base pairs have linear dichroism similar to the base pairs themselves. However, the dichroism of groove binders is frequently opposite to that of the base pairs, since they bind along the edge of the base pairs. Thus, LD is a useful spectroscopy for assessing the binding mode of a drug to DNA.

In practice, the use of LD in combination with CD, particularly ICD, allows to distinguish among the different types of drug-DNA interactions. The principal modes of binding of small molecules to ds-DNA have been shown in Figure 2. All these interactions belong to the group of reversible interactions (non-covalent) whereas the covalent interactions mean an unbreakable bond formation between the two molecules.

4.5 Fluorescence emission spectroscopy

The mode of binding of drugs to DNA can be determined by high-resolution structural techniques like X-ray diffraction or NMR, but fluorescence spectroscopy and the various analytical tools based on fluorescence emission can also provide particularly useful information. The orientation of fluorophoric ligands and their proximity to the DNA pairs of bases can be studied by fluorescence anisotropy or fluorescence resonance energy transfer. Fluorescence quenching experiments afford additional information concerning the localization of the drugs and their mode of interaction with DNA.

Fluorescence emission is very sensitive to the environment, and hence the fluorophore transfer from high to low polarity environments usually causes spectral shifts (10-20 nm) in the excitation and emission spectra of drugs (Suh & Chaires, 1995). Moreover, the effective interaction with DNA usually causes a significant enhancement of the fluorescence intensity as a consequence of different factors. Thus, in the case of intercalating drugs, the molecules are inserted into the base stack of the helix. The rotation of the free molecules favours the radiationless deactivation of the excited states, but if the drugs are bound to DNA the deactivation via fluorescence emission is favoured, and a significant increase in the fluorescence emission is normally observed. Interestingly, a decrease in the fluorescence intensity of drugs was observed in the presence of DNA for different derivatives of quinolizinium salts (Martín et al., 1988 and 2002). The quenching behaviour did not fit the Stern-Volmer equation, suggesting that two possible quenching mechanisms (static and dynamic) could be coexisting (Figure 6A). Nevertheless, the quenching effect observed, in many cases is adjusted to the Stern-Volmer equation (Kumar et al., 1993) (Figure 6B). Thus, for the interaction of amino derivatives of ethidium bromide a fluorescence quenching was observed in the presence of calf thymus DNA. The quenching effect shows a good adjustment to the Stern-Volmer equation with K_{SV} constants of 8.4 x 10^6 and 4.6 x 10^6. Studies concerning temperature on the quenching effect showed that K_{SV} decreased when temperature was increased and the authors suggest a static mechanism for the quenching

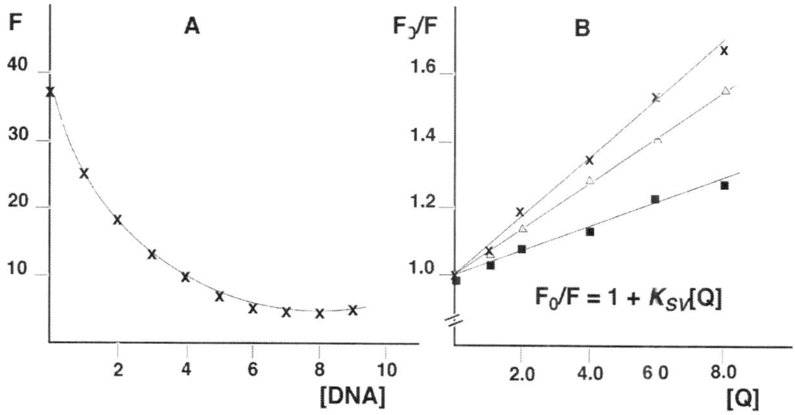

Fig. 6. Fluorescence quenching studies of drug-DNA interactions.(A) Quenching effect by increasing concentrations of DNA (mM) on the native fluorescence of drug. (B) Stern-Volmer plots obtained for drug quenching by halide anions (quencher, mM) in the presence of different concentrations of DNA: (X) 0.0 mM, (△) 10.0 mM and (■) 20 0 mM

effect (Akbay et al., 2009). Other studies concerning the interaction of ethidium bromide analogues with DNA have shown that the presence of weak electron-donating substituents on phenantridinium moiety favours a significant fluorescence quenching (Prunkl et al., 2010). In the case of groove binding agents, electrostatic, hydrogen binding or hydrophobic interactions are involved and the molecules are close to the sugar-phosphate backbone, being possible to observe a decrease in the fluorescence intensity in the presence of DNA (Li et al., 1997).

The use of well-established quenchers, i.e. halide ions, provides further information about the binding of drugs to DNA. The groove binders are more sensitive to the quenching effect by halides than the intercalating agents, because the pairs of bases hamper the accessibility of the drug by the quenchers. Besides, the electrostatic repulsive forces among phosphate groups on DNA and anionic quenchers collaborate to protect the drug from the quencher effects. Thus, in the case of intercalating agents a considerable reduction in the K_{SV} values is observed in the presence of DNA.

Fluorescence polarization measurements afford useful information related to molecular mobility, size, shape and flexibility of the molecules, and also on the fluidity and viscosity of the surroundings of the fluorescent molecules. Thus, a fluorophore in homogeneous solution excited by linearly polarized radiation will emit totally or partially depolarized fluorescence. The emission of non-polarized light is due to torsion vibrations, Brownian motion, transfer of the excitation energy to other molecules with different orientation as well as non-parallel absorption and emission transition moments. In the presence of DNA, the fluorophores that interact with the macromolecules show a enhancement in the fluorescence polarization. This is due to the fact that the torsion vibrations and rotational motions are restricted. The *polarization ratio* (*p*) and *emission anisotropy* (*r*) can be determined as shown in Figure 7. The interaction with DNA causes an increase in the polarization ratio and emission anisotropy (Δp≈0.001-0.2 and Δr≈0.001-0.3) similar to those obtained in high viscosity media and at low temperature.

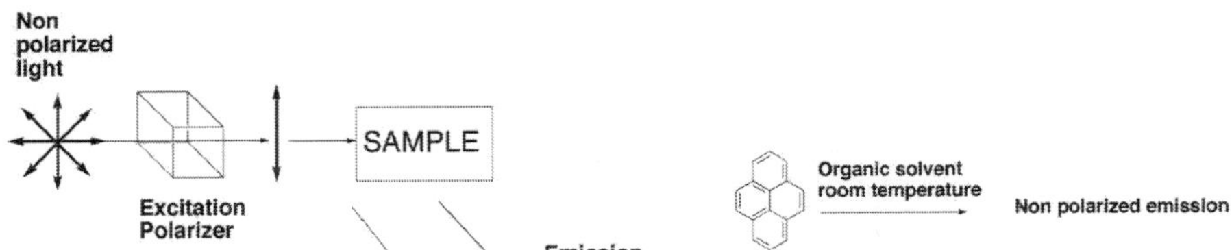

Fig. 7. Scheme of the configuration for fluorescence polarization measurements.

As previously mentioned for the quenching experiments, the changes observed in polarization ratio for DNA intercalating agents should be higher than the ones corresponding to groove-binding agents, but this general rule does not always hold. For instance, in the case of Hoechst 33258 (Suh & Chaires, 1995) and other groove-binding model molecules a significant increase in the polarization values is obtained because the molecules are immobilized and their free rotation is hampered after complexation with DNA.

Fluorescence resonance energy transfer (FRET) is a phenomenon that can be observed when the emission spectrum of the donor molecules (D) is overlapped with the excitation spectrum of the acceptor molecules (A). Under adequate experimental conditions (concentration and distance), the fluorescence observed when using the excitation wavelength of the donor corresponds to the acceptor because the emission energy of the donor is transferred to the acceptor (Figure 8). The efficiency of energy transfer depends not only on the overlapping of acceptor excitation and donor emission spectra but also on the quantum yield of the donor and the orientation of the transition dipoles of donor and acceptor. Besides, donor and acceptor should be in close proximity, i.e. at a distance of 60-100 Å according to Förster's theory (Gianetti et al., 2006). The dependence of FRET phenomenon with distance makes it possible to use these experiments to measure distances between donor and acceptor in macromolecules. Furthermore, different isoforms in proteins or supercoiled and relaxed forms of DNA can be evidenced on the basis of FRET measurements.

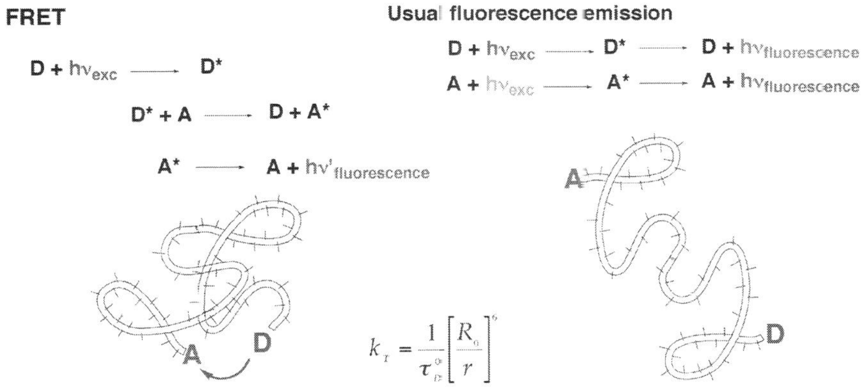

Fig. 8. Scheme of the FRET process in macromolecules depending on their conformations.

The *energy transfer* proceeds during the lifetime of the donor excited state (τ_D^0). Thus, the equilibrium constant for energy transfer (k_T) varies inversely with the distance (r) between donor and acceptor. R_0 is the Förster critical radius, defined as the distance at which transfer and spontaneous decay of the excited state of donor present the same probability, and therefore $k_T = 1/\tau^0$. Energy transfer allows studying drug-DNA and proteins-DNA interactions (López-Crapez et al., 2008) and also differentiating the nature of the interaction for intercalating and grooving agents. Thus, in the case of fluorescent intercalating agents, the UV energy absorbed by DNA pair bases can be efficiently transferred to the intercalated fluorescent drug. In the case of the groove interacting agents no FRET is observed because of the greater distance and also due to the fact that orientation of dipoles is not adequate for the energy transfer. FRET exhibits a great variety of applications, not only to determine the

distances between fluorophores in macromolecules (Valeur, 2001) but also due to its potential in the design of DNA arrays and genosensors as will be described in the Section 6.
To end this Section devoted to fluorescence spectroscopy, it is important to note that equilibrium constants can be deduced by the increase/decrease in fluorescence intensity as a consequence of the presence of DNA. Other methodologies involve the competitive displacement of a model interacting agent. In this procedure, ethidium bromide is bound to DNA and the addition of the drug under study causes a decrease in the fluorescence intensity because free ethidium bromide is less fluorescent than bound one. In the case of groove interacting agents the same procedure is employed using Hoechst 33258 as reference compound. This methodology is not adequate to study fluorescent drugs due to possible spectral interferences between the drug and the displaced probe. The competitive displacement assay can be developed under classical or high throughput screening (HTS) conditions (Tse & Boger, 2004). The latter employs a 96-well format or higher density formats and the fluorescence measurements are carried out with an optical fiber in connection to the fluorescence spectrophotometer. In one assay different DNA types (from different species, ds-DNS, ss-DNA, variable nucleotide sequences with increased AT or CG contents,...) can be studied in a reduced analysis time and in an automatized fashion (Figure 9). Additionally, the drug-DNA association constant values can be easily determined. Several reference agents possessing variable DNA affinities like ethidium bromide or thiazole orange as intercalanting agents and netropsine, dystamicin A or Hoechst 33258 as minor groove binding compounds can be assayed simultaneously. In these assays the fluorescence emission of the probe (ethidium or others) decreases proportionally with the concentration of drug bound to DNA.

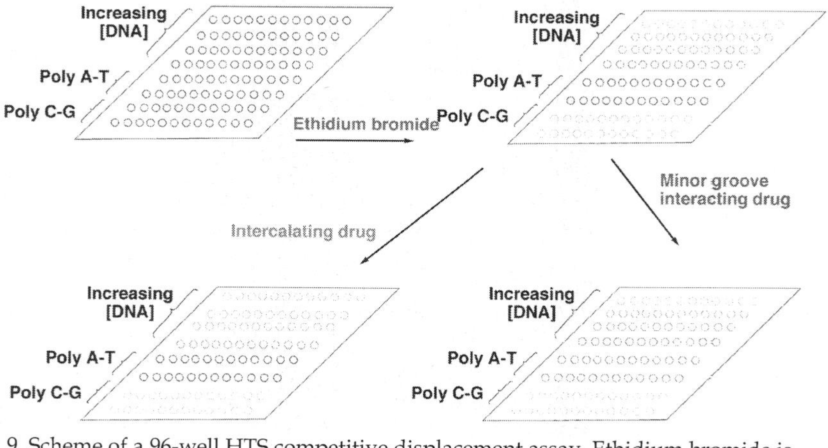

Fig. 9. Scheme of a 96-well HTS competitive displacement assay. Ethidium bromide is displaced in the case of intercalating agents but not for the minor groove-interacting drugs.

4.6 Metal enhanced fluorescence (MEF)

MEF is a new research field still at an early development stage. It provides the concepts and methods to dramatically improve the performance of fluorophores in a surprising whole new way. MEF can be achieved by building appropriated nano-scaled physicochemical systems and it does not need instruments different from those required for classic fluorescence measurements. Some of the main advantages of MEF are the largely increased sensitivity, photo-stability, directionality of emission, *resonance energy transfer* (RET) distances and signal-to-background ratio with regard to conventional fluorescence.

Metals are well-known fluorescence quenchers. The use of cobalt (Co^{2+}), nickel (Ni^{2+}), gold (Au^{+}) or silver (Ag^{+}) to quench the emission of different fluorophores is widely extended in the literature. Nevertheless, when properly engineered, metals like silver or gold can also dramatically improve the fluorescence behaviour of fluorophores. It is important to remark that in this section the word "metals" does not refer to metal oxides or cations in solution, but to metal colloids, islands or films, acting as conducting surfaces. Fluorescence is classically observed in the far-field after emission of a fluorophore in an homogeneous non conducting medium. Radiative decay rate (Γ) from the excited state after light absorption depends on the extinction rate of the fluorophore (the oscillator strength of the electronic transition). This parameter is only dependent, and very weakly, on the solvent. Opposite to that, in MEF the interactions of the fluorophores with metal surfaces in the near-field (sub-wavelength distances) leads to additional radiative decay rates (Γ_m) (Lakowicz, 2001). The new radiative decay rate Γ_m not only increases the quantum yield but also decreases the lifetime (Figure 10). This last fact has two implications: the first one is that it makes easier to distinguish the fluorophore from the background by using time-resolved fluorescence; the second one is that the photo-stability of the fluorophore becomes significantly improved as it remains less time in excited state (Lakowicz et al., 2002).

It is interesting to remark that in MEF we are not observing the phenomenon of metal surfaces acting as mirrors reflecting the photons emitted by the fluorophore. A reflection takes place *after* light has been emitted. Instead, we are considering how metals alter the *free space* condition for the fluorophores *before* emission. In this idea, there are two main interactions allowing MEF that occur between fluorophores and metal surfaces at sub-wavelength distance. The first one is the increased excitation rate. Electromagnetic fields "bend" and concentrate around metallic particles, so a fluorophore in the vicinity of such particles will be exposed to an increased local field (*Lightening Rod Effect*). This will result in a larger excitation rate of the fluorophore compared to being excited in the free-space. This effect may lead to apparent quantum yields larger than 1, when compared to control solutions in the absence of metal surfaces. The second one is that the oscillating excited state dipole of the fluorophore can excite plasmons on the surface of the metal. This phenomenon results in emission from a complex moiety formed by the fluorophore and the metal, called *plasmophore* or *fluoron*. The emission coming from plasmophores retains features from both the fluorophore and the metal: it has the spectral shape of the fluorophore, but it is p-polarized and directional as corresponds to radiating plasmons. So, when speaking about MEF, light emission should not be considered to arise from the fluorophore itself but from the *plasmophore* (Zhang et al., 2010).

Several general considerations about MEF should be taken into account (Lakowicz et al., 2008). First, at distances under 5 nm from the metal, quenching of the fluorophore is always observed due to energy transfer to those metals. Then, an optimal distance of around 10 nm has been established for an efficient MEF process. Second, MEF allows a higher improvement of the quantum yields of fluorophores with low intrinsic quantum yields or even almost non-fluorescent chromophores. A third relevant consideration is about the size and shape of metal particles employed to produce MEF. It has been observed that ellipsoids with an aspect ratio of 1.75 yield the best results. The improvement of the fluorescence is also related to the orientation of the fluorophore relative to the metal particle. Parallel orientation will lead to the dipole in the metal particle to cancel the dipole in the fluorophore. A perpendicular orientation, instead, will cause both dipoles to add.

Subwavelength features or patterns imprinted in metal layers can be used for *Surface Plasmon-Coupled Emission* (SPCE), a phenomenon which affords a highly directional fluorescence emission. One example is the use of silver *nanogratings* allowing a controlled separation of the emission angles for every wavelength coming from the fluorophore. Other example is the use of *nanohole arrays*, thick metal layers with nanoholes of a certain diameter

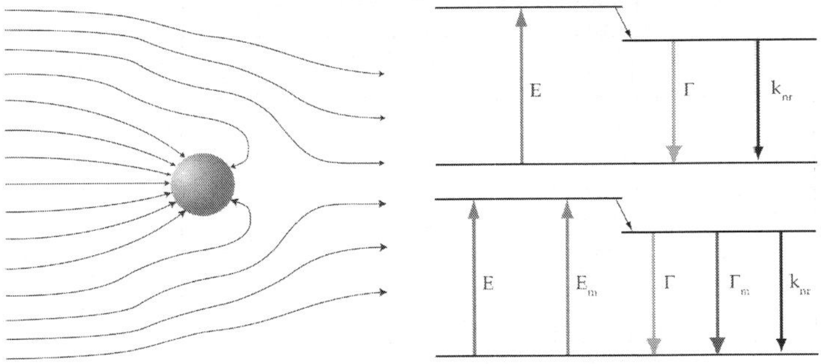

Fig. 10. *Lightening Rod Effect* on a metal particle. Energy transitions and radiative and non-radiative decay rates in absence and presence of metal surfaces.

and spacing. These arrays present a high transmission of a single wavelength in a narrow directional beam, thus monochromating and focusing emission in a very particular way. As the advantages provided by this kind of nanostructures come from the way in which plasmons propagate in them, these devices are said to produce *plasmon controlled fluorescence* (PCF) (Lakowicz et al., 2008).

Recent applications of MEF in the field of detection of specific gene sequences include the development of easy-to-prepare arrays capable of selectively and "label-free" detect DNA sequences in concentrations lower than 100 pM before optimization of the system (Peng et al., 2009). It has recently been described that Au and Ag nanoparticles coated with silicon-carbon alloy layers allow real-time monitoring of the hybridization process of a specific DNA labeled oligonucleotide at concentrations down to 5 fM (Touahir et al., 2010).

4.7 Surface plasmon resonance (SPR)-based techniques

Surface plasmon resonance-based measurements have become one of the fastest-growing analytical techniques in the last decade. The many advantages of SPR, together with the commercial availability of instruments and sensing surfaces, have made it the technique of choice for many kinetic and steady-state studies (Schasfoort & Tudos, 2008).

SPR instruments allow the real-time measurement of the changes occurring on the mass garnered on a functionalized metal layer as a consequence of the binding or unbinding of a certain (macro)molecule (de Mol & Fisher, 2010). This mass variation implies an alteration of the refractive index (and thus of the dielectric constant) of the medium closest to the surface. Such changes can be continuously observed by monitoring the value of the optimum angle for exciting surface plasmons on the metal layer.

Free electrons inside a conductor can be displaced away from a point by an incident electromagnetic field. The remaining electrons may be attracted by the unshielded positive background and thus create a region of increased negative charge density. Then, Coulomb repulsion will push these electrons back to restore the charge neutrality in the region. The resultant of these two forces will set up longitudinal oscillations of the free electrons plasma. A quantum of these oscillations is known as a *plasmon*. These plasmons are supported by metal-dielectric interfaces and then are referred to as *surface plasmons*.

Direct light cannot excite surface plasmons at a metal-dielectric interface, because the propagation constant of surface plasmons in metal is greater than the one of the light wave in the dielectric medium (Sharma et al., 2007). To solve this problem, surface plasmons are generated by coupling them to an evanescent field. Most SPR systems are based on a *Kretschmann-arranged* coupling device. This consists on a prism coated with a very thin (~50 nm) gold layer on its base. On the other side of the gold layer is the aqueous medium where experiments are to be carried out (the dielectric). When a p-polarized light beam shines into the prism with an angle greater than the *critical angle*, attenuated total reflection occurs. A part of the energy of the light is reflected, but another part generates an evanescent wave on the prism-gold interface, radiating to the aqueous medium. The nature of this wave is able to excite surface plasmons on the gold surface. The more efficiently plasmons are excited, the less light is reflected. In addition, this evanescent field penetrates further (~200 nm) than the gold layer, and gets into the experimental medium being strongly affected by changes on its refractive index, or dielectric constant.

There is a preferential incidence angle for the light beam at which most of the energy of the radiation is used to excite surface plasmons by means of the evanescent field. This angle can be measured because it is the angle at which least light is reflected due to the absorption of the plasmons. As changes on the dielectric constant of the experimental medium due to mass binding/unbinding will change the nature of the evanescent field, it will turn out in a change of the optimal angle of incidence of the excitation light, as shown by Equation 3:

$$\frac{\omega}{c}\sqrt{\varepsilon_p}\sin\theta = \frac{\omega}{c}\sqrt{\frac{\varepsilon_m\varepsilon_s}{\varepsilon_m + \varepsilon_s}} \tag{3}$$

Where c is the velocity of light, ω is the frequency of incident light, ε are the dielectric constants and θ is the optimum incidence angle for surface plasmon resonance; subscripts refer to *p*rism, *m*etal, and working *s*olution.

SPR instruments are built up from three main parts (Schasfoort & Tudos, 2008): 1) optical system, or *dry section*, able to measure the SPR angle changes; 2) liquids handling unit, or *wet section*, in charge of buffers and samples delivery; 3) sensor chip, where the experiments take place, and which acts as a barrier between the *wet* and *dry sections*.

The main component of the optical system is the coupling device. As mentioned above, it usually consists of a prism in Kretschmann arrangement (Figure 11), although other possibilities exist (grating couplers, fiber-optics and optical waveguides are less common). Most common setups use a diode array to detect the reflected intensities at different angles, but some systems have a mobile light source capable of scanning several degrees of excitation angles. Most advanced SPR *imaging* systems (SPRi) use CCD cameras and more complicated optics to simultaneously follow the events happening on hundreds of spots on an array, so many different experiments can be carried out in parallel mode (Steiner, 2004). With this concept, an array of oligonucleotide ligands can be "spotted" on the sensor

surface, and the SPR angle variation recorded for every spot. These systems open the door to high throughput screening based on SPR (Scarano et al., 2010).
Liquid handling is a vital part of SPR instruments. Liquids are flown in order to functionalize, condition and regenerate the sensing surface, and also to deliver samples. Stability of the flow is critical specially when performing kinetic studies. Liquid handling systems can be ascribed to three main categories: flow cells, cuvettes and microfluidic chips. Cuvette systems are less frequent, but they are useful for liquid samples with suspended particles (e. g. blood or culture media). Another advantage is that the whole sample can be easily recovered after measurement. As drawbacks, evaporation can occur, and a continuous homogenization system is required (Ŝpringer et al., 2010). Another component is the sensor chip. This is the place in whose functionalized surface the binding of the analyte takes place. Metal surface is functionalized by using gold-thiol chemistry. Carboxymethyl-dextran (CMD) is commonly employed to cover the gold layer. CMD provides a notable advantage: it constitutes a three-dimensional matrix which provides more depth so more ligand molecules can be immobilized, then more analyte per surface unit can be bound and this results in an increased sensitivity of the assay. Typically, mass changes in the order of pg mm^{-2} can be measured (Harding & Chowdhry, 2001).

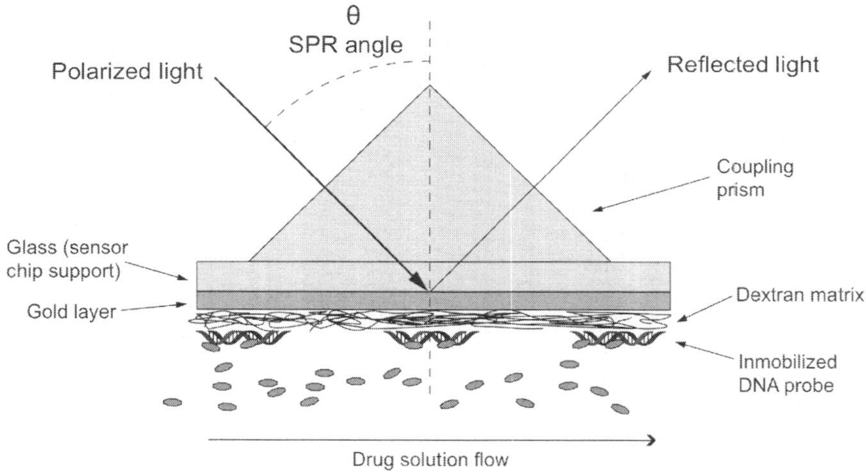

Fig. 11. Typical prism in Kretschmann arrangement used for SPR analysis. Example of detection of sample drugs in fluids based on SPR phenomena and after recognition by the immobilized ds-DNA.

For a drug-DNA binding study, it is necessary to decide the entity to be immobilized: the drug or the DNA. As SPR-based instruments measure changes in the mass on the sensing surface, immobilizing the drug on the CMD and flowing the DNA molecules as analyte would provide a more sensitive assay, since a single DNA molecule will increase the mass on the sensor surface *much more* than a drug molecule. Nevertheless, in order to minimize the diffusion phenomena, the common choice is to immobilize the heaviest element and flow the lighter one (Nguyen et al., 2006). It is possible to monitor the binding of very small molecules (MW < 200) by using DNA hairpins of 10,000 Da.

Injections of the analyte at different concentrations allow the calculation of the binding constant (K_{ass}) and thus, the strength of the interaction between drugs and DNA sequences can be inferred. Determination of binding constant (K_{ass}) through the CMD matrix will distort the results for association rates faster than 10^6 M^{-1} s^{-1}. Because of this, limitations have to be considered when developing such experiments (Harding & Chowdhry, 2001).

SPR experiments are not optimal for concentration assays, however it is possible to perform concentration measurements by generating calibration curves. Development of arrays allowing for multiple measurements to be carried at the same time should solve the problems relative to concentration assays and the long equilibration periods demanded.

Recently, several applications of such techniques have proven that it is possible to detect the presence of specific gene sequences without the need for PCR amplification or labelling of the sample. Gold nano-particles on a sensor chip are able to detect specific DNA sequences in 4.1 x 10^{-20} M concentration despite the presence of much higher amounts of interfering DNA (D'Agata et al., 2010).

5. Enzimatic methods: footprinting

Footprinting is a method for determining the sequence selectivity of DNA-binding compounds (Cardew & Fox, 2010; Hampshire et al., 2007). It was first used (Galas & Schmitz, 1978) to study the interaction between proteins and DNA, and since then, it has been employed for identifying the sequence-specific interaction of many drugs with DNA. It is based on the fact that the binding of a drug to a region of DNA protects this site of the macromolecule against cleavage by different agents. A ds-DNA fragment labelled to one end of one strand is digested by a cleavage agent in the presence and absence of a ligand. The cleavage products are resolved on denaturing polyacrylamide gels. DNA-regions where the ligand is bound are not cleavaged, and a gap or footprint appears in the ladder of cleavage products (Figure 12). The method requires that each DNA strand is cleaved just once on the average, and it is desirable that the agent does not show sequence selectivity in order to ensure an even distribution of cleavage products.

As cleavage agents several enzymes and chemicals have been employed, but the most widely used ones are hydroxyl radicals and, specially, DNases. DNase I is the most commonly used, due to its low cost and ease of use, but it generates an uneven ladder of cleavage products, as the efficiency of the enzyme is affected by the global and local DNA structure. DNase is a monomeric glycoprotein with a molecular weight of about 30,400. It is a double strand-specific endonuclease, that requires the presence of divalent cations (Ca^{2+}, Mg^{2+}) and introduces single strand nicks by hydrolysis of the C3'-P bond in the phosphodiester backbone to release 5'-phosphorylated products. DNase I binds to about 10 base pairs in the minor groove of the DNA duplex, so the enzyme overestimates the size of drug binding sites. Hydroxyl radicals are generated by the Fenton reaction between Fe(II) and H_2O_2. They are highly reactive species and generate a much more even ladder of cleavage products.

The DNA fragments employed for the reaction are usually between 50 and 200 base pair long. They are restriction fragments obtained from plasmids or synthetic oligonucleotides, which should include the sequence which the ligand under study can recognize. The assay begins with a natural fragment to gain a general idea of the binding site, followed by the use of synthetic fragments containing probable binding sequences. Labelling of DNA substrate is commonly by radio-labelling either in 3' or 5'-ends using ^{32}P.

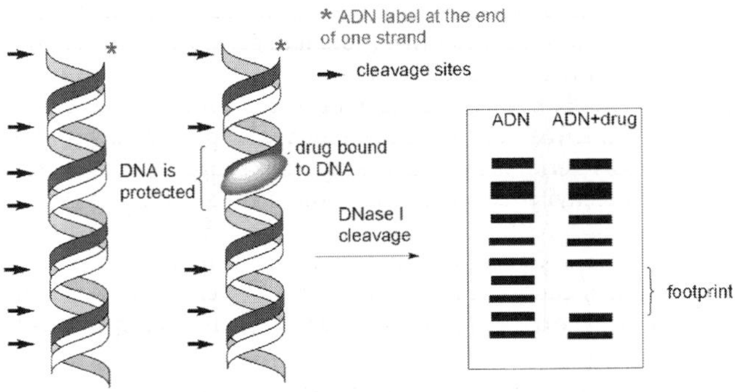

Fig. 12. Scheme of footprinting experiment. DNase I can cleave labelled DNA molecules except for drug-bound sequence. The cleavage products of both samples are resolved on a denaturing polyacrylamide gel and missing fragments are the footprint of the drug corresponding to the protected DNA region.

6. Genosensors

A *genosensor* is any device capable for the selective and sensitive detection of a specific gene, or more specifically, a particular alele of a gene (Teles & Fonseca, 2008). This chapter has shown that many techniques provide a way to set up such a device, and currently optical methods and PCR-electrophoresis techniques are the most widely employed to reveal the detection of specific DNA sequences. Among optical methods, fluorescence-based techniques are by far the most common and versatile. Fluorescence, fluorescence quenching, RET or anisotropy are only a few examples of fluorescence related techniques widely used to reveal the presence of a specific DNA sequence by pairing them to electrophoresis, PCR, real-time/quantitative PCR, molecular beacons or DNA arrays. SPR and MEF-based methods are also promising tools readily pointing towards the target of the single molecule detection.

Nevertheless, over the past few years the term *genosensor* has been narrowed to the field of electrochemical sensors intended to detect DNA presence or hybridization, or the binding of molecules to DNA. This section is devoted to describe different devices (biosensors, biochips, microarrays, molecular beacons, electrochemical DNA sensors) that use DNA as selective recognition element. The union with the complementary DNA chain causes a change in the optical or electrochemical properties to be measured, and thus the target to be detected can be analyzed.

6.1 Electrochemical genosensors

DNA sensors are a class of electrochemical sensors in which the molecular recognition is achieved by using DNA oligomers. As the recognition is in charge of a biological molecule, they are classified as *biosensors* since the 1990 decade. The signal originated on the recognition surface is then *transduced* into an electrical signal. Both *amperometric* or *potentiometric* measurements can be carried out. In amperometric measurements, an external potential is applied to oxidize or reduce an electrochemically active compound at its intrinsic redox potential. The current produced in the process is monitored. In potentiometric methods, an equilibrium is reached on the sensor surface without the need of an external potential. The *membrane potential* (potential generated between the electrode and the measured solution) is then recorded.

In amperometric measurements, the choice of the working potential provides some selectivity to the method, as the potential can be set at the specific redox value of the analyte of interest. Nevertheless, interferences in the sample can share the same potential value with the analyte. As this selectivity is not enough, the surface of the electrode needs to be functionalized.

For amperometric studies, Cottrel's equation takes into account the mass transport restrictions in the solution, and if the system is kept under continuous stirring, the intensity of the current depends on the concentration of analyte as follows (Equation 4):

$$I = nFA\frac{D}{L}C \tag{4}$$

Where A is the area of the electrode, D and C are the diffusion coefficient and concentration of the analyte and L is the thickness of the diffusion layer closest to the surface.

This equation can be simplified as $I = KC$, and then it can be witnessed that the measured intensity is proportional to the concentration of the analyte in the solution.

The electrode used as transducer element can be made up from different materials (Lucarelli et al., 2004). Platinum, gold, vitrified carbon or pyrolytic graphite are commonly employed. The use of *composites* (solid conductors dispersed into polymeric nonconducting matrices) is growing over the last years. As mentioned before, in electrochemical biosensors, the electrode is the transducer but a specific recognition step has been previously carried out by a biological macromolecule. Most extended electrochemical biosensors use enzimes or antibodies as recognizing molecules, but *genosensors* use DNA. DNA molecules afford two remarkable advantages over proteins: they are much more chemically stables and they can be easily synthesized with high purity.

DNA can be immobilized on the electrode surface using different techniques. 1) Physical adsorption, 2) electrochemical adsorption, due to the phosphate backbone of DNA, 3) avidin (or streptavidin) / biotin to immobilize the DNA probes on the surface of the electrode, 4) covalent electrode-DNA binding. This method depends strongly on the nature of the electrode, 5) pyrrole or other monomers can be electropolymerized on the surface of an electrode. If this process is conducted in the presence of the DNA probe, the polymer constitutes a matrix that traps the DNA molecules binding them to the electrode.

Once the DNA has been immobilized, the recognition step can take place. This event must result on an electrochemical phenomenon measurable by the electrode. Different strategies can be followed (Kerman et al., 2004).

For the detection of electroactive DNA binding agents, non-specific double-stranded DNA can act as recognizing biomolecules. After the compound binds to the DNA, it can be oxidized or reduced at its redox potential and the current can be monitored. Any electroactive DNA binding molecule will be detected, the selectivity only determined by the different intrinsic redox potential of every substance. This method allows the estimation of drug-DNA binding mode and binding constants (Tian et al., 2008).

For the detection of a specific DNA sequence, the most common approach is to immobilize the single-stranded DNA complementary sequence on the electrode. Then, the hybridization of the target sequence to the probe on the electrode's surface can be monitored by two main ways. The most widely used is adding to the solution an electroactive substance which only binds to the hybrid dsDNA, but not to the ssDNA alone. Myriads of substances have been employed with this aim: cationic metal complexes like $Co(phen)_3^{3+}$ and $Co(bpy)_3^{3+}$ or intercalating organic molecules like antramines or daunomycin are only a few examples. Commercial systems exist based on this approach (Motorola's eSensor™ and Toshiba's Genelyzer™). The second method to detect the hybridization is *label free* and relies on the redox properties of guanine. The intrinsic redox potential of this base on ssDNA (+1.03 V) decreases when hybridization to form dsDNA happens. This change can be monitored to detect hybridization of the probe and the target sequence. Nevertheless, this change is small and hard to detect, so more complex techniques are required. Furthermore, this method cannot be applied if the probe sequence itself posses guanine bases that would be quickly oxidized. To bypass this problem, probes with inosine instead of guanine can be synthesized. Inosine peak can be easily distinguished from guanine. It is also possible to use other labelling methods to detect the binding to the DNA probes such as metal nanoparticles or enzimes, but their uses are less frequent, although growing.

For the last years, the use of nanostructured materials is spreading in the field of nanosensors. This class of materials such as metal nanoparticles, magnetic nanoparticles or carbon nanotubes possesses very attractive features. The high surface and very characteristic conducting properties make them of interest to achieve better response times, higher sensitivity and improved specificity (Abu-Salah et al., 2010). Aligned carbon nanotubes were recently employed to detect a DNA sequence characteristic for genetically modified organisms with sensitivity in the nanomolar range (Berti et al., 2009). A combination of magnetic beads for immunomagnetic separation and a later detection step using magnetic graphite-epoxy composite electrode has been recently employed for the detection of *Salmonella* in milk with limit of detection from 5 to 7.5 x 10^3 CFU mL^{-1} in a short time (50 minutes) (Liébana et al., 2009).

6.2 Optical genosensors

Microarray technology has been developed due to the necessity of accurate and sensitive methodologies to make use of knowledge afforded by the Human Genome Project. This configuration offers a massive parallel analysis platform for hybridization reactions. According to Leher (Leher et al., 2003) microarrays are ordered two-dimensional spatial arrangements of small structures (oligonucleotides) on a solid support. The oligonucleotides are bounded or adsorbed on the solid support as the selective recognition element. When the complementary sample sequence is recognized, the optical properties of the probe bound to DNA changes and this fact results in a sensitive response. Different optical responses can be processed i.e. UV-Vis absorption, or fluorescence emission properties, and other optical events in connection with plasmon resonance phenomena. Among the different alternatives, fluorescence techniques (emission, total or partial reflection fluorescence and scanning fluorescence techniques) offer advantageous features due to its sensitivity (about 10^{-8} M of the probe and sub-microliter volumes) joint to the fact that a large number of fluorescent probes are able to react with DNA. Thus, the contact of the sample DNA with the sensor microarray during the readout process allows monitoring the continuous binding of molecules present in the sample and, then, interacting with the genosensor surface. Another advantage of optical genosensors (microarrays, biochips) is the possibility of repeated cycles of hybridization and denaturation with a single genosensor surface, where a large number of experiments with different targets and probe sequences under various experimental conditions can be developed. Figure 13 shows an example of detection of pathogens or genetically modified seeds using an optical genosensor based on the fluorescence enhancement.

Different fluorescence phenomena (spectral shifts, intensity enhancement or quenching, RET, anisotropy variations, life-time changes…) may be observed after hybridization as a consequence of the specific recognition of a sequence of DNA. Two main formats of experiments can be developed. The oligonucleotides adsorbed on the support (microarray) can be labelled with an appropriate fluorescent probe (Figure 13B) and the target DNA to be recognized reacts with them. In the second possibility, the DNA extracted from the cells under study (pathogens, i. e. *Salmonella sp., Helicobacter pylori, Escherichia coli*... or genetically modified seeds) is bounded to the fluorescent probe (Figure 13A) and then the hybridization is produced and the organisms are detected (Leung et al., 2007).

Different devices for detection can be employed, such as scanning fluorescence microscope, laser excitation combined with CCD-TV, or fluorescence spectrophotometry coupled to fiber optical devices (Schäferling & Nagl, 2006).

An important number of optical genosensors for selective detection of specific nucleic acid sequences use fluorescent intercalating and groove binding agents to evidence the hybridization of DNA, and many of them are commercially available in suitable kits. The fluorescence emission of the probes is enhanced or quenched in the presence of the hybridized DNA. Ethidium bromide is considered the fluorescent standard for detection of DNA hybridization, however thiazole orange and other derivatives become in an attractive alternative to other traditional fluorescent probes (Hanafi-Bagby et al., 2000). The offer covers from the traditional fluorescent probes to the promising fluorescent nanoparticles.

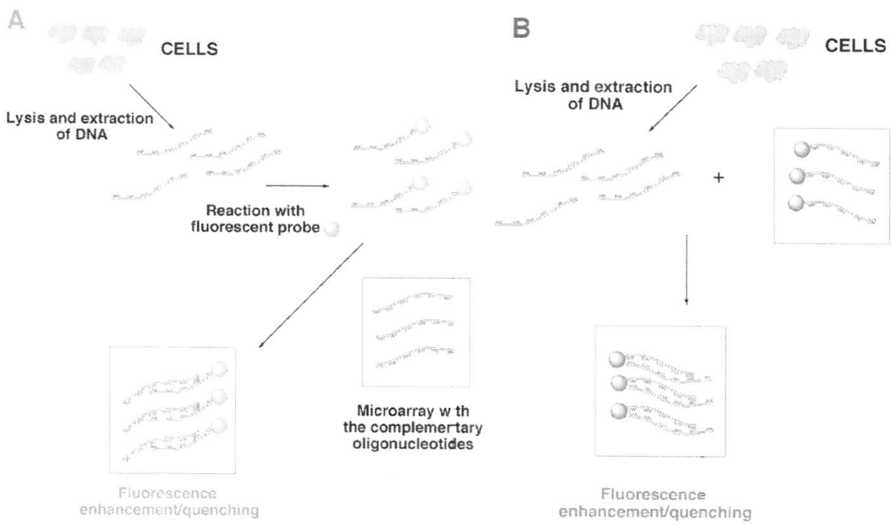

Fig. 13. Detection of pathogens or genetic disorders by the use of optical genosensors.

7. Conclusion

The study of the interaction of small molecules with DNA is a field of high topical interest, and we hope to have provided a clear, concise introduction to this fascinating area at the boundary between chemistry and biology. The detailed knowledge of these interactions can be used as the basis for the rational design of new DNA ligands with potential application in a variety of fields, *e.g.* as anticancer drugs and DNA probes allowing *in vitro* and *in vivo* monitoring of genetic diseases. Special relevance can be attached to the analysis of drugs, genetically modified organisms and environmentally toxic compounds capable to induce important DNA changes employing these innovative strategies. The design of suitable high throughput systems will improve the performance of these analytical challenges. This is a rapidly evolving topic, and devices able to recognize and bind to DNA are certain to find a host of additional applications in the near future.

8. Acknowledgements

Financial support from Ministerio de Ciencia e Innovación (Spain) through grants CTQ 2009-11312-BQU and CTQ 2009-12320-BQU, as well as from Grupos de Investigación UCM (920234), is gratefully acknowledged. The authors are also grateful to MEC for the award of a FPU research fellowship to V. González-Ruiz.

9. References

Abu-Salah, K. M.; Alrokyan, S. A.; Khan, M. N. & Ansari, A. A. (2010) Nanomaterials as Analytical Tools for Genosensors. *Sensors*, 10, 1, (January 2010), 963-993, 1424-8220

Akbay, N.; Seferoglu, Z. & Gök, E. (2009) Fluorescence Interaction and Determination of Calf Thymus DNA with Two Ethidium Derivatives, *Journal of Fluorescence*, 19, 6, (November 2009) 1045-1051, 1053-0509

Anker, J. N.; Hall, W. P.; Lyandres, O.; Shah, N. C.; Zhao, J. & Van Duyne, R. P. (2008). Biosensing with plasmonic nanosensors. *Nature materials*, 7, 6, (June 2008) 442-453, 1476-1122

Araya, F.; Huchet, G.; McGroarty, I.; Skellern, G.G.& Waigh R.D. (2007). Capillary electrophoresis for studying drug-DNA interactions. *Methods*, 42, 2, (June 2007) 141-149, 1046-2023.

Aslan, K.; Lakowicz, J. R.; Szmacinski, H. & Geddes, C. D. (2004). Metal-enhanced fluorescence solution-based sensing platform. *Journal of Fluorescence*, 14, 6, (November 2004) 677-679, 1053-0509

Baba, Y. (1999). Capillary affinity gel electrophoresis: new technique for specific recognition for DNA sequence and the mutation detection on DNA. *Journal of biochemical and biophysical methods*, 41, 2-3, (November 1999) 91-101, 0165-022X.

Banyay, M.; Sarkar, M. & Gräslund, A. (2003). A library of IR bands of nucleic acids in solution. *Biophysical Chemistry*, 104, 2, (June 2003) 477-488, 0303-4622.

Barber, J.; Cross, H. F. & Parkinson, J. A. (1993). High-Resolution NMR of DNA and Drug-DNA Interactions. In: *Methods in Molecular Biology, Spectroscopic Methods and Analyses: NMR, Mass Spectrometry, and Metalloprotein Techniques, Vol 17*, Jones, C.; Mulloy, B. & Thomas, A. H. (Eds.). Humana Press Inc, 978-1-59259-504-4, Totowa, NJ.

Berti, F.; Lozzi, L.; Palchetti, I.; Santucci, S. & Marrazza, G. (2009) Aligned carbon nanotube thin films for DNA electrochemical sensing. *Electrochimica Acta*, 54, 2, (September 2009), 5035-5041, 0013-4686

Blackburn, G. M.; Gait, M. J.; Loakes, D. & Williams, D. M. (2006) *Nucleic Acids in Chemistry and Biology*, The Royal Society of Chemistry, 978-0-85404-654-6, Cambridge.

Cardew, A. T. & Fox, K. R. (2010). DNase I Footprinting, In: *Methods in Molecular Biology. Drug-DNA Interaction Protocols,* K. R. Fox (ed.), 2nd Ed., Chapter 10, 153-172, Humana Press, 978-1-60327-417-3, Southampton.

D'Agata, R.; Corradini, R.; Ferretti, C.; Zanoli, L.; Gatti, M.; Marchelli, R & Spoto, G. (2010). Ultrasensitive detection of non-amplified genomic DNA by nanoparticle-enhanced surface plasmon resonance imaging. *Biosensors and Bioelectronics,* 25, 9, (May 2010) 2095-2100, 0956-5663.

De Mol, N. J. & Fisher, M. J. E. (Eds.) (2010). *Surface Plasmon Resonance Methods and Protocols,* Humana Press / Springer Science+Business Media, 978-1-60761-669-6, New York.

Eriksson, M. & Nordén, B. (2001). Linear and Circular Dichroism of Drug-Nucleic Acid Complexes. In : *Methods in Enzymology, Drug-Nucleic Acid Interactions, Vol. 340,* Chaires, J. B. & Waring M. J. (Eds.). Academic Press, 0-12-182241-9, San Diego.

Galas, D. J. & Schmitz, A. (1978). DNAase footprinting- simple method for detection of protein-DNA binding specificity. *Nucleic Acids Research,* 5, 9, 3157-3170, 1362-4962.

Giannetti, A.; Citti, L.; Domenici, C.; Tedeschi, L.;Baldini, F.; Wabuyele, M. B. & Vo-Dinh, T. (2006) FRET-based protein-DNA binding Assay for Detection of Active NF-kB, *Sensors and Actuators B: Chemical*, 113, 2 (February 2006) 649-654, 0925-4005

Hampshire, A. J.; Rusling, D. A.; Broughton-Head, V. J. & Fox, K. R. (2007). Footprinting: A method for determining the sequence selectivity, affinity and kinetics of DNA-binding ligands. *Methods,* 42, 2, (June 2007) 128-140, 1046-2023.

Hanafi-Bagby, D.; Piunno, P. A. E.; Wust, C. C. & Krull, U. J. (2000) Concentration Dependence of a Thiazole Orange Derivative that is Used to Determine Nucleic Acid Hybridization by an Optical Biosensor, *Analytica Chimica Acta,* 411, 1-2, (May 2000) 19-30, 0003-2670

Harding, E. S. & Chowdhry, B. Z. (Eds.) (2001). *Protein-ligand interactions: hydrodynamics and calorimetry, a practical approach,* Oxford University Press, 0-19-963746-6, New York.

Islam, M. M.; Chowdhury, S. R. & Kumar, G. S. (2009) Spectroscopic and Calorimetric Studies on the Binding of Alkaloids Berberine, Palmatine and Coralyne to Double Stranded RNA Polynucleotides, *Journal of Physical Chemistry B,* 113, 4, (January 2009), 1210-1224, 1520-6106

Jangir, D.K.; Tyagi, G.; Mehrotra, R. & Kundu, S. (2010). Carboplatin interaction with calf-thymus DNA: A FTIR spectroscopic approach. *Journal of Molecular Structure,* 969, 1-3, (April 2010) 126-129, 0022-2860.

Kerman, K.; Kobayashi, M. & Tamiya, E. (2004) Recent trends in electrochemical DNA biosensor technology. *Measurement Science and Technology,* 15, 2, (February 2004) R1-R11, 0957-0233

Koster, D.A.; Czerwinski, F.; Halby, L.; Crut, A.; Vekhoff, P.; Palle, K.; Arimondo, P.B. & Dekker, N.H. (2008). Single-molecule observations of topotecan-mediated TopIB activity at a unique DNA sequence. *Nucleic Acids Research,* 36, 7, (April 2008) 2301-2310, 0305-1048

Kral, T.; Leblond, J.; Hof, M.; Scherman, D.; Herscovici, J. & Mignet, N. (2010). Lipopolythiourea/DNA interaction: a biophysical study. *Biophysical Chemistry*, 148, 1-3, (May 2010) 68-73, 0301-4622

Krylova, S.M.; Wegman, D.W. & Krylov, S.N. (2010). Making DNA hibridization assays in capillary electrophoresis quantitative. *Analytical Chemistry*, 82, 11, (June 2010) 4428-4433, 0003-2700

Kumar, C. V.; Turner, R. S. & Asuncion, E. H. (1993) Groove Binding of a Styrylcyanine Dye to the DNA Double Helix: the Salt Effect, *Journal of Photochemistry and Photobiology A: Chemistry*, 74, 2-3, (September 1993) 231-238, 1010-6030

Lehr, H.-P.; Reimann, M.; Brandenburg, A.; Suiz, G. &Klapproth, H. (2003) Real Time Detection of Nucleic Acid Interactions by Total Internal Reflection Fluorescence, *Analytical Chemistry*, 75, 10, (May 2003) 2414-2420, 0003-2700

Lakowicz, J. R. (2001) Radiative decay engineering: biophysical and biomedical applications. *Analytical Biochemistry*, 301, 2, (February 2002) 261-277, 0003-2697

Lakowicz, J. R.; Shen, Y.; D'Auria, S.; Malicka, J.; Fang, J.; Gryczynski, Z. & Gryczynski, I. (2002) Radiative Decay Engineering 2: effects of silver island films on fluorescence intensity, lifetimes, and resonance energy transfer. *Analytical Biochemistry*, 298, 1, (November 2001) 1-24, 0003-2697

Lakowicz, J. R.; Ray, K.; Chowdhury, M.; Szmacinski, H.; Fu, Y.; Zhang, J. & Nowaczyk, K.; (2008) Plasmon-controlled fluorescence: a new paradigm in fluorescence spectroscopy. *The Analyst*, 133, 10, (October 2008) 1308-1346, 0003-2654

Lane, A. N. (2001). Nuclear Magnetic Resonance Studies of Drug-DNA Complexes in Solution. In : *Methods in Enzymology, Drug-Nucleic Acid Interactions, Vol. 340*, Chaires, J. B. & Waring M. J. (Eds.). Academic Press, 0-12-182241-9, San Diego, USA.

Leung, A.; Shankar, P. M. & Mutharasan, R. (2007) A Review of Fiber-Optic Biosensors, *Sensors and Atuators B: Chemical*, 125, 2 (August 2007) 688-703, 0925-4005

Li, W.-Y.; Xu, J.- G.; Guo, X.-Q.; Zhu, Q.-Z. & Zhao, Y. B. (1997) Study of the Interaction Between Rivanol and DNA and its Application to DNA Assay, *Spectrochimica Acta A*, 53, 5 (May 1997) 781-787, 1386-1425

Liébana, S.; Lermo, A.; Campoy, S.; Barbé, J.; Alegret, S. & Pividori, M. I. (2009) Magneto Immunoseparation of Pathogenic Bacteria and Electrochemical Magneto Genosensing of the Double-Tagged Amplicon, *Analytical Chemistry*, 81, 14, (July 2009), 5812-5820, 0003-2700

Lopez-Crapez, E.; Maligne, J.-M.; Gatchitch, F.; Casano, L.;Langlois, T.; Pugnière, M.; Roquet, F.; Mathis, G. & Bazin, H. (2008) A homogeneous Resonance Energy Transfer-Based Assay to Monitor MutS/DNA interactions, *Analytical Biochemistry*, 383, 12, (December 2008) 301-306, 0003-2697

Lucarelli, F.; Marrazza, G.; Turner, A. & Mascini, M. (2004) Carbon and gold electrodes as electrochemical transducers for DNA hybridisation sensors. *Biosensors and Bioelectronics*, 19, 6, (January 2004), 515-530, 0956-5663

Mandeville, J. S.; N'soukpoé-Kossi, C. N.; Neault, J. F. & Tajmir-Riahi, H. A. (2010). Structural analysis of DNA interaction with retinol and retinoic acid. *Biochemistry Cell Biology*, 88, 3, (June 2010) 469-477, 1208-6002.

Martín, M. A.; del Castillo, B. & Lerner, D. A. (1988) Study of the Luminescence Properties of a New Series of Quinolizinium Salts and Their Interaction with DNA, *Analytica Chimica Acta.*, 205, 1-2, (February 1988) 105-115, 0003-2670

Martín, M. A.; Bouin, A. S.; Muñoz-Botella, S. & del Castillo, B. (2002) Study of the Interaction of Azaquinolizinium Salts with DNA, *Polycyclic Aromatic Compounds*, 22, 1, (February 2002) 37-53, 1040-6638

Neault, J. F. & Tajmir-Riahi, H. A. (1996). Diethylstilbestrol-DNA Interaction Studied by Fourier Transform Infrared and Raman Spectroscopy. *Journal of Biological Chemistry,* 271, 14, (April 1996) 8140-8143, 0021-9258

Nguyen B.; Tanious, F. A. & Wilson, W. D. (2007). Biosensor-surface plasmon resonance: Quantitative analysis of small molecule-nucleic acid interactions. *Methods,* 42, 2, (June 2007) 150-161, 1046-2023

Paul, P.; Hossain, M.; Yadav, R. C. & Kumar, G. S. (2010) Biophysical Studies on the Base Specificity and Energetics of the DNA Interaction of Photoactive Dye Thionine: Spectroscopic and Calorimetric Approach, *Biophysical Chemistry,* 148, 1-3 (May 2010), 93-103, 0301-4622

Peng, H. I.; Strohsahl, C. M., Leach, K. E.; Krauss, T. & Miller, B. L. (2009) Label-free DNA detection on nanostructured Ag surfaces. *ACS nano,* 3, 8, (August 2009) 2265-2273, 1936-0851

Prunkl, C.; Pichlmaier, M.; Winter, R.; Kharlanov, V.; Rettig, W. & Wagenknecht, H.-A. (2010) Optical, Redox and DNA-Binding Properties of Phenanthridinium Chromophores: Elucidating the Role of the Phenyl Substituent for Fluorescence Enhancement of Ethidium in the Presence of DNA, *Chemistry - A European Journal,* 16, 11 (March 2010), 3392-3402, 0947-6539

Rodger, A. (2010). Circular and Linear Dichroism of Drug-DNA Systems. In: *Drug-DNA Interaction Protocols, Methods in Molecular Biology. Vol. 613* , Fox, K. R. (Ed.). Humana Press, 978-1-60327-417-3, Southampton.

Scarano, S.; Mascini, M., Turner, A. P. F. & Minunni, M. (2010). Surface plasmon resonance imaging for affinity-based biosensors. *Biosensors and Bioelectronics,* 25, 5, (January 2010) 957-966, 0956-5663

Schäferling, M. & Nagl, S. (2006) Optical Technologies for the Read out Quality Control of DNA and Protein Microarrays. *Analytical and Bioanalytical Chemistry,* 385, 2 (January 2006) 500-517, 1618-2642

Schasfoort, R. B. M. & Tudos, A. J. (Eds.) (2008). *Handbook of Surface Plasmon Resonance,* The Royal Society of Chemistry, 978-0-85404-267-8, Cambridge.

Serganov, A. & Patel, D. J. (2006). Structural Features of the Specific Interactions between Nucleic Acids and Small Organic Molecules, In: *Sequence-Specific DNA Binding Agents,* Waring, M. (Ed.), 233-252, The Royal Society of Chemistry, 978-0-085404-370-5, Cambridge.

Sharma A. K.; Jha, R. & Gupta, B. D. (2007). Fiber-Optic Sensors Based on Surface Plasmon Resonance: A comprehensive Review. *IEEE Sensors Journal,* 7, 8, (August 2007) 1118-1129, 1530-437X

Ŝpringer, T.; Piliarik, M. & Homola, J. (2010). Surface plasmon resonance sensor with dispersionless microfluidics for direct detection of nucleic acids at the low femtomole level. *Sensors and Actuators B,* 145, 1, (March 2010) 588-591, 0925-4005

Steiner G. (2004). Surface plasmon resonance imaging. *Analytical and Bioanalytical Chemistry*, 379, 3, (June 2004) 328-331, 1618-2642

Su, X.; Kong, L.; Lei, X.; Hu, L.; Ye, M. & Zou, H. (2007a). Biological fingerprinting analysis of trditional Chinese medicines with targeting ADME/Tox property for screening of bioactive compounds by chromatographic and MS methods. *Mini-Reviews in Medicinal Chemistry*, 7, 1, (January 2007) 87-98, 1389-5575.

Su, X.; Qin, F.; Kong, L.; Ou, J.; Xie, C. & Zou, H. (2007b). Characterization of enantioselective binding of racemic natural tetrahydropalmatine to DNA by chromatographic methods. *Journal of Chromatography B*, 845, 1, (January 2007) 174-179, 1570-0232.

Suh, D. & Chaires, J. B. (1995). Criteria for the Mode of Binding of DNA Binding Agents, *Biorganic and Medicinal Chemistry*, 3, 6, (June 1995) 723-728, 0968-0896

Teles, F. R. R. & Fonseca, L. P. (2008) Trends in DNA biosensors. *Talanta*, 77, 2, (December 2008), 606-623, 0039-9140

Tian, R.; Xu, S.; Lei, X.; Jin, W.; Ye, M. & Zou, H. (2005). Characterization of Small-Molecule-Biomacromolecule Interactions: from Simple to Complex, *Trends in Analytical Chemistry*, 24, 9 (October 2005), 810-825, 0165-9936

Tian, X.; Song, Y.; Dong, H. & Ye, B. (2008) Interaction of anticancer herbal drug berberine with DNA immobilized on the glassy carbon electrode. *Bioelectrochemistry*, 73, 1, (June 2008), 18-22, 1567-5394

Touahir, L.; Galopin, E.; Boukherroub, R.; Gouget-Laemmel, A. C.; Chazalviel, J. N.; Ozanam, F. & Szunerits, S. (2010) Localized surface plasmon-enhanced fluorescence spectroscopy for highly-sensitive real-time detection of DNA hybridization. *Biosensors and Bioelectronics*, 25, 2, (August 2010) 2579-2585, 0956-5663

Tse, W. C. & Boger D. L. (2004). A Fluorescent Intercalator Displacement Assay for Establishing DNA Binding Selectivity and Affinity, *Accounts of Chemical Research*, 37, 1 (January 2004), 61-69, 0022-2313

Valeur, V. (2001). Resonance Energy Transfer and its Applications, In: *Molecular Fluorescence Principles and Applications*, Valeur, V., 247-272, Wiley-VCH, 3-527-29919-X, Weinheim

Wu, F.-Y.; Xiang Y.-L.; Wu, Y.-M. & Xie, F.-Y. (2009). Study of the Interaction of a Fluorescent Probe with DNA, *Journal of Luminescence*, 129, 11 (November 2009), 1286-1291, 0022-2313

Yang, B.; Lu, N.; Qi, D.; Ma, R.; Wu, Q.; Hao, J.; Liu, X.; Mu, Y.; Reboud, V.; Kehagias, N.; Sotomayor-Torres, C. M.; Boey, F. Y. C.; Chen, X. & Chi, L. (2010). Tuning the intensity of metal-enhanced fluorescence by engineering silver nanoparticle arrays. *Small*, 6, 9, (May 2010) 1038-1043, 1613-6829

Zhang, Y.; Padhyay, A.; Sevilleja, J. E.; Guerrant, R. L. & Geddes, C. D. (2010) Interactions of Fluorophores with Iron Nanoparticles: Metal-Enhanced Fluorescence. *The Journal of Physical Chemistry C* (May 2010) 114, 17, 7575-7581, 1932-7447

Zoriniants, G. & Barnes, W. L. (2008). Fluorescence enhancement through modified dye molecule absorption associated with the localized surface plasmon resonances of metallic dimers. *New Journal of Physics*, 10, 10, (October 2008) 105002-105013, 1367-2630

4

Specific Applications of Vibrational Spectroscopy in Biomedical Engineering

Sylwia Olsztyńska-Janus[1],
Marlena Gąsior-Głogowska[1,4], Katarzyna Szymborska-Małek[2],
Bogusława Czarnik-Matusewicz[3] and Małgorzata Komorowska[1,4]
[1]Institute of Biomedical Engineering and Instrumentation, Wrocław University of Technology,
[2]Institute of Physical and Theoretical Chemistry, Wrocław University of Technology,
[3]Faculty of Chemistry, University of Wrocław,
[4]Regional Specialist Hospital in Wrocław, Research and Development Centre, Wrocław, Poland

1. Introduction

Nucleic acids such as proteins, amino acids, lipids and carbohydrates are located, as the basic components of animal cells, plant cells and microorganisms, in many cellular organelles. In eukaryotic organisms, deoxyribonucleic acid (DNA) is found in the cell nucleus, mitochondria and chloroplasts, while ribonucleic acid (RNA) occurs mainly in the cytoplasm of the cell. In prokaryotes such as bacteria and archaea, DNA is also found in the cytoplasm of the cell. Nucleic acids play an important role in storage, transfer and incorporation of genetic information into the cell. DNA contains the genetic codes to make RNA, while RNA contains the codes for the primary sequence of amino acids for protein synthesis, which plays a fundamental role for living creatures (Campbell & Farrell, 2009).

Fundamental vital processes occur at the molecular level, therefore research methods allowing for investigation of molecular processes are crucial in their understanding. Vibrational (Infrared and Raman) Spectroscopy is used to obtain both structural and conformational information of biological systems, including amino acids, proteins and lipids (Barth, 2007; Byler & Susi, 1986; Cieślik-Boczula et al., 2007; Murawska et al., 2010; Murayama et al., 2001; Szwed et al., 2010; Szyc et al., 2008; Wolpert & Heellwig, 2006; Wu et al., 2002). Raman spectroscopy seems also to be a very powerful tool for the study of stress-induced molecular changes in both natural and synthetic polymers (Amer, 2009; Koening, 2001). This technique has been applied for such tissues as tendon, blood vessel walls and skin. Simple correlation between the Raman spectroscopic data and mechanical relations can be established (Hanuza et al., 2009; Winchester et al., 2008).

Temperature, pH, presence of salts, electromagnetic radiation exposure and organic solvents modify biological compounds, inducing specific conformational changes which are relevant for the understanding of their functions (Parker, 1983). Vibrational spectroscopy has been applied to study cells or molecules in tissues changed by various factors. It is therefore frequently used as a diagnostic tool in pharmacy (Wartewig & Neubert, 2005), in cancer research (Amharref et al., 2007; Li et al., 2005), in neurological disorders and diseases of the cardiovascular system (Pysz et al., 2010) and in bone diseases (Fuchs et al., 2008), as well as in Alzheimer's disease (Griebe et al., 2007). It allows the progress of these diseases and the effectiveness of therapy to be monitored. It is necessary to use measuring techniques which make it possible to reach the micro- and even nanoareas of tissue or enable the structure and properties of single molecules to be examined.

One of the most important infrared spectroscopy methods used in studies of biological systems is Attenuated Total Reflection (ATR) Fourier Transform Infrared (FTIR). The ATR accessory operates by measuring the absorption when a totally internally reflected infrared beam comes into contact with a sample. This technique provides a powerful and sensitive approach able to reveal changes in the biochemical properties of biomedical samples studied at the molecular level (Olsztynska et al., 2006a; Olsztynska et al., 2001). It enables study of the relative concentrations of individual components of tissue and inter- or intramolecular interactions between them. Many substances in the solid and liquid state can be characterized, identified and also quantified by FTIR-ATR spectroscopy (Heise et al., 2002). Studies of tissue can be carried out on thin sections with a thickness of several micrometers. In the case of liquid samples a few micro litres of fluid are sufficient for measurements. Typically, tissue samples are collected during a biopsy, endoscopy or puncture, or from intraoperative material used for this purpose. One of the key advantages of FTIR-ATR is that studies can be conducted on a small amount of biomedical material. Another is not needing to use additional reagents or biological markers, which significantly reduces sample preparation time and reduces the cost of analysis. Research material downloaded without fixation, dyeing and additional chemical treatment can be almost immediately analysed. FTIR with an ATR accessory has shown to be a very valuable tool in pharmaceutical (McAuley et al., 2009) and polymer (Licoccia et al., 2005) applications. Tissue or tissue components having been characterized by FTIR-ATR spectroscopy are human hair (Chan et al., 2005), biological fluids including blood (Damm et al., 2007; Heise et al., 1989), and cancer tissue (Sun et al., 2003).

2. Vibrational spectroscopy of macromolecules; amino acids, proteins and DNA

2.1 Amino acids

Amino acids (AAs) are the basic building blocks of peptides and proteins. As they belong to the simplest class of biomolecules, detailed investigation of their properties and interactions is essential for understanding the behaviour of macromolecules in different circumstances. Despite the fact that physiological processes occur in the aqueous phase, measurements of AAs are often performed in the solid state (Medien, 1998), which does not provide information about effects occurring in aqueous solutions. Even a newly developed dissolution-spray-deposition infrared technique (Cao & Fischer, 1999) is no help in understanding biological processes at the molecular level. AAs are not easily studied by vibrational spectroscopy, in that the vibrational bands of AAs in aqueous solution are usually broad, overlapped or even incomplete as a result of strong solvent absorption, particularly that arising from water, and solute-solvent interactions. It is well known that AAs may exist in various protonation states, which are clearly reflected in the vibrational spectra. Wolpert and Hellwig (Wolpert & Hellwig, 2006) have presented spectra of AA head groups in different protonation states and made detailed assignments for the 20 alpha AAs in aqueous solution in the range 1800-500 cm^{-1}. The IR spectra of glycine in aqueous solutions obtained in the pH range 0.2-14 allow charge distribution on the molecule to be determined (Max et al., 1998).

For example, presented in Figure 1 are the FTIR-ATR spectra of different AAs, i.e. L-glycine (Gly), L-alanine (Ala) and L-phenylalanine (Phe), in aqueous solution obtained in the region 1800–800 cm^{-1}. Tentative assignments of the main infrared bands of these three AAs are summarized in Table 1.

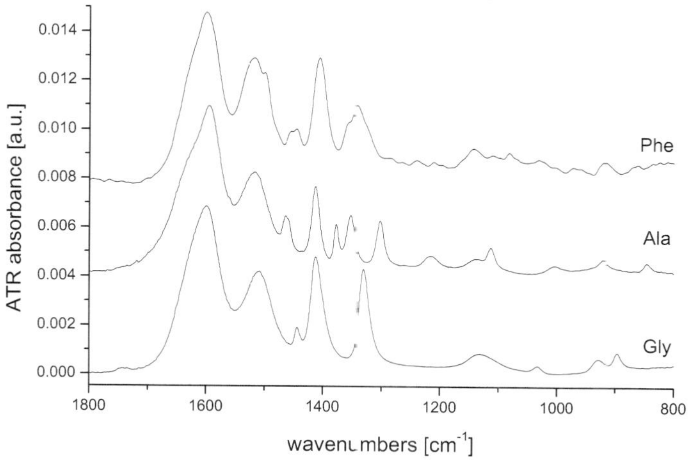

Fig. 1. FTIR-ATR spectra of L-glycine (Gly), L-alanine (Ala) and L-phenylalanine (Phe) in aqueous solution obtained in the region 1800–800 cm^{-1}. The spectra are shifted in absorbance for clarity.

Gly	Ala	Phe	Assignments*
1614 sh	1620 sh	1628 sh	$\beta_{as}(NH_3^+)$
1601	1597	1583	$\nu_{as}(CO_2^-)$
1509	1516	1528	$\beta_s(NH_3^+)$
		1448	$\beta_s(CH_2)$
1412	1412	1408	$\nu_s(CO_2^-$
	1373	1364	$\beta_s(CH_2)$
	1353		$\beta_s(CH_2)$
1331		1340	$\beta_s(CH_2)$
1131	1138	1131 sh	$\rho(NH_3^+)$
929	919	913	$\gamma(CH_2)$

*Abbreviations: ν, stretching; β, in-plane bending; γ, out-of-plane bending; ρ, rocking; s, symmetrical; as, asymmetrical; sh, shoulder.

Table 1. Major positions (in cm^{-1}) and tentative assignment of IR bands of aqueous Gly, Ala and Phe.

2.2 Proteins

There are several experimental methods available for determination of protein secondary structure, such as circular dichroism (CD) (Shanmugam & Polavarapu, 2006), nuclear magnetic resonance (NMR) (Sun et al., 2005), X-ray scattering and diffraction (Sun et al., 2005), calorimetry and fluorescence (Gelamo et al., 2002), diffuse reflectance (DR) (Ishida & Griffiths, 1993), electron paramagnetic resonance ESR (Gelamo et al., 2004), Raman (Bolton & Scherer, 1989), near infrared (NIR) (Wu et al., 2000) and IR spectroscopy (Cai & Singh, 1999; Grdadolnik & Maréchal, 2001a & 2001b; Jackson et al., 1989; Maréchal, 2004 & 2003; van de Weert et al., 2001; Zhang & Yan, 2005). The last has for many years been a promising technique for the determination of the secondary structure of proteins in that some peptide vibrations are sensitive to conformation (Harris & Chapman, 1992; Jackson & Mantsch, 1995). In particular, FTIR-ATR has recently been applied for rapid analysis (Jeyachandran et al., 2009; Pevsner & Diem, 2001; Smith et al., 2002; Wang et al, 2003).

Of particular interest in interpreting infrared spectra of proteins are the amide I, II and III bands. These can be described as a function of backbone coordinates, as shown in Table 2. The three amide bands are usually a superposition of several individual components of the different secondary structure elements. It is possible to identify them only with the mathematical procedures for band resolution, i.e. derivative spectroscopy (Zhang & Yan, 2005) and Fourier self-deconvolution (Byler & Susi, 1986). The component bands can be assigned to specific secondary structures, such as α helix, β sheet, β turns or random coil (Byler & Susi, 1986). Frequencies of amide I vibrations for the most popular secondary structures are collected in Table 3.

Designation		Approximate frequency (cm^{-1})	Assignment and PED*
Amide	A	3300-3230	ν(NH) 100%
	B	~ 3100	ν(NH) 100%
	I	1700-1600	ν(CO) 70-85% ν(CN) 10-20%
	II	1580-1510	δ(NH) 40-60% ν(CN) 18-40%; ν($C^{\alpha}C^{sch}$) ~10%
	III	1400-1200	δ(NH) 10-40% ν(CN) 0-40%; ν($C^{\alpha}C^{sch}$) 0-20%

*Abbreviations: PED, potential energy distribution; ν, stretching; δ, in-plane bending; sch, side chain.

Table 2. Summary of the characteristic bands associated with the peptide group.

Most methods used to determine the secondary structure of peptides and proteins concentrate on an analysis of the amide I (Dong et al., 1990), amide I and II (Dousseau & Pézolet, 1990), or amide III bands (Cai & Singh, 2004; Fabian & Mäntele, 2002; Fu et al., 1994).

Selected as a model protein was bovine serum albumin (BSA), which belongs to a major class of animal proteins. BSA is free of prosthetic groups and other complicating factors, and its primary, secondary and tertiary structure has been well-characterized. When FTIR-ATR spectroscopy is combined with derivative and difference spectroscopy procedures, it is possible to monitor even small changes in the conformation of a BSA protein in aqueous solution affected by any factor. The FTIR-ATR spectra of BSA in an aqueous solution with concentrations of 10 wt % are presented in Figure 2 in the range of the three amide bands.

Secondary structure	Position of Amide I band (cm^{-1}) v(C=O)
α helix	1660-1648
β sheet	1640-1625 (strong absorption) 1690 (weak absorption)
β turns	1685-1660
random coil	1660-1652
β turns (3_{10}-helix)	1670-1660
aggregated	1628-1610

Table 3. Frequencies of amide I vibrations for different secondary structures.

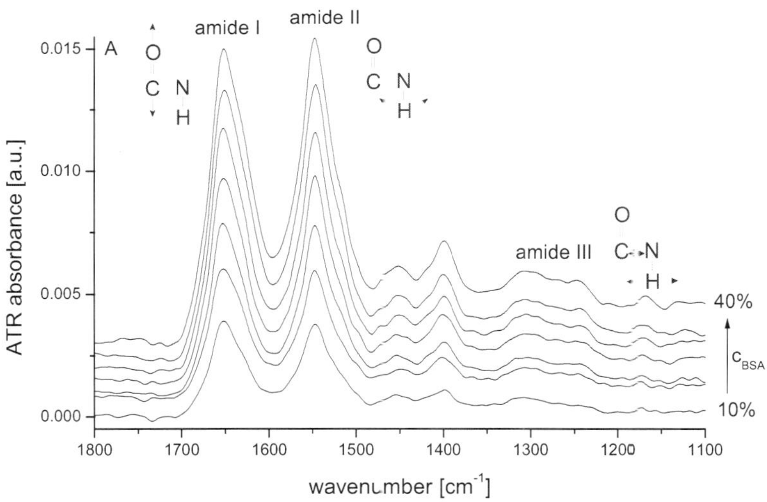

Fig. 2. FTIR-ATR spectra in the region 1800–1100 cm^{-1} of BSA in aqueous solutions at different concentrations (10, 15, 20, 25, 30, 35 and 40 wt %). The spectra were constructed using the water spectrum as the background. The spectra are shifted in absorbance for clarity.

FTIR-ATR spectroscopy was applied to study the effect of pH and metal ions on the conformation of BSA in aqueous solution (Qing et al., 1996). Small effects of binding with metal ions can also be detected by the splitting of the conformation-sensitive amide I band (Ahmed & Tajmir-Riahi 1993; Prestrelski et al., 1991). Ozaki's group investigated pH and heat-induced changes in the secondary structures of human serum albumin (HSA) and in the hydrogen bondings of side chains by two-dimensional/ATR correlation spectroscopy (Wu et al., 2002; Murayama et al., 2001). The ATR technique has been also used for investigation of protein films, including thin hydrated films of soluble and membrane protein in a phospholipid bilayer (Goormaghtigh et al., 1990).

2.3 DNA

Raman and IR spectroscopies can be used to examine both short oligonucleotides and large structures of DNA. It is possible to study DNA samples in a solution, dehydrated fibre, film or crystalline form (Prescott et al., 1984; Taillandier et al., 1989; Taillandier & Liquier, 1992). Different factors, such as temperature, pH (Tajmir-Riahi et al., 1995), varying hydration (Falk et al., 1963; Lee et al., 2004; Pevsner & Diem, 2003; Tao et al., 1989) and ionic strength (Keller & Hartman, 1986; Taillandier et al., 1989, Taillandier & Liquier, 1992), affect the physical state of DNA samples.

2.3.1 IR spectroscopy

Vibrational spectroscopy is one of the main methods used to determine the secondary structures of A, B, C, D and Z-DNA forms (Banyay et al., 2003; Pohle & Fritzsche, 1980; Rauch et al., 2005; Taboury et al., 1985; Taillandier et al., 1989). IR spectroscopy can also be used successfully to study conformational changes during B→A and B→Z transitions (Adam et al., 1986; Pilet & Brahms, 1973; Taboury et al., 1985; Taillandier et al., 1989; Taillandier & Liquier, 1992) and DNA denaturation (Banyay et al., 2003; Lee et al., 2004). The IR spectra of DNA show many characteristic bands, which are sensitive to denaturation, dehydration and conformational transition. Table 4 shows the main IR absorption bands observed during the melting of DNA and transformation between B and A (or Z) forms. IR also allows single-stranded, double-stranded and triple-stranded chains of DNA to be distinguished (Banyay et al., 2003; Taillandier & Liquier, 1992). In the literature there are plenty of data on the conformational changes induced by pH or temperature changes (Lee et al., 2004; Tajmir-Riahi et al., 1995), dehydration (Falk et al., 1963; Lee et al., 2004) and interaction with metal ions such as Mn^{2+}, Co^{2+}, Ni^{2+}, Cu^{2+}, Cd^{2+}, Mg^{2+} and Pt^{2+} (Hackl et al., 2005; Matsui et al., 2009). IR spectroscopy is also a powerful technique in investigating the interaction of DNA with drugs (Taillandier & Liquier, 1992).

The IR spectrum can be divided into four characteristic spectral ranges. Absorbed in the range 1800-1500 cm^{-1} are bands related to the C=O, C=N, C=C and N-H stretching vibrations of bases. These bands are sensitive to changes in the base stacking and base pairing interactions. Bands occurring in the interval 1500-1250 cm^{-1} assigned to vibrations of the bases and base-sugar connections are strongly related to the conformational changes of the backbone chain and glycosidic bond rotation. The range 1250-1000 cm^{-1} involves sugar-phosphate vibrations, such as PO_2^- symmetric and asymmetric stretching vibrations and C-O stretching vibrations. These vibrations show high sensitivity to conformational changes in the backbone. The range 1000-800 cm^{-1} is characteristic for bands associated with vibrations of sugars which correlate with the various nucleic acid sugar puckering modes (C2'-endo and C3'-endo) (Adam et al., 1986; Banyay et al., 2003; Lee et al., 2004; Parker, 1983; Pevsner & Diem, 2003; Taillandier et al., 1989; Taillandier & Liquier, 1992).

It is worth mentioning that IR spectroscopy applied to nucleic acids gives structural information comparable to that obtained from X-ray crystallography or high resolution NMR. In addition, this method compared to the aforementioned techniques allows examination of the samples in various states.

B form	Bands observed for melting	Bands characteristic for B→A transition	Bands characteristic for B→Z transition	Assignments*
1715	-1690	1708	1690	ν(C=O), ν(C=C), ν(C=N), β(N-H)
1664	-1649	1664	1664	
1610	-1607	1605	1610	
			1433	dA syn
1425	-1410			dC2′-endo
		1418	1408	dC3′-endo
1375	+1362	1375		d purine/anti
			1355	d purine/syn
1292	disappears			$\nu(C4NH_2)$ of C
1280	disappears	1275		β(CN3H) of dT
			1265	dC, dG
1225	-1241	1240	1212	$\nu_{as}(PO_2^-)$
		1188		ν(C-O)b
1088	-1096	1088	1085, 1060	$\nu_s(PO_2^-)$
1052	+1069	1052		ν(C-O)d
970	-957	975, 970, 953	969, 951, 925	ν(C-C)b
894	-883	899, 877, 864	928	δd
840	-819	807	838	ν(O-P-O)b

*Abbreviations: ν, stretching; β, in-plane bending; δ, in-plane bending (ring); s, symmetrical; as, asymmetrical; dA, deoxyadenosine; dC, deoxycytidine; dG, deoxyguanosine; dT, thymidine; d, deoxyribose; b, backbone.

Table 4. Changes in the position of IR bands observed for melting of DNA, B→A and B→Z transitions. A plus (or minus) sign indicates a band which gained (or lost) appreciable intensity during melting.

2.3.2 Raman spectroscopy

Raman spectroscopy allows study of the structure of individual groups of atoms and provides information on the conformational changes taking place in macromolecules. Moreover, it is possible to monitor the denaturing processes (transition from ordered double stranded to a disordered single-stranded helix) and the B→A and B→Z conformational changes (Duguid et al., 1996; Erfurth & Peticolas, 1975; Prescott et al., 1984; Taillandier et al., 1989). Collected in Table 5 are the main Raman lines observed during the melting process and the B→A (Z) transitions. This technique also enables examination of the structural changes of DNA caused by radiation (Synytsya et al., 2007), temperature and pH change (Duguid et al., 1996; Erfurth & Peticolas, 1975; O'Connor et al., 1982) and the addition of metal ions or organic compounds (Duguid et al., 1993; Langlais et al., 1990; Martin et al., 1978; Martin et al., 1982).
The Raman spectrum can be divided into characteristic spectral regions. The dominated band in the range 1800-1600 cm^{-1} at 1668 cm^{-1} is assigned to coupled C=O stretching and N-H deformation modes of dT, dG and dC, which is very sensitive to the denaturation process. Located in the interval 1600-1200 cm^{-1} are bands associated with purine and pyrimidine ring vibrations. The bands are shaped by conformational transition and melting

process. In addition, they are perturbed by metal binding at ring sites and are sensitive indicators of electronic structure changes of the ring.

B form	Bands observed for melting	Bands characteristic for B→A transition	Bands characteristic for B→Z transition	Assignments*
1688	+1654, +1684	1688		ν(C=O), δ(NH2) of dT, dG, dC
1610	+1597	1603		dC
1578	+1572, -1582	1574	1577	dG, dA
1534	+1528	1533		dC
1511	+1504	1512	1521	dA, dC
1489	+1481, -1494	1483	1491	dG, dA
1421	+1412			d purine/syn
		1396		d(CH_2 δ), dG
1376	+1365, -1381	1374	1362	dT, dA, dG
1339	+1324, -1343	1336	disappears	dA, dG
1320	+1320	1322		dG
			1314	d purine/syn
1304	+1308	1301		dA
1292	+1289		1292	dC
1257	+1257		1257	dC, dA
1238	+1238	1243	1238	dT
1218	+1218	1209	1220	dT
1186	+1183	1186	1186	dT, dC
1142	disappears	1145		ν(C-C)
1094	-1094	1099	1094	$\nu_s(PO_2^-)$
1054	+1060		1051	ν(C-O)
895	+872			d
835	-828	806	810	ν(O-P-O)
781	+773, -792		746	dC
750	+738	748	748	dT
729	+725	727	715	dA
		704		d
682	-682	682		dG C2′-endo/anti
			625	dG C3′-endo/syn

*Abbreviations: ν, stretching mode; δ, deformation mode; s, symmetrical; dA, deoxyadenosine; dC, deoxycytidine; dG, deoxyguanosine; dT, thymidine; d, deoxyribose; b, backbone.

Table 5. Changes in the position of IR bands observed for melting of DNA, B*A and B*Z transitions. Plus (or minus) sign indicates that the band has gained (or lost) appreciable intensity as a result of DNA melting

The symmetric PO_2^- band near 1092 cm^{-1} is correlated with changes in the electrostatic environment of the phosphate group. The bands in the range 1100-800 cm^{-1} characterize the backbone geometry and secondary structure. The region 800-600 cm^{-1} includes bands which are sensitive to nucleoside conformation. The transition near 750 cm^{-1} is assigned to C2'-endo/anti conformers of thymidine (Duguid et al., 1993; Erfurth & Peticolas, 1975; Prescott et al., 1984; Taillandier et al, 1989).

Raman spectra of nucleic acids in aqueous solution are not perturbed by water absorption, thus Raman spectroscopy can be used successfully to study both solids and aqueous solutions of DNA.

2.4 The primary and secondary action of Near Infrared Radiation on biological materials. Spectrophotometric study

2.4.1 Introduction

Phototherapy is one of the oldest therapeutic methods; initially known as solar therapy, later light therapy and low power laser therapy. Light therapy has been used for more than forty years to promote healing, reduce pain and inflammation and prevent tissue death. Light irradiation as a local phototherapeutic modality is characterized by its ability to induce non-thermic, nondestructive photobiological processes in cells and tissues. A variety of studies both *in vivo* and *in vitro* have shown that light irradiation has a significant influence on cell functional state. The response of light action is biphasic following irradiation both *in vitro* and *in vivo*. The so-called Arndt-Schultz curve of energy dose versus the response reveals that low doses of energy stimulate cell and tissue processes, while high energy doses reverse the stimulation and lead to inhibition.

Results of experiments *in vitro* and *in vivo* on isolated cells as well as on animals and humans are ambiguous. Despite many investigations on the subject, the therapy remains controversial largely due to uncertainties about the fundamental molecular and cellular mechanisms responsible for transducing signals from the photons incident on the cells to the biological effects that take place in the tissues illuminated. Different explanations based on light absorption by primary endogenous chromophores (mitochondrial enzymes, cytochromes, flavins and porphyrins) have been proposed to describe the biological effects of light. However, a precise theory concerning the therapeutic effects of light biostimulation has not been developed.

NIR radiation is widespread in medicine, both in therapy and diagnostics. It is recognized that NIR light is used to accelerate wound healing processes, reduce inflammations, support central nervous system regeneration, promote vascular and lymphatic microcirculation, stimulate the immune system and reduce and control pain (Eells et al., 2004; Posten et al., 2005; Sieron et al., 1994). Between 600 and 1200 nm is the so-called "therapeutic window" used in phototherapy. Radiation from this region is absorbed mainly by several tissue components, including water, glucose, hemoglobin, lipids, amino acids, proteins and nucleic acids (Olsztynska-Janus et al., 2008).

The effect of NIR radiation on biological systems was investigated using the example of erythrocytes and liposomes (Chludzińska et al , 2005; Komorowska et al., 2002a; Komorowska et al., 2002b; Komorowska & Czyżewska, 1997). Radiation in this range reduces the ability of cells and liposomes to aggregate. Exposure to NIR decreases the rate of hemolysis with increasing resistance of the membranes, which in turn is associated with increased flexibility and mechanical strength of erythrocyte membranes. NIR radiation protects them from oxidative stress, and thus affects the stabilization of the aging process of erythrocytes.

We attempted to resolve the molecular mechanism of the photochemical and therapeutic action of light in the NIR region *in vivo* and *in vitro* on the basis of results from spectrophotometric study of such molecules as amino acids, proteins and DNA.

2.4.2 NIR action on the amino acid phenylalanine

In order to explain the process undergone following exposure to NIR, a simple object was studied, in this case phenylalanine amino acid (Olsztynska-Janus et al., 2009; Olsztynska-Janus et al., 2008). The FTIR-ATR spectra of L-phenylalanine aqueous solutions were measured between 4000 and 700 cm^{-1}. Quantum chemical calculations, performed in parallel, made it possible to propose the primary and secondary process induced by the NIR irradiation. According to the results obtained, the interaction between two identical amino acids involves hydrogen bonding -C=O···HOOC-, which leads to cyclic dimers analogous to those formed by carboxylic acids (Olsztynska et al., 2003). The dimer formation is preceded by conformational changes of the amino acid. The greatest possible is the *trans/cis* transition. As a consequence of dimer formation, the p*K*a values of the amino acid can be shifted (Figure 3, Table 6) (Olsztynska et al., 2006b).

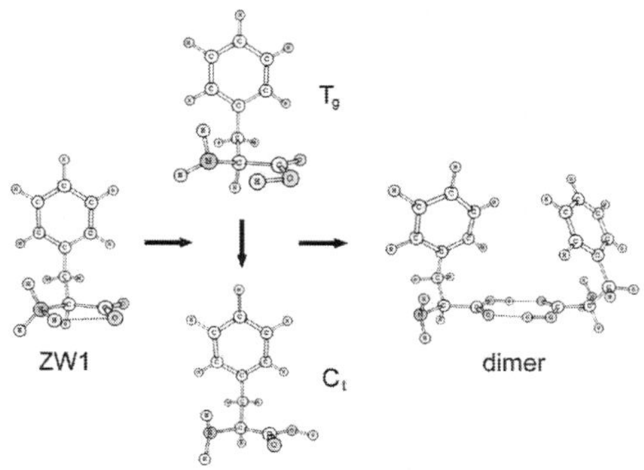

Fig. 3. NIR effect on conformational changes of phenylalanine zwitterion (ZW) due to *trans/cis* isomerization (T_g/C_t), dimer formation and shifts of p*K*a values (see Table 6).

	Dark Phe	NIR Phe	ΔpK_a
pK_1	2.31	2.79	+0.48
pK_2	9.28	8.66	–0.62

Table 6. p*K*a values of phenylalanine before (dark) and after NIR irradiation. Δ p*K*a is the difference between p*K*a ($pKa_{Phe(NIR)}$ - $pKa_{Phe(Dark)}$).

2.4.3 NIR action on DNA

2.4.3.1 Mathematical techniques used to study changes in spectroscopic data

2.4.3.1a Principal components analysis (PCA)

According to Brereton, "PCA is probably the most widespread multivariate chemometric technique … that most significantly changed the chemist's view of data analysis." (Brereton,

2003). In the literature there are many examples of application of PCA as an efficient tool supporting medical diagnosis, where the DNA bands have important contributions (Ly et al., 2009; Owen et al., 2006; Petrich, 2001; Wood et al., 2000).

PCA is an abstract transformation of the original data X matrix with m rows and n columns, and with each wavenumber (variable) being a column and each spectrum (sample) a row, into a sum of k $t_1$and p_1 vectors.

$$X = t_1 p_1^T + t_2 p_2^T + \ldots + t_k p_k^T + E \tag{1}$$

The t_1 vectors are known as scores and contain information on how the samples relate to each other. The p_1 vectors are known as loadings and contain information on how the variables relate to each other. The t_1, p_1 pair captures the greatest amount of variation in the data, where as each subsequent pair captures the greatest possible amount of variance remaining after subtracting $t_1 p_1^T$ from X. The number of principal components (PCs) that can adequately describe variations in the raw data X is equal k. In general, the raw data can be adequately described using far fewer factors than original variables. The reduction of the large amount of original data to a much smaller, more manageable dataset is a major advantage of PCA. This method provides great potential for the visualization of relations between samples and variables against PCs. Score plots allow many different questions on the relationships between objects to be answered. Loading plots provide detailed information about which wavenumbers are most associated with which object. PCA also provides an answer to the question of grouping samples into clusters. Measurements of distances between samples allow the number of clusters and similarity of objects inside the clusters to be determined.

2.4.3.1b *Two-dimensional correlation spectroscopy*

To the question "Vibrational spectroscopy: a 'vanishing' discipline? Meier answers that "... compared to the past, a shift in applications has taken place, bringing new opportunities. This is partly due to the introduction of new features, including ... 2D correlation spectroscopy (Meier, 2005). Specific applications of vibrational spectroscopy in biomedical engineering can be also enhanced substantially by application of the 2D correlation technique, which will be shown in the next section. A detailed introduction to the subject of 2D correlation spectroscopy is beyond scope of this work and therefore is kept to a minimum. Readers interested in this technique are referred to the monograph published in 2004 (Noda & Ozaki, 2004) which remains as the most authoritative reference source in this field. Recently, to mark the Fifth International Symposium on Two-Dimensional Correlation Spectroscopy (2DCOS-5) held in Wrocław, Poland in August 2009, a comprehensive review on research aided by 2D correlation spectroscopy was compiled by Noda (Noda, 2010). It covers the period between 2007 and 2009, with many different examples discussed, also analysis of which was substantially improved thanks to application of the 2DCOS method.

Generally speaking, the 2DCOS is recognized as a very efficient procedure for enhancement of the spectral resolution of a broad absorption envelope that hides bands assigned to vibrations having a different response to a perturbation applied. The 2DCOS calculations begin with arrangement of the measured data into the X matrix. In the majority of cases the 2D calculations are preceded by subtraction of the reference spectrum of the system from the raw-pretreated data. The result of the subtraction is called the dynamic spectrum ($\tilde{Y}$) because it presents the response of the system perturbed to the perturbation applied. If an averaged spectrum is chosen as the subtrahend, the dynamic spectra are identical to the mean-centered spectra and synchronous 2D correlation intensities ($\Phi(v_1,v_2)$) have the same sense as covariance matrix ($\mathrm{cov}(\tilde{Y})$).

$$\Phi(v_1,v_2)=\frac{1}{m-1}\tilde{Y}(v_1)^T\times\tilde{Y}(v_2)=\mathrm{cov}(\sim\tilde{Y}) \tag{2}$$

The discrete form of an asynchronous 2D spectrum $\Psi(v_1,v_2)$ is obtained by multiplying the data matrix $\tilde{Y}$ by the orthogonal counterpart of $\tilde{Y}$, obtained using the Hilbert transformation (N).

$$\Psi(v_1,v_2)=\frac{1}{m-1}\tilde{Y}(v_1)^T\times N\times\tilde{Y}(v_2) \tag{3}$$

Much useful information is available from synchronous and asynchronous spectra analyzed according to the guidelines popularly known as Noda's rules (Noda & Ozaki, 2004). Some of the most important information provided is the sequential order of events observed using the spectroscopic technique along the external perturbation. It finds excellent application in many studies, allowing, for example, the evolution of the unfolding mechanism of polypeptides (Ashton et al., 2006) and proteins to be investigated (Czarnik-Matusewicz et al., 2009). Whenever the correlated wavenumbers come from different spectral ranges the method is known as a heterospectral 2D correlation. Such modification of 2D correlation spectroscopy enhances the content and quality of spectral information in relation to that obtained with 2D homospectral correlation (Jung et al., 2000).

2.4.3.1c Combined PCA-2DCOS analysis of the DNA films

Our previous research performed for aqueous solutions of herring sperm DNA irradiated by NIR light for periods of 5, 10 and 20 minutes revealed distinct differences for melting profiles obtained from UV and FTIR-ATR measurements (Szymborska-Małek et al., 2009a, b). Most probably, properties of the water comprising a shell around DNA are modified during the irradiation in a manner dependent on the dose of NIR light exposure. According to results already obtained, the NIR-reshaped hydration shell leads to liposomes being more able to agglomerate (Komorowska et al., 2006) and to aggregation of L-phenylalanine (Olsztynska-Janus et al., 2009). The aim of the present research is an analysis of the phenomenon for DNA with limited water content. The measurements were therefore performed for thin film samples obtained from solutions of DNA following water evaporation to a constant level. The effect of the NIR radiation is hard to discuss in detail without application of some pattern recognition method due to minute absorbance changes caused by temperature increase, as shown in Figure 4. The profiles were so common across the four sets of data that it was not possible to distinguish differences between them by way of ordinary analysis.

The spectra presented above are results of pretreatments performed in the following order:

- denoising by means of the coif-5 mother wavelet with a five-level decomposition and soft thresholding criterion;
- the second order baseline correction at the same three anchor points;
- the offset at 1810 cm^{-1};
- normalization over the integral area calculated in the range analyzed, i.e. 1810-867 cm^{-1}.

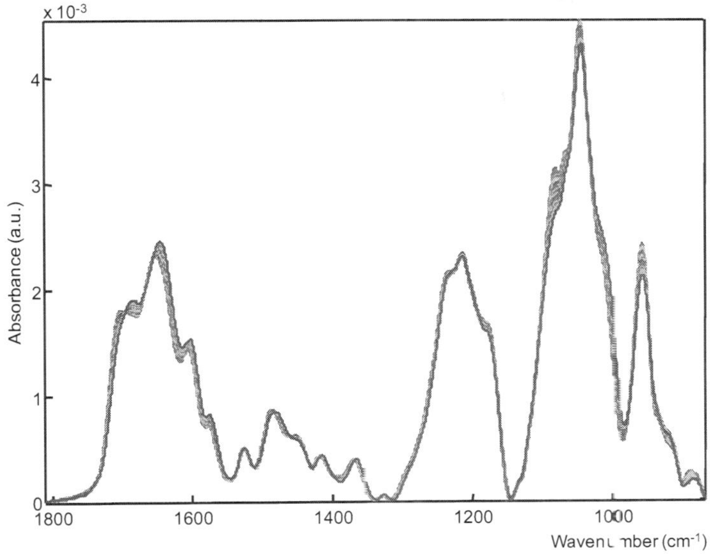

Fig. 4. FTIR-ATR temperature-dependent spectra recorded for DNA film obtained from solution unexposed to NIR radiation. Measurement was performed within the temperature range 25-90°C (for colour see www.intechweb.org).

It is very important to apply the same procedures of pretreatment to all spectra subjected to PCA and 2DCOS calculations, which was strictly respected in the research presented.

Applying PCA, the pattern between samples arising independently from temperature and NIR radiation can be successfully investigated The bands sensitive to effects of base pairing and base stacking which are strongly overlapped and difficult to assign due to the wide-type of measured DNA can be resolved substantially by 2DCOS analysis.

Here the main concepts of PCA and 2DCOS will be illustrated by the analysis of the four sets of the FTIR-ATR temperature-dependent spectra collected for the films of DNA samples obtained from DNA-buffer solutions irradiated for 5, 10 and 20 minutes by NIR light. The non-irradiated solution, treated as the control, was also subjected to the same temperature studies. For clarity the notations 5^{NIR}, 10^{NIR}, 20^{NIR} and 0^{NIR} will be used, respectively, for the samples. The spectral range selected for the PCA analysis is composed of many strongly overlapped bands attributed to different moieties of the DNA film which undergo very small variations with temperature increase. The primary purpose of the research has been to provide information on the influence of NIR radiation on DNA structure. In particular, the research was conducted for film samples where there is no absorption from water which very strongly overlaps with that originating from vibrations of different nucleobases. The bands are extremely sensitive to base stacking and base pairing interactions and are changed substantially during the thermal denaturation process. One of the main advantages of using PCA is its ability to convert the multivariate data to a simple graphical presentation. Among the many ways of visualizing PCs one of the simplest is that of the score of one PC against the other.

Figure 5 illustrates the PC plot for the first two PCs, which together capture 86% of the spectral variance for the matrix comprising all of the four sets of data. The first PC captures the largest amount of variations in the data set, i.e. 73%, which are independent of the 13% of variations captured by the second PC. For the system studied, the two principal components adequately describe all of the variation in the spectra measured induced by both temperature changes and NIR radiation. Each circle in the loading plot represents the location of a spectrum projected into the plane defined by the pairs of first two principal component axes. The circles are differently colored to assist in distinguishing the samples exposed to NIR radiation at different periods of time. The loading plot very clearly show that the first PC captures the major absorbance changes induced by temperature increase, whereas the second PC captures the minor absorbance changes caused by NIR radiation. They are almost 6 times smaller than those induced by temperature.

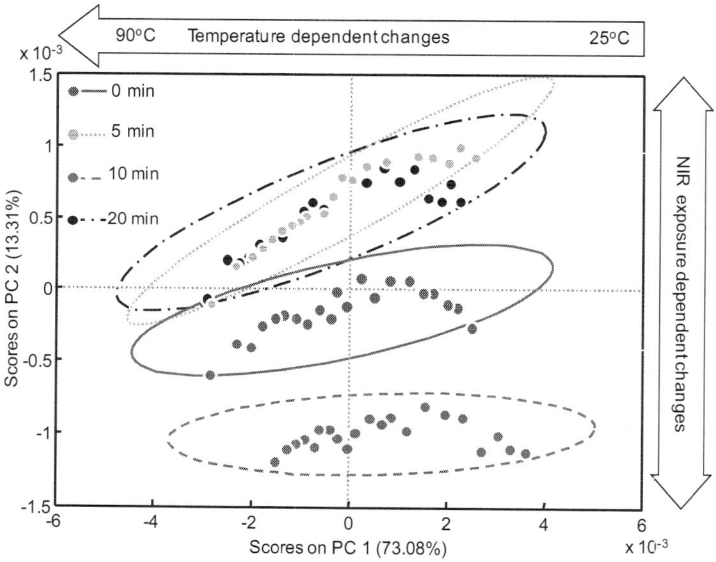

Fig. 5. Score plot of the spectra for the four systems combined into one matrix for the first two PCs (for colour see www.intechweb.org).

Analyzing the distribution of the samples against the first PC makes it easily noticeable that the 5^{NIR}, 20^{NIR} and 0^{NIR} for temperatures between 25°C and 62°C are characterized by positive scores, while negative scores relate to measurements performed at temperatures above 62°C. For the 10^{NIR} sample the border between positive and negative scores is shifted from 62 to 68°C. Distribution of scores against PC1 reveals that all samples undergo a very similar process of structural change due to temperature increase, excepting the fact that the extent of the change induced for the 10^{NIR} sample is smaller than for the others.

The second PC that captures the remaining changes, not described by PC1, correlates with the period of NIR radiation. According to the analysis of the distribution of samples against the PC2, i.e. along the vertical axis, the whole data set should be divided into three clusters. The 10^{NIR} sample has more negative scores on PC2, the 0^{NIR} sample is almost uncorrelated with the period of NIR radiation, whereas the 5^{NIR} and 20^{NIR} are characterized by positive scores. Moreover, the slopes of the clusters reveal that the influence of NIR radiation on the absorbance changes decreases with temperature elevation, except in the case of the 10^{NIR} sample.

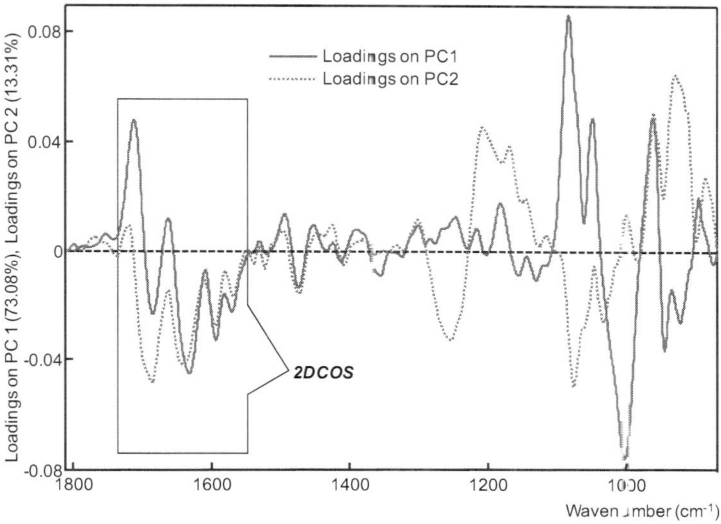

Fig. 6. Loading plot of the spectra for the four systems combined into one matrix for PC1 (solid line) and PC2 (dotted line). The grey box contains a marked range selected for 2DCOS calculations (for colour see www.intechweb.org).

The next step of PCA always involves examination of the loading plot to see which variables fulfil the conditions described by subsequent scores. Analysis of the loading plot shown in Figure 6 analyzed in the context of PC1 enable discrimination between absorbance changes at the two stages of heating resolved by scores values. This allows it to be determined that at the initial steps of heating, beginning at 25°C, the more active bands are those at 1081, 1711, 1047 and 959 cm^{-1}. According to the literature data (Banyay et al., 2003; Parker, 1983;), the first is attributed to the $\nu_s(PO_2^-)$ vibration and is sensitive to the changes in hydration pattern around the phosphate groups, whereas that at 1711 cm^{-1} relates to changes in base pairing as it arises from in-plane stretching modes of the C=O groups of paired bases. The band at 1047 cm^{-1} also reflects changes in hydration of backbone as it is mainly attributed to C-O skeletal vibrations of ribose. The last band at 959 cm^{-1} is assigned to ribose-phosphate skeletal motions. All of the changes indicate that a temperature increase from 25°C to 60°C causes changes in backbone configuration and in base pairing interaction for the low hydrated films. For higher temperatures it is mainly changes at 1000, 1632, 942, and 919 cm^{-1} which are manifested on the loadings distribution against PC1. All of the bands, except that at 1632 cm^{-1}, are characteristic of ribose-phosphate main chain vibration. The other arises from combined C=N and C=C vibration of base residues. The separation of the bands into the two groups according to sign of loadings reveals the separate character of conformational changes in the DNA dehydrated film at lower and higher temperatures. The phosphate groups generally very sensitive to changes in hydration properties also in dehydrated conditions undergo perturbation accompanied by base-pairing interaction changes. This process evolves below 60°C, whereas above the temperature another begins, embracing the phosphodiester moieties and the aromatic rings of bases. An important fact is that the band assigned to the $\nu_{as}(PO_2^-)$ vibration is almost totally insensitive to temperature changes.

The loading plot reflects very clearly the differences in response of the symmetric and antisymmetric stretching vibrations for the PO_2^- group with the temperature increase and the NIR radiation effect. The $\nu_{as}(PO_2^-)$ band is sensitive to both varying hydration and orientation of the phosphate group, whereas the $\nu_s(PO_2^-)$ is sensitive to orientation only (Parker, 1983) and changes in the dielectric environment around the phosphate group which are responsible more for its intensity variations than its shift (Pevsner & Diem, 2003). As a consequence of their different sensitivity to hydration, the $\nu_{as}(PO_2^-)$ is a characteristic marker for backbone conformational changes between B- and A-form, as the B-A transition is strictly correlated with deficiency of water in the hydration sphere of the phosphate groups. For the $\nu_s(PO_2^-)$ its insensitivity to hydration involves a lack of influence on its position by the B-A transition, but its intensity could be influenced by subtle changes in the local polarity.

Examination of the loading plot against the second PC2 allows bands for which absorbance is correlated with dose of NIR radiation to be selected. For the 10^{NIR} sample most characteristic are the two stretching bands arising from vibration of the PO_2^- group and bands assigned to the in-plane base vibrations. Moreover, from combined observation of loadings for PC2 against PC1 it can be stated that in the case of the $\nu_s(PO_2^-)$ vibrations at 1074 cm^{-1} the NIR effect is better distinguished at lower temperatures, whereas for the $\nu_{as}(PO_2^-)$ vibration at 1253 cm^{-1} this effect is manifested at higher temperatures. This means that in the case of the 10^{NIR} sample that due to the NIR radiation both on the hydrational, orientational properties of the phosphate groups as well as the local dielectric constant in vicinity of PO_2^- are modified. The absorbance changes at 1686, 1641, 1593 and 1569 cm^{-1} which arise from the in-plane base vibrations dominate at temperatures above 70°C. This means that for the thin film samples the NIR-dependent alternations in base pairing and base stacking interactions, more strongly manifested at higher temperatures, are preceded by variations in the NIR-modified hydration layer which is sensitive to temperature changes at lower range. For the 5^{NIR} and 20^{NIR} samples the phosphate symmetric and in-plane base vibrations are not affected by NIR. However, the band at 1207 cm^{-1}, attributed to the $\nu_{as}(PO_2^-)$ vibration, is 46 cm^{-1} red shifted relative to the band at 1253 cm^{-1} for the 10^{NIR} sample, which indicates better hydration of the phosphate groups for 5^{NIR} and 20^{NIR}. The band at 1168 cm^{-1}, as a marker of A-form, reveals a different degree of B-A transition for the two groups of samples. Also the bands at 958 and 927 cm^{-1} sensitive to the changes in the B-A transition are well resolved in the loadings plotted against PC2. Based on the PCA results presented, we are able to suggest that due to NIR radiation mainly hydration pattern around the phosphate groups is modified and the extent of the changes can be modulated by the period of the NIR radiation.

The advantages arising from using 2DCOS in analysis of spectra composed from many overlapped bands will be presented for a selected range of 1850-1550 cm^{-1} contributed by several in-plane base vibrations. The changes in base-stacking and helical stability are evidenced by the complex intensity changes of their bands. Also the synchronous spectra in Figure 7 obtained for the four data sets confirm that the changes developed in the 1850-1550 cm^{-1} range for the 10^{NIR} sample (see Fig. 7C) have a pattern different from those for the other three systems.

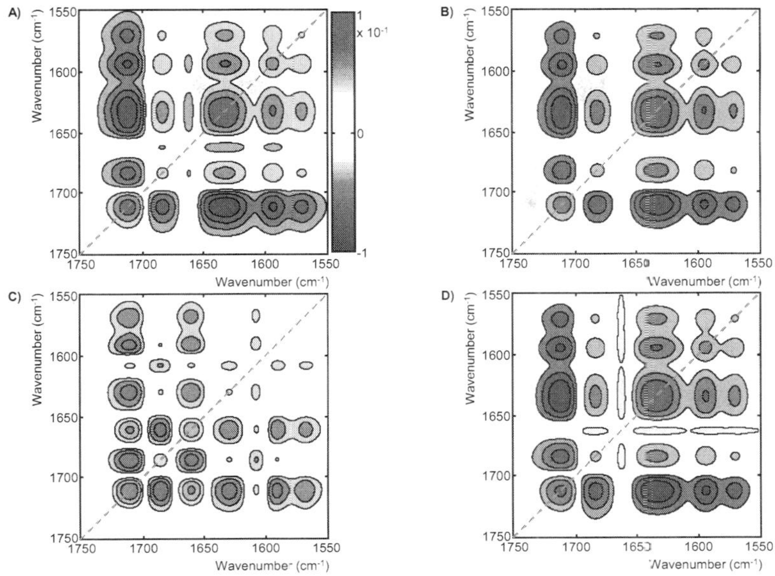

Fig. 7. Synchronous 2D FTIR-ATR correlation spectra obtained from the temperature-perturbed measurements for the 0^{NIR} (A), 5^{NIR} (B), 10^{NIR} (C) and 20^{NIR} (D) systems (for colour see www.intechweb.org).

For the synchronous map an important feature is the sign of the ($\Phi(v_1,v_2)$) peaks which represents the simultaneous or coincidental changes of two separate spectral intensity variations measured at v_1 and v_2 during the temperature changes from 25 to 90°C. Positive cross peaks, i.e. peaks outside the diagonal, indicate that their correlated intensities are either increasing or decreasing with the function of the temperature increase, whereas negative peaks indicate that the correlated changes are in opposite directions. The positions and signs of the ($\Phi(v_1,v_2)$) peaks from Figures 7A, B and D allow identification of only one peak at 1712 cm⁻¹, the intensity of which decreased with temperature, and four peaks at 1684, 1634, 1594 and 1570 cm⁻¹, the intensity of which increased with temperature elevation. In the literature, there is a large diversity in assignments of the bands for the ν(C=O) vibrations. According to the most comprehensive review of this topic available to date (Banyay et al., 2003), in the range of the ν(C=O) vibrations, a double strand (*ds*) to single strand (*ss*) transition results in a decrease in intensity of the bands at higher frequencies with a concomitant increase in intensity of the bands at lower frequencies. In addition, bands arising from the in-plane stretching modes of the C=C and C=N groups of bases and the NH_2 scissoring vibrations, located below 1650 cm⁻¹, gain in intensity at the *ds* to *ss* transition. In accordance with these facts are the changes developed for the 0^{NIR} (Fig. 7A), 5^{NIR} (Fig. 7B) and 20^{NIR} (Fig. 7D) systems, whereas for the 10^{NIR} system (Fig. 7C) the 2D synchronous map has an additional two peaks of different sign. The peak at 1660 cm⁻¹ arising from the ν(C=O) vibration loses intensity with temperature increase, while the peak at 1607 cm⁻¹ is amplified.

Figure 8 presents the power spectra extracted from the synchronous maps. The peaks are located at diagonal positions and their intensity is a measure of the overall extent of spectral intensity variations due to temperature elevation from 25 to 90°C. As Figure 8 shows, for the 10^{NIR} system the in-plane ring vibrations from the C=C and C=N are less perturbed than the C=O vibrations during the heating process. This could mean that for the system irradiated for 10 minutes during heating the changes in base pairing predominate over the changes in base stacking. For the other system the two kinds of interaction change to a similar extent with temperature increase.

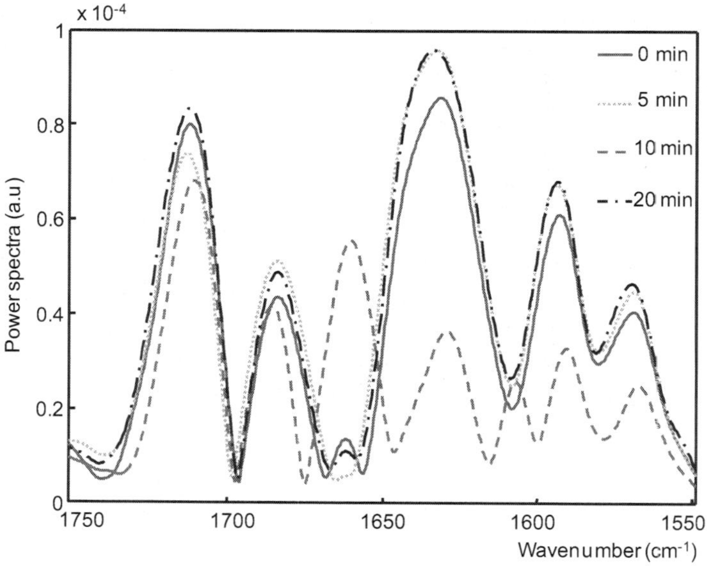

Fig. 8. The power spectra extracted from the synchronous maps (for colour see www.intechweb.org).

The pattern of peaks at the asynchronous spectra in Figure 9 confirms the different behavior of the 10^{NIR} system during the temperature destruction of the *ds* structure. The asynchronous peaks develop at frequencies at which the intensities are changing in an uncorrelated manner. Their sign provides useful information on the sequential order of the processes developed in the course of the temperature changes from 25 to 90°C which are detected by FTIR-ATR spectroscopy. For the 0^{NIR} system most asynchronous are the peaks that combine different ν(C=O) vibrations and the ν(C=O) vibrations with the in-ring. This same is true for the 5^{NIR} and 20^{NIR} systems. For the 10^{NIR} system the bands attributed to the ν(C=O) vibrations are asynchronously correlated only with the in-plane ring. This confirms that the base pairing and base stacking interactions are differently modified by NIR radiation. For all of the systems the changes in the base pairing interaction are ahead of the changes in base stacking. These findings are in good agreement with the available scenarios for the melting of *ds*DNA where pairing and stacking are treated as separate, non-cooperative processes (Gonzales et al., 2009).

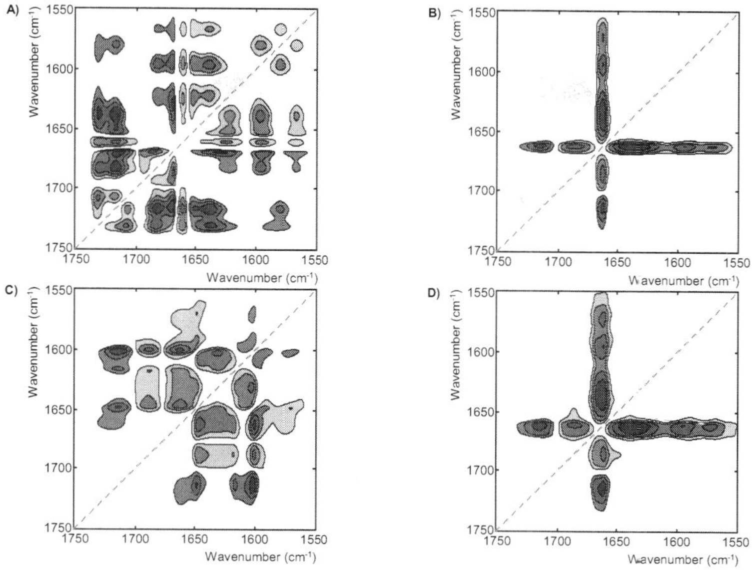

Fig. 9. Asynchronous 2D FTIR-ATR correlation spectra obtained from the temperature-perturbed measurements for the 0^{NIR} (A), 5^{NIR} (B), 10^{NIR} (C) and 20^{NIR} (D) systems (for colour see www.intechweb.org).

2.4.4 Stress/strain measurements in soft matters by Raman spectroscopy

Raman spectroscopy is a very powerful tool for the study of stress-induced molecular changes in natural and synthetic polymers (Amer, 2009; Koening, 2001). The application of stress leads to changes in interatomic distances and consequently shifts the positions of the bands. Such effects have been observed in silk, wool and collagen fibre analysis (Church et al., 1998; Colomban et al., 2008; Sirichaisit et al., 2000; Wang et al., 2000).

For unstrained wool fibres, the maximum of amide I band was found at 1652 cm^{-1} (typical for α helical proteins) and shifted to 1672 cm^{-1} (β-pleated sheet conformation) in the spectrum for stretched fibres. An intensity of peak observed at 1239 cm^{-1} (amide III, β-pleated sheet structure) increases during stretching, which confirms information obtained from amide I band analysis (Church et al., 1998). The α-β transition caused by stretching silk fibres was also reported (Colomban et al., 2008). The significant, almost linear, stress-induced shift was observed for ν(C-C) band at 1095 cm^{-1} in the silk Raman spectrum. Elongation of polypeptide backbone occurs when the fibre is stretched (Sirichaisit et al., 2000). Deformation of protein backbone was also noticed for rat tail collagen (Wang et al., 2000).

The Raman spectrum of soft tissues is dominated by the structural protein bands: $\delta(CH_2, CH_3)$ (~1450 cm^{-1}), $\nu(C_\alpha\text{-}C)$ (~940 cm^{-1}) and amide bands. Amide I and III bands for triple-helical collagen structure are observed near 1668 and 1248 cm^{-1}, respectively. Elastin exhibits bands in positions typical for unordered proteins, i.e. at 1662 cm^{-1} and 1250 cm^{-1}. Apart from protein, in skin and aorta spectra, weaker intensity lipid bands (1100-1150 cm^{-1}) are to be seen. The tendon has a hierarchical structure and is composed of collagen molecules, fibrils, fibre bundles, fascicles and tendon units that run parallel to the tendon's long axis. The diameter of the fibril depends on species, age and location. Tendon also contains small amounts of elastin (~2%) (Penteado et al., 2006; Silver et al., 2003; Wang et al., 2000).

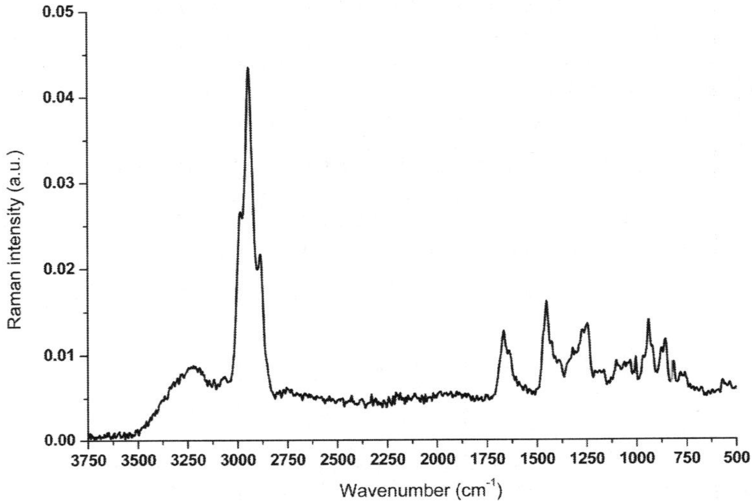

Fig. 10. Representative Raman spectrum of pig tail tendon.

Peak position (cm^{-1})	Assignments
3225	ν(NH), ν(OH)
2940	ν(CH_2)
1666	ν(C=O), amide I, collagen, elastin
1451	δ(CH_2, CH_3)
1266	ν(CN), δ(NH), amide III, non-polar triple helix of collagen
1248	ν(CN), δ(NH), amide III, polar triple helix of collagen, elastin
1004	ν(CC), phenylalanine
940	ν(C_α-C), α-helix
922	ν(CC), proline
875	ν(CC), hydroxyproline
856	ν(CC), proline
815	ν(CC), protein backbone

Table 6. Major bands identified in tendon spectra (Gąsior-Głogowska et al., 2010).

The major peaks in tendon spectra, shown in Figure 10, are attributed to the proteins: ν(CH_2) (~2942 cm^{-1}), δ(CH_2, CH_3) (~1450 cm^{-1}), ν(C_α-C) (~940 cm^{-1}) and amide bands, with maxima of 1666 cm^{-1} (amide I) and 1249 cm^{-1} (amide III). The amide I band in the unstrained tendon

spectrum is strongly asymmetric and its deconvolution allowed identification of few components within 1600-1700 cm^{-1}: collagen (1631 and 1666 cm^{-1}), hydrated water (1641 cm^{-1}), elastin (1653, 1675 and 1683 cm^{-1}) and aromatic amino acids (1606, 1617 and 1698 cm^{-1}). In the amide III region bands assigned to unordered (1248 cm^{-1}) and triple-helical (1266 cm^{-1}) collagen structure are observed. The weak shoulder of the amide III band at 1239 cm^{-1} is due to elastin. The bands near 875, 856 and 922 cm^{-1} can be assigned to ν(C-C) modes of amino acids characteristic for collagen, i.e. hydroxyproline and proline. The band near 1004 cm^{-1} is assigned to the phenyl ring breathing mode of phenylalanine. Table 6 lists the wavenumbers of the observed bands and their assignment (Dong et al., 2004; Gąsior-Głogowska et al., 2010; Penteado et al., 2006; Wang et al., 2000).
When a pig tail tendon sample is subjected to increased levels of macroscopic strain, noticeable changes in the position of amide III bands in several stages are noted as shown in Figure 11. The observed variations mean protein backbone alternation. A significant shift for C_{α}-C stretching vibrations at 940 cm^{-1} also took place.

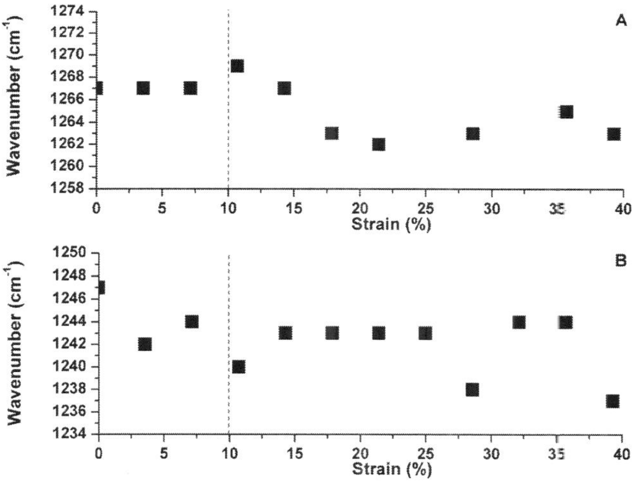

Fig. 11. Raman spectra of the tendon as a function of strain: A) proline-rich triple helix of collagen; B) proline-poor triple helix of collagen and elastin (Gąsior-Głogowska et al., 2010).

The amount and distribution of elastin and collagen fibres determine the mechanical properties of the soft tissues. Spectroscopic analysis shows differing tension thresholds for rich collagen material (ligaments, tendons) and tissues containing a high amount of elastin (blood vessel walls, skin). Moreover, the stress–strain plots and the Raman spectra recorded for the circumferentially and longitudinally oriented samples of aortic wall show significant differences (Hanuza et al., 2009).

3. Affiliation

This chapter is part of project "Wrovasc – Integrated Cardiovascular Centre", co-financed by the European Regional Development Fund, within Innovative Economy Operational Program, 2007-2013.

4. References

Adam, S.; Liquier, J.; Taboury, J.A. & Taillandier, E. (1986). Right- and left-handed helixes of poly[d(A-T)].cntdot.poly[d(A-T)] investigated by infrared spectroscopy. *Biochemistry*, Vol. 25, No. 11, 3220-3225.

Ahmed, A. & Tajmir-Riahi, H.A. (1993). Interaction of toxic metal ions Cd2+, Hg2+, and Pb2+ with light+harvesting proteins of chloroplast thzlakoid membranes. An FTIR spectroscopic study. *J. Inorg. Biochem.*, Vol. 50, No. 4, 235-243.

Amer, M.S. (2009). *Raman Spectroscopy for Soft Matter Applications*, John Wiley & Sons, Inc., ISBN 978-0-470-45383-4, Hoboken, New Jersey.

Amharref, N.; Beljebbar, A.; Dukic, S.; Venteo, L.; Schneider, L.; Pluot, M. & Manfait, M. (2007). Discriminating healthy from tumor and necrosis tissue in rat brain tissue samples by Raman spectral imaging. *Biochim. Biophys. Acta*, Vol. 1768, No. 10, 2605-2615.

Ashton, L.; Barron, L.D.; Czarnik-Matusewicz, B.; Hecht, L.; Hyde, J. & Blanch, E.W. (2006). Two-dimensional correlation analysis of Raman optical activity data on the α-helix-to-β-sheet transition in poly(L-lysine). *Mol. Phys.*, Vol. 104, No. 9, 1429- 445.

Banyay, M., Sarkar, M. & Gräslund, A. (2003). A library of IR bands of nucleic acids in solution. *Biophys. Chem.*, Vol. 104, No. 2, 477-488.

Barth, A. (2007). Infrared spectroscopy of proteins. *Biochim. Biophys. Acta*, Vol. 1767, No. 9, 1073-1101.

Bolton, B.A. & Scherer, J.R. (1989). Raman spectra and water absorption of bovine serum albumine. *J. Phys. Chem.*, Vol. 93, No. 22, 7635-7640.

Brereton, R.G. (2003). *Chemometrics: Data Analysis for the Laboratory and Chemical Plant*, Wiley, ISBN 0-471-48978-6, Chichester.

Byler, D.M. & Susi H. (1986). Examination of the secondary structure of proteins by deconvolved FTIR spectra. *Biopolymers*, Vol. 25, No. 3, 469-487.

Cai, S. & Singh B.R. (2004). A distinct utility of the amide III infrared band for secondary structure estimation of aqueous protein solutions using partial least squares methods. *Biochemistry*, Vol. 43, No. 9, 2541-2549.

Cai, S. & Singh B.R. (1999). Identification of beta-turn and random coil amide III infrared bands for secondary structure estimation of proteins. *Biophys. Chem.*, Vol. 80, No. 1, 7-20.

Cambpell, M.K. & Farrell, S.O. (2009). Biochemistry, Brooks Cole; 6th edition, ISBN-13: 9780495390411, 1-36, 235-260, Belmont

Cao, X. & Fischer, G. (1999). New infrared spectra and the tautomeric studies of purine and αl-alanine with an innovative sampling technique. *Spectrochim. Acta A*, Vol. 55, No. 11, 2329-2342.

Chan, K.L.A.; Kazarian, S.G.; Mavraki, A. & Williams, D.R. (2005). Fourier transform infrared imaging of human hair with a high spatial resolution without the use of a synchrotron. *Appl. Spectrosc.*, Vol. 59, No. 2, 149-155.

Chludzińska, L.; Jarosławska, E. & Komorowska, M. (2005). Near-infrared radiation protects the red cell membrane against oxidation. *Blood Cells, Mol. Dis.*, Vol. 35, No. 1, 74-79.

Church, J.S., Corino, G.L.; Woodhead, A.L. (1998). The effect of stretching on wool fibres as monitored by FT-Raman spectroscopy. *J. Mol. Struct.*, Vol. 440 No. 1-3, 15-23.

Cieślik-Boczula, K.; Czarnik-Matusewicz, B.; Perevozkina, M.; Filarowski, A.; Boens, N.; De Borgraeve, W.M. & Koll, A. (2007). ATR-IR spectroscopic study of the structural changes in the hydraophobic region of an ICPAN/DPPC bilayers. *J. Mol. Struct.*, Vol. 878, No. 1-3, 162-168.

Colomban, P.; Dinh, H.M.; Riand, J.; Prinsloo, L.C. & Mauchamp, B. (2008). Nanomechanics of single silkworm and spider fibres: a Raman and micro-mechanical *in situ* study of the conformation change with stress. *J. Raman Spectrosc.*, Vol. 39, No. 12, 1749-1764.

Czarnik-Matusewicz, B., Kim, S.B. & Jung, Y.M. (2009). A Study of Urea-dependent Denaturation of β-Lactoglobulin by Principal Component Analysis and Two-dimensional Correlation Spectroscopy. *J. Phys. Chem. B.*, Vol. 113, No. 2, 559–566.

Damm, U.; Kondepati, V.R. & Heise, H.M. (2007). Continuous reagent-free bed-side monitoring of glucose in biofluids using infrared spectrometry and micro-dialysis. *Vib. Spectrosc.*, Vol. 43, No. 1, 184–192.

Dong, A., Huang P. & Caughey W.S. (1990). Protein Secondary Structures in Water from Second-Derivative Amide I Infrared Spectra. *Biochemistry*, Vol. 29, No. 13, 3303-3308.

Dong, R.; Yan, X.; Pang, X. & Liu, S. (2004). Temperature-depended Raman spectra of collagen and DNA, *Spectrochim. Acta Part A*, Vol. 60, No. 3, 557-561.

Dousseau, F. & Pézolet M. (1990). Determination of the Secondary Structure Content of Proteins in Aqueous Solutions from Their Amide I and Amide I1 Infrared Bands. Comparison between Classical and Partial Least-Squares Methods. *Biochemistry*, Vol. 29, No. 37, 8771-8779.

Duguid, J.G.; Bloomfield V.A.; Benevides, J.M. & Thomas Jr, G.J. (1993). Raman spectroscopy of DNA-metal complexes. I. Interactions and conformational effects of the divalent cations: Mg, Ca, Sr, Ba, Mn, Co, Ni, Cu, Pd, and Cd. *Biophys. J.*, Vol. 65, No. 5, 1916-1928.

Duguid, J.G.; Bloomfield V.A.; Benevides, J.M. & Thomas Jr, G.J. (1996). DNA melting investigated by differential scanning calorimetry and Raman spectroscopy. *Biophys. J.*, Vol. 71, 3350-3360.

Eells, J.T; Wong-Riley, M.T.T.; VerHoeve, J.; Henry, M.; Buchman, E.V.; Kane, M.P.; Goulds, L.J.; Das, R.; Jett, M.; Hodgson, B.D.; Margolis, D. & Whelan, H.T. (2004). Mitochondrial signal transduction in accelerated wound and retinal healing by near-infrared light therapy. *Mitochondrion*, Vol. 4, No. 5-6, 559–567.

Erfurth, S.C. & Peticolas, W.L. (1975). Melting and premelting phenomenon in DNA by laser Raman scattering. *Biopolymers*, Vol. 14, No. 2, 247-264.

Fabian, H. & Mäntele, W. (2002). Infrared Spectroscopy of Proteins, in: *Handbook of Vibrational Spectroscopy*, Chalmers, J.M. & Griffiths, P.R. (Eds.). Vol. 5, 3399-3425, John Wiley & Sons, ISBN 978-0471988472, Chichester.

Falk, M.; Hartman, K. & Lord K. (1963). Hydration of Deoxyribonucleic Acid. II. An Infrared Study. *J. Am. Chem. Soc.*, Vol. 85, No. 4, 387–391.

Fu, F.-N.; DeOliveira, D.B.; Trumble, W.R.; Sarkar, H.K. & Singh, B.R. (1994). Secondary structure estimation of proteins using the amide III region of Fourier Transform

Infrared Spectroscopy: Application to analyze calcium-binding-induced structural changes in calsequestrin. *Appl. Spectrosc.*, Vol. 48, No. 11, 1432-1441.

Fuchs, R.K.; Allen, M.R.; Ruppel, M.E.; Diab, T. ; Phipps, R.J; Miller, L.M. & Burr, D.B. (2008). In situ examination of the time-course for secondary mineralization of Haversian bone using synchrotron Fourier transform infrared microspectroscopy. *Matrix Biol.*, Vol. 27, No. 1, 34-41.

Gąsior-Głogowska, M.; Komorowska, M.; Hanuza, J.; Mączka, M.; Będziński, R.; Kobielarz, M. (2010). Structural alteration of collagen fibers - spectroscopic and mechanic studies. *Acta Bioeng. Biomech.* In preparation.

Gelamo, E.L.; Itri, R.; Alonso, A.; da Silva, J.V. & Tabak, M. (2004). Small-angle X-ray scattering and electron paramagnetic resonance study of the interaction of bovine serum albumin with ionic surfactants. *J. Coll. Interface Sci.*, Vol. 277, No. 2, 471-482.

Gelamo, E.L.; Silva, C.H.T.P.; Imasoto, H. & Tabak, M. (2002). Interaction of bovine (BSA) and human (HSA) serum albumins with ionic surfactants: spectroscopy and modelling. *Biochim. Biophys. Acta*, Vol. 1594, No. 1, 84-99.

Gonzalez, R., Zeng, Y., Ivanov, V. & Zocchi, G. (2009). Bubbles in DNA melting. *J. Phys.: Condens. Matter*, Vol. 21, No. 3, 034102 (9pp).

Goormaghtigh, E.; Cabiaux, V. & Ruysschaert, J.-M. (1990). Secondary structure and dosage of soluble and membrane proteins by attenuated total reflection Fourier-transform infrared spectroscopy on hydrated films. *Eur. J. Biochem.*, Vol. 193, No. 2, 409-420.

Grdadolnik, J. & Maréchal, Y. (2001a). Bovine serum albumin observed by infrared spectrometry. I. Methodology, structural investigation, and water uptake. *Biopolymers (Biospectroscopy)*, Vol. 62, No. 1, 40-53.

Grdadolnik, J. & Maréchal, Y. (2001b). Bovine serum albumin observed by infrared spectrometry. II. Hydration mechanisms and interaction configurations of embedded H(2)O molecules. *Biopolymers (Biospectroscopy)*, Vol. 62, No. 1, 54-67.

Griebe, M.; Daffertshofer, M.; Stroick, M., Syren M., Ahmad-Nejad P., Neumaier M., Backhaus J., Hennerici M.G. & Fatar, M. (2007). Infrared spectroscopy: A new diagnostic tool in Alzheimer disease. *Neurosci. Lett.*, Vol. 420, No. 1, 29-33.

Hackl, E.V.; Kornilova, S.V. & Blagoi, Y.P. (2005). DNA structural transitions induced by divalent metal ions in aqueous solutions. *Int. J. Biol. Macromol.*, Vol. 35, No. 3-4, 175-191.

Hanuza J.; Mączka M.; Gąsior-Głogowska M.; Komorowska M.; Będziński R.; Szotek S.; Maksymowicz K. & Hermanowicz K. (2009). FT-Raman spectroscopic study of thoracic aortic wall subjected to uniaxial stress. *J. Raman Spectrosc., Vol.* 40. In Press.

Harrick, N.J. (1979). *Internal Reflection Spectroscopy*, Vol. 30, Harrick Scientific Corp., ISBN 0933946139, Ossining, New York.

Harris, P.I. & Chapman, D. (1992). Does Fourier-transform infrared spectroscopy provide useful information on protein structures? *Trends Biochem. Sci.*, Vol. 17, No. 9, 328-333.

Heise, H.M.; Küpper, L. & Butvina, L.N. (2002). Bio-analytical applications of mid-infrared spectroscopy using silver halide fiber-optic probes. *Spectrochim. Acta B*, Vol. 57, No. 10, 1649–1663.

Heise, H.M.; Marbach, R.; Janatsch, G. & Kruse-Jarres, J.D. (1989). Multivariate determination of glucose in whole blood by attenuated total reflection infrared spectroscopy. *Anal. Chem.*, Vol. 61, No. 18, 2009-2015.

Ishida, K.P. & Griffiths, P.R. (1993). Comparison of the Amide I/II intensity ratio of solution and solid-state proteins sampled by Transmission, Attenuated Total Reflectance, and Diffuse Reflectance Spectrometry. *Appl. Spectrosc*, Vol. 47, No. 5, 584-589.

Jackson, M. & Mantsch, H.H. (1995). The use and misuse of FTIR spectroscopy in the determination of protein structure. *Crit. Rev. Biochem. Mol. Biol.*, Vol. 30, No. 2, 95-120.

Jackson, M.; Harris, P.I. & Chapman, D. (1989). Fourier transform infrared spectroscopic studies of lipids, polypeptides and proteins. *J. Mol. Struct.*, Vol. 214, 329-355.

Jeyachandran, Y.L.; Mielczarski, E.; Rai, B. & Mielczarski, J.A. (2009). Quantitative and qualitative evaluation of adsorption/desorption of bovine serum albumin on hydrophilic and hydrophobic surfaces. *Langmuir*, Vol. 25, No. 19, 11614-11620.

Jung, Y.M., Czarnik-Matusewicz, B. & Ozaki, Y. (2000). Two-Dimensional Infrared, Two-Dimensional Raman, and Two-Dimensional Infrared and Raman Heterospectral Correlation Studies of Secondary Structure of β-Lactoglobulin in Buffer Solutions. *J. Phys. Chem. B*, Vol. 104, No. 32, 7812–7817.

Keller, P.B. & Hartman, K.A. (1986). Structural forms, stabilities and transitions in double-helical poly(dG-dC) as a function of hydration and NaCl content. An infrared spectroscopic study. *Nucleic Acids Res.*, Vol. 14, No. 20, 8167-8182.

Koening J.L. (2001). *Infrared and Raman Spectroscopy of Polymers.* Rapra Review Reports, Vol. 12, No. 2, Report 134, 2001, iSmithers Rapra Publishing, ISBN 978-1-85957-284-9.

Komorowska, M.; Cuissot, A.; Czarnołęski, A. & Białas, W. (2002a). Erythrocyte response to near-infrared radiation. *J. Photochem. Photobiol., B: Biology*, Vol. 68, No. 2-3, 93-100.

Komorowska, M. & Czyżewska, H. (1997). The effect of Near Infrared radiation on erythrocyte membranes; ESR study. *Nukleonika*, Vol. 42, No. 2, 379-386.

Komorowska, M.; Gałwa, M.; Herter, B. & Wesłowska, U. (2002b). Hydration effects under near-infrared radiation. *Colloids Surf., B.*, Vol. 26, No. 3, 223-233.

Langlais, M.; Tajmir-Riahi, H.A. & Savoie, R. (1990). Raman spectroscopic study of the effects of Ca2+, Mg2+, Zn2+, and Cd2+ ions on calf thymus DNA: binding sites and conformational changes. *Biopolymers*, Vol. 30, No. 7-8, 743-752.

Lee, S.; Debenedetti, P.; Errington, J.; Pethica, B. & Moore, D. (2004). A Calorimetric and Spectroscopic Study of DNA at Low Hydration. *J. Phys. Chem. B*, Vol. 108, No. 9, 3098–3106.

Li, Q.-B.; Sun, X.-J.; Xu, Y.Z.;Yang, L.-M.; Zhang, Y.-F.; Weng, S.-F.; Shi, J.-S. & Wu, J.-G. (2005). Diagnosis of gastric inflammation and malignancy in edoscopic biopsies based on Fourier Transform Infrared Spectroscopy. *Clin. Chem.*, Vol. 51, No. 2, 346-350.

Licoccia, S.; Trombetta, M; Capitani, D.; Proietti, N.; Romagnoli, P. & Di Vona, M.L. (2005). ATR-FTIR and NMR spectroscopic studies on the structure of polymeric gel electrolytes for biomedical applications. *Polymer*, Vol. 46, No. 13, 4670-4675.

Ly, E. Piot, O.; Wolthuis, R.; Durlach, A.; Bernard, P. & Manfait, M. (2008). Combination of FTIR spectral imaging and chemometrics for tumour detection from paraffin-embedded biopsies. *Analyst,* Vol. 133, No. 2, 197–205.

Maréchal, Y. (2004). Observing the water molecule in macromolecules using infrared spectrometry: structure of the hydrogen bond network and hydration mechanism. *J. Mol. Struct.*, Vol. 700, No. 1-3, 217-223.

Maréchal, Y. (2003). Observing the water molecule in macromolecules and aqueous media using infrared spectrometry. *J. Mol. Struct.*, Vol. 648, No. 1-2, 27-47.

Martin, J.C.; Wartell, R.M. & O'Shea, D.C. (1978). Conformational features of distamycin-DNA and netropsin-DNA complexes by Raman spectroscopy. *Proc. Natl. Acad. Sci. USA,* Vol. 75, No. 11, 5483-5487.

Martin, J.C. & Wartell, R.M. (1982). Changes in raman vibrational bands of calf thymus DNA during the B-to-A transition. *Biopolymers,* Vol. 21, No. 3, 499-512.

Matsui, H.; Toyota, N.; Nagatori, M.; Sakamoto, H. & Mizoguchi, K. (2009). Infrared spectroscopic studies on incorporating the effect of metallic ions into a M-DNA double helix. *Phys. Rev. B.,* Vol. 79, 235201-1-235201-8.

Max, J.-J.; Trudel, M. & Chapados, C. (1998). Infrared titration of aqueous glycine. *Appl. Spectrosc.,* Vol. 52, No. 2, 226-233.

McAuley, W.J.; Mader, K.T.; Tetteh, J; Lane, M.E. & Hadgraft, J. (2009). Simultaneous monitoring of drug and solvent diffusion across a model membrane using ATR-FTIR spectroscopy. *Europ. J. Pharmac. Sci.,* Vol. 38, No. 4, 378-383.

Medien, H.A.A. (1998). Spectrophotometric method for determination and kinetics of amino acids through their reaction with syringaldehyde. Spectrochimica Acta A, Vol. 54, No. 2, 359-365.

Meier, R.J. (2005). Vibrational spectroscopy: a 'vanishing' discipline? *Chem. Soc. Rev.,* Vol. 34, 743–752.

Murawska, A.; Cieślik-Boczula, K. & Czarnik-Matusewicz, B. (2010). Interactions in two-component liposomes studied by 2D correlation spectroscopy. *J. Mol. Struct.,* Vol. 974, No. 1-3, 183–191.

Murayama, K.; Wu, Y.; Czarnik-Matusewicz, B. & Ozaki, Y. (2001). Two-Dimensional/Attenuated Total Reflection Infrared Correlation Spectroscopy Studies on Secondary Structural Changes in Human Serum Albumin in Aqueous Solutions: pH-Dependent Structural Changes in the Secondary Structures and in the Hydrogen Bondings of Side Chains. *J. Phys. Chem. B,* Vol. 105, No. 20, 4763-4769.

Noda, I. & Ozaki, Y. (2004). *Two-dimensional Correlation Spectroscopy – Applications in Vibrational and Optical Spectroscopy,* Wiley, ISBN 0-471-62391-1, Chichester.

Noda, I. (2010). Two-dimensional correlation spectroscopy — Biannual survey 2007–2009. *J Mol. Struct.,* Vol. 974, No. 1-3, 3-24.

O'Connor, T.; Mansy, S.; Bina, M.; McMillin, D. R.; Bruck, M.A. & Tobias, R.S. (1982). The pH-dependent structure of calf thymus DNA studied by Raman spectroscopy. *Biophys. Chem.,* Vol. 15, No. 1, 53-64.

Olsztynska-Janus, S.; Szymborska, K.; Komorowska, M. & Lipinski, J. (2009). Conformational changes of L-phenylalanine – Near infrared-induced mechanism of dimerization: B3LYP studies. *J. Mol. Struct. (THEOCHEM)*, Vol 911, No. 1-3, 1-7.

Olsztynska-Janus, S.; Szymborska, K.; Komorowska, M. & Lipinski, J. (2008), Usefulness of spectroscopy for biomedical engineering. *Acta Bioeng. Biomech.*, Vol. 10, No. 3, 45-49.

Olsztynska, S.; Dupuy, N.; Vrielynck, L. & Komorowska, M. (2006a). Water evaporation analysis of L-phenylalanine from initial aqueous solutions to powder state by vibrational spectroscopy. *Appl. Spectrosc.*, Vol. 60, No. 9, 1040-1053.

Olsztynska, S.; Komorowska, M. & Dupuy, N. (2006b). Influence of Near-Infrared Radiation on the pK_a values of L-phenylalanine *Appl. Spectrosc.*, Vol. 60, No. 6, 1040-1053.

Olsztynska, S.; Domagalska B.W. & Komorowska, M. (2003). Aggregation of L-phenylalanine amino acid, [in:] *Surfactants and dispersed systems in theory and practice*, Wilk, K.A. (ed.), Oficyna Wydawnicza Politechniki Wrocławskiej, Wrocław, ISBN 83-7085-701-9, 405-409.

Olsztynska, S.; Komorowska, M.; Dupuy. N. & Vrielynck, L. (2001). Vibrational spectroscopic study of L-phenylalanine: Effect of pH. *Appl. Spectrosc.*, Vol. 55, No. 7, 901-907.

Owen, C.A.; Notingher, I.; Hill R.; Stevens, M. & Hench, L.L. (2006). Progress in Raman spectroscopy in the fields of tissue engineering, diagnostics and toxicological testing. *J. Mater. Sci.: Mater. Med.*, Vol. 17, 1019–1023.

Parker, F.S. (1971). Application of infrared spectroscopy in biochemistry, biology and medicine, Plenum Press, ISBN 978-0306305023, New York.

Parker, F.S., (1983). Nucleic Acids and Related Compounds, In: *Applications of Infrared, Raman, and Resonance Raman Spectroscopy in Biochemistry*, 349-398, Plenum Press, ISBN 0-306-41206-3, New York.

Penteado, S.G.; Meneses, C.S; de Oliveira Lobo, A.; Martin, A.A. & da Silva Martinho, H. (2006). Diagnosis of rotator cuff lesions by FT-Raman spectroscopy: a biochemical study. *Presented on SPEC 2006 Shedding Light on Disease: Optical Diagnosis for the New Millenium*, 4th International Conference, 20-24th May, 2006, Heidelberg, Germany

Petrich, W. (2001). Mid-Infrared and Raman Spectroscopy for Medical Diagnostics. *Appl. Spectrosc. Rev.*, Vol. 36, No. 2&3, 181-237.

Pevsner, A. & Diem, M. (2001). Infrared spectroscopic studies of major cellular components. Part I: The effect of hydration on the spectra of proteins. *Appl. Spectrosc.*, Vol. 55, No. 6, 788-793.

Pevsner, A. & Diem, M. (2003). IR spectroscopic studies of major cellular components. III. Hydration of protein, nucleic acid, and phospholipid films. *Biopolymers*, Vol. 72, No. 4, 282-289.

Pilet, J. & Brahms, J. (1973). Investigation of DNA structural changes by infrared spectroscopy. *Biopolymers*, Vol. 12, No. 2, 387-403.

Pohle, W. & Fritzsche, H. (1980). A new conformation-specific infrared band of A-DNA in films. *Nucleic Acids Res.*, Vol. 8, No. 11, 2527–2535.

Posten, W.; Wronde, D.A.; Dover, J.S.; Arndt, K.A.; Silapunt, S. & Alam, M. (2005). Low-level laser therapy for wound healing: mechanism and efficacy. *Dermatol. Surg.*, Vol. 31, No. 3, 334-340.

Prescott, B.; Steinmetz, W. & Thomas Jr, G.J. (1984). Characterization of DNA structures by laser Raman spectroscopy. *Biopolymers*, Vol. 23, No. 2, 235-256.

Prestrelski S.J.; Byler, D.M. & Thompson, M.P. (1991). Effect of metal ion binding on the secondary structure of bovine α-lactalbumin as examined by infrared spectroscopy. *Biochemistry*, Vol. 30, No. 36, 8797-8804.

Pysz, M.A.; Gambhir, S.S. & Willmann, J.K. (2010). Molecular imaging: current status and emerging strategies. *Clin. Radiol.*, Vol. 65, No. 7, 500-516.

Qing, H; He Yanlin, H.; Fenlin, S. & Zuyi, T. (1996), Effect of pH and metal ions on the conformation of bovine serum albumin in aqueous solution. An attenuated total reflection (ATR) FTIR spectroscopic study. *Spectrochim. Acta A*, Volume 52, No. 13, 1795-1800.

Rauch, C.; Pichler, A.; Trieb, M.; Wellenzohn, B.; Liedl, R.K. & Mayer, E. (2005). Z-DNA's Conformer Substates Revealed by FT-IR Difference Spectroscopy of Nonoriented Left-Handed Double Helical Poly(dG-dC). *J. Biomol. Struct. Dyn.*, Vol. 22, No. 5, 595-614.

Shanmugam, G. & Polavarapu, P.L. (2006). Structures of intact glycoproteins from vibrational circular dichroism. *Proteins*, Vol. 63, No. 4, 768-776.

Sieroń, A.; Cieślar, G, & Adamek, M. (1994). *Magnetotherapy and lasertherapy*, Polish ed., Silesian Academy of Medicine, ISBN 8390110776, Katowice.

Silver, F.H.; Freeman, J.W. & Seehra, G.P. (2003). Collagen self-assembly and the development of tendon mechanical properties. *J. Biomech., Vol.* 36, No. 10, 1529-1553.

Sirichaisit, J.; Young, R.J. & Vollrath, F. (2000). Molecular deformation in spider dragline silk subjected to stress. *Polymer*, Vol. 41, No. 3, 1223-1227.

Smith, B. M.; Oswald, L. & Franzen, S. (2002). Single-Pass Attenuated Total Reflection Fourier Transform Infrared Spectroscopy for the Prediction of Protein Secondary Structure. *Anal. Chem.*, Vol. 74, No. 14, 3386-3391.

Sun, X.-J.; Su, Y.-L.; Soloway, R.D.; Zhang, L.; Wang, J.-S.; Ren, Y.; Yang L.-M.; Zheng, A.-G.; Zhang, Y.-F; Xu, Y.-Z.; Weng, S.-F.; Shi, J.-S.; Xu, D.-F. & Wu, J.-G. (2003). Rapid, intraoperative detection of malignancy using attenuated total reflectance (ATR) and mobile Fourier transform infrared (FT-IR) spectroscopy. *Gastroenterology*, Vol. 124 (Suppl.), No. 4, Suppl.1, A420-A421.

Sun, C.; Yang, J.; Wu, X.; Huang, X.; Wang F. & Liu, S. (2005). Unfolding and refolding of bovine serum albumin induced by cetylpyridinium bromide. *Biophys. J.*, Vol. 88, No. 5, 3518-3524.

Synytsya, A.; Alexa, P.; de Boer, J.; Loewe, M.; Moosburger, M.; Wurkner, M. & Volka, K. (2007). Raman spectroscopic study of calf thymus DNA: an effect of proton- and γ-irradiation. *J. Raman Spectr.*, Vol. 38, No. 14, 1406-1415

Szwed, J.; Cieślik-Boczula, K.; Czarnik-Matusewicz, B.; Jaszczyszyn, A., Gąsiorowski, K.; Świątek, P. & Malinka, W. (2010). Moving-window 2D correlation spectroscopy in studies of fluphenazine–DPPC dehydrated film as a function of temperature. *J. Mol. Struct.*, Vol. 974, No. 1-3, 192–202.

Szyc, Ł.; Pilorz, S. & Czarnik-Matusewicz, B. (2008). FTIR-ATR investigations of an alpha-helix to beta-sheet conformational transition in poly(L-lysine) *J. Mol. Liq.*, Vol. 141, No. 3, 155-159.

Szymborska-Małek, K.; Czarnik-Matusewicz, B. & Komorowska M. (2009a). Two-dimensional correlation analysis in studies of influence of NIR radiation on thin film of DNA measured by FTIR-ATR spectroscopy. *Book of Abstracts of The Fifth International Symposium on Two-Dimensional Correlation Spectroscopy*, pp. 54, Wroclaw, August 2009, Poland; and article in preparation.

Szymborska-Małek, K.; Czarnik-Matusewicz, B. & Komorowska M. (2009b). Study of influence of NIR radiation on herring sperm DNA by ATR-FTIR, UV spectroscopies and DSC. *Book of Abstracts of XIII European Conference on the Spectroscopy of Biological Molecules*, pp. 53, Palermo, August 2009, Italy; and article in preparation.

Taboury, J. A.; Liquier, J. & Taillandier, E. (1985). Characterization of DNA structures by infrared spectroscopy: double helical forms of poly(dG–dC) • poly(dG–dC), poly(dD8G–dC) • poly(dD8G–dC), and poly(dG–dm5C) • poly(dG–dm5C). *Can. J. Chem.*, Vol. 63, No. 7, 1904–1909.

Taillandier, E.; Liquier, J. & Ghomi, M. (1989). Conformational transitions of nucleic acids studied by IR and Raman spectroscopies. *J. Mol. Struct.*, Vol. 214, 185-211.

Taillandier, E. & Liquier, J. (1992). Infrared spectroscopy of DNA. *Methods Enzymol.*, Vol. 211, 307-335.

Tajmir-Riahi, H. A.; Ahmad, R.; Naoui, M. & Diamantoglou S. (1995). The effect of HCl on the solution structure of calf thymus DNA: a comparative study of DNA denaturation by proton and metal cations using Fourier transform IR difference spectroscopy. *Biopolymers*, Vol. 35, No. 5, 493-501.

Tao, N.; Lindsay, S. & Rupprecht, A. (1989). Structure of DNA hydration shells studied by Raman spectroscopy. *Biopolymers*, Vol. 28, No. 5, 1019-1030.

Van de Weert, M.; Harris, P.I.; Hennink, W.E. & Crommelin, D.J.A. (2001). Fourier Transform Infrared Spectrometric Analysis of Protein Conformation: Effect of Sampling Method and Stress Factors. *Anal. Biochem.*, Vol. 297, No. 2, 160-169.

Wang Y.-N.; Galiotis C. & Bader D.L. (2000). Determination of molecular changes in soft tissues under strain using laser Raman microscopy. *J. Biomech.*, Vol. 33, No. 4, 483-486.

Wang, S.-L.; Wei, Y.-S. & Lin, S.-Y. (2003). Subtractive similarity method used to study the infrared spectra of proteins in aqueous solution. *Vib. Spectrosc.*, Vol. 31, No. 2, 313-319.

Wartewig, S. & Neubert, R.H. (2005). Pharmaceutical applications of Mid-IR and Raman spectroscopy. *Adv. Drug Deliv. Rev.*, Vol. 57, No. 8, 1144-1170.

Winchester M.W., Winchester L.W., Chou N.Y. (2008). Application of Raman Scattering to the Measurement of Ligament Tension. *Conference Proceedings: Engineering in Medicine and Biology Society*, pp.3434–3437, 30th Annual International Conference of the IEEE, 14th October, 2008, Vancouver.

Wolpert, M. & Hellwig, P. (2006). Infrared spectra and molar absorption coefficients of the 20 alpha amino acids in aqueous solutions in the spectral range from 1800 to 500 cm^{-1}. *Spectrochim. Acta A*, Vol. 64, No. 4, 987-1001.

Wood, B.R.; Tait B. & Mcnaughton, D. (2000). Fourier Transform Infrared Spectroscopy as a Method for Monitoring the Molecular Dynamics of Lymphocyte Activation. *Appl. Spectrosc.*, Vol. 54, No. 3, 353-359.

Wu, Y.; Murayama, K.; Czarnik-Matusewicz, B. & Ozaki, Y. (2002). Two-Dimensional Attenuated Total Reflection/Infrared Correlation Spectroscopy Studies on Concentration and Heat-Induced Structural Changes of Human Serum Albumin in Aqueous Solutions. *Appl. Spectrosc.*, Vol. 56, No. 9, 1186-1193.

Wu, Y.; Czarnik-Matusewicz, B.; Murayama, K. & Ozaki, Y. (2000). Two-Dimensional Near-Infrared Spectroscopy Study of Human Serum Albumin in Aqueous Solutions: Using Overtones and Combination Modes to Monitor Temperature-Dependent Changes in the Secondary Structure. *J. Phys. Chem. B*, Vol. 104, No. 24, 5840-5847.

Zhang, J. & Yan, Y.-B. (2005). Probing conformational changes of proteins by quantitative second derivative infrared spectroscopy. *Anal. Biochem.*, Vol. 340, No. 1, 89-98.

5

Application of Micro-Fluidic Devices for Biomarker Analysis in Human Biological Fluids

Heather Kalish
National Institute of Biomedical Imaging and Bioengineering, National Institutes of Health USA

1. Introduction

The current interest in microanalysis has heightened over the past years with the development of capillary electrophoresis (CE) followed by the development of commercially available micro-fluidic devices such as micro -mixers, CE chips and micro-reaction vessels or plates. This has made basic micro-fluidic analysis more readily available and has extended their use to biomedical analysis, especially clinically relevant biomarkers and field studies. Here the advantages of such devices are their relative speed of analysis, lower reagent costs, smaller sample requirements, and the potential for high-throughput. These factors become important when special situations arise such as the analysis of precious, archival, or field samples, monitoring surgical procedures, assessing newborns, analyzing specific areas from biopsy materials, measuring the functional aspects of single cells isolated from biological fluids or monitoring contamination of environmental factors.

The combination of antibody-mediated isolation techniques with micro - and nano-scale electrokinetic separations has great potential for analyzing defined analytes in complex biological matrices. In chip-based formats, such systems can recover and measure up to 25 analytes in a reasonably rapid time frame. Further, such devices require sub-microlitre amounts of sample to perform the analyses. Coupling these devices to laser-induced fluorescence greatly enhances the sensitivity of the analysis allowing certain analytes such as protein, peptides, and toxins to be measured in the sub-picogram/mL range. Further, coupling micro-analysis to mass spectrometry adds in the characterization of many significant biomarkers. The combination of fast binding, bio-engineered antibodies requiring relatively short reaction time with rapid desorption and electrophoretic separation with on-line detection can make the analysis almost "real-time".

Today, chip-based analyses are performed on a variety of devices ranging from simple micro-sample plates, to micro-mixers, and chip-based CE, many of which are commercially available. However, more complicated devices such as the "lab-on-a-chip" still require intricate design and specialized facilities. These latter devices hold the potential for automation and involve procedures that utilize both chromatographic and electrophoretic driving mechanisms. Additionally, a lab-on-a-chip can involve the integration of hyphenated techniques in order to achieve the desired analysis, including the integration of a highly sensitive detection system capable of measurement in the femtomolar or attomolar range. The need for such sensitivity often arises from the extremely small sample size obtained for the analysis.

Current work in the literature has focused on the development of micro -fluidic devices for measuring important biomarkers in a number of bio-medically important areas, ranging from the assessment of head trauma patients, assessing the immune status of newborns, especially those at risk from intra-uterine infections and inflammation to exposure to toxic or environmental factors. A biomarker may be defined as "a characteristic, which is objectively measured and evaluated as an indicator of a normal or a pathogenic biological process or even a pharmacological response to a therapeutic intervention." (Atkinson, et al. 2001) This chapter will be a review of current technologies and methodologies in the field of micro-fluidic devices, their application to biomarker analysis and current challenges facing the development of new technologies.

2. Capillary electrophoresis

Capillary electrophoresis is considered one of the analytical tools that started the field of microfluidics. There have been several recent reviews written on the technique and it's applications in numerous research areas. (Siminonato et al., 2010; Ryan et al., 2010; El Rassi, 2010; Mikus & Maráková, 2009) The term capillary electrophoresis is a broad term used to refer to a variety of techniques that exploit the application of a voltage across a capillary to achieve separation of analytes. CE systems are both lab built and commercially available from numerous companies and can be coupled to a wide variety of detectors, such as mass spectrometry (MS), UV/Vis and laser induced fluorescence (LIF). However, improvements in separation media, sample preparation and detection still need to be overcome if CE is to realize its full potential in analytical research. (El Rassi, 2010)

The simplest form of CE is capillary zone electrophoresis, CZE, which separates analytes based on their charge-to-size ratio. (Kalish & Phillips, 2009) Traditional gel electrophoresis has been modified and adapted to a capillary in capillary gel electrophoresis (CGE). This technique is used when analytes that have similar charge to mass ratios need to be separated, based on just their size. (Holovics et al., 2010) The technique of choice when studying protein mixtures is capillary isoelectric focusing (CIEF). Over the past 20 years CIEF has proven to be a fast, high resolution, pI-based technique for the separation of amphoteric compounds, e.g. proteins and peptides. (Silvertand et al., 2009) Micellar microemulsion electrokinetic chromatography (MEEKC) is a mode of CE, which utilizes microemulsions as separation media and allows for separation of neutral as well as charged analytes. (Ryan et al., 2010) Capillary electrochromatography is a hybrid of CE and high performance liquid chromatography, which provides both selectivity and efficiency. (Suntornsuk, 2010) Using capillary isotachophoresis (cITP), sample components are separated based on their electrophoretic mobilities and can be concentrated 2-3 orders of magnitude. (Korir et al., 2006)

CE can be used with numerous different detection instruments, each with their advantages and disadvantages. Laser induced fluorescence (LIF), UV/Vis and mass spectrometry (MS) are the three most common instruments used for detection; however, electrochemical detection, nuclear magnetic resonance (NMR) and conductivity has been used as well. LIF is a very common method of detecting analytes separated by CE. It has a large range of sensitivity and is fairly easy to operate. However analytes need to be pre-labeled either before injection or on the column. UV/Vis requires no prior workup of the compounds of interest and is one of the most popular and useful detectors. (Olędzka et al., 2009) However, analytes must possess natural chromophores that absorb in the UV/VIS region and the limits of detection for UV/Vis are often higher than other detection methods. Both LIF and

UV/Vis allow for identification of compounds only if standards of each analyte have been previously characterized individually. Electrochemical detection offers excellent selectivity and sensitivity and the ability to modify microelectrodes to gain further selectivity for targeted analysis. (Mukherjee & Kirchhoff, 2009) Capacitively coupled contactless conductivity detection (C^4D) offers further acceleration and simplification of CE analyses. It detects analytes in their native state and does not require time-consuming sample derivatization. (Tuma, et al. 2010)

In order to identify new compounds or elucidate structural information, MS or NMR detectors must be used in conjunction with CE separation. MS is the detector of choice when trying to identify unknown compounds. CE-MS can be used as a fully automated high-throughput, high-resolution, and highly reproducible system for the analysis of clinical samples. (Kaiser et al. 2004) A detection method that is rarely used in combination with CE but offers superb specificity is NMR, as seen in Figure 1. Besides providing powerful structural information, NMR has the capability to reveal dynamic information useful in understanding various processes such as diffusion and binding. (Korir et al., 2006) All of these detection methods offer a range of sensitivity, and can be used in conjunction with both traditional bench top CE and microchip CE systems. The challenge to overcome with any of the detectors is effectively coupling the detector to the CE system.

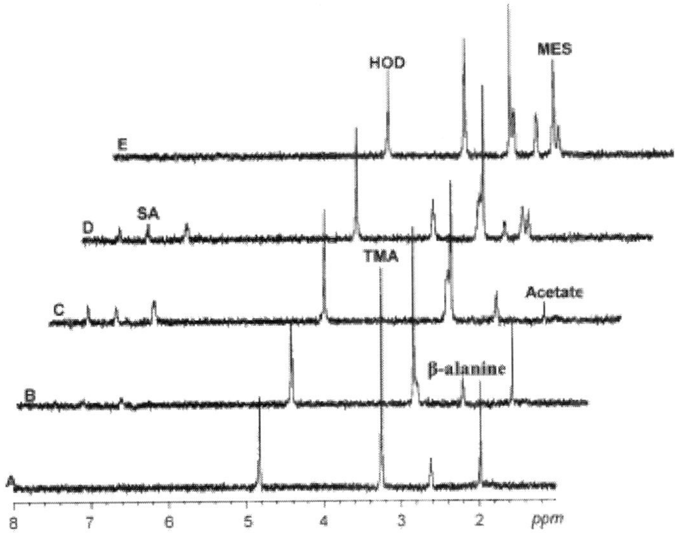

Fig. 1. Profile of the migration of ions in the course of an anionic cITP-NMR experiment. The buffers used were 160 mM DCl/80 mM β-alanine/20 mM TMA acetate (LE) and 160 mM MES (TE). The analyte is 250 μM salicylate. Spectrum A contains the resonances of the LE only (TMA acetate and β-alanine). In spectrum B, the salicylate resonances (SA) begin to emerge in the aromatic region of the spectrum and become more intense in spectra C and D. The TE resonances (MES) begin to emerge in spectrum D, becoming more intense in E. Note that the acetate resonances are detected only up to spectrum C. Reprinted with permission from *Analytical Chemistry*, 2006, 78, 7078-7087. Copyright 2006 American Chemical Society.

3. Microchip Capillary Electrophoresis

Further miniaturization of CE has placed the entire process on a microchip. Micro-CE has all the benefits of traditional CE and further lends itself towards portability and automation. Microchips for CE have been made out of glass, PDMS, polymers and even plastic, which means they are disposable. One dilemma to overcome is that chips need to be onetime use only, but at the same time have to provide all the steps necessary for complex analysis. Analysis of physiological fluids and tissues using microfluidic devices presents a special challenge, both in terms of sensitivity and fouling of microchannels by matrix components. (Coyler et al., 1997)

Microchips have been made with various configurations of channels, allowing for mixing, labeling, separation and detection all within the chip. Perhaps one of the most important factors in the successful resolution of any compound mixture is the design of the chip. (Kalish & Phillips, 2009) Obstacles to overcome in chip design include reproducibility of injection volume, separation length which can be increased by moving from straight channels to meandering ones as seen in Figure 2, and delivery of the analytes to the detector. Sample volume on a microchip ranges in the order of nanoliters to picoliters, so the successful resolution and detection of the isolated compounds remains one of the largest obstacles in the field of micro- CE.

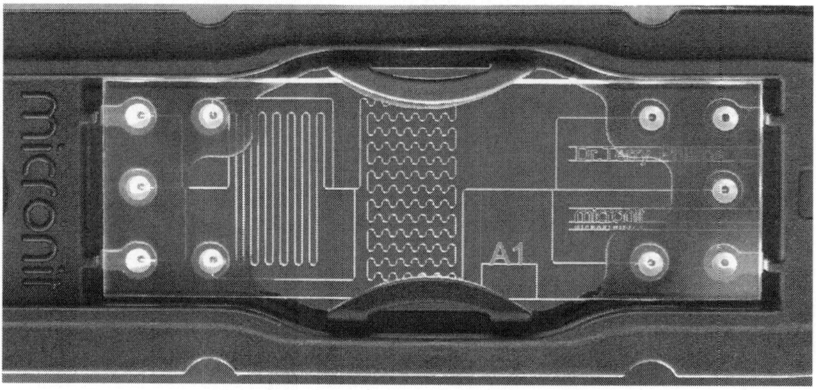

Fig. 2. A Micronit microchip (Netherlands) with a serpentine channel for longer separation and a wavy channel to allow for sample mixing.

Microchips which can incorporate the purification and pre-concentration of samples are becoming more common place as the move towards systems that can be used in point-of-care settings gains momentum. Many processing steps including desalting, labeling and extraction have been successfully performed in microchip systems. (Yang et al., 2010) The integration of an affinity column and capillary electrophoresis channels within a microdevice for the isolation and quantitation of a panel of proteins has been demonstrated by Yang et al. (Yang et al., 2010) Using this microdevice, it was possible to selectively extract and analyze four proteins in spiked human blood and the system has the potential to be expanded to 30 biomarkers using additional antibodies in the affinity columns. This device is but one example of numerous new micro-fluidic devices that incorporate multiple analytical steps onto a microchip platform.

Improvements will be required in detectability, reproducibility, and ease of fabrication, together with integration of different functional operations, to enable Micro-CE for protein separation to provide comprehensive solutions for applications in the fields of proteomics, glycomics, and biomarker detection for diagnosis. (Tran et al., 2010)

4. Immunoaffinity Capillary Electrophoresis (ICE)

Immunoaffinity techniques use immune complexes to capture specific analytes from complex samples, such as human blood or serum, and then use CE to separate and detect the analytes. Sensitivity is greatly enhanced by this technique as the signal to noise ratio for the analytes is greater. Additionally small samples can be reused over and over as analytes of interest are withdrawn and the remaining sample can be recycled. Derivatizing the capillary with antibodies to allow for the selective capture and analysis of specific analytes makes ICE a very practical analytical technique. (Kalish & Phillips, (b) 2009) This technique can allow for the simultaneous measurement of numerous analytes with little sample pre-treatment and fairly small increases in overall analysis time.

Antibodies can also be immobilized to substances other than capillary walls to carry out immunoaffinity capture. Using immobilized recombinant cytokine receptors, Phillips modified the ICE technique to measure only bioactive cytokines in skin biopsies. (Phillips et al., 2009) The immobilized cytokine receptors were bound to a silanized glass filter and were employed as pre-separation affinity selectors in order to capture only those cytokines that were bioactive at the time of biopsy. By comparing cytokines present in normal skin biopsies to cytokines in lesions in the same skin biopsies, the severity and outcome of inflammatory episodes was predicted. Magnetic beads are another solid support to which antibodies can be bound easily and used for immunoaffinity capture.

Chen and co workers covalently bound antibodies to magnetic beads and then held them in place within the capillary walls by two magnets positioned outside the capillary walls. (Chen et el., 2008)

Caulum and co-workers present an immunoaffinity- based CE assay referred to as the cleavable tag immunoassay (CTI). (Caulum et al., 2007) The technique used is similar to ICE, but rather than measure the analytes released by the antibody, a fluorescent tag is cleaved from the detection antibody and imaged, as shown in Figure 3. This technique offers an improvement in resolution over traditional ICE as the cleaved tags can be altered if resolution improvement is necessary, whereas ICE is limited to the structures of the captured analytes.

5. Sample analysis

Human biofluids that can be analyzed by CE, micro-CE and ICE include blood/plasma/serum/dried blood spots, urine, sweat, amniotic fluid, cerebral spinal fluid (CSF), saliva, and vitreous and aqueous fluids. Many biological matrices contain high concentrations of salts and proteins, both of which can cause problems in CE analysis. Thus the composition of any biological sample plays a significant role in determining the choice of which CE analytical approach to take. (Lloyd, 2008)

A. Urine

Urine is a human fluid that is non-invasive to obtain. Samples can be easily collected and usually there is an abundance of sample available. However, samples may be so dilute that preconcentration or other preparation steps may be necessary to observe analytes present in small quantities.

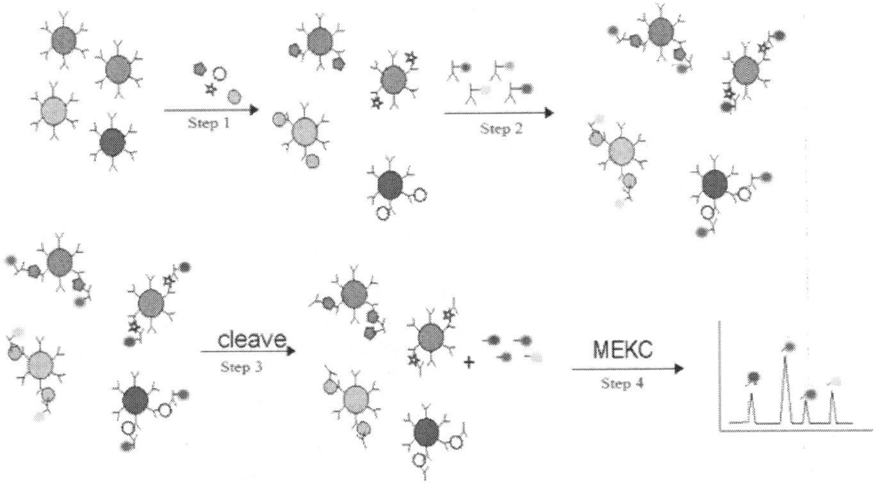

Fig. 3. CTI chemistry. Step 1: sample is added and biomarkers bind to capture antibodies immobilized on the particle surface. Step 2: detection antibodies are added. Step 3: tags are cleaved from immobilized assay. Step 4: separation and detection using MEKC with fluorescence. Reprinted with permission from (2007) *Analytical Chemistry*, 79, 14, 5249-5256. Copyright 2009 American Chemical Society.

Human urine samples from both healthy individuals and patients with various chronic kidney diseases were analyzed by CE-MS by Good, et al. to produce a peptidome analysis of naturally occurring human urinary peptides and proteins. (Good et al. 2010) The advantages of using CE-MS as a proteomic tool for profiling the peptides/proteins include the insensitivity of CE towards interfering compounds, the ability to detect both large and small highly charged molecules, and the lack of interference by precipitates.

The identification and validation of urinary biomarkers as an indicator of patients suffering from anti-neutrophil cytoplasmic antibody associated vasculitis was carried out by Haubitz and co-workers. (Haubitz et al., 2009) Using CE- coupled with MS, the group was able to identify 113 potential biomarkers and changes in these biomarkers could be observed during periods when the patients were undergoing immunosuppressive therapy. This allowed for a non-invasive kidney monitoring and potentially non-invasive diagnosis of patients with anti-neutrophil cytoplasmic antibody associated vasculitis.

Liu and co-workers were able to increase the limits of detection for human urinary proteins by tagging the proteins with gold nanoparticles, which amplifies the mass spectrometry signal, and increase the techniques overall sensitivity. (Liu et al., 2010) Changes in the cholinergic system may be indicative of neuronal degradation in diseases like Alzheimer's and related dementia.

Biomarkers of the cholinergic system are choline and acetylcholine, which Mukherjee and Kirchhoff detected and quantified using CE coupled with electrochemical detection. (Mukherjee & Kirchhoff, 2009) This sensitive system was able to detect biomarkers in the range of fmol to atmol, which far exceeds previous detection limits and makes the system particularly applicable to the detection of these neuronal biomarkers in human samples.

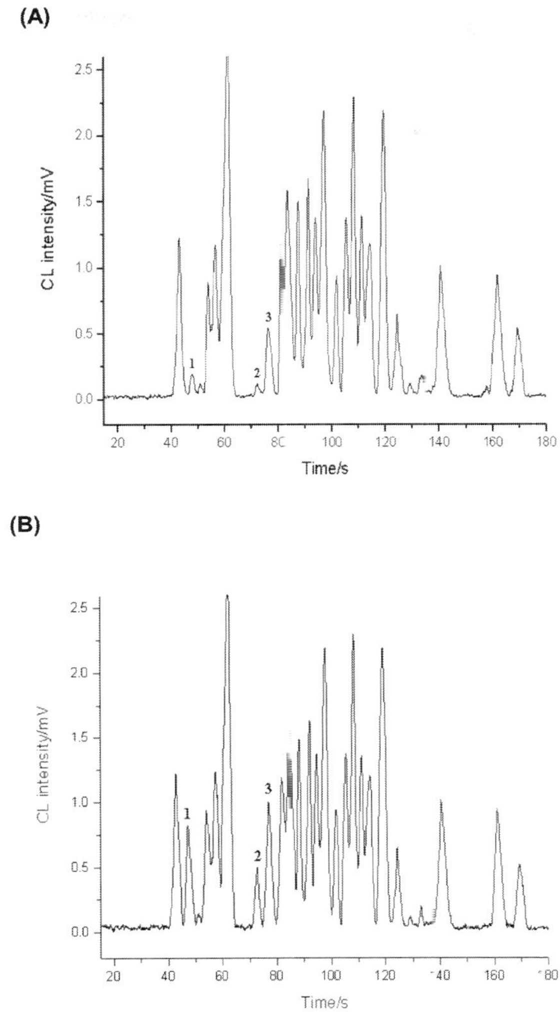

Fig. 4. Electropherograms obtained from the separation of a human urine sample (A) and the sample spiked with Agm, E and DA at 3.5 x 10^{-6} M each (B). The experimental conditions were: Electrophoretic electrolyte was 20 mM phosphate buffer (pH 10.0) containing 10 µM HRP and 25 mM SDS. The oxidizer solution was 20 mm phosphate buffer (pH 11.0) containing 110 mM H_2O_2. Peaks: 1. Agm(Agmatine); 2. E (epinephrine); 3. DA (dopamine). 'Reprinted from Journal of Chromatography A, 1216, Zhao, S.; Huang, Y.; Shi, M. & Liu, Y.M. Quantification of biogenic amines by microchip electrophoresis with chemiluminescence detection. 5155-5159, Copyright 2009, with permission from Elsevier.

The measurement of free cortisol in urine was carried out by Olędzka et al. (Olędzka et al., 2010) Using a solid phase extraction (SPE)- coupled MEKC with UV detection, free cortisol was detected and quantified with a limit of quantification in the 5 ng/mL range. This non-invasive measurement of cortisol was fast, precise and detected changes due to stress situations.
Biogenic amines are naturally formed by the enzymatic decarboxylation of natural amino acids, however certain levels have been shown to promote adverse effects on human health. Using micro- CE coupled with chemiluminescence detection, Zhao et al. were able to quantify biogenic amines in human urine samples, as seen in Figure 4. (Zhao et al., 2009) By pre-labeling the samples, the assay sensitivity was increased and three biogenic amines were able to be identified in human urine samples.

B. Saliva

Saliva is another non-invasive biofluid that can be used to investigate biomarkers. It is readily obtained, constantly reproduced by patients and produced in sufficient quantities for analysis. For patients, the non-invasive collection method of oral fluid sampling reduces anxiety and discomfort. However, the sample matrix is more heterogeneous, and because of the low levels of salivary biomarkers, it sometimes becomes difficult to distinguish between background and target- specific signal in these low concentration samples. (Jokerst et al., 2009)
Saliva from both healthy controls and patients suffering from oral, breast and pancreatic cancers were collected by Sugimoto et al. (Sugimoto et al. 2010) and analyzed by CE-MS to develop a metabolic profile specific to each of the diseases. The samples were used without pretreatment other than centrifugation to remove any solid particles and dilution of the cancer patient samples, due to high electrolyte content.
A panel of 28 biogenic amino acids (AA) were separated and identified by Tůma and co-workers. (Tůma et al., 2010) Using a minimum capillary length on a bench top CE with C^4D detection, a decrease in analysis time and an increase in sensitivity resulted in the identification of 23 of the 28 amino acids in saliva. The decreased separation times and low limits of detection make it applicable to analysis of a variety of human biofluids.
Amino acids were also separated and analyzed from human saliva by Jiang et al. (Jiang et al., 2009) Using copper ions in the running media and an online sweeping enrichment technique, pictured in Figure 5, two of the most prevalent amino acids in human saliva were separated and identified using a CE with UV detection and no sample pretreatment.
A third examination of amino acid neurotransmitters present in human saliva samples was done by Deng and co workers. (Deng et al., 2008) N-Hydroxysuccinimidyl fluorescein-O-acetate, a fluorescein-based dye, was used to derivatize saliva that was centrifuged and diluted with water. Six analytes were recovered from native and spiked saliva samples using CE-LIF to perform the separation and detection steps.
Bradykinin, a vasoactive nonapeptide, and its metabolites were identified using CE-LIF by Chen et al. (Chen et al., 2009) Using transient isotachophoresis preconcentration, 3 bradykinin metabolites were recovered with close to 90% recovery rates from saliva of both a healthy female and a male suffering from hypertension and coronary disease. The method was also applied to human plasma, which showed similar recovery rates of 2 bradykinin metabolites.
The presence of four hormones in saliva was evaluated by Wellner and Kalish using a standard double T microchip. (Wellner & Kalish, 2008) By placing disposable immunoaffinity disc into the sample port, 4 hormones were removed and concentrated from human urine. Samples were compared with no pretreatment and pretreatment cleanup and results indicated that urine analysis yielded false positives when no pretreatment was preformed.

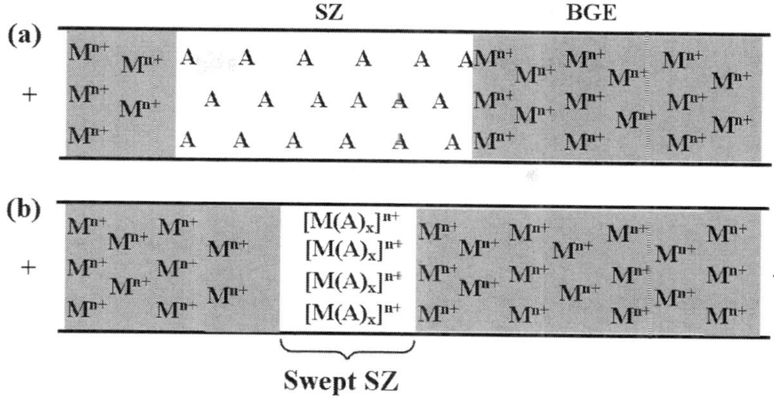

Fig. 5. Schematic diagram of coordination sweeping. (a) is the situation before voltage applied, and (b) is the situation of sweeping after voltage applied. SZ, sample zone; BGS, background solution. "A" represents the free analytes, amino acids, and "M^{n+}" represents transition ions contained in the CE running medium, copper ions. Jiang, X.; Xia, Z.; Wei, W. & Gou, Q. (2009) Direct UV detection of underivatized amino acids using capillary electrophoresis with online sweeping enrichment. *Journal of Separation Science*, 32, 11, 1927-1933. Copyright Wiley-VCH Verlag GmbH & Co. KGaA. Reproduced with permission.

C. Cerebrospinal fluid

CSF is contained primarily in the spinal canal, the ventricles of the brain and in the subarachnoid space at a total volume of about 125-150 mL. With a low protein concentration compared to other biofluids, CSF may be considered more analysis friendly matrix than plasma. (Lloyd, 2008) However, due to the invasive nature of sampling this fluid, analyses are limited.

Steinberg et al. used CE to investigate the role of nitric oxide (NO) in cluster headaches, by measuring their oxidation products, nitrite and nitrate in CSF. (Steinberg et al., 2010) The CSF samples were able to be processed with little pre analytical cleanup and provided a sample that was closer to the areas affected by the disease then previously studied plasma samples. Their results found that NO appears to be involved in pathology of cluster headaches, but increased levels of NO do not appear to directly promote them.

The use of CE to separate and quantitate five amyloid peptides considered as potential biomarkers of Alzheimer's disease was undertaken by Verpillot, et al. (Verpillot et al., 2008) A novel CZE method using a dynamic coating sufficiently separated the five amyloid peptides with minimal adsorption by the capillary wall. However the technique was not sensitive enough with UV detection to measure peptides directly from CSF without preconcentration.

Using noncovalently coated capillaries, Ramautar et al. were able to use CE-UV and CE-MS to analyze CSF for organic acids. (Ramautar et al., 2008) The CE-MS system was able to distinguish the metabolic profile of a healthy individual from the metabolic profile of an individual suffering from complex regional pain syndrome. However, a large set of samples from both groups needs to be analyzed to determine conclusive differences.

In order to establish a quantitative protein profile for CSF samples from patients suffering from traumatic brain injury, Zuberovic et al. used CE coupled with MALDI-TOF. (Zuberovic et al., 2009) To minimize protein wall interaction, capillaries were coated and samples were also prelabeled with isobaric tags. A total of 43 unique proteins were identified and their concentration levels varied over time with the progression of the brain injury.

Microchip CE lends itself to CSF analysis due to the small amount of sample necessary for analysis. CSF samples collected from patients with cephalitis, brain tumors and surgical brain damage with analyzed by CE with chemiluminescence by Zhao and co workers. (Zhao et al., 2009) Three carnosine- related peptides were separated and identified using the micro CE-CL method; however the sensitivity limits were only low enough to detect one of the analytes in actual human CSF samples.

Microchip CE with LIF was used to determine the levels of D-Asp and D-Glu in human CSF samples by Huang, Shi and Zhao. (Huang et al., 2009) Samples were prederivatized with FITC to allow for detection with LIF and analysis took place in a cross T chip. While D-Asp was detected by this method, D-Glu was not. The absence might be due to the lack of D-Glu in CSF samples or amounts that are unable to be detected by the method used.

D. Blood/ Plasma/ Serum/ Dried Blood Spots

Blood is the most accessible biofluid to analyze. It is relatively non-invasive to obtain, is not easily contaminated by external factors, like urine or saliva, and can often be used with little or no pretreatment.

The quantitative analysis of IgG in human serum can be valuable to detect disease and monitor disease progression. However the detection of IgG in human serum can be complicated by the abundant amounts of other proteins and high abundance of human serum albumin. Wu and co-workers improved upon a MEKC-UV method to determine the IgG in human serum, by using solid phase extraction for the removal of human serum albumin and on-column preconcentration to improve sensitivity. (Wu et al., 2010)

IgE in human serum was also measured by Chen and co workers. (Chen et al., 2008) While IgE has the lowest concentration its role in the development of allergy and parasitic diseases has focused attention on this immunoglobulin and driven Chen et al. to develop an immunoassay CE technique that can rapidly detect IgE from only 1 μL of human serum. This technique could be further modified by modifying the magnetic beads and determining different IgE antigens specific for certain allergens.

To evaluate the correlation between neurotrophins and clinical diagnosis of traumatic brain injury, Kalish and Phillips used ICE to measure the concentrations of five different neurotrophins from patient's sera with mild, moderate or severe traumatic brain injury,as seen in Figure 6. (Kalish & Phillips, 2010) Five neurotrophins were simultaneously identified and measured from a small sample in about 40 minutes from serum samples, which are easier to obtain in a clinical setting than samples directly at the site of the brain injury.

Increased levels of α-1-acid glycoprotein (AGP) have been related to cancer and comparing its isoforms between healthy and diseased individuals might provide valuable information about diagnosis. Ongay et al. purified AGP from human serum by different procedures and analyzed the samples by CZE-UV and CZE-ESI-TOF-MS to evaluate which purification method worked best. (Ongay et al., 2009) Overall they obtained a higher yield of AGP using a method without acidic precipitation, but neither preparation affected glycosylation of AGP.

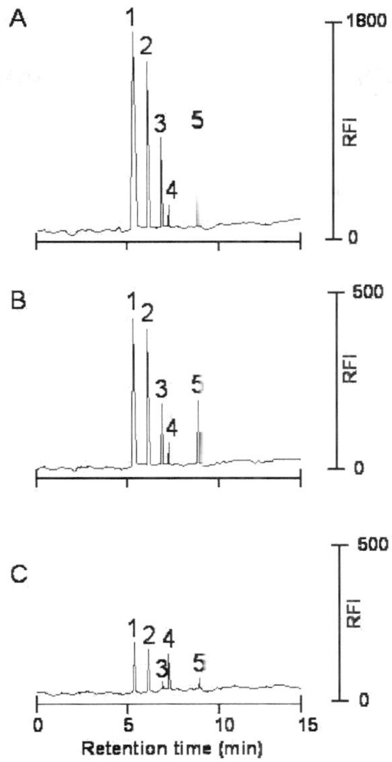

Fig. 6. Electropherograms from ICE analyses of unspiked serum samples of patients suffering from (A) mild, (B) moderate, and (C) severe head trauma. Analyses were performed under the conditions described in Section 2.6. Peak identification: 1. BDNF(brain-derived neurotrophic factor), 2. CNTF(ciliary neurotrophic factor), 3. NT 3(neurotrophin-3), 4. NT-4(Neurotrophin-4), 5. β-NGF(β-nerve growth factor). ' Reprinted from Journal of Chromatography B, 878, Kalish, H. & Phillips, T.M. Analysis of neurotrophins in human serum by immunoaffinity capillary electrophoresis following traumatic head injury, 194-200, Copyright 2010, with permission from Elsevier.

Newborn blood spots were analyzed for inborn errors of metabolism (IEM) by Chalcraft and McKibbin. (Chalcraft & Britz-McKibbin, 2009) Using CE-ESI-MS, dried blood spots from healthy volunteers were extracted and analyzed to determine levels of metabolites in healthy adults. Twenty underivatized metabolites associated with IEM were detected by this new method without chemical derivatization, sample desalting or complicated sample handling.

Both plasma and carotid plaque samples were analyzed by Zinellu et al. to measure thiols in patients undergoing carotid endarterectomy. (Zinellu et al., 2009) CZE-LIF was conducted on both sets of samples to determine if the distribution of thiols differed. Three thiols showed correlation between levels in plasma and plaques, while others were higher or lower in plaques than in plasma. Therefore, evaluating both the plaque and plasma might provide a more complete picture of the plaque progression and fate.

A microchip-CE based noncompetitive immunoassay technique was used for assaying a tumor marker in human serum. Ye et al. coupled LIF detection with microchip based CE to analyze the serum of normal and cancer patients for the cancer biomarker, carcinoembryonic antigen (CEA). (Ye et al., 2010) Using a double T chip and offline incubation of human serum with CEA monoclonal antibody, the CEA levels of normal patients and patients with different cancers were quantified. In all cases the cancer patients showed a higher level of CEA than normal patient levels.

E. Amniotic and follicular fluid

There are very few examples of analyses on these fluids, however they can be very valuable in assessing the health of both the mother and fetus. Amniotic fluid is accessible if the mother undergoes an amniocentesis; however, this is a single time point in the timeline of a fluid that changes on a daily basis. Examination of follicular fluid may lead to a better understanding of reproductive health in a woman.

The proteome of normal amniotic fluid (AF) and disease biomarkers, which may serve as predictions of birth outcomes, are starting to be reported in the literature. Gao and co-workers have used CE to analyze both the major components of amniotic fluid and to determine if any of the components might relate to birth outcome. The concentrations of albumin, IgG, transferrin and uric acid at 15 weeks gestation were measured by CE and it was determined that room temperature storage or multiple freeze thaw cycles revealed no detectable changes to the major components. (Gao et al., 2009)

CE was also used by Gao et al. to determine that higher levels of transferrin and uric acid in second trimester amniotic fluid correlated strongly with both birth weight and gestational age. (Gao et al., 2008)

Follicular fluid may contain biomarkers or proteins which can assist in reproductive medicine. Wen et al. used CZE coupled with UV/Vis to examine proteins found in follicular fluid of women undergoing controlled ovarian hyperstimulation. (Wen et al., 2009) Proteins from follicular fluid were resolved and all but one showed a decrease in concentration as the diameter of the follicle increased. Protein removal may assist researchers in examining follicular fluid closer and identifying smaller peaks.

A combination of analytical techniques can be used to profile the components in complex biological fluids. Hanrieder and co workers, used isoeletric focusing followed by tryptic digestion and CE coupled off line to MALDI-TOF MS/MS, as shown in Figure 7 to analyze human follicular fluid. (Hanrieder et al., 2009) This complex analysis led to the identification of 73 unique proteins, including several proteins known to be involved in human reproduction.

F. Sweat and vitreous fluid

There are very few publications dealing with analysis of these biofluids. Due to the difficulty of collecting vitreous fluid, it is not surprising that there are few publications dealing with its analysis. It is somewhat surprising that there are not more publications dealing with the analysis of sweat. Sweat is an analytically friendly biofluid, with very low protein concentrations. (Lloyd, 2008).

The analysis of sweat for cations, amines and amino acids was carried out by Hirokawa et al. (Hirokawa et al., 2007) While CE coupled with UV detection was used to detect alkali and alkaline earth cations and other target analytes in three male samples, there was variability in the results, which were dependent on the individual and the sampling spots samples were obtained from.

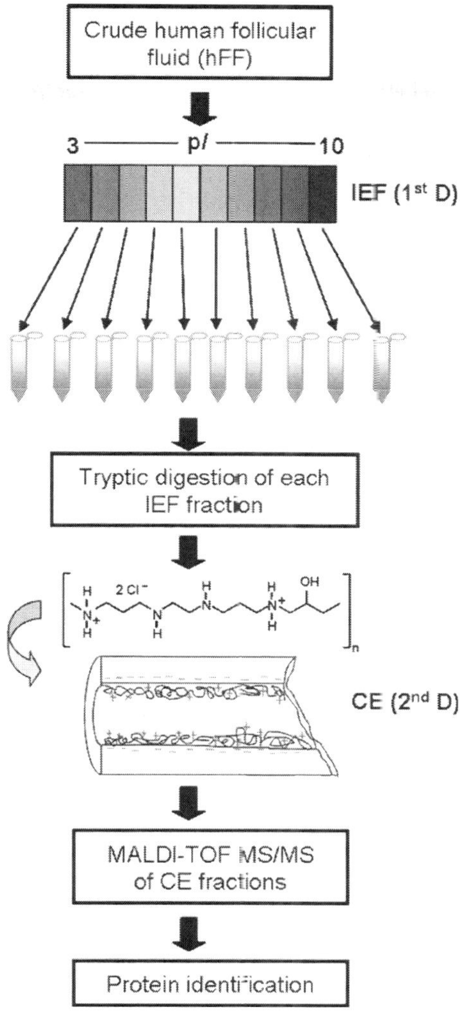

Fig. 7. Experimental overview of the liquid-phase 2D electrophoretic separation and MS profiling of the protein content in human follicular fluid, hFF. Sample prefractionation in microscale IEF was followed by separation and fractionation of tryptically digested peptides in PolyE-323 modified capillaries by CE, interfaced off-line to MALDI tandem time-of-flight MS. " Reprinted from Journal of Chromatography A, 1216,Hanrieder, J.; Zuberovic, A. & Bergquist, J. Surface modified capillary electrophoresis combined with in solution isoelectric focusing and MALDI-TOF/TOF MS: A gel-free multidimensional electrophoresis approach for proteomic profiling—Exemplified on human follicular fluid, 3621-3628., Copyright 2009, with permission from Elsevier.

Amino acid levels were also measured in vitreous fluid of patients with retinal detachment by Bertram and coworkers. (Bertram et al., 2008) Using CE coupled with LIF, patient samples were collected and analyzed for the presence of 9 amino acids. When compared to control samples, patients with retinal detachment had higher levels of glutamate than those of the controls.

Analysis of amino acids in vitreous fluid of patients with proliferative diabetic retinopathy (PDR) was also carried out by CE. Lu et al. used MEKC coupled with LIF to quantitate the differences in amino acid levels in healthy controls and patients with PDR. (Lu et al., 2007) This new method allowed for faster separation and better resolution of amino acids and showed an elevation in glutamate and arginine in PDR patient samples.

Gao et al. also used rapid CE analysis to evaluate the vitreous fluid in samples of patients suffering from PDR. (Gao et al., 2007) Using a laboratory built CE coupled to a UV/Vis detector, nitrate was measured in vitreous fluid. In PDR patients the nitrate peak is found to be significantly higher than that of the control group, suggesting NO might be involved in the disease course of PDR patients.

6. Future direction

Lab on a chip devices offer the potential of bedside analysis with very little wait time and require little to no skilled labor to operate the process. While CE lends itself to microchip format, other laboratory methods are being miniaturized as well. Sun et al. detail a miniature 96 sample ELISA- lab on a chip device that is coupled to a charge coupled device camera for detection. (Sun et al. 2010) The system is portable, sensitive enough to detect concentrations as low as 0.1 ng/mL, and flexible to adapt the system to several sample configurations.

Bed side analysis of endothelial progenitor cells detected in small volumes of white blood cells samples have been achieved using a novel microfluidic system developed by Ng and co workers. (Ng et al., 2010) The detection of clinically relevant sample volumes of CD34+ cells in a relatively short amount of time was demonstrated using label-free impedance detection on an MEA chip surface.

Slab—gel immunoblotting is an invaluable technique in immunology, however the process is extremely manual labor intensive and time consuming. He and Herr have designed, fabricated and validated an automated immunoblotting assay that relies on high-resolution polyacrylamide (PA) gel photopatterning in a two dimensional (2D) microfluidic architecture to yield polyacrylamide gel electrophoresis (PAGE), transfer, and antibody-functionalized blotting regions. (He & Herr, 2010) Using this micrfluidic immunoassay, He and Herr were able to obtain a complete native immunoblot of free prostate specific antigen (fPSA) extracted from human seminal fluid, as seen in Figure 8. This assay was carried out in fewer than 5 minutes with less consumption of antibodies, reagents and manual labor than the traditional bench-top technique.

Microfluidic devices are further being reduced in size to accommodate nanofluidic measurements. Many of these devices incorporate traditional assays such as sandwich assays on a microchip format and use new technologies to increase sensitivity. Jokerst and co workers incorporate quantum dots onto a nano-bio-chip in order to analyze serum and saliva samples. The multiplexed and programmable nano-bio-chip system has clinically demonstrated advantages including intense signal, low LODs necessary for saliva analysis and short assay times. (Jokerst et al., 2009)

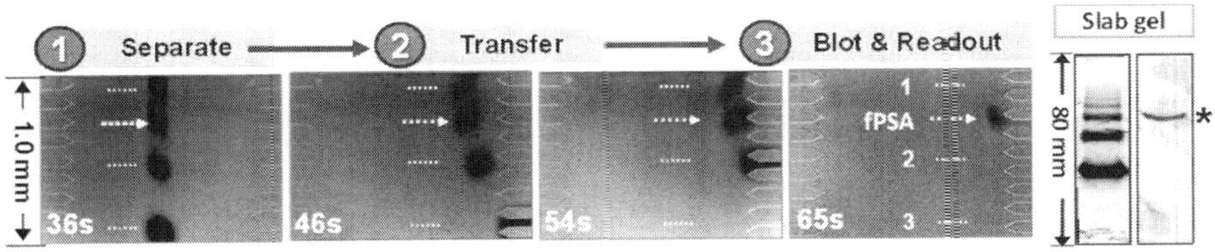

Fig. 8. On-chip immunoblotting of native fPSA extracted from human seminal fluid is rapid and automated. Fluorescence CCD images show the PA gel patterned chamber during: separation, transfer, and blot. A conventional native slab mini-gel blot allows comparison (inverted grayscale, * marks fPSA, numerals 1-3 mark non-fPSA sample peaks). Reprinted with permission from *Journal of the American Chemical Society*, 2010, 132, 8, 2512-2513.

The applications of micro- fluidic and eventually nano-fluidic devices to the analysis of human biofluids are fields that are in their infancy. In order for the fields to realize their full potential much work must be done in transferring the work out of the academic research laboratories and into the commercial sector.

7. References

Atkinson, A. J., Jr.; Colburn, W. A.; DeGruttola, V. G.; DeMets, D. L.; Downing, G. J.; Hoth, D. F.; Oates, J. A.; Peck, C. C.; Schooley, R. T.; Spilker, B. A.; Woodcock, J.& Zeger, S. L. (2001) Biomarkers and surrogate endpoints: Preferred definitions and conceptual framework. *Clinical Pharmacology and Therapeutics*, 69, 3, 89–95.

Bertam, K.M.; Bula, D.V.; Pulido, J.S.; Shippy, S.A.; Gautam, S.; Lu, M.J.; Hatfield, R.M.; Kim, J.H.; Quirk, M.T. & Arroyo, J.G. (2008) Amino-acid levels in subretinal and vitreous fluid of patients with retinal detachment. *Eye*, 22, 4, 582-589.

Caulum, M.M.; Murphy, B.M.; Ramsay, L.M. & Henry, C.S. (2007) Detection of cardiac biomarkers using micellar electrokinetic chromatography and a cleavable tag immunoassay. *Analytical Chemistry*, 79, 14, 5249-5256.

Chalcraft, K.R & Britz-Mckibbin, P. (2010) Newborn screening of inborn errors of metabolism by capillary electrophoresis-electrospray ionization-mass spectrometry: a second-tier method with improved specificity and sensitivity. *Analytical Chemistry*, 81, 1, 307-314

Chen, H.; Busnel, J.; Peltre, G.; Zhang, X & Girault, H. H. (2008) Magnetic beads based immunoaffinity capillary electrophoresis of total serum IgE with laser induced fluorescence detection. *Analytical Chemistry*, 80, 24, 9583-9588.

Chen, Y.; Zhang, L.; Xu, L.; Lin, J. & Chen, G.(2009) Assay of bradykinin metabolites in human body fluids by CE-LIF coupled with transient ITP preconcentration. *Electrophoresis*, 30, 13, 2300-2306.

Coyler, C.L.; Tang, T.; Chiem, N. & Harrison, D.J. (1997) Clinical potential of microchip capillary electrophoresis systems. *Electrophoresis*, 18, 10, 1733-1741.

Deng, Y.H.; Wang, H. & Zhang, H.S. (2008) Determination of amino acid neurotransmitters in human cerebrospinal fluid and saliva by capillary electrophoresis with laser-induced fluorescence detection. *Journal of Separation Science*, 31, 16-17, 3088-3097.

El Rassi, Z. (2010) Electrophoretic and electrochromatographic separation of proteins in capillaries: an update covering 2007-2009. *Electrophoresis*, 31, 1, 174-191.

Gao, L.; Pulido, J.S.; Hatfield, R.M.; Dundervill, R.F.; McCannel, C.A. & Shippy, S.A. (2007) Capillary electrophoresis assay for nitrate levels in the vitreous of proliferative diabetic retinopathy. *Journal of Chromatography B*, 847, 2, 300-304.

Gao, T.; Zablith, N.R.; Burns, D.H.; Skinner, C.D. & Koski, K.G. (2008) Second trimester amniotic fluid transferrin and uric acid predict infant birth outcomes. *Prenatal Diagnosis,* 28, 9, 810-814.

Gao, T.; Zablith, N.; Burns, D.H.; Koski, K.G. & Skinner, C.D. (2009) Identification and quantitation of human amniotic fluid components using capillary zone electrophoresis. *Analytical Biochemistry,* 388, 1, 155-157.

Good, D. M.; Zurbig, P.; Argiles, A.; Bauer, H. W.; Behrens, G.; Coon, J. J.; Dakna, M.;Decramer, S.; Delles, C.; Dominiczak, A. F.; Ehrich, J. H.; Eitner, F.; Fliser, D.; Frommberger, M.; Ganser, A.; Girolami, M. A.; Golovko, I.; Gwinner, W.; Haubitz, M.; Herget-Rosenthal, S.; Jankowski, J.; Jahn, H.; Jerums, G.; Julian, B. A.; Kellmann, M.; Kliem, V.; Kolch, W.; Krolewski, A. S.; Luppi, M.; Massy, Z.; Melter, M.; Neususs, C.; Novak, J.; Peter, K.; Rossing, K.; Rupprecht, H.; Schanstra, J. P.; Schiffer, E.; Stolzenburg, J. U.; Tarnow, L.; Theodorescu, D.; Thongboonkerd, V.; Vanholder, R.; Weissinger, E. M.; Mischak, H. & Schmitt-Kopplin, P. (2010) Naturally occurring human urinary peptides for use in diagnosis of chronic kidney disease, *Molecular and Cellular Proteomics,* Ahead of Print.

Hanrieder, J.; Zuberovic, A. & Bergquist, J. (2009) Surface modified capillary electrophoresis combined with in solution isoelectric focusing and MALDI-TOF/TOF MS: A gel-free multidimensional electrophoresis approach for proteomic profiling—Exemplified on human follicular fluid. *Journal of Chromatography A,* 1216, 17, 3621-3628.

Haubitz, M.; Good, D.M.; Woywodt, A.; Haller, H.; Rupprecht, H.; Theodorescu, D.; Dakna, M.; Coon, J.J. & Mischak, H. (2009) Identification and Validation of Urinary Biomarkers for Differential Diagnosis and Evaluation of Therapeutic Intervention in Anti-neutrophil Cytoplasmic Antibody-associated Vasculitis. *Molecular and Cellular Proteomics*, 8, 10, 2296-2307.

He, M. & Herr, A E. (2010) Polyacrylamide gel photopatterning enables automated protein immunoblotting in a two-dimensional microdevice. *Journal of the American Chemical Society,* 132, 8, 2512-2513.

Hirokawa, T.; Okamoto, H.; Gosyo, Y.; Tsuda, T. & Timerbaev, A.R. (2007) Simultaneous monitoring of inorganic cations, amines, and amino acids in human sweat by capillary electrophoresis. *Analytica Chimica Acta,* 581, 1, 83-88

Holovics, H. J.;He, Y.;Lacher, N. A. & Ruesch, M. N. (2010) Capillary gel electrophoresis with laser-induced fluorescence of plasmid DNA in untreated capillary, *Electrophoresis,* 31,14, 2436-2441.

Huang, Y.; Shi M. & Zhao, S. (2009) Quantification of D-Asp and D-Glu in rat brain and human cerebrospinal fluid by microchip electrophoresis. *Journal of Separation Science,* 32, 17, 3001-3006.

Jiang, X.; Xia, Z.; Wei, W. & Gou, Q. (2009) Direct UV detection of underivatized amino acids using capillary electrophoresis with online sweeping enrichment. *Journal of Separation Science,* 32, 11, 1927-1933

Jokerst, J.V.; Raamanathan, A.; Christodoulides, N.; Floriano, P.N.; Pollard, A.A.; Simmons, G.W.; Wong, J.; Gage, C.; Furmaga, W.B.; Redding, S.W. & McDevitt, J.T. (2009) Nano-bio-chips for high performance multiplexed protein detection: Determinations of cancer biomakers in serum and saliva using quantum dot bioconjugate labels. *Biosensors and Bioelectronics.* 24, 12, 3622-3629

Kaiser, T.; Wittke, S.; Just, I.; Krebs, R.; Bartel, S.; Fliser, D.; Micchak, H. & Weissinger, E.M. (2004) Capillary electrophoresis coupled to mass spectrometer for automated and robust polypeptide determination in body fluids for clinical use. *Electrophoresis,* 25, 13, 2044-2055.

Kalish, H. & Phillips, T.M. (2009) The application of micro-analytical techniques to biomedical analysis. *Current Pharmaceutical Analysis,* 5, 3, 208-228, 1573-4129.

(b) Kalish, H. & Phillips, T.M. (2009) Application of immunoaffinity capillary electrophoresis to the masurements of secreted cytokines by cultured astrocytes. *Journal of Separation Science,* 32, 10, 1605-1612.

Kalish, H. & Phillips, T.M. (2010) Analysis of neurotrophins in human serum by immunoaffinity capillary electrophoresis following traumatic head injury. *Journal of Chromatography B,* 878, 2, 194-200.

Kasicka, V. (2010) Recent advance in CE and CEC of peptides, (2007-2009), *Electrophoresis,* 31, 1, 122-146.

Korir, A.K.; Almeida, V.K. & Larive, C.K. (2006) Visualizing ion electromigration during isotachophoretic separations with capillary isotachophoresis-NMR, *Analytical Chemistry,* 78, 20, 7078-7087, ISSN.

Lloyd, D.K. (2008) Capillary electrophoresis analysis of biofluids with a focus on less commonly analyzed matrices. *Journal of Chromatography B,* 866, 1-2, 154-166.

Liu, J.M.; Li, Y.; Jiang, Y. & Yan, X.P. (2010) Gold Nanoparticles Amplified Ultrasensitive Quantification of Human Urinary Protein by Capillary Electrophoresis with On-Line Inductively Coupled Plasma Mass Spectroscopic Detection, *Journal of Proteome Research,* 9, 7, 3545-3550.

Lu, M.J.; Pulido, J.S.; McCannel, C.A.; Pulido, J.E.; Hatfield, R.M.; Dundervill, R.F. & Shippy, S.A. (2007) Detection of elevated signaling amino acids in human diabetic vitreous by rapid capillary electrophoresis. *Experimental Diabetes Research,* 2007, 39765.

Mikus, P. & Maráková,K (2009) Advanced CE for chiral analysis of drugs, metabolites, and biomarkers in biological samples, *Electrophoresis,* 30, 16, 2773-2802, ISSN.

Mukherjee, J. & Kirchhoff, J.R. (2009) Electrocatalytic microelectrode detectors for choline and acetylcholine following separation by capillary electrophoresis, *Analytical Chemistry,* 81, 16, 6996-7002.

Ng, S.Y.; Reboud, J.; Wang, K.Y.P.; Tang, K.C.; Zhang, L.; Wong, P.; Moe, K.T.; Shim W. & Chen, Y. (2010) Label-free impedance detection of low levels of circulating endothelial progenitor cells for point-of-care- diagnosis. *Biosensors and Bioelectronics,* 25, 5, 1095-1101.

Olędzka, I.; Plenis, A.; Konieczna, L.; Kowalski, P. & Bączek, T. (2010) Micellar electrokinetic chromatography for the determination of cortisol in urine samples in view of biomedical studies. *Electrohporesis,* 31, 14, 2356-2364.

Ongay, S.; Neusüβ, C.; Vaas, S.; Díez-Masa, J.C & de Frutos, M. (2010) Evaluation of the effect of the immunopurification-based procedures on the CZE-UV and CZE-ESI-TOF-MS determination of isoforms of intact a-1-acid glycoprotein from human serum. *Electrophoresis,* 31, 11, 1796-1804.

Phillips, T.M; Kalish, H. & Wellner, E. (2009) Receptor affinity CE for measuring bioactive inflammatory cytokines in human skin biopsies. *Electrophoresis,* 30, 22, 3947-3954.

Ramautar, R.; Mayboroda, O.A.; Deelder, A.M.; Somsen, G.W. & de Jong, G.J. (2008) Metabolic analysis of body fluids by capillary electrophoresis using noncovalently coated capillaries. *Journal of Chromatography B,* 871, 2, 370-374

Ryan, R.; Donegan, S.; Power, J. & Altria, K (2010) Advances in the theory and application of MEEKC. *Electrophoresis,* 31, 5, 755-767.

Sanchez, L.; Gonzalez, R.; Crego, A.L. & Cifuentes, A. (2007) A simple capillary gel electrophoresis approach for efficient and reproducible DNA separations. Analysis of genetically modified soy and maize. *Journal of Separation Science,* 30, 4, 579-585.

Silvertand, L. H.; Torano, J. S.; de Jong, G. J. & van Bennekom, W. P. (2009) Development and characterization of cIEF-MALDI-TOF MS for protein analysis, *Electrophoresis,* 30,10, 1828-35.

Simionato, A.V.C.; Carrilho, E. & Tavares, M.F.M (2010) CE-MS and related techniques as a valuable tool in tumor biomarker research. *Electrophoresis,* 31, 7, 1214-1226.

Steinberg,A.; Wiklund, N.P; Brundin, L. & Remahl, A.I.M.N. (2010) Levels of Nitric Oxide metabolites in cerebrospinal fluid in cluster headache. *Cephalalgia,* 30, 6, 696-702.

Sugimoto, M.; Wong, D.T.; Hirayama, A.; Soga, T. & Tomita, M. (2010) Capillary electrophoresis mass-spectrometry-based saliva metabolomics identified oral, breast and pancreatic cancer-specific profiles. *Metabolomics,* 6, 1,78-95.

Sun, S.; Yang, M.; Kostov, Y. & Rasooly, A. (2010) ELISA-LOC: lab-on-a-chip for enzyme-linked immunodetection. *Lab on a Chip.* 10,16, 2093-2100.

Suntornsuk, L. (2010) Recent advances in capillary electrophoresis in pharmaceutical analysis. *Analytical and Bioanalytical Chemistry.* 398, 1, 29-52

Tran, N.T.; Ayed, I.; Pallandre, A. & Taverna, M. (2010) Recent innovations in protein separation on microchips by electrophoretic methods: An update. *Electrophoresis,* 31, 1, 147-173.

Tůma, P.; Málková, K.; Samcová, E & Štulík, K. (2010) Rapid monitoring of arrays of amino acids in clinical samples using capillary electrophoresis with contactless conductivity detection. *Journal of Separation Science,* 33, 16, 1-8

Verpillot, R.; Otto, M.; Klafki, H. & Taverna, M. (2008) Simultaneous analysis by capillary electrophoresis of five amyloid peptides as potential biomarkers of Alzheimer's disease. *Journal of Chromatography A,* 1214, 1-2, 157-164.

Wellner, E.F & Kalish, H. (2008) A chip-based immunoaffinity capillary electrophoresisassay for assessing hormones in human biological fluids. *Electrophoresis,* 29, 16, 3477-3483

Wen, X.; Pereet, D.; Patel, P.; Li, N.; Docherty, S.M.; Tozer, A.J. & Iles, R.K. (2009) Capillary electrophoresis of human follicular fluid. *Journal of Chromatography B,* 877, 31, 3946-3952

Wu, Y.; Liu, J.; Deng, Z.; Zhang, J.; Jiang, F.; Xiong, K. & Zhang, H. (2010) MEKC determination of IgG in human serum via a pH-mediated acid stacking method. *Journal of Separation Science,* ahead of print.

Yang, W.; Yu, M.; Sun, X. & Woolley, A.T. (2010) Microdevices integrating affinity columns and capillary electrophoresis for multibiomarker analysis in human serum. *Lab on a Chip,* 10, 19, 2527-2533.

Ye, F.; Shi, M.; Huang, Y. & Zhao, S. (2010) Noncompetitive immunoassay for carcinoembryonic antigen in human serum by microchip electrophoresis for cancer diagnosis. *Clinica Chimica Acta,* 411, 15-16, 1058-1062.

Zhao, S.; Huang, Y.; Shi, M. & Liu, Y.M. (2009) Quantification of biogenic amines by microchip electrophoresis with chemiluminescence detection. *Journal of Chromatography A,* 1216, 26, 5155-5159.

Zhao, S.; Huang, Y.; Shi, M.; Huang, J. & Liu, Y.M. (2009) Quantification of carnosine-related peptides by microchip electrophoresis with chemiluminescence detection. *Analytical Biochemistry,* 393, 1, 105-110.

Zinellu, A.; Lepedda, A. Jr; Sotgia, S.; Zinellu, E.; Scanu, B.; Turrini, F.; Spirito, R.; Deiana, L.; Formato, M, & Carru, C. (2009) Evaluation of low molecular mass thiols content in carotid atherosclerotic plaques. *Clinical Biochemistry,* 42, 9, 796-801.

Zuberovic, A.; Wetterhall, M.; Hanrieder, J. & Bergquist, J. (2009) CE MALDI-TOF/TOF MS for multiplexed quantification of proteins in human ventricular cerebrospinal fluid. *Electrophoresis,* 30, 10, 1836-1843.

6

Detection of Stem Cell Populations Using in Situ Hybridisation

Virginie Sottile
Wolfson STEM Centre, School of Clinical Sciences, The University of Nottingham, UK

1. Introduction

RNA in situ hybridisation (RISH) on tissue sections allows the detection of mRNA expressed in discrete populations within a tissue. Based on the use of a specific riboprobe complementary to the target sequence, RISH enables the detection of individual cells present within an organ whose structure and organization are maintained.

Originally developed with radiolabelled probes, RISH now mostly relies on non-radioactive detection techniques, using nucleotide tags such as fluorescein or digoxigenin (DIG) as discussed below. Such non-radioactive labelling can both reduce the risks to health and the environment, and offer higher sensitivity with lower probe detection time (Wilkinson, 1995, Moorman et al., 2001).

The fact that RISH on tissue sections provides information on both cell number and cell distribution makes it an important technique for the study of stem cell populations, with a range of applications including identifying endogenous populations through the detection of stem cell markers' mRNAs, characterising the in vivo behaviour of endogenous stem cells, or following the transplantation of exogenous cells in animal studies. The analysis of stem cell populations after they have been injected into an animal model, whether embryonic or adult, is particularly amenable to RISH: using a probe specific for the injected cells, such as for example an anti-GFP probe for labelled stem cells, the number and distribution of injected cells in the host tissue can be analysed on tissue sections. Since probe specificity will directly affect the success of the experiment, the choice and design of the probe represent critical aspects of the preparation which should be determined before starting the RISH.

2. RISH technique for the detection of stem cells within a host organ

2.1 Principle and preparation

The detection of the target sequence involves 3 phases: (i) preparation of the sections, (ii) hybridisation of the probe, and (iii) post-hybridisation detection of the probe. The probe can be detected through fluorescence or enzymatic methods. Fluorescence methods can have more limited sensitivity than enzymatic methods.

Probes labelled by incorporation of DIG-labelled ribonucleotides can be detected by anti-DIG antibodies which are coupled with an enzyme such as alkaline phosphatase (fig. 1). The enzyme is then used to trigger a colour reaction in situ within the cells in which the DIG-labelled probe has bound to the target RNA. Different methods and kits for probe labelling and preparation are available from commercial sources (www.roche-applied-science.com/dig, Gandrillon et al., 1996). One method routinely used relies on the prior sub-cloning of a partial or entire cDNA fragment of the gene of interest, and the in vitro transcription carried out in the presence of DIG-labelled nucleotides (fig. 2).

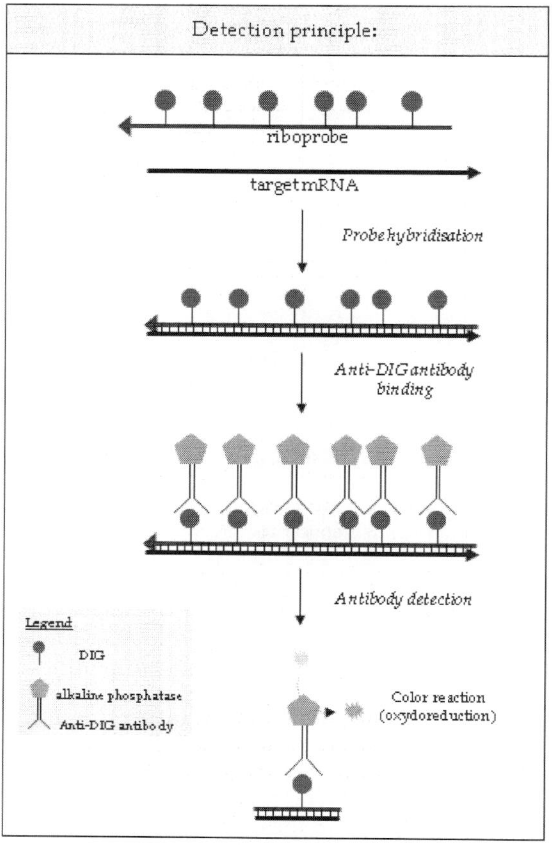

Fig. 1. Principle of the probe hybridisation-based detection of the target sequence using an enzymatic-based colour reaction.

Detection of the target sequence requires a stepwise protocol which can run over 3 to 6 days depending on the level of expression of the gene of interest and on the target tissue. The method described here is used for the successful detection of target mRNA in frozen sections using DIG labelled probe. However, several steps may need to be optimized by the user for optimal results, as indicated throughout. This technique requires organization in order to prepare all necessary supplies and solutions ahead of the procedure (see section 3), and care in order to avoid degradation of the sample's RNA by contaminating nucleases.

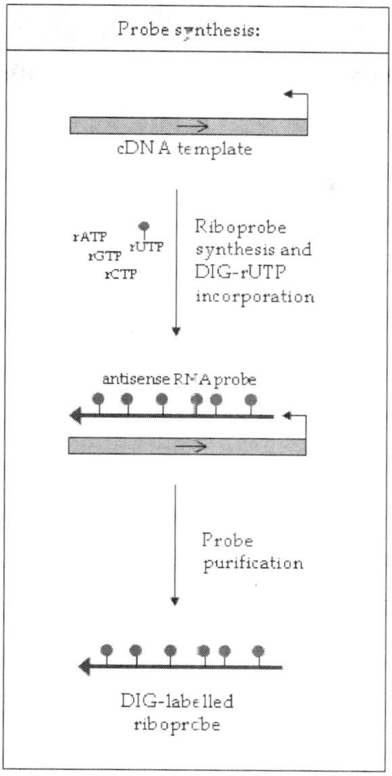

Fig. 2. Principle underlying the preparation of the DIG-labelled antisense probe used to detect a target sequence.

2.2 Slide preparation

RISH on frozen tissue section provides reliable results and high sensitivity with minimal tissue damage. The tissue of interest should be dissected and processed with care and diligence following the protocol presented below (fig. 3) to avoid structural damage and degradation of the mRNA which will impair the experimental outcome.

Following the harvesting of the appropriate tissue, the sample is washed in PBS for 5min at room temperature ('RT'). The tissue is then fixed in 4% ice-cold paraformaldehyde (PFA), for a period ranging from 30min to overnight depending on the size and density of the tissue (this parameter needs to be optimised by the user for each type of tissue). The sample should remain at 4°C throughout. Following fixation, the PFA should be removed and the sample washed in PBS for 5min at RT.

Before cryoembedding, the sample should be transferred to a 15% sucrose solution kept at 4°C until it sinks to the bottom of the vessel (this may require overnight incubation depending on the size of the sample). This is repeated by transfer to a 30% sucrose solution at 4°C until the tissue sinks to the bottom of the vessel (this may also require overnight incubation, depending on the size of the sample).

Sucrose-equilibrated samples are then washed once with OCT for 5min at RT, before being transferred to an appropriate mould (plastic or foil) filled with OCT, the tissue is orientated according to the plane of sectioning to be used. The mould is placed in a plastic beaker containing cold isopentane, and the beaker dipped into a vessel containing liquid nitrogen. The mould content progressively becomes opaque as it freezes over a few seconds. Care should be taken to remove the sample as soon as its content is frozen to avoid cracks in the sample. Cryopreserved samples can be stored at -20°C until sectioning. The cryostat will then be used to generate 10 to 12µm thick tissue sections, following manufacturer's instructions, and the sections produced will be stored at -20°C until in situ hybridisation.

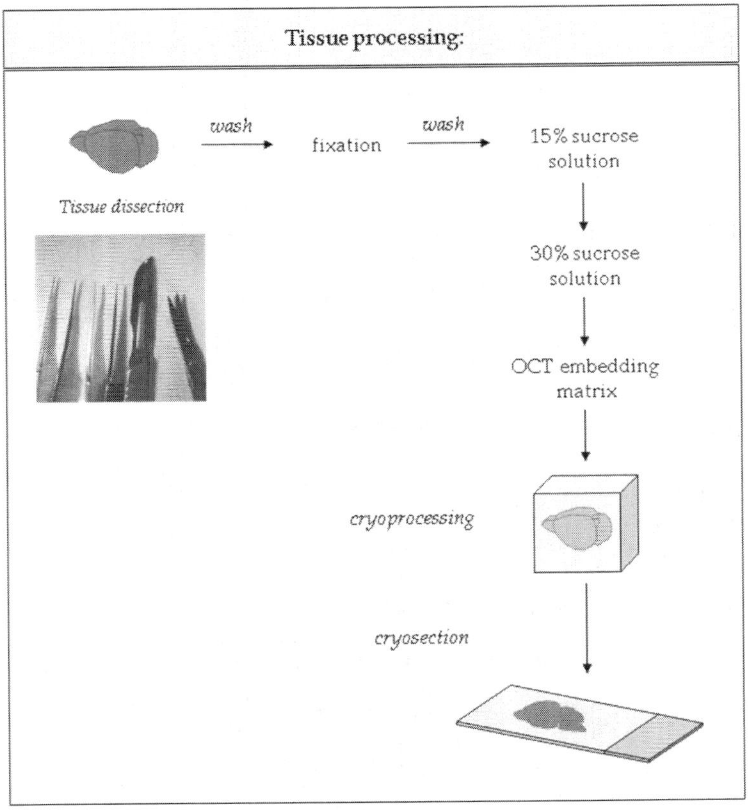

Fig. 3. Preparation of tissue cryosections for RISH.

2.3 Probe hybridization

Work with riboprobes requires significant precautions to minimize exposure of the slides to contaminating RNases, which can degrade both the probe and target sequence before the hybridisation step is completed. All steps described below (fig. 4) must therefore be carried out in a clean working area, using gloves and RNAse-free solutions.

Before starting with the pre-hybridisation treatment, the slides need to be immersed in PBS for 3min at RT in order to remove the residual OCT matrix. Each slide is then re-fixed with 1ml of PFA and incubated 10min at RT (*NB: this step needs to be carried out in a fume cupboard to minimise exposure to fixative).* During this incubation step, the Proteinase K solution should be pre-warmed at 37°C.

After 3 brief washes with PBST (for 5min each), each slide is then covered with 500µl of prewarmed Proteinase K solution for 5min at RT to permeabilise the sample. After a series of 3 PBST washes for 3min each, sections are PFA-fixed again for 20min to maintain their integrity following permeabilisation, and washed again 3 times in PBST.

Before adding the riboprobe to the samples, the probe solution is pre-heated at 68°C for 5min in Hybridisation solution to reduce secondary structure. The probe solution is added to each slide, covered with a hybrid-slip. The sections are placed in a hermetic box humidified with a solution made of 50% formamide and 5x SSC and incubated overnight in the hybridisation oven at 70°C. The temperature and length of hybridisation need to be optimized by the user, as the nature of the sequence and the tissue can affect the efficiency of this procedure.

2.4 Probe detection

2.4.1 Posthybridisation washes and antibody binding:

Following the hybridisation step, extensive washing is crucial to ensure signal specificity and low background. The wash Solutions 1 and 2 need to be pre-warmed before the start of these post-hybridisation washes. Slides will then undergo (i) 3 washes in Wash Solution 1 at 70°C, for 30min each ; (ii) 3 washes in Wash Solution 2 at 65°C, for 30min each ; (iii) 3 washes in Wash Solution 3 at RT, for 5min each (fig.4).

Once the unbound probe has been removed by serial washes, slides are prepared for the probe detection, which is carried out using an anti-DIG antibody. Before the antibody is applied, slides are exposed to 500µl of Block solution for 1 hour to decrease unspecific signal. Slides are then covered with 500µl anti-DIG antibody solution, covered with parafilm and placed in a humidified box placed overnight at 4°C.

2.4.2 Antibody washes and colour detection:

After the antibody has been in contact with the tissue sections, extensive washing is required to remove the unbound antibody. Slides are washed 3 times in Wash Solution 3, for 20min each time, and twice in Detection buffer, for 5min each time.

The final step in the detection of the DIG-labelled probe is carried out through an enzymatic reaction which will highlight the cells containing the target sequence (fig. 1). To initiate the detection of the bound antibody in the tissue sections, each slide is overlaid with 300µl Colour solution, covered with a coverslip and incubated in the dark until the desired staining intensity is achieved. This step can take minutes to days, depending on the level of expression of the target RNA, and the quality of the sample. As a rule, fresh colour solution can be replaced every 8-10hours to prolong the reaction and minimise unspecific darkening of the tissue.

When the coloration is satisfactory (fig.5), the reaction is stopped by incubating the slide in TE buffer for 5min at RT. Slides can then be mounted with a coverslip for microscope examination, using a mounting medium such as Vectashield (following manufacturer's instructions).

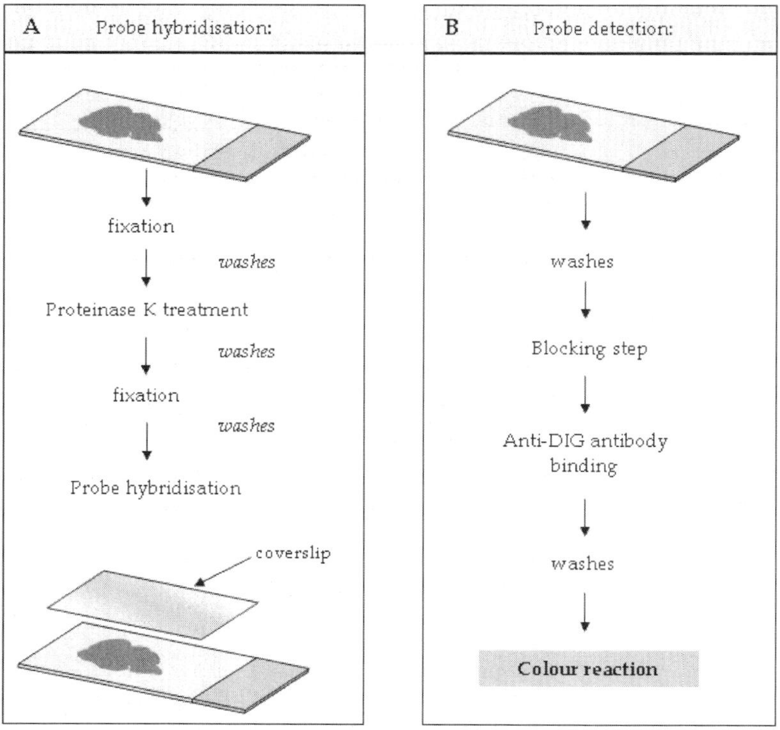

Fig. 4. Experimental steps for signal detection. (A) Preparation for the probe hybridisation phase. (B) Principle of signal detection after hybridisation of the probe.

3. Reagents and solutions

The section below describes the equipment and supplies used to carry out RISH on frozen tissue sections (Table1). A description of the different buffers and solutions used as described in the previous sections is also provided (Table2).

Supplies:	**Equipment:**
Hybrid-slips	Cryostat
Coplin jars	Microscope
Superfrost slides	Waterbath
Forceps	Hybridisation oven
Scissors	Heatblock
Glass coverslips	Hermetic slide box
Parafilm	Liquid nitrogen vessel

Table 1. Equipment and supplies used in the protocol.

Solution:	Composition:
Paraformaldehyde	Dilute 4g of paraformaldehyde in 100ml PBS, and incubate in 65°C until dissolved. Bring pH to 7.4 and aliquote. Store at -20°C
Sucrose solutions	Dilute the necessary amount of Sucrose (7.5g for 15%, 15g for 30%) in 50ml PBS.
PBST	Add 1μl/ml of Tween20 to PBS and mix well.
Proteinase K solution:	Dilute Proteinase K powder in PBST to a final concentration of 1μg/ml.
20x SSC solution:	Dilute 175.3g/l NaCl and 88.2g/l NaCitrate in H_2O, adjust pH to 4.5 and autoclave.
10% SDS	Dilute 100g/l SDS powder (follow manufacturer's instructions) in H_2O, and adjust pH to 7.2.
Wash solution 1	Prepare the following solution in H_2O: 0.5x Formamide, 1% SDS, 5x SSC
Hybridisation solution	Prepare solution as described for Wash solution 1 and add tRNA (50μg/ml) and Heparin (50μg/ml).
Wash solution 2	Prepare the following solution in H_2O: 0.5x Formamide, 2x SSC
Wash solution 3	Prepare the following solution in H_2O: 8g/l NaCl, 0.1M Tris (pH7.5), 10μl/ml Tween20.
Block solution	Dilute 100μl/ml of Sheep serum in Wash solution 3.
Anti-DIG solution	Dilute 10μl/ml of Sheep serum and 0.2μl/ml anti-DIG antibody in Wash solution 3.
Detection buffer	Prepare the following solution in H_2O: 0.1M NaCl, 50mM MgCl2, 0.1M Tris (pH9.5), 10μl/ml Tween20.
Colour solution	Prepare the following solution in Alkaline phosphatase buffer: 4.5μl/ml NBT, 3.5μl/ml BCIP.
TE buffer	Prepare the following solution in H_2O: 10mM Tris (pH7.5), 1mM EDTA (pH8).

Table 2. Solutions required for the protocol.

4. Optimisation and general advice

4.1 Integrity of the sample:

The quality of the results obtained will depend on the preservation of the sample integrity throughout the procedure, from tissue harvest to target detection. Because the technique relies on detection of mRNA, careful handling of the samples in RNAse free conditions is essential for the 1st part of the procedure (until hybridisation). Gloves must be worn at all times, bench surfaces and equipment must be cleaned with RNase zap. It is also preferable to use a dedicated set of glassware and pipettes for RISH, and to use filter tips until the post-hybridisation stages.

Another critical factor comes from the fact that the hybridisation step takes place in a limited volume, over a long time and at high temperature. Evaporation is therefore a potential problem which could cause the sections to dry and become unusable. To ensure the slides do not dry up during this step, it is critical to maintain the slides in a humidified atmosphere in the hybridisation box, by including soaked tissue and carefully sealing the box.

As the length and relative complexity of the RISH procedure can be detrimental to the tissue, which is exposed to serial incubations and washes in stringent conditions, the quality, reproducibility and sensitivity of RISH can be significantly enhanced by the use of an automated slide processor (such as the BioLane™ HTI). The use of such automation can significantly reduce variability and preserve the integrity of precious samples, while allowing higher throughput for the batch processing of sections by RISH.

4.2 Signal intensity:

The length of the colour development phase can vary significantly (from minutes to several days) depending on the level of expression of the gene of interest, the nature of the probe, and the quality of the tissue. The optimal length of development needs to be determined on a case by case basis. It is crucial to regularly monitor the slides during this phase, and replace the colour solution to avoid drying of the slide as well as unspecific deposition of the substrate over time.

Some detection problems may also arise if the target tissue is likely to exhibit endogenous alkaline phosphatase activity, as this would cause background staining during the colour reaction. This can be avoided by adding levamisole to the colour reaction, which can inhibit endogenous activity (Ponder & Wilkinson, 1981).

4.3 Analysis and quality control methods:

Positive controls: Although it can be useful to use a probe for a housekeeping gene as a control for RISH detection, the interpretation can sometimes be difficult between ubiquitous staining and unspecific background staining. Therefore, using a control probe and tissue previously shown to give specific staining is usually the best way to validate the technique in the lab. Comparison with the expression pattern obtained by immunostaining, whenever possible, can provide assurances that the RISH signal obtained is specific. Above all, reproducibility of the staining in independent RISH runs is essential.

Negative controls: The 2 sets of controls described below are required to enable the evaluation of possible false positive staining on the tissue sections:

(i) Sense control: The parallel handling of a slide hybridised with a sense probe is a common method to ascertain the specificity of the probe. The sequence of the sense probe is identical to that of the target mRNA (whereas the antisense probe is complementary to it), thus the sense probe does not hybridise with the target transcript. Any signal detected in the sense control is therefore considered to result from unspecific binding of the probe or antibody, and allows the relative assessment of the antisense results (fig. 5).

(ii) Alkaline phosphatase control: A slide processed in parallel but not exposed to the anti-DIG antibody can provide another type of negative control, by measuring the contribution of endogenous alkaline phosphatase signal in the target tissue. Based on the results of this test, levamisole may be added to the Detection buffer to decrease background alkaline phosphatase activity in the tissue section (see section 4.2).

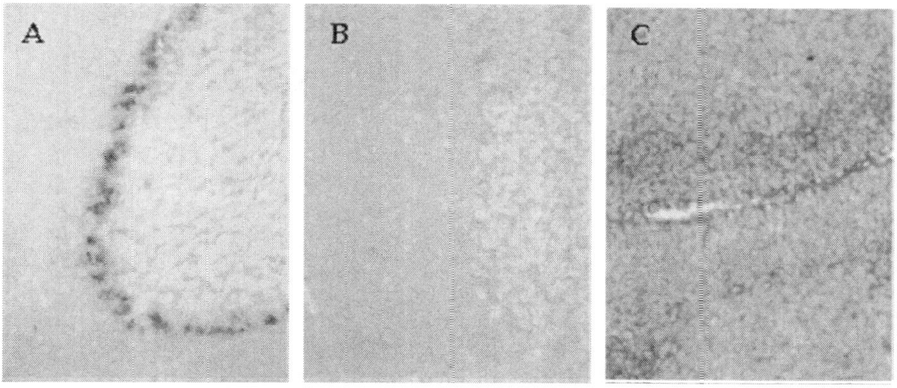

Fig. 5. Examples of RISH detection on mouse brain tissue. (A) Specific signal obtained with an antisense probe shows clear cell labelling on the tissue section with little background. (B) Negative control using a sense probe shows no unspecific signal in the tissue. (C) Example of unspecific background coloration observed throughout the tissue.

5. Related procedures and future research

5.1 Related methods:

The detection method described here is amenable to several variations and amendments. In addition to cryopreserved tissues, RISH can be performed on wax-embedded samples (Moorman et al., 2001). This can help preserve the tissue if its structure is likely to be damaged by freezing, however the signal obtained by RISH can be lower than when using cryosections.

RISH as described here can be adapted to detect more than one target using probes labelled with different tags. The detection of target sequences also recently benefited for the availability of custom made locked nucleic acid ('LNA') oligonucleotides which can provide increased sensitivity and improved hybridisation affinity (Thomsen et al., 2005). LNAs are particularly used to study miRNA expression in cells and tissues (Kloosterman et al., 2006).

The RISH approach described in this chapter is also compatible with subsequent immunodetection of specific antigens by immunofluorescence for instance (Sottile et al., 2006). The combination of multiple markers, at the RNA and protein levels, enables a more elaborated characterisation of target cell populations and their interaction with other cell types within the tissue of interest.

5.2 Stem cell research:

As discussed in the introduction, RISH can give access to a range of information for the study of stem cell-specific transcripts: whether there are any cells in the tissue expressing these markers, how many cells are positive, where they are located within the tissue (Alcock & Sottile, 2009).

In addition to the identification of stem cell populations in a tissue through the use of probes specific for stem cell markers, RISH offers another prime application: the study of exogenous stem cell populations in xenograft models. Careful design of the probe can offer species-specificity, allowing donor-derived transcripts to be specifically detected using differences in sequence.

RISH is also useful to study stem cells in ex vivo models. As described here for the analysis of stem cells within tissue sections, RISH is a technique which is also effective for the analysis of stem cell-derived organoids generated in vitro such as embryoid bodies, neurospheres or mammospheres. Cell aggregates can be embedded in agarose first for easier manipulation at the cryopreservation stage, and the agarose mass can then be processed as a piece of tissue following to the protocol presented above. RISH can equally be used to study gene expression changes in cellularised scaffolds loaded with stem cell populations. Although the sample sectioning steps may require optimisation depending on the nature of the scaffold and properties of the biomaterial used, the RISH technique can be expected to occupy a significant place in the study of novel stem cell-based tissue engineering approaches.

6. Acknowledgements:

VS is grateful to the Anne McLaren Fellowship scheme (University of Nottingham) and to the Alzheimer's Society for their support, past and present.

7. References

Alcock, J. & Sottile, V. (2009) Dynamic distribution and stem cell characteristics of Sox1-expressing cells in the cerebellar cortex. *Cell Res.* 19(12):1324-33.

Gandrillon, O., Solari, F., Legrand, C., Jurdic, P., Samarut, J. (1996) A rapid and convenient method to prepare DIG-labelled RNA probes for use in non-radioactive in situ hybridization. *Mol Cell Probes.* 10(1):51-5.

Kloosterman, W.P., Wienholds, E., de Bruijn, E., Kauppinen, S., Plasterk, R.H. (2006) In situ detection of miRNAs in animal embryos using LNA-modified oligonucleotide probes. *Nat Methods* 3(1):27-9.

Moorman, A.F., Houweling, A.C., et al. (2001) Sensitive nonradioactive detection of mRNA in tissue sections: novel application of the whole-mount in situ hybridization protocol. *J Histochem Cytochem.* 49(1):1-8.

Ponder, B.A. & Wilkinson, M.M. (1981) Inhibition of endogenous tissue alkaline phosphatase with the use of alkaline phosphatase conjugates in immunohistochemistry. *J Histochem Cytochem.* 29(8):981-984.

Sottile, V., Li, M., Scotting, P. (2006) Stem cell marker expression in the Bergmann glia population of the adult mouse brain. *Brain Res.* 12,1099(1):8-17

Thomsen, R., Nielsen, P.S., Jensen, T.H. (2005) Dramatically improved RNA in situ hybridization signals using LNA-modified probes. *RNA* 11(11):1745-1748.

Wilkinson, D.G. (1995) RNA detection using non-radioactive in situ hybridization. Curr *Opin Biotechnol.* 6(1):20-3.

Part 3

Clinical Advances in Diagnosis

7

Clinical Application of Automatic Gene Chip Analyzer (WEnCA-Chipball) for Mutant KRAS Detection in Peripheral Circulating Tumor Cells of Cancer Patients

Suz-Kai Hsiung[1,2], Shiu-Ru Lin[1,2], Hui-Jen Chang[1,2], Yi-Fang Chen[3], and Ming-Yii Huang[4,5]

[1]*Department of Medical Research, Fooyin University Hospital, Pingtung,*
[2]*School of Medical and Health Science, Fooyin University, Koahsiung,*
[3]*Gene Target Technology Co.Ltd, Koahsiung,*
[4]*Department of Radiation Oncology, Kaohsiung Medical University Hospital,Kaohsiung,*
[5]*Department of Radiation Oncology, Faculty of Medicine, College of Medicine, Kaohsiung Medical University, Kaohsiung*
Taiwan, ROC

1. Introduction

KRAS is an important oncogene that participates in the mitogen-activated protein kinase (MAPK) pathway. The MAPK pathway is involved in various cellular functions, including cell proliferation, differentiation and migration. Mutations in KRAS are found in many types of malignancies including lung cancer (Fong et al., 1998; Slebos & Rodenhuis, 1989; Chen et al., 2003; Siegfried et al., 1997), colorectal cancer (Calistri et al., 2006; Weijenberg et al., 2008; Wang et al., 2007), and pancreatic cancer (Smit et al., 1988; Gocke et al., 1997). As early as 1989, Slebos *et al.* have identified that the KRAS mutation status can be used for lung cancer detection or prognosis prediction (Slebos & Rodenhuis, 1989). In 1995, Yakubovskaya *et al.* detected 12 different KRAS mutations in nearly 60% of tissue specimens of non-small cell lung cancer (NSCLC) patients (Yakubovskaya et al., 1995). As for pancreatic, stomach and breast cancers, there have been a number of studies reporting KRAS mutations (Smit et al., 1988; Gocke et al., 1997; Deramaudt & Rustgi, 2005; Carstens et al., 1988; Lee et al., 2003; Shen et al., 2008). The predictive value of KRAS mutation in metastatic colorectal cancer patients treated with cetuximab plus chemotherapy has recently been shown in that patients with tumor KRAS mutation were resistant to cetuximab and had shorter progression survival and overall survival times compared with patients without mutation (Lievre et al., 2006; Lievre et al., 2008). Additionally, NCCNClinical Practice Guidelines in Oncology Version 3, 2008, strongly recommends KRAS genotyping of tumor tissue (either primary tumor or metastasis) in all patients with metastatic colorectal cancer before treatment with epidermal growth factor receptor (EGFR) inhibitors. KRAS mutational analysis has advantages over attempts to predict responsiveness to anti-EGFR antibodies.

To date, detection of KRAS mutations are limited to traditional techniques. The traditional techniques such as direct sequencing, polymerase chain reaction and restriction fragment length polymorphism are complicated and can easily be used only in tissue samples, which limits KRAS mutation detection in clinical applications. In order to improve the mutant KRAS detection efficiency, we successfully developed an Activating KRAS Detection Chip and colorimetric membrane array (CLMA) technique capable of detecting KRAS mutation status by screening circulating carcinoma cells in the surrounding bloodstream (Chen et al., 2005; Wang et al., 2006; Chong et al., 2007; Yang et al., 2009; Yen et al., 2009; Yang et al., 2010). However, the sensitivity still needs further improvement. In addition, the digoxigenin enzyme used on the colorimetric gene chip platform is too costly for routine laboratory diagnosis, and the high criteria of the operation techniques have prevented its widespread availability for clinical applications. Therefore, we have developed the next generation gene chip operation platform named the weighted enzymatic chip array (WEnCA), as shown in figure 1. The technical difference between the WEnCA and CLMA system includes the different weighted value for each gene target on the gene chip of the WEnCA system, dependent on the importance of each gene during the cancer development process. Furthermore, the conventional digoxigenin system was replaced by the biotin-avidin enzyme system to lower the cost. The manual operation process of the WEnCA system has been successful established and published (Tsao et al., 2010; Yen et al., 2010). The proposed platform may benefit post-operative patients or facilitate patient follow-ups, and also bring breakthrough improvements in the prediction and evaluation of the therapeutic effects of anti-EFGR drugs. However, as the technical threshold of chip array remained relatively high, human errors during clinical examinations were commonly seen, and the propagation of associating operations somehow became restricted.

The analysis of gene overexpression has led to fundamental progress and clinical advances in the diagnosis of disease (Chen et al., 2005; Wang et al., 2006). The techniques that are commonly used to study gene overexpression include Northern blot, reverse transcriptase *polymerase chain reaction* (RT-PCR), and real-time PCR (Chong et al., 2007; Yen et al., 2009; Yanget al., 2009). Since Northern blot involves complex steps and a large numbers of samples, its application is limited to research instead of clinical diagnosis. On the other hand, since RT-PCR and real-time PCR are performed through a series of simple steps, they are applied extensively for the detection of a single gene, as with the hepatitis virus and infectious pathogens (Yang et al., 2010; Tsao et al., 2010). Although the invention of PCR ranks as one of the greatest discoveries of all time, most PCR techniques have a few common problems: (1) contamination, i.e., false positive results from oversensitive detection of, say, aerosolized DNA or previous sample carry-over; (2) RT-PCR is regarded as only semi-quantitative, since it is difficult to control the efficiency of sequence amplification when comparing different samples; and (3) interference is caused by annealing between the primers. RT-PCR or real-time PCR is used extensively in the detection of a single-gene target (Yen et al., 2010; Harder et al., 2009; Sheu et al., 2006). For the detection of multiple targets or gene clusters, PCR-related techniques tend to have the disadvantages of being time-consuming, cumbersome and costly.

The rapid development of biotechnology in recent years has made gene chips an important tool in clinical diagnosis or drug efficacy evaluation (Popovtzer et al., 2008). Our previous study has developed and evaluated a membrane array-based method for simultaneously detecting the expression levels of multiple mRNA markers from circulating cancer cells in the peripheral blood for cancer diagnosis (Chen et al., 2006). In those studies, the expression levels of molecular markers were simultaneously evaluated by RT-PCR and membrane array. Data obtained from RT-PCR and membrane array were subjected to linear regression analysis, revealing a high degree of correlation between the results of these two methods (r=0.979, P<0.0001) (Chen et al., 2006). However, even though the array-based chip technology has proven to be a powerful platform for gene overexpression analysis, some drawbacks still exists and may hinder its practical applications. Two of the critical issues are its tedious sample pretreatment and time-consuming hybridization process. Sample pretreatment process including cell lysis, DNA/RNA extraction and several tedious washing process requiring well-trained personnel and specific instruments, which indicate that the array methods can be only operated in a central lab or medical center, and also limited its applicability for clinical diagnosis. Besides, the manual operation may cause the fragile RNA samples to be degraded by the surrounding RNases (Chirgwin et al., 1979; Chomczynski, 1993). Recently, magnetic bead-based extraction has been widely employed for high-quality RNA extraction. When compared with the conventional methods, the high-quality RNA samples can be stably extracted by simply applying an external magnetic field. Regarding to the hybridization process, it is another time-consuming process due to slow diffusion between target and immobilized probes for conventional array technology. It has been reported that proper mixing is important to achieve an efficient hybridization (Southern et al., 1999). The rotation of the array was reported to be effective in reduction of hybridization time (Chee et al., 1996). Regarding to the above-mentioned issues, there is a great need to develop a rapid and automatic sample pretreatment platform to isolate specific RNA samples from cells and efficient hybridization for array-based methods.

With the rapid advancements in the field of fluid manipulation technology, and especially biomedicine development in recent years, automated and rapid biomedical analysis is now considered to offer the greatest potential and market value (Chen et al., 2003; Siegfried et al., 1997). In terms of biomedical applications, the automatic biomedical analysis system that integrated of several fluid manipulation device including transportation, mixing and heating, which based on the "Lab-on-a-chip" concept, has the advantages of high detection sensitivity, portability, low sample/test sample consumption, low power consumption, compact size, and low cost. Compared to the conventional analysis techniques, it represents a significant breakthrough. With a variety of innovative techniques, a wide range of precision fluid manipulation devices have been integrated to control biological fluids such as whole blood, reagents and buffers, to reduce the size of the biochemical analytical instruments, and integrate the processes into a one-step automated system that facilitates the rapid conducting of biomedical analysis from samples to results (Calistri et al., 2006). In this research, the integrated fluid manipulation technology is adopted to operate the WEnCA platform (figure 1), significantly reduce detection time and errors arising from human operation. Thus, the bottleneck that was preventing the commercialization of the chip detection technique has been overcome. In the current study, we developed an automatic gene chip analyzer which named Chipball (as shown in Fig. 3b), and we have introduced an automatic WEnCA operating platform to improve the manual operations. The system is designated the 'WEnCA-Chipball system', as shown in figure 2. In order to understand the difference between test results obtained by operating the WEnCA-Chipball and WEnCA-manual systems, and to assess the clinical applications of the WEnCA-Chipball system a number of screenings were evaluated. The WEnCA-Chipball platform can be automatically operated to effectively reduce the manual errors and limitations due to current technical criteria.

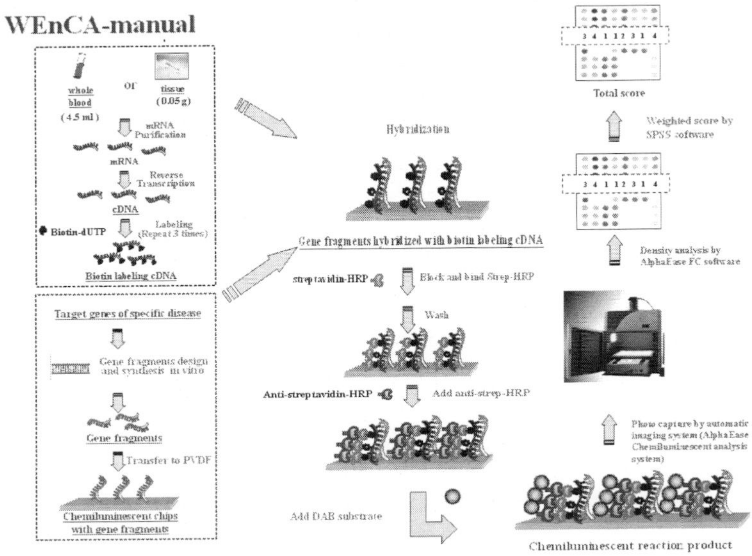

Fig. 1. The manual operation platform of Weighted Enzymatic Chip array (WEnCA) (Hsiung, et al., 2009).

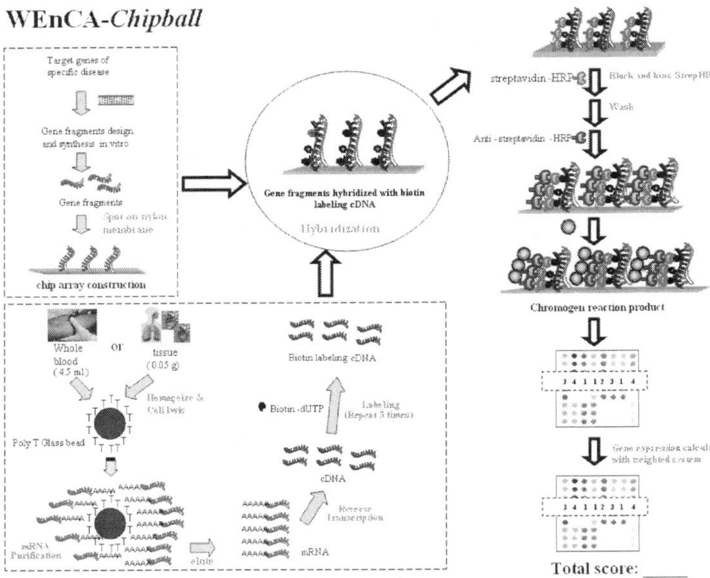

Fig. 2. The automatic WEnCA-*Chipball* operation platform (Hsiung, et al., 2009).

In addition, the activated KRAS expression in blood samples of 209 lung cancer patients was determined according to the experimental procedure shown in Figure 3 and then analyzed by both WEnCA-manual and WEnCA-Chipball; the results were compared and the clinical applicability of WEnCA-Chipball was defined. Further comparisons were performed on the sensitivity, the specificity and the accuracy of the WEnCA-manual and WEnCA-Chipball; the application, the operation time, and the cost of the two platforms were investigated to evaluate the clinical applicability potential of WEnCA-Chipball.

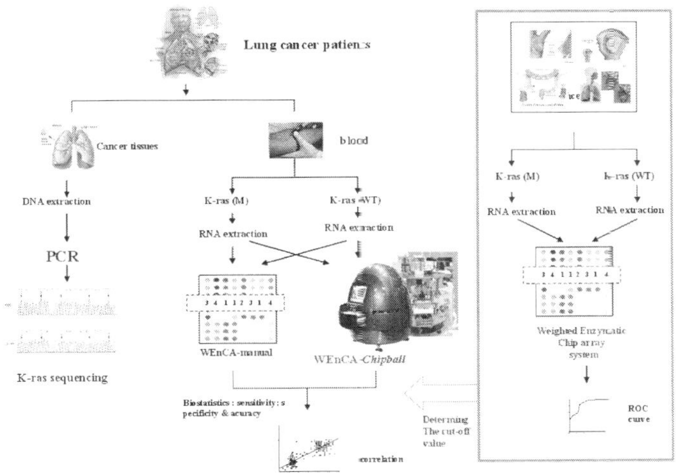

(a)

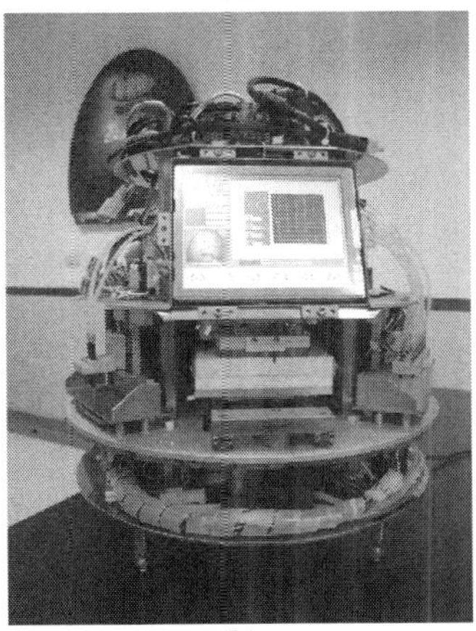

(b)

Fig. 3. (a) The research flow chart of current study (Hsiung, et al., 2009). (b) Photograph of the proposed automatic gene chip analyzer.

2. Materials and methods

2.1 Specimens collection

Initially, cancer tissues from two hundreds selected cancer patients including 85 patients with breast cancer, 64 patients with colorectal cancer (CRC), and 51 patients with non-small cell lung cancer (NSCLC) cancer who had undergone surgical resection or biopsy between January 2007 and December 2008 were enrolled into this study. The data from the 200 cancerous patients were used for the analysis of sensitivity, specificity and diagnostic accuracy of WEnCA-*Chipball*. Tissue samples from various cancer patients were divided into two groups, one group of 100 cancer tissues with *KRAS* mutation including 32 CRCs, 51 breast cancers and 17 NSCLCs and the other group of 100 cancer tissues without *KRAS* mutation including 32 CRCs, 34 breast cancers and 34 NSCLCs were used to determine the cut-off-value of weighted enzymatic chip array method for further circulating tumor cells (CTCs) analysis of 209 lung cancer patients. In order to clinically evaluate and compare both two systems, CLMA and WEnCA-Chipball; blood specimens were collected within test tubes containing anticoagulant sodium citrate from 209 lung cancer patients. To avoid contamination of skin cells, the blood sample was taken via an intravenous catheter, plus the first few milliliters of blood were discarded. Total RNA was immediately extracted from the peripheral whole blood, and then served as a template for cDNA synthesis. Sample acquisition and subsequent usage were approved by the Institutional Review Boards of three hospitals. Written informed consent was obtained from all participants.

2.2 Total RNA isolation and cDNA synthesis

Total RNA was isolated from the collected cancer tissue specimens using the acid - quanidium-phenol-chloroform (AGPC) method according to the standard protocol. The RNA concentration was determined spectrophotometrically based on the absorbance at 260 nm. First-strand cDNA was synthesized from total RNA using the Advantage RT-PCR kit (Promega, Madison, WI) and then reverse transcription was performed in a reaction mixture consisting of Transcription Optimized Buffer, 25 mg=mL Oligo (dT)15, Primer, 100mM=L PCR Nucleotide Mix, 200 mM=L MLV Reverse Transcriptase, and 25 mL Recombinant RNasin Ribonuclease Inhibitor. The reaction mixtures were incubated at 42°C for 2 h, heated to 95°C for 5 min, and then stored at 48°C until the analysis.

2.3 Establishment of membrane array-based method

The rapid development of biotechnology in recent years has made gene chips an important tool in clinical diagnosis or drug efficacy assessment (Popovtzer et al., 2008). Visual OMP3 (Oligonucleotide Modeling Platform, DNA Software, Ann Arbor, MN) was used to design probes for each target gene and β-actin, the latter of which was used as an internal control. The probe selection criteria included strong mismatch discrimination, minimal or no secondary structure, signal strength at the assay temperature, and lack of cross-hybridization. The oligonucleotide probes were then synthesized according to the designed sequences, purified, and controlled before being grafted onto the substracts. The newly synthesized oligonucleotide fragments were dissolved in distilled water to a concentration of 20 mM, applied to a BioJet Plus 3000 nL dispensing system (BioDot, Irvine, CA), which blotted the selected target oligonucleotides and TB (Mycobacterium tuberculosis) and the β-actin control sequentially (0.05 μL per spot and 1.5 mm between spots) on SuPerCharge nylon membrane (Schleicher and Schuell, Dassel, Germany) in triplicate. Dimethyl sulfoxide

(DMSO) was also dispensed onto the membrane as a blank control. In addition, the housekeeping gene was β-actin while the bacterial gene was derived from Mycobacterium tuberculosis. Both served as positive and negative controls, respectively, and blotted on the membrane. After rapid drying and cross-linking procedures, the preparation of membrane array for target genes expression was accomplished. Our previous study developed and evaluated a membrane array-based method simultaneously detecting the expression levels of multiple mRNA markers from circulating cancer cells in peripheral blood for cancer diagnosis (Wang et al., 2006; Yen et al., 2009; Tsao et al. 2010). We have carried out membrane array analysis using normal human adrenal cortical cells with KRAS mutation, and obtained 22 upregulated genes most closely related to the KRAS oncogene through bioinformatic analysis. The Activating KRAS Detection Chip for detecting the activated KRAS from peripheral blood was successfully constructed. Although this method is a convenient way of directly using peripheral blood for detecting KRAS activation, and has achieved major breakthroughs in clinical applications, the sensitivity of this technique is only about 84% (Chen et al., 2005).

The colorimetric membrane array (CLMA) was reported in clinical applications for diagnosis of cancer (Harder et al., 2009; Sheu et al., 2006). By the CLMA method, the interpretation importance of each gene is equally included in the diagnosis and each gene is calculated by the same value; this does not evaluate or differentiate the importance of each gene for specific disease diagnosis. That is a major limitation of this technique in clinical application (Tsao et al., 2010). In addition, the cost of the digoxigenin enzyme used on the CLMA platform was too high for routine laboratory diagnosis, and the high criteria of the operation techniques prevented its widespread availability for clinical applications.

Therefore, as mentioned above, our team developed a new generation gene chip operation platform designated as WEnCA. The technical difference between the WEnCA system and the conventional membrane array includes the different weighted value for each gene target on the gene chip, dependent on the importance of each gene during the carcinogenesis of cancer. Furthermore, the conventional digoxigenin system was replaced by the biotin-avidin enzyme system to lower costs.

2.4 Configuration of integrated automatic gene chip analyzer

In order to realize the concept of automatic performing the gene chip operation procedure from samples to images, an integration system composed of several modules including fluid manipulation, temperature controlling, magnetic controlling, actuation, image acquiring and operation platform was investigated, which can perform the critical procedure of array-based gene chip operation such as sample pretreatment, DNA/mRNA purification, reverse transcription, probe labeling and hybridization process, and the image of the gene chip can be acquired automatically after the hybridization as well. The framework of the proposed automatic gene chip analyzer was shown in Fig. 4. Regarding to the Lab-on-chip concept, we have designed an operation platform to provide the interaction fields of the fluid such as samples and reagents, and gene chip operation. The operation platform also was considered as an interface between the sample/reagents and instrument, so that the fluid can be manipulated by utilizing the external devices. In addition, a vessel device contains corresponding reagents to specific process was included in the system. Briefly, the major functions of the proposed system were samples/reagents manipulation, cell lysis, mRNA collection/purification, reverse transcription, probe labeling, and gene chip hybridization.

The images of gene expression can be acquired accordingly. As mentioned above, several modules were designed to achieve these functions. For sample/reagents transporting, samples and reagents can be manipulated and transported through the micro piezoelectric pump device, the volume can be controlled precisely and the operation process can be performed in sequence. By utilizing the fluid manipulation device, the reagents can be sucked and transported from the vessel to the operation platform in specific area, and the reactants can be manipulated between the reaction chambers, the wasted fluid also can be excluded from the operation platform accordingly. Since the temperature control is the critical issue for the gene chip operation, the temperature of each operation process such as cell lysis and hybridization can also be controlled by embedded heaters and thermal sensors, the temperatures, heating/cooling rates and thermal distribution can be well controlled. Compare to the time-consuming and instrument-intensive conventional method of mRNA purification, the commercial magnetic beads were utilized to realize the automatic mRNA purification in this system, and a magnetic controlling device was designed for the magnetic beads manipulation, so that the mRNA can be collected accordingly. Furthermore, for the purpose of interaction enhancing, an active mixing device for shaking mechanism was added into the system. By utilizing the simplified design, the operation platform can be rotated to generate the mixing effect of the samples and reagents inside the operation platform. Finally, the images of the gene chip representing the gene expression can be obtained after all the operation process, and the images can be recorded by the image acquiring device, which including the CCD (Charged-couple device) and image analysis software. The image data can be stored and transmitted to the central laboratory via internet.

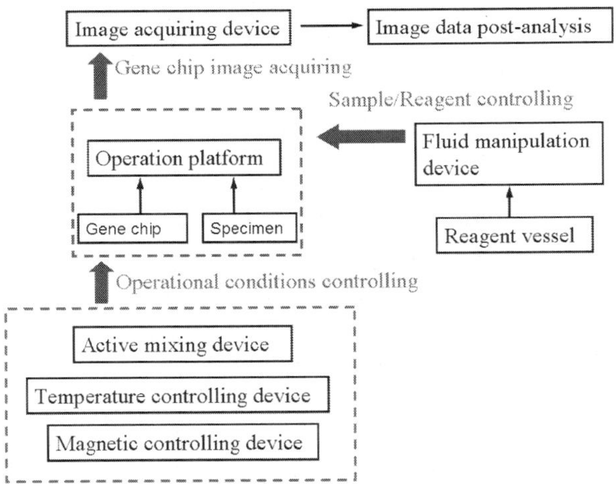

Fig. 4. The framework of the proposed automatic gene chip analyzer.

2.5 Design of the operation platform

In this study, for the purpose to provide the interface between sample/reagents and modules which can control the critical parameters of each process, an operation platform has been designed to perform the sample manipulation and gene analysis. For easy fabrication and low cost, the material utilized for the operation platform was Polymethylmethacrylate (PMMA), the width and length of the substrate was 10 cm each, and the thickness was 1 cm. As shown in Fig. 5, we have divided the platform into four chambers for specific operation process, including sample pretreatment area, sample purification area, transcription and probe labeling area, and hybridization area. The four areas were fabricated by a micro-milling machine, the diameter and depth of each chamber has been calculated precisely to ensure the volume was sufficient for each process. Initially, a membrane array device with specific gene probes was first integrated into the hybridization area, and then the operation platform was placed onto a telescopic loading tray structure, which was designed in this system for the orientation and operation of the platform with external controlling device. Each area on the platform was corresponding to an external module for its specific operation process. For instance, a temperature controlling device embedded onto the tray structure including a set of heater and thermal sensor was placed underneath the sample pretreatment area for cell lysis application. We have set up three temperature controlling device corresponding to area I, III and IV for the adjustment of operation temperature, and a simple design of magnet lift-up mechanism to control the magnetic force and collect the magnetic beads in area II for mRNA purifying application. In order to transport the reagents into the operation chamber and manipulate the sample/reagents between the chambers, several commercial piezoelectric pumps were utilized. Sets of sucking needles were inserted into the reagent vessels and operation chamber before the piezoelectric pumps were activated, and corresponding samples/reagents can be transported to the specific chamber by activating specific pump. After the samples/reagents transportation in each chamber, a mixing mechanism was required for the sample interactions. The tray structure and operation platform can be clockwise rotated simultaneously by utilizing a cam and electric motor device. The rotation speed can be adjusted within a dynamic range from 50 to 200 rpm. As shown in fig. 5, the

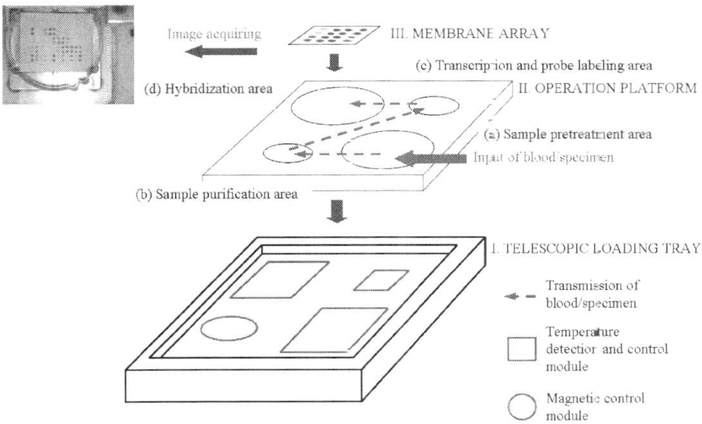

Fig. 5. Illustration of the fluidic operation platform, which divided into four areas, the blood/specimen can be operated sequentially through the four operation process. The membrane array device was firstly integrated into the hybridization area, and then the operation platform was placed onto the telescopic loading tray for further external control.

image of the gene expression on the gene chip can be obtained after finished all operation process. The darkness of each probe can reveal the interaction between pretreated DNA/RNA sample and probe with specific sequence on gene chip. The image can be recorded by a CCD, and then the recorded image can be sent to the commercial image analysis software for further analysis. The darkness of each probe can reveal the expression of specific sequence for the gene information analysis.

2.6 Operating procedure of automatic gene chip analyzer

Firstly, a sample pretreatment process from whole blood to mRNA was required, as shown in Fig. 6. In order to breakdown the sample cells and isolate mRNA from the specimen, the fluid manipulation device delivers the whole blood and lysis buffer to the first reaction chamber (sample pretreatment area), as shown in Fig. 6(a). The fluid manipulation device also delivered the magnetic beads, binding buffer, and washing buffer from reagent vessel to the first reaction chamber (Fig. 6b). The samples were then mixed by the active mixing device to ensure that the samples react effectively and to enhance the mRNA conjugation with the magnetic beads. As shown in Fig. 6(c), biotin poly dT and streptavidin magnetic beads were used to isolate the mRNA. The reacted samples and the beads that have conjugated mRNA onto the surface can then be delivered to the second reaction chamber (sample purification area) by the fluid manipulation device. In this area, magnetic controlling device was utilized to manipulate magnetic beads and to separate the target mRNA samples from the surroundings (Fig. 6d). The mRNA-conjugated magnetic beads can be collected by the external magnet and then washing buffer can be transported into the area by the fluid manipulation device for further washing process (as Fig. 6e). The remaining waste fluid excluding the mRNA-conjugated beads can be transported by the fluid manipulation device to the waste collection area. The elution buffer was then delivered through the fluid manipulation device to the reaction chamber for the further mixing reaction. The mRNA-conjugated magnetic beads were demagnetized and suspended in the elution buffer after the external magnet descended. As shown in Fig. 6(f), after the mixing and elution process, the magnet activated again to separate the beads and target mRNA samples. Hence the buffer contained the purified mRNA samples that have been extracted and released were then delivered through the fluid manipulation device to the third reaction chamber (transcription and probe labeling area). The required temperature for the transcription can be regulated by the temperature controlling device allowing the mRNA to be converted into stable cDNA for chromogen labeling for the bio-molecular test target. The reacted samples and buffer solution were then delivered by the fluid manipulation device to the hybridization area for the hybridization process. Meanwhile, prior to deliver the samples to the hybridization area, the gene chip was placed in the hybridization area for the pre-hybridization procedure. The labeled cDNA samples then entered the reaction chamber contained the Express Hyb hybridization solution where the required temperature for the hybridization reaction was regulated by the temperature controlling device. Subsequently, samples and reagents including biotin-labeling mixture, washing buffer, blocking buffer, strepavidin conjugation, detection buffer, DAB, and ddH_2O were delivered into the chamber through the fluid manipulation device. Finally, after all processes of the hybridization reaction were completed, the image of gene chip can be obtained and acquired by the image acquiring device and image/information processing system for the further gene expression information analysis. A detailed operation process can be seen in Table 1. As the result, the overall operation time can be decreased less than 8 hours, which was shorten by 70%

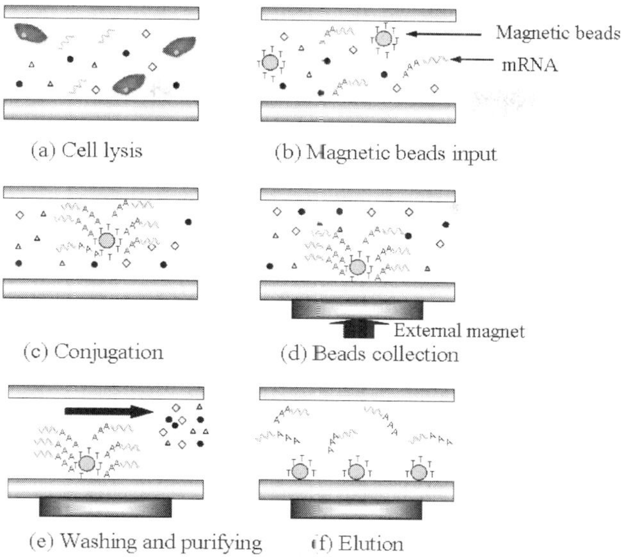

Fig. 6. Illustration of the purifying and separation process from whole blood to mRNA samples.

Areas	Reagents	Volume (ml)	Time (min)	Temperature (°C)
Sample Pretreatment Area	Lysis Solution	1.02	15	60
	Whole Blood	4		
	Magnetic Beads	0.25	1	Room Temperature
	Binding Solution	0.25	4	
Sample Purification Area	Washing Buffer I	0.25	3	
	Washing Buffer II	0.25	3	
	Elution Solution	0.25	5	
Transcription and Probe Labeling Area	RT Reagents	0.25	40/5	42/75
	DIG-Labeling solution	0.25	60	37
Hybridization Area	Hybridization solution	3	30	42
	Washing Buffer I	2	10	
	Washing Buffer II	2	10	Room Temperature
	Washing Buffer III	2	10	
	Blocking Buffer	2	10	
	Anti-DIG AP Buffer	5	10	
	Detection Buffer	2	10	
	NBT/BCIP	1	3	

Table 1. Detailed operation process of the automatic gene chip analyzer.

when compared to the conventional manual method, and also represented the great potentials and advantages of the proposed automatic gene chip analyzer for gene diagnosis applications.

3. Results

3.1 Comparison between colorimetric membrane array and weighted enzymatic chip array method

In order to verify the sensitivity, specificity and accuracy of the activating KRAS detection chip, we enrolled 209 NSCLC patients (pathologically proved) to detect the activating KRAS from their peripheral blood specimens. All specimens were tested by both the CLMA and WEnCA methods. We also analyzed tissue samples of 209 cases of patients with KRAS mutations by a traditional PCR-combing direct sequencing method to be a standard reference. Experimental results indicated that there were 71 cases with KRAS mutations by sequencing analysis, and a total of 59 patients tested positive by the CLMA, while the WEnCA tested positive in a total of 66 cases. Moreover, in 138 NSCLC cases without KRAS mutation, CLMA detected 133 cases as negative, and WEnCA detected 130 cases as negative. After statistical analysis, the CLMA sensitivity was 83%, specificity 96%; and WEnCA sensitivity could be raised to be 93%, while the specificity still is maintained at around 94%. The examinational comparison results also compared the ability of peripheral blood detection results of two technology platforms where 3 cancer cells /cc blood were detected by the WEnCA, and 5 cancer cells /cc blood by the CLMA. These findings suggest that the WEnCA platform has a higher detection rate for activated KRAS oncogene, and great potential for further investigation and clinical application.

To determine the cutoff value of the Activating KRAS Detection Chip by the WEnCA method, we analyzed 200 cancer tissues of which 100 had the KRAS mutation and the others had wild-type KRAS. The 200 tissues collected underwent mRNA extraction and first cDNA labeling before reacting to the Activating KRAS Detection Chip by the WEnCA-manual method. After signal development, each gene spot density was normalized using the density of β-actin on the same chip. Next, the result obtained from the cancer tissue with KRAS mutation was divided by the normalized value obtained from the sample spot of the tissue without mutant KRAS to obtain the ratio. A ratio higher than 2 was defined as being positive for gene overexpression. In terms of analysis using WEnCA, to determine the weighted value of each gene spot, we divided the percentage of each gene overexpression in the 100 cancer tissues with the activating KRAS mutation to provide four classes. The gene spot that showed overexpression in over 80 cancer tissues had a weighted value of 4 (3 in 70−80 cancer tissues, 2 in 60−70 cancer tissues, and 1 in 50−60 cancer tissues). After the reaction through WEnCA, the positive gene spots were multiplied by their respective weighted values to obtain the total score of the chip. Then underwent analysis using the receiver operating characteristic curve can be obtained with a positive reaction cutoff value of 20. Results showed that the sensitivity reached 96% and the specificity reached 97%.

3.2 Detection limitation of the WEnCA-manual and WEnCA-Chipball assay

Evaluating the detection limitation of WEnCA-manual and WEnCA-Chipball system, with the addition of 100, 25 and 12 cancer cells that possessed the activated mutant KRAS into 5cc of blood, which obtained total scores higher than the cutoff value 20 in both systems. In addition, when only 6 cells were added, in which case the total score equaled 8 in WEnCA-manual and 5 in WEnCA-Chipball system, which are both lower than 20. Therefore, no significant difference was found between the detection limitations of the two systems.

3.3 Clinical assessment of the accuracy of WEnCA-manual and WEnCA-chipball system

To further understand the practical clinical detection of the WEnCA-Chipball system, we obtained blood samples of 209 pathology-proven lung cancer patients and analyzed the KRAS pathway-related genes overexpression in those blood specimens by previously constructed Activated KRAS Detection Chip using both the WEnCA-manual and WEnCA-Chipball systems. The paired cancer tissue with KRAS mutational status then served as the reference standard. As shown in Table 2, the results are as follows: 74 cases of the 209 clinical samples were identified with activated KRAS by the WEnCA-manual method, and the WEnCA-Chipball system test results showed in a total of 71 cases. Among them, 66 were positive through WEnCA-manual and 63 through WEnCA-Chipball. Moreover, among the 138 paired cancer tissues with wild type KRAS, 130 were negative through both WEnCA-manual and WEnCA-Chipball system. According to the results, we can obtain the sensitivity, specificity and accuracy of WEnCA-manual were 93%, 94% and 94%; the sensitivity, specificity and accuracy of WEnCA-Chipball were 89%, 94%, and 92%, respectively. As the results in Table 3, using WEnCA-Chipball, the average total score of the positive sample was 6.1 lower and the average total score of the negative sample was 3.9 lower while the overall average total score was 4.7 lower than the WEnCA-manual. Regarding to the operation time, the WEnCA-Chipball system takes 7.5 h to complete all tasks, while the operation time of the WEnCA-manual system is around 72 h, which was approximately 9 folds than the time required for the automatic system. The operating cost of the WEnCA-manual system was approximately 5 times more expensive than that incurred for the WEnCA-Chipball system. There was no difference in the detection limitation between the two systems. We believe that the WEnCA-Chipball operating system has considerable potential in clinical medicine applications.

		WEnCA-Chipball (WEnCA-manual)		
		Negative	Positive	Total
KRAS	Wild Type	130 (130)	8(8)	138
	Mutation	8 (5)	63(66)	71
Total		138 (135)	71(74)	209

Table 2. The sensitivity, specificity and accuracy of WEnCA-Chipball and WEnCA-manual system

Method / Mean score	WEnCA-manual	WEnCA-Chipball	Difference **(Chipball- Manual)**
Positive specimens	46.1	40	-6.1
Negative specimens	13.8	9.9	-3.9
Total specimens	25.2	20.6	-4.7

Table 3. Comparing the total score of Activating KRAS Detection Chip analyzed by WEnCA-manual and WEnCA-Chipball system

4. Discussion

In recent years, target therapy has rapidly developed. Research and development for the targeted therapy drugs, such as Iressa and Cetuximab, have been proven efficient in advanced NSCLC (Thatcher, 2007; Chang, 2008). Many studies report that KRAS mutations are highly-specific independent predictors of response to single-agent EGFR tyrosine kinase inhibitors (Iressa) in advanced NSCLC; and, similarity to anti-EGFR monoclonal antibodies (Cetuximab) alone (Rossi et al., 2009; Tiseo et al., 2010). However, at the present time, therapeutic targets such as HER2/neu, EGFR, KRAS, Raf, etc., are analyzed using RT-PCR combining direct sequencing, fluorescence in situ hybridization (FISH), real-time PCR, and other methods (Hilbe et al., 2003; Cappuzzo et al., 2007; Akkiprik et al., 2008). The above methods have disadvantages such as inadequate sensitivity, and the need to collect patients' cancer tissues as specimens, which make medicinal effect evaluations prior to clinical treatment cumbersome. RT-PCR and real-time PCR are applied for the detection of single genes, and most PCR techniques have a few common problems: (1) contamination, such as false-positive results from oversensitive detection of aerosolized DNA or previous sample carry-over; (2) RT-PCR is regarded as only semi-quantitative, since it is difficult to control the efficiency of sequence amplification when comparing different samples; and, (3) interference is caused by annealing between the primers. RT-PCR or real-time PCR is used extensively in the detection of a single-gene target. For the detection of multiple targets or gene clusters, PCR-related techniques tend to be time-consuming, labor-intensive, and costly. Therefore, the current study successfully developed the WEnCA-Chipball to effectively address and solve those problems.

In the WEnCA-Chipball system, the total operation time from input of samples to completion of the image analysis was about 7.5 h, which is a substantial decrease in time when compared to the three days required for the original manually operated membrane array, and significantly minimizes the occurrence of human errors. The WEnCA-Chipball system not only provides an innovative automatic system for clinical target therapy efficacy evaluation, but also improves the clinical usability and accuracy compared to the manual method. Thus, it has been proven to be a practical means to assess the drug efficacy of clinical target treatment.

The WEnCA-Chipball system developed by this research team not only retains the advantages of the Lab-on-a-chip, but also overcomes the problem of the microfluidic chip's unsuitability for continuous operation and linkage to an interpretation system. As the world's first automatic chip analyzer, it will be useful in the future for the molecular diagnosis of infectious diseases, the detection of CTC through chip replacements, or the assessment of drug efficacy.

5. Future trends

Medical automation technology is the future trend that can reduce labor, operation errors, and time-consumption. WEnCA-Chipball is suited for clinical application to detect mutant KRAS in CTCs before target therapy. The specialized automatic gene chip detecting system would be designed for the fast and accurate detection of KRAS in CTCs in each human cancer specimen. This is the challenge to meet for the years ahead.

The WEnCA-Chipball system, through a built-in computer system, will not only instantly produce the results of the chip analysis but also connect to a global network. The detection results can be transmitted locally in any operation area and stations around the world through common software used in data transmission and interpretation. The station networks around the world can be completed through the prevalent WEnCA-Chipball system. The WEnCA-Chipball system is believed to be capable for extensive applications in clinical medicine, and holds great potential for future development.

6. References

Akkiprik, M.; Celikel, C.A.; Dusunceli, F.; Sonmez, O.; Gulluoglu, B.M.; Sav, A. & Ozer, A. (2008). Relationship between overexpression of ras p21 oncoprotein and K-ras codon 12 and 13 mutations in Turkish colorectal cancer patients. *Turk J Gastroenterol.*, Vol. 19, No. 1, 22-27.

Calistri, D.; Rengucci, C.; Seymour, I.; Leonardi, E.; Truini, M.; Malacarne, D.; Castagnola, P. & Giaretti, W. (2006). KRAS, p53 and BRAF gene mutations and aneuploidy in sporadic colorectal cancer progression *Cell Oncol.*, Vol. 28, No. 4 ,161-166.

Carstens, C.; Messe, E.; Zang K.D. & Blin, N. (1988). Human KRAS oncogene expression in meningioma. *Cancer Lett.*, Vol. 43, No. 1-2, 37-41.

Cappuzzo, F.; Ligorio, C.; Janne, P.A.; Toschi, L.; Rossi, E.; Trisolini, R.; Paioli, D.; Holmes, A.J.; Magrini, E. & Finocchiaro, G (2007). Prospective study of gefitinib in epidermal growth factor receptor fluorescence in situ hybridization-positive/phospho-Akt-positive or never smoker patients with advanced non-small-cell lung cancer: the ONCOBELL trial. *J. Clin. Oncol.,*, Vol. 25, No. 16, 2248-2255.

Chang, A.Y. (2008). The role of gefitinib in the management of Asian patients with non-small cell lung cancer. *Expert Opin. Investig. Drugs*, Vol. 17, No. 3, 401-411.

Chen, C.C.; Hou, M.F.; Wang, J.Y.; Chang, T.W.; Lai, D.Y.; Chen, Y.F.; Hung, S.Y. & Lin, S.R. (2006). Simultaneous detection of multiple mRNA markers CK19, CEA, c-Met, Her2/neu and hMAM with membrane array, an innovative technique with a great potential for breast cancer diagnosis. *Cancer Lett.*, Vol. 240, No. 2, 279-288.

Chen, C.C.; Chang, T.W.; Chen, F.M.; Hou, M.F.; Hung, S.Y.; Chong, I.W.; Lee, S.C.; Zhou, T.H. & Lin, S.R. (2006). Combination of multiple mRNA markers (PTTG1, Survivin, UbcH10 and TK1) in the diagnosis of Taiwanese patients with breast cancer by membrane array. *Oncology*, Vol. 70, No. 6, 438-446.

Chen, Y.F.; Chiu, H.H.; Wu, C.H.; Wang, J.Y.; Chen, F.M.; Tzou, W.H.; Shin, S.J. & Lin, S.R. (2003). Retinoblastoma protein (pRB) was significantly phosphorylated through a Ras-to-MAPK pathway in mutant K-ras stably transfected human adrenocortical cells. *DNA Cell Biol.*, Vol. 22, No. 10, 657-664.

Chen, Y.F.; Wang, J.Y.; Wu, C.H.; Chen, F.M.; Cheng, T.L. & Lin, S.R. (2005). Detection of circulating cancer cells with K-ras oncogene using membrane array. *Cancer Lett.*, Vol. 229, No. 1, 115-122.

Chee, M.; Yang, R.; Hubbell, E.; Berno, A.; Huang, X.C.; Stern, D.; Winkler, J.; Lockhart, D.J.; Morris, M.S. & Fodor, S.P. (1996). Accessing genetic information with high-density DNA arrays. *Science*, Vol. 274, No. 5287, 610-614.

Chirgwin, J.M.; Przybyla, A.E.; MacDonald, R.J. & Rutter, W.J. (1979). Isolation of biologically active ribonucleic acid from sources enriched in ribonuclease. *Biochemistry*, Vol. 18, No. 24, 5294-5299.

Chong, I.W.; Chang, M.Y.; Sheu, C.C.; Wang, C.Y.; Hwang, J.J.; Huang, M.S. & Lin, S.R. (2007). Detection of activated K-ras in non-small cell lung cancer by membrane array: a comparison with direct sequencing. *Oncol. Rep.*, Vol. 18, No. 1, 17-24.

Chomczynski, P. (1993). A reagent for the single-step simultaneous isolation of RNA, DNA and proteins from cell and tissue samples. *Biotechniques*, Vol. 15, No. 3, 532-534.

Deramaudt, T. & Rustgi, A.K. (2005). Mutant KRAS in the initiation of pancreatic cancer. *Biochim. Biophys. Acta*, Vol. 1756, No. 2, 97-101.

Fong, K.M.; Zimmerman, P.V. & Smith, P.J. (1998). KRAS codon 12 mutations in Australian non-small cell lung cancer. *Aust. N. Z. J. Med.*, Vol. 28, No. 2, (184-189).

Gocke, C.D.; Dabbs, D.J.; Benko, F.A. & Silverman, J.F. (1997). KRAS oncogene mutations suggest a common histogenetic origin for pleomorphic giant cell tumor of the pancreas, osteoclastoma of the pancreas, and pancreatic duct adenocarcinoma. *Hum. Pathol.*, Vol. 28, No. 1, 80-83.

Harder, N.; Mora-Bermudez, F.; Godinez, W.J.; Wunsche, A.; Eils, R.; Ellenberg, J. & Rohr, K. (2009). Automatic analysis of dividing cells in live cell movies to detect mitotic delays and correlate phenotypes in time. *Genome Res.*, Vol. 19, No. 11, 2113-2124.

Hilbe, W.; Dlaska, M.; Duba, H.C.; Dirnhofer, S.; Eisterer, W.; Oberwasserlechner, F.; Mildner, A.; Schmid, T.; Kuhr, T. & Woll, E. (2003). Automated real-time PCR to determine K-ras codon 12 mutations in non-small cell lung cancer: comparison with immunohistochemistry and clinico-pathological features. *Int. J. Oncol.*, Vol. 23, No. 4, 1121-1126.

Hsiung, S.K.; Chang, H.J.; Yang, M.J.; Chang, M.S.; Tsao, D.A.; Chiu, H.H.; Chen, Y.F.; Cheng, T.L. & Lin, S.R. (2009). A novel technique for detecting the therapeutic target, KRAS mutant, from peripheral blood using the automatic chipball device with weighted enzymatic chip array. *Fooyin J. Health Sci.*, Vol. 1, No. 2, 72-80.

Lee, S.H.; Lee, J.W.; Soung, Y.H.; Kim, H.S.; Park, W.S.; Kim, S.Y.; Lee, J.H.; Park, J.Y.; Cho, Y.G. & Kim, C.J. (2003). BRAF and KRAS mutations in stomach cancer. *Oncogene*, Vol. 22, No. 44, 6942-6945.

Lievre, A.; Bachet, J.B.; Le Corre, D.; Boige, V.; Landi, B.; Emile, J.F.; Cote, J.F.; Tomasic, G.; Penna, C. & Ducreux, M. (2006). KRAS mutation status is predictive of response to cetuximab therapy in colorectal cancer. *Cancer Res.*, Vol. 66, No. 8, 3992-3995.

Lievre, A.; Bachet, J.B.; Boige, V.; Cayre, A.; Le Corre, D.; Buc, E.; Ychou, M.; Bouche, O.; Landi, B. & Louvet, C. (2008). KRAS mutations as an independent prognostic factor in patients with advanced colorectal cancer treated with cetuximab. *J. Clin. Oncol.*, Vol. 26, No. 3, 374-379.

Popovtzer, R.; Neufeld, T.; Popovtzer, A.; Rivkin, I.; Margalit, R.; Engel, D.; Nudelman, A.; Rephaeli, A.; Rishpon, J. & Shacham-Diamand, Y. (2008). Electrochemical lab on a chip for high-throughput analysis of anticancer drugs efficiency. *Nanomedicine*, Vol. 4, No. 2, 121-126.

Rossi, A.; Galetta, D. & Gridelli, C. (2009). Biological prognostic and predictive factors in lung cancer. *Oncology*, Vol. 77, No. 1, 90-96.

Sheu, C.C.; Yu, Y.P.; Tsai, J.R.; Chang, M.Y.; Lin, S.R.; Hwang, J.J. & Chong, I.W. (2006). Development of a membrane array-based multimarker assay for detection of circulating cancer cells in patients with non-small cell lung cancer. *Int. J. Cancer*, Vol. 119, No. 6, 1419-1426.

Shen, C.H.; Chen, H.Y.; Lin, M.S.; Li, F.Y.; Chang, C.C.; Kuo, M.L.; Settleman, J. & Chen, R.H. (2008). Breast tumor kinase phosphorylates p190RhoGAP to regulate rho and ras and promote breast carcinoma growth, migration, and invasion. *Cancer Res.*, Vol. 68, No. 19, 7779-7787.

Slebos, R.J. & Rodenhuis, S. (1989). The molecular genetics of human lung cancer. *Eur. Respir. J.*, Vol. 2, No. 5, 461-469.

Southern, E.; Mir, K. & Shchepinov, M. (1999). Molecular interactions on microarrays. *Nat. Genet.*, Vol. 21, 5-9.

Siegfried, J.M.; Gillespie, A.T.; Mera, R.; Casey, T.J.; Keohavong, P.; Testa, J.R. & Hunt, J.D. (1997). Prognostic value of specific KRAS mutations in lung adenocarcinomas. *Cancer Epidemiol. Biomarkers Prev.*, Vol. 6, No. 10, 841-847.

Smit, V.T.; Boot, A.J.; Smits, A.M.; Fleuren, G.J.; Cornelisse, C.J. & Bos, J.L. (1988). KRAS codon 12 mutations occur very frequently in pancreatic adenocarcinomas. *Nucleic Acids Res.*, Vol. 16, No. 16, 7773-7782.

Thatcher, N. (2007). The place of targeted therapy in the patient management of non-small cell lung cancer. *Lung Cancer*, Vol. 57, No.2, S18-23.

Tiseo, M.; Rossi, G.; Capelletti, M.; Sartori, G.; Spiritelli, E.; Marchioni, A.; Bozzetti, C.; De Palma, G.; Lagrasta, C. & Campanini, N. (2010). Predictors of gefitinib outcomes in advanced non-small cell lung cancer (NSCLC): study of a comprehensive panel of molecular markers. *Lung Cancer*, Vol. 67, No. 3, 355-360.

Tsao, D.A.; Yang, M.J.; Chang, H.J.; Yen, L.C.; Chiu, H.H.; Hsueh, E.J.; Chen, Y.F. & Lin, S.R. (2010). A fast and convenient new technique to detect the therapeutic target, K-ras mutant, from peripheral blood in non-small cell lung cancer patients. *Lung Cancer*, Vol. 68, No. 1, 51-57.

Weijenberg, M.P.; Aardening, P.W.; de Kok, T.M.; de Goeij, A.F. & van den Brandt, P.A. (2008). Cigarette smoking and KRAS oncogene mutations in sporadic colorectal cancer: results from the Netherlands Cohort Study. *Mutat. Res.*, Vol. 652, No. 1, 54-64.

Wang, J.Y.; Hsieh, J.S.; Lu, C.Y.; Yu, F.J.; Wu, J.Y.; Chen, F.M.; Huang, C.J. & Lin, S.R. (2007). The differentially mutational spectra of the APC, K-ras, and p53 genes in sporadic colorectal cancers from Taiwanese patients. *Hepatogastroenterology*, Vol. 54, No. 80, 2259-2265.

Wang, J.Y.; Yeh, C.S.; Chen, Y.F.; Wu, C.H.; Hsieh, J.S.; Huang, T.J.; Huang, S.Y. & Lin, S.R. (2006). Development and evaluation of a colorimetric membrane-array method for the detection of circulating tumor cells in the peripheral blood of Taiwanese patients with colorectal cancer. *Int. J. Mol. Med.*, Vol. 17, No. 5, 737-747.

Yakubovskaya, M.S.; Spiegelman, V.; Luo, F.C.; Malaev, S.; Salnev, A.; Zborovskaya, I.; Gasparyan, A.; Polotsky, B. & Machaladze, Z. & Trachtenberg, A.C. (1995). High frequency of K-ras mutations in normal appearing lung tissues and sputum of patients with lung cancer. *Int. J. Cancer*, Vol. 63, No. 6, 810-814.

Yang, M.J.; Hsu, C.K.; Chang, H.J.; Yen, L.C.; Tsao, D.A.; Chiu, H.H.; Huang, Y.T.; Chen, Y.F.; Wang, J.Y. & Lin, S.R. (2009). The KRAS mutation is highly correlated with EGFR alterations in patients with non-small cell lung cancer. *Fooyin J. Health Sci.*, Vol. 1, No. 2, 65-71.

Yen, L.C.; Yeh, Y.S.; Chen, C.W.; Wang, H.M. Tsai, H.L.; Lu, C.Y.; Chang, Y.T.; Chu, K.S.; Lin, S.R. & Wang, J.Y. (2009). Detection of KRAS oncogene in peripheral blood as a predictor of the response to cetuximab plus chemotherapy in patients with metastatic colorectal cancer. *Clin. Cancer Res.*, Vol. 15, No. 13, 4508-4513.

Yen, L.C.; Uen, Y.H.; Wu, D.C.; Lu, C.Y.; Yu, F.J.; Wu, I.C.; Lin, S.R. & Wang, J.Y. (2010). Activating KRAS mutations and overexpression of epidermal growth factor receptor as independent predictors in metastatic colorectal cancer patients treated with cetuximab. *Ann. Surg.*, Vol. 251, No. 2, 254-260.

Yang, M.J.; Hsu, C.K.; Chang, H.J.; Yen, L.C.; Tsao, D.A.; Chiu, H.H.; Huang, Y.T.; Chen, Y.F.; Wang, C.Y. & Lin, S.R. (2009). TheKRAS mutation is highly correlated with EGFR alterations in patients with non-small cell lung cancer. *Fooyin J. Health Sci.*, Vol. 1, No. 2, 65-71.

Yang, M.J.; Chiu, H.H.; Wang, H.M.; Yen, L.C.; Tsao, D.A.; Hsiao, C.P.; Chen, Y.F.; Wang, J.Y. & Lin, S.R. (2010). Enhancing detection of circulating tumor cells with activating KRAS oncogene in patients with colorectal cancer by weighted chemiluminescent membrane array method. *Ann. Surg. Oncol.*, Vol. 17, No. 2, 624-633.

8

Statistical Analysis for Recovery of Structure and Function from Brain Images

Michelle Yongmei Wang, Chunxiao Zhou and Jing Xia
University of Illinois at Urbana-Champaign
U.S.A.

1. Introduction

Brain imaging has the potential to advance our understanding of human health and to improve diagnosis and treatment of neurological diseases. Inspired by key questions in neuroscience and medicine, it becomes extremely important to develop statistical methods that can accurately and efficiently recover useful quantitative information from large amounts of brain images. The underlying computational issues are challenging and often hampered by uncertainties in imaging acquisition parameters, the variability of human anatomy and physiology, as well as the nature of the imaging data to be handled such as the presence of noise and correlation, and the sample and data sizes, and so on.

Structural and Functional MRI (sMRI and fMRI) Among the varieties of brain imaging modalities, magnetic resonance imaging (MRI) is primarily a noninvasive imaging technique used in radiology to visualize the brain's structure and function. Two main forms of MRI include: Structural MRI (sMRI) images the anatomy and strucure of the brain (Symms et al., 2004) and provides detailed pictures of the brain's size and shape; functional MRI (fMRI) identifies active regions, patterns of functional connectivities during either tasks specifically designed to study various aspects of brain fundtion or during the resting state (Martijn et al., 2010). The MRI machine is, in essence, a big magnet. As the subject lies in its magnetic field, invisible radio waves are released around the subject. This will result in harmless radio waves bouncing off the different substances that make up the brain. The radio waves are then detected by a computer, which transforms the data into images of the brain's structure and activity. In fMRI, as the subject lies in the MRI machine, simple tasks are given; the MRI then maps what parts of the brain are most active during those tasks compared with activity while the brain is at rest. This allows researchers to understand how the brain functions. This information is used together with the data from the sMRI data to reveal a comprehensive picture of brain structure and function that fit in the overall studies or to allow us to understand how the healthy brain works. The informaiton and fusion of structural and functional MRI can also improve our understanding and the treatment of neurodegenerative diseases and mental disorders such as Alzheimer's disease and schizophrenia.

Brain Morphometry Analysis with Hypothesis Testing from Structural MRI Structural MRI (sMRI), or simply called MRI, scans are usually stored in the format of three-dimensional (3D) voxels. There are several procedures for MRI post-processing, and the two important ones are registration and segmentation. The registration maps an MRI scan to a pre-defined template (i.e. matches anatomical landmarks from different MRI images); this makes the exploration of group differences achievable. The segmentation classifies the voxels of an MRI scan as gray matter, white matter, cerebrospinal fluid, background, or region of interest (ROI); it serves as a foundation form for many analytical tools, including voxel-based morphometry, shape-based morphometry, and cortical thickness measuring, etc.

Volumetry analysis of the whole brain (Buckner et al., 2004) and ROIs (Jack et al., 1997; Wang et al., 2003) have been traditionally used to obtain the measurements of anatomical volumes and to investigate normal or abnormal tissue structure. However, pure volume measures of the brain or ROIs do not reveal the localized regional morphometry of brain structures. In addition, it is based on the definition of regions according to some a prior hypothesis, which, in practice, is not always available. Thus, in general, it limits the ability of a study to identify new and previously unexplored relationships between structural changes. The localization limitation of volumetry analysis can be overcome by methods generally referred to as high-dimensional morphologic analysis, such as voxel-based morphometry (VBM) (Ashburner and Friston, 2000; Chung et al., 2001; Davatzikos, et al., 2001), or surface-based (i.e. shape-based) morphometry (SBM) that examines the corresponding surface vertex locations or shape differences (Shen et al., 2005; Styner et al., 2005; Thompson et al., 2004). The outputs from these methods are statistical parametric maps of the 3D brain volume or the 3D surface of the ROIs, showing differences at each voxel (in VBM) or vertex (in SBM) between the comparison groups. Thus, the subsequent inference of differences among the groups is usually performed through hypothesis testing at each voxel or at each vertex.

The standard parametric test, such as *t*-test or *F*-test, could be used in brain morphometry analysis for simplicity with the assumption that the data to be tested are independent, identically, and normally distributed, for small or medium size samples. When the sample size is large enough, this assumption is not that strict any more. However, in practical neuroimage analysis, the distribution of the data is typically unknown and sample size is quite small, in which case, the nonparametric randomization or permutation tests can be applied for improved accuracy. Permutation tests obtain *p*-values from permutation distributions of a test statistic, rather than from parametric distributions. They belong to the nonparametric "distribution-free" category of hypothesis testing and are thus flexible, and have been used successfully in biomedical image analysis (Nichols & Holmes, 2001; Pantazis, et al., 2004; Zhou et al., 2009). One way to construct the permutation distribution is through exact permutation which enumerates all possible arrangements. Another way is to construct an approximate permutation distribution based on random sampling from all possible permutations (i.e. random permutation). The computational cost is the main disadvantage of exact permutation. Random permutation has the problem of replication and causes more Type I errors. When a large number of repeated tests are needed, it is also computationally expensive to achieve satisfactory *p*-value accuracy. In Section 2, we present our novel moments-based permutation methods, which take advantage of the parametric and nonparametric features for both efficiency and accuracy.

Brain Connectivity Analysis from Functional MRI fMRI is a powerful technique that noninvasively measures and characterizes brain functions in humans under various cognitive and behavioral tasks. One of the most common forms of fMRI is the Blood Oxygen Level-Dependent (BOLD) imaging (Ogawa et al., 1990), measuring the magnetic resonance properties of the blood. As neurons do not have direct energy sources but only get energy from blood, more active neurons will need to be supplied with energy from the blood at a higher rate. Therefore, this BOLD contrast, is able to show which parts of the brain are more active. At a number of different time points over the course of an expeirment, fMRI provides a set of scans (at different depths through the brain) constituting a volume. fMRI data is a time-course of the BOLD intensity for each voxel in the brain.

During fMRI data acquisition, even a light move of a subject's head can cause severe irregularities within the acquired data. To account for these potential movements, a realignment or motion correction procedure needs to be performed on the data (Lindquist, 2008). This usually entails looking for six parameters - three rotations and three translations, that lead the volumes maximally aligned. The next pre-processing step is normalization: each complete set of volumes is normalized to a canonical brain, or the same stereo-tactic space. This is especially useful in multiple subjects studies to account for differences in brain size. Moreover, in order to improve the data signal to noise ratio, a spatial smoothing is often carried out by comvolving a Gaussin kernel with the fMRI data.

A number of analytic methods have been developed for detecting brain activity patterns and how these patterns change in patients with cognitive disorders (Calhoun et al., 2001; McIntosh & Lobaugh, 2004; Worsley & Friston, 1995). A thorough understanding of the neural mechanisms not only requires the accurate delineation of activation regions ("functional segregation or specification") but demands precise description of function in terms of the information flow across networks of areas ("functional integration"). That is, our brain is a newtork: it consistes of spatially distributed, but functionally linked regions that continuously share information with each other. Various approaches have been proposed to extract association information from fMRI datasets, most of which rely on either functional or effective connectivity (Horwitz, 2003). Functional connectivity has been identified as "temporal correlations between spatially remote neurophysiological events" (Friston et al., 1993). In Section 3, we present a novel and general statistical framework for robust and more complete estimation of functional connectivity or brain networks.

Overview In this chapter, we will present the statistical methods we have developed for the problems in the realms of brain morphometry and connectivity from analyzing structural and functional MRI data. The integration of the recovered structure and function from these imaging data may be able to provide complementary information and thus enhance our understanding of how the brain works and how its diseases occur. We will provide an explaination of the problem areas, a description of the statistical techniques involved and a demonstration of results on simulated and real imaging data using these statistical methods.

2. Brain shape morphometry analysis using novel permutation methods

There is increasing evidence that surface shape analysis of brain structures provides new information which is not available by conventional analysis. A critical issue in surface morphometry is the shape description and representation. Various strategies have been investigated recently in the literature, such as (Brechbühler et al., 1995; Thompson et al., 2004; Wang & Staib, 2000). The spherical harmonics (SPHARM) approach using spherical harmonics as basis functions for a parametric surface description was proposed in (Brechbühler et al., 1995). The correspondence across different surfaces is established by aligning the parameterizations via the first order ellipsoid. The present work employs the SPHARM-PDM shape description (Styner et al., 2006), which leads to corresponding location vectors across all surfaces for our subsequent statistical analysis of surface shape. At each corresponding position on the surfaces, we test whether there is a significant mean vector difference between location vectors of two groups. If a hypothesis test leads to a p-value smaller than the pre-chosen α-level, we reject the null hypothesis and conclude that a significant shape difference exists at this surface location. In this chapter, we focus on the surface shape analysis for two groups, though our method can be extended to the multi-group case.

Since the distribution of the location vectors is unknown, only a limited number of subject samples are available, and the same tests are repeated on thousands of locations, we propose to use our hybrid or moments-based permutation approach to the brain shape analysis. This approach takes advantage of nonparametric permutation tests and parametric Pearson distribution approximation for both efficiency and accuracy/flexibility. Specifically, we employ a general theoretical method to derive moments of permutation distribution for any linear test statistics. Here, the term "linear test statistic" refers to a linear function of test statistic coefficients, instead of that of data. An extension of the method to the general weighted v-statistics has also been developed recently in (Zhou et al., 2009). The key idea is to separate the moments of permutation distribution into two parts, permutation of test statistic coefficients and function of the data. We can then obtain the moments without any permutation since the permutation of test statistic coefficients can be derived theoretically. Given the first four moments, the permutation distribution can be well fitted by Pearson distribution series. The p-values are then estimated without any real permutation. For multiple comparison of two-group difference, given the sample size $n_1 = 21$ and $n_2 = 21$, the number of tests is $m = 2000$. $m\times(n_1+n_2)!/\ n_1!/\ n_2! \approx 1.1\times10^{15}$ permutations are needed for an exact permutation test. Even for 20,000 random permutations per test, 4×10^7 permutations are still required. Alternatively, our hybrid or moments-based permutation method using Pearson distribution approximation only involves the calculation of analytically derived first four moments of exact permutation distributions while achieve high accuracy. Instead of calculating the test statistics in factorial scale with exact permutation, our permutation using mean difference test statistic only require $O(n)$ computation cost, where $n = n_1+n_2$.

2.1 Hypothesis

Classical Hypothesis Given registered location vectors across all subjects, surface shape morphometry analysis becomes a two-sample test for equality of means at each surface location. The hypothesis is typically constructed as:

$$H_0:\ \underset{\sim}{\mu_A} = \underset{\sim}{\mu_B} \quad \text{vs.} \quad H_a:\ \underset{\sim}{\mu_A} \neq \underset{\sim}{\mu_B} \tag{1}$$

where $\underset{\sim}{\mu_A} = [\mu_A^{(x)}\ \mu_A^{(y)}\ \mu_A^{(z)}]^T$ and $\underset{\sim}{\mu_B} = [\mu_B^{(x)}\ \mu_B^{(y)}\ \mu_B^{(z)}]^T$ are three dimensional mean vectors of group A and B.

Bioequivalence Hypothesis In many applications, statistical significance is not equivalent to practical significance since smaller differences of two group location vectors can be more statistically significant than the larger ones. Statistical significance means that the observed difference is not a consequence of sampling error. Practical significance indicates whether the difference is large enough to be of value in a practical sense. Statistical significance does not necessarily indicate practical significance because extremely small and non-notable differences can be statistically significant. For example, there are two pairs of observed mean location vectors $(\underset{\sim}{\mu}_{A1}, \underset{\sim}{\mu}_{B1})$ at location 1 and $(\underset{\sim}{\mu}_{A2}, \underset{\sim}{\mu}_{B2})$ at location 2, with $\underset{\sim}{\mu}_{A1} = [1,1,1]^T$, $\underset{\sim}{\mu}_{B1} = [0.999,0.999,0.999]^T$, $\underset{\sim}{\mu}_{A2} = [1,1,1]^T$, and $\underset{\sim}{\mu}_{B2} = [0.7,0.7,0.7]^T$. We assume that the variance of location vectors at location 2 is much larger than that at location 1, and their p-values of the observed mean differences are $p_1 = 0.001$ and $p_2 = 0.01$ respectively. The mean difference at location 1 is physically very small, although it is more statistical significant than the one at location 2. In this case, it is more reasonable to identify practical or physical shape difference at location 2 rather than at location 1. In order to achieve this, we propose to use the multivariate bioequivalence hypothesis test for our surface morphometry analysis:

$$\begin{aligned} H_0: &\ \max\{\left|\mu_A^{(s)} - \mu_B^{(s)}\right|\} \le \Delta, s \in \{x,y,z\} \text{ bioequivalence} \\ H_a: &\ \max\{\left|\mu_A^{(s)} - \mu_B^{(s)}\right|\} > \Delta, s \in \{x,y,z\} \text{ bioinequivalence} \end{aligned} \tag{2}$$

where Δ is the desired threshold. That is, the shape difference is detected as significant if the mean vector difference is large enough in either x, y or z direction. Bioequivalence tests were originally introduced in the pharmaceutical industry to determine the bioequivalence (Brown et al., 1997). Here, we employ bioequivalence concept though for detecting bioinequivalence as in Eq. (2) we constructed, instead of bioequivalence as in the standard pharmaceutical studies.

A permutation test is valid if the observations are exchangeable under the null hypothesis. However, the condition of exchangeability under null hypothesis is not satisfied in hypothesis Eq. (2). We thus propose to utilize a two-step permutation test.

Step 1: $H_0^{(1)}: \ \mu_A^{(s)} = \mu_B^{(s)} + \Delta, s \in \{x,y,z\}$

$$H_a^{(1)}: \ \mu_A^{(x)} > \mu_B^{(x)} + \Delta \ or \ \mu_A^{(y)} > \mu_B^{(y)} + \Delta \ or \ \mu_A^{(z)} > \mu_B^{(z)} + \Delta \tag{3}$$

Step 2: $H_0^{(2)}: \ \mu_A^{(s)} = \mu_B^{(s)} - \Delta, \ s \in \{x,y,z\}$

$$H_a^{(2)}: \ \mu_A^{(x)} < \mu_B^{(x)} - \Delta \ or \ \mu_A^{(y)} < \mu_B^{(y)} - \Delta \ or \ \mu_A^{(z)} < \mu_B^{(z)} - \Delta \tag{4}$$

If a hypothesis test of significance in step 1 (Eq. (3)) or in step 2 (Eq. (4)) gives a p-value lower than the $\alpha/2$-level, we reject the null hypothesis and significant shape difference exists. The total significance level in this case is still α due to the involved two steps in Eq. (3) and Eq. (4). Note that the classical hypothesis is a special case of the bioequivalence hypothesis when $\Delta = 0$. Classical hypothesis is used in applications where statistical and practical significances are consistent. Otherwise bioequivalence test is preferred if there is any non-negligible difference between practical significance and statistical significance.

2.2 New Permutation Approach

Pearson Distribution Series The Pearson distribution series (Pearson I ~ VII) are a family of probability distributions that are more general than the normal distribution (Hubert, 1987). As shown in Fig. 1 (Hahn & Shapiro, 1967), it covers all distributions in the (β1, β2) plane including normal, beta, gamma, log-normal and etc., where distribution shape parameters β1, β2 are the square of the standardized skewness and kurtosis measurements, respectively. Given the first four moments, the Pearson distribution series can be utilized to approximate the permutation distribution of the test statistic without conducting real permutation.

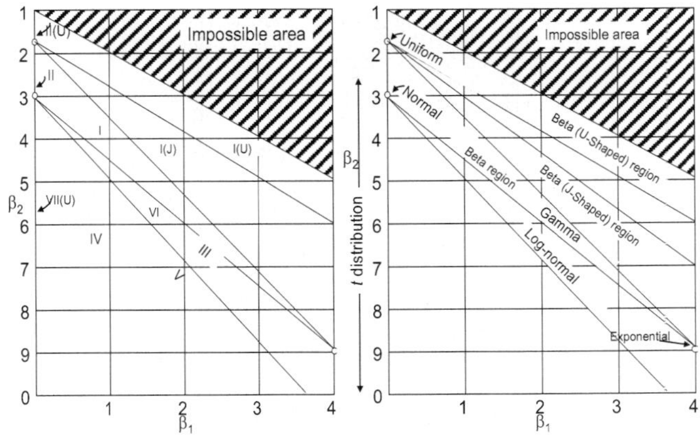

Fig. 1. Left: Regions in $(\beta1, \beta2)$ plane for various types of Pearson distribution series; Right: Regions in $(\beta1, \beta2)$ plane for various types of parametric distributions (Hahn & Shapiro, 1967).

Theoretical Derivation of Moments In order to approximate the permutation distribution with Pearson distribution, the moments of the exact permutation distribution need to be computed. Let $X = [x_1, x_2, ..., x_n]^T$ be the one dimensional data, and $T = C^T PX$ denotes the linear test statistic for permutation test. $C = [c_1 \cdots c_n]^T$ is the linear test statistic coefficients vector. The permutation matrix P is a matrix that has exactly one entry 1 in each row and each column and 0's elsewhere. A permutation matrix is a matrix obtained by permuting the rows of an identity matrix according to some permutation of the numbers 1 to n. For example, let $P = \begin{bmatrix} 0 & 0 & 1 \\ 1 & 0 & 0 \\ 0 & 1 & 0 \end{bmatrix}$, $X = [x_1\ x_2\ x_3]^T$ and $C = [c_1\ c_2\ c_3]^T$, thus $PX = [x_3\ x_1\ x_2]^T$ and $T(X,\pi) = C^T PX = c_2 x_1 + c_3 x_2 + c_1 x_3 = \sum_i c_{\pi(i)} x_i$, where $(\pi(1), \pi(2), \pi(3)) = (2,3,1)$ denotes a permutation of vector data by row. Then the linear test statistic can be denoted as $T(X,\pi) = C^T PX = \sum_i c_{\pi(i)} x_i$. The r-th conditional moment can be derived as:

$$E(T^r(X,\pi)|X) = E((C^T PX)^r) = \frac{1}{n!}\sum_{\pi}\sum_{i_1,\cdots i_r}(\prod_{k=1}^{r} c_{\pi(i_k)} x_{i_k})$$

$$= \frac{1}{n!}\sum_{\pi}\sum_{i_1,\cdots i_r}(\prod_{k=1}^{r} x_{i_k} \prod_{k=1}^{r} c_{\pi(i_k)}) = \sum_{i_1,\cdots i_r}(\prod_{k=1}^{r} x_{i_k} \frac{1}{n!}\sum_{\pi}\prod_{k=1}^{r} c_{\pi(i_k)}) \tag{5}$$

To compute $\frac{1}{n!}\sum_{\pi}\prod_{k=1}^{r}c_{\pi(i_k)}$, it is natural to partition the index space $U=\{1\,2\cdots n\}^r$ into $\bigcup_{(\lambda_1,\lambda_2,\cdots,\lambda_q)\in L} U^{(\lambda_1,\lambda_2,\cdots,\lambda_q)}$, where $L=\{(\lambda_1,\lambda_2,\cdots,\lambda_q):\lambda_1,\lambda_2,\cdots,\lambda_q\in Z^+;\ \lambda_1\le\lambda_2\le\cdots\le\lambda_q;\ \lambda_1+\lambda_2+\cdots+\lambda_q=r\}$. $U^{(\lambda_1,\lambda_2,\cdots,\lambda_q)}$ means that all r indices are permuted into q different numbers. Each number corresponds to λ_i indices. When $r=3$, $U=U^{(1,1,1)}\bigcup U^{(1,2)}\bigcup U^{(3)}$, where $U^{(1,1,1)}$ is the set of $\{i_1\ne i_2\ and\ i_1\ne i_3\ and\ i_2\ne i_3\}$ with $q=3$ and $\lambda_1=\lambda_2=\lambda_3=1$, $U^{(1,2)}$ is the set of $\{i_1=i_2\ne i_3\ or\ i_1=i_3\ne i_2\ or\ i_2=i_3\ne i_1\}$ with $q=2$ and $\lambda_1=1,\lambda_2=2$, and $U^{(3)}$ is the set of $\{i_1=i_2=i_3\}$ with $q=1$ and $\lambda_1=3$. Since permutation is equally related to all r indices, $\frac{1}{n!}\sum_{\pi}\prod_{k=1}^{r}c_{\pi(i_k)}$ is invariant in each category, we define $\frac{1}{n!}\sum_{\pi}\prod_{k=1}^{r}c_{\pi(i_k)}$ as moment coefficient, $a_{(\lambda_1,\lambda_2,\cdots,\lambda_q)}$, if $(i_1\,i_2\cdots i_r)\in U^{(\lambda_1,\lambda_2,\cdots,\lambda_q)}$. Eventually, the r-th conditional moment is:

$$E(T^r(X,\pi)|X)=\sum_{\lambda_1,\lambda_2,\cdots,\lambda_q}a_{(\lambda_1,\lambda_2,\cdots,\lambda_q)}\sum_{(i_1,\cdots i_r)\in U^{(\lambda_1,\lambda_2,\cdots,\lambda_q)}}(\prod_{k=1}^{r}x_{i_k}) \qquad (6)$$

Eq. (6) separates the permutation from the data. To get the moments, we only need to derive the permutation of the coefficients of pre-chose test statistics and calculate the summation terms of data. Due to the simple pattern of the coefficients of test statistics which is the same for repeated tests, we can derive the moments of permutation distribution without permutation of the data. Alternatively, all a s can also be calculated by computer simulation without analytical derivation. In addition, the discussed approach can be easily extended to the multivariate case (Zhou & Wang, 2008).

Mean Difference Test Statistic In surface shape analysis, we use mean vector difference as test statistic, and $T = [TX, TY, TZ]^T = [CPX^*, CPY^*, CPZ^*]^T$, where the mean difference vector $C=[\frac{1}{n_1}1_{1\times n_1},\frac{-1}{n_2}1_{1\times n_2}]$, $X^*=X+[0_{1\times n_1},1_{1\times n_2}]^T\Delta$, $Y^*=Y+[0_{1\times n_1},1_{1\times n_2}]^T\Delta$, $Z^*=Z+[0_{1\times n_1},1_{1\times n_2}]^T\Delta$. Δ is the desired threshold for bioequivalence test, and is equal to zero in classical hypothesis test case. The detailed and complete formulas of corresponding a s are derived and listed in (Zhou & Wang, 2008). For the mean difference test statistic, the computation cost of data summation terms for the r-th moment in each index subspace can be reduced to $O(n)$ from $O(n^r)$.

Multiple Comparison via Adaptive ROI Constrained FDR Determining whether a location on the brain surface has significant group shape difference or not corresponds to performing a described hypothesis test at that position. Clearly, the location-wise p-values are spatially dependent. The significance rule, applied in the conventional False Discovery Rate (FDR) approach is defined as the expected proportion of false positives among the declared significant results. It is more powerful and less stringent than the Family-Wise-Error-Rate (FWER) approach. We adopt the adaptive concept of the FDR (Benjamini et al., 2006) and develop a ROI constrained adaptive FDR in (Zhou & Wang, 2008). This adaptive FDR control is more powerful than the conventional one. It can find more significant areas while preserving the same desired FDR rate.

2.3 Experiments and results

Simulated Data In this experiment, we generated six different simulated data sets to evaluate our hybrid permutation tests. In case #1 and case #2, two group data are normal distributed with different mean and variance (Normal(0,1) vs. Normal(1,0.5)) in balanced design (n_1 = n_2 = 10) and unbalanced design (n_1 = 6, n_2 = 18), respectively. Each group has gamma distribution in case #3 (Gamma(3,3) vs. (Gamma(3,2), n_1 = n_2 = 10) and case #4 (Gamma(3,3) vs. (Gamma(3,2), n_1 = 6, n_2 = 18). In case #5 and case #6, two group data have beta distribution with different parameters (Beta(0.8,0.8) vs. Beta(0.1,0.1)) in balanced design (n_1 = n_2 = 10) and unbalanced design (n_1=6, n_2=18).

	Case #1	Case #2	Case #3	Case#4	Case#5	Case#6
t_HP	0.0113	0.0113	0.0123	0.0137	0.0172	0.0018
t_RP	1.1584	1.1438	1.1369	1.1250	1.1262	1.1384
t_EP	4.4389	4.2795	4.2983	4.3240	4.1320	4.2948
p_HP	0.0499	0.1314	0.0010	0.0249	0.0908	0.0805
p_RP	0.0495	0.1269	0.0012	0.0242	0.0889	0.0818
p_EP	0.0498	0.1301	0.0010	0.0250	0.0925	0.0803

Table 1. Comparison of computation costs and p-value accuracy for three permutation test methods. (HP: hybrid permutation; RP: random permutation; EP: exact permutation.). t_HP, t_RP and t_HP denote the respective computation time (in seconds) per test; p_HP, p_RP and p_EP are the respective p-value measurements by the three permutation methods.

Table 1 indicates the high accuracy of our hybrid permutation technique, especially for the tail area (Note: the exact permutation results are considered as ground truth.) Furthermore, comparing with exact permutation or random 20,000 permutations, the hybrid permutation tests reduce more than 99% computation cost and can further save computation time as the sample size increases. In order to demonstrate the robustness of our method, we repeated the simulation for 10 times in each case, and calculate the mean and variance of the absolute biases of p-values of both hybrid permutation and random permutation, treating the p-values of exact permutation as gold standard. In most cases, hybrid permutation is less biased and more stable than random permutation (Table 2), which demonstrates the robustness and accuracy of our method.

We also generated a synthetic dataset to demonstrate that bioequivalence test plays an important role in identifying practical significance. There are 12 surfaces in group A and 9 in group B, which were generated by adding two types of Gaussian noises to the two flat patches, a (5×5) top patch and a (21×21-5×5) bottom patch. For group A, Gaussian noise with mean zero and standard deviation σ_b = 0.01 was added to the bottom patch with z = 0; Gaussian noise with mean zero and standard deviation σ_t = 0.09 is added to the top patch with z = 1. The 9 surfaces in group B were generated with the same noise patterns as in group A but to different bottom patch z = 0.01 and top patch z = 0.9. Since the differences between the bottom patches of the two groups are very small (z = 0 vs. z = 0.01), the practical group differences should only occur on the top patch (z = 1 vs. z = 0.9). Fig. 2(c) shows that

	Case #1	Case #2	Case #3	Case #4	Case #5	Case #6
Mean_ABias_HP	8.79e-5	8.97e-6	9.54e-5	2.16e-4	6.79e-4	4.53e-4
Mean_ABias_RP	2.82e-4	6.64e-5	2.14e-4	1.30e-3	2.78e-4	5.99e-4
VAR_ABias_HP	5.99e-8	1.34e-7	2.10e-6	3.66e-7	9.55e-7	9.78e-6
VAR_ABias_RP	1.98e-6	1.42e-7	1.41e-6	5.34e-6	1.05e-5	1.00e-5

Table 2. Robustness and accuracy comparison of hybrid (moments-based) permutation and random permutation across 10 simulations, considering the p-values of exact permutation as gold standard. Mean_ABias_HP and VAR_ABias_HP are the mean and variance of the absolute biases of p-values of hybrid permutation; Mean_ABias_RP and VAR_ABias_RP are the mean and variance of the absolute biases of p-values of random permutation, respectively.

many significance locations on both the top and bottom patches are detected by the classical hypothesis tests. Also, the non-practical significances can not be revealed with a more conservative significance level (i.e., lower α) because not all p-values on the top patch are lower than those of the bottom patch (see Fig. 2(d)). Using bioequivalence tests, we are able to precisely identify the practical significances that occur at the top patch (Fig. 2(e)).

Real Data of the Human Brain The MRI hippocampi used in this experiment were semi-automatically segmented by human expert raters and manually grouped into 2 groups with 21 subjects in group A and 15 in group B (see the following site for details: *http://www.ia.unc.edu/dev/download/shapeAnalysis/*). This dataset serves as a testing dataset for methodology validation for all users of the SPHARM-PDM software. Evaluation of our bioequivalence test using hybrid permutation with the mean difference test statistics on this hippocampus dataset is shown in Fig. 3. It can be seen that the Pearson distribution approximation based on the first four moments leads to an accurate approximation to the real permutation distribution and thus p-values (Fig. 3(c) vs. Fig. 3(d)). At the same significance level α = 0.05, there are differences (Fig. 3(e)) between the results of classical test

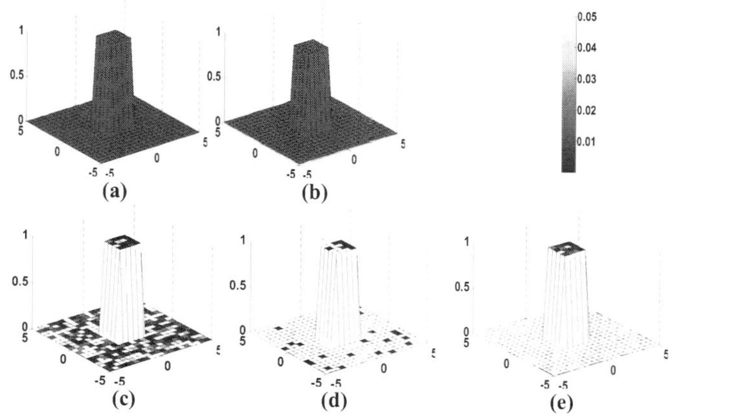

Fig. 2. (a): Mean shape of group A. (b): Mean shape of group B. (c) and (d): Results using conventional hypothesis tests with α = 0.05 (c) and with α = 0.001 (d). (e) Results using bioequivalence tests with α = 0.05 and Δ = 0.025.

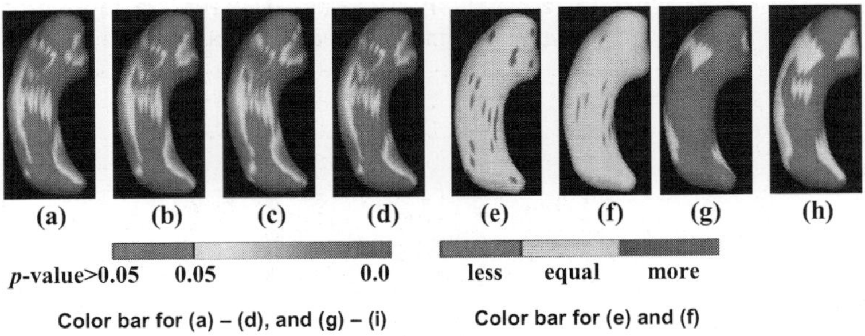

Fig. 3. (a) and (b): Raw p-value maps from classical hypothesis test using Pearson approximation, at $\alpha = 0.05$ (a), and at $\alpha = 0.035$ (b). (c) and (d): Raw p-value maps from bioequivalence test at $\alpha = 0.05$ (without correction), through real permutation ((c); number of permutations = 10,000), and using Pearson approximation (d). (e): The difference between (a) and (d), locations in red showing significances in (a) but not in (d). (f): The difference between (b) and (d), locations in blue showing significances in (d) but not in (b). (g): Our ROI constrained adaptive FDR corrected p-map for (d). (h): Our ROI constrained adaptive FDR corrected p-map for (a).

(Fig. 3(a)) and bioequivalence test (Fig. 3(d)). In addition, at a lower significance level, ($\alpha = 0.035$, Fig. 3(b)) both the non-notable differences and some practical significances that we would like to detect are shown as non-significant (see Fig. 3(f)). This indicates that simply decreasing the significance level in a standard hypothesis test may not lead to practical significances, which can only be achieved through the proposed bioequivalence test. The false positive error control results are shown in Fig. 3 (g) and (h).

3. Brain connectivity analysis from functional MRI

For functional connectivity studies, a common approach is to calculate the temporal correlation coefficients of a fMRI signal from a selected voxel or region (so called "seed", or "seed region") in a region of interest with all other voxels in the brain (Worsley et al., 2005). Each correlation map is resulting from the cross-correlation of only one seed region. However, when areas with quite different time series patterns are used as seed regions for brain connectivity inference, they should not be grouped as a single region; in some applications, functional co-activation to multiple seeds rather than a single one would be of particular interest. Multiple seeds can be chosen to calculate multiple correlation maps to separately discover the functional connectivity to different seeds. But how to reasonably integrate multiple connectivity maps for brain function inference is still unresolved and ambiguous. Furthermore, it is often unrealistic to examine all pair-wise correlations. Therefore, it is desirable to have a single correlation map resulting from the cross-correlation of two or more seed regions simultaneously.

Dynamic connections in fMRI are thought to be reflected by high temporal correlations of the time series. The strong correlation between the time series of each region in the network with that of another distant region implied by the functional interactions may be related to the spatially structured noise in fMRI (Cordes, et al., 2002). The spatial correlations of the noise must therefore be taken into account when dealing with sensitive and reproducible estimation of the network. Furthermore, brain functional connectivity based on marginal correlation can be dominated by the stimulus-locked responses. For example, if visual and auditory stimuli are presented concurrently, the stimulus-locked neural responses would cause increases in the BOLD signal in the primary auditory cortex (A1) and the primary visual cortex (V1) simultaneously. Correlation between A1 and V1 would thus be high, though not due to any intrinsic task-induced functional couplings but due to the responses in both regions to externally driven stimuli. Partial correlation is the conditional correlation which estimates any remaining correlation between time series after taking into account the relationship of each to one or more reference time series. The stimulus-locked responses can then be accounted for by choosing the reference functions to model the external stimuli. This allows us to measure any additional task-induced, but not stimulus-locked relation over brain regions. Recently, methods using partial correlation (or coherence) have been proposed (Sun et al., 2004; Marrelec et al., 2006), though they are for pair-wise correlation (or coherence) analysis and not applicable to multiple seeds. How to apply the partial correlation concept to multiple seed regions to brain connectivity study while considering spatial partial correlations in noise to those seed regions is challenging. Here, we propose a novel procedure to achieve this as one of the goals of this work.

3.1 Functional connectivity using multiple correlations

Estimating Temporal/Sample Multiple Correlations Let T be the total number of time points of the fMRI data. The temporal or sample multiple correlation coefficient considers the fMRI time series correlation between a given voxel X and a combination of seed regions, $S_1, S_2, \cdots S_p$. Its estimation is based on the variance-covariance matrix:

$$\hat{\boldsymbol{\Sigma}}_{tem} = \begin{bmatrix} \hat{\text{var}}_X & \hat{\text{cov}}_{X,S_1} & \cdots & \hat{\text{cov}}_{X,S_p} \\ \hat{\text{cov}}_{S_1,X} & \hat{\text{var}}_{S_1} & \cdots & \hat{\text{cov}}_{S_1,S_p} \\ \vdots & \vdots & \vdots & \vdots \\ \hat{\text{cov}}_{S_p,X} & \hat{\text{cov}}_{S_p,S_1} & \cdots & \hat{\text{var}}_{S_p} \end{bmatrix} = \begin{bmatrix} \hat{\text{var}}_X & \hat{\mathbf{cov}}_{XS}' \\ \hat{\mathbf{cov}}_{XS} & \hat{\boldsymbol{\Sigma}}_{SS} \end{bmatrix},$$

where var(X) and var_{S_p} are the time series variances for voxel X and seed S_p ($p = 1, 2, \cdots P$), respectively; and cov_{X,s_p} is their covariance. The temporal multiple correlation coefficient $\hat{R}_{tem}$ between voxel X and the multiple seeds $[S_1, S_2, \cdots S_P]'$ can be calculated as (Anderson, 2003):

$$\hat{R}_{tem} = \sqrt{\frac{\hat{\mathbf{cov}}_{XS}' \cdot \hat{\boldsymbol{\Sigma}}_{SS}^{-1} \cdot \hat{\mathbf{cov}}_{XS}}{\hat{\text{var}}_X}}.$$

Estimating Spatial Multiple Correlations in Noise The factors contributing to the spatial correlation of the noise include fMRI data preprocessing, the point spread function, which causes data from an individual voxel to contain some signal from the tissue around that voxel, an effect compounded by motion correction techniques, and the smoothness introduced by interpolation in motion correction (Woolrich et al., 2004). Despite the strategies and efforts to reduce such structured noise (Wang et al., 2003; Wang, 2005), some residual and further corrections are still essential for robust fMRI data analysis.

Voxel-based Spatial Correlograph of Noise. We assume the spatial noise is stationary and has a multivariate Gaussian distribution with variance-covariance matrix $\mathbf{\Sigma} = \left(\sigma_{i,j}\right)_{i,j=1}^{M}$, where M is the total number of voxels; σ_i and σ_j are positive standard deviations for voxels X_i and X_j. The spatial correlations in noise then depend only on the spatial distance between voxels: $\sigma_{ij} = \sigma_i\sigma_j\rho\left(\|i-j\|\right)$, where $\|i-j\|$ denotes the spatial distance or lag between X_i and X_j; and ρ is the spatial correlogram, a real-valued function that satisfies $\rho(0)=1$ and is bounded by -1 and 1. Since it is unknown what voxels or regions are predominantly influenced by the noise, the entire set $D_h = \left\{\left(X_i, X_j\right) \mid \|i-j\| = h\right\}$ of pairs of voxels at lag h over the whole brain area is considered for the non-parametric estimate based on the median: $\hat{\rho}(h) = median\left\{r_{ij},\ \left(X_i, X_j\right) \in D_h\right\},$, where r_{ij} is the Pearson's linear correlation between the time series of the two voxels. As in general the empirical estimator $\hat{\rho}$ of the correlogram does not provide a positive-definite correlation matrix, we focus on a parametric class of valid matrices, based on the empirical values $\hat{\rho}$ estimated from the fMRI data. The rational-quadratic model $\rho_{\mathbf{\theta}}(h)$ in (Cressie, 1993; Wang & Xia, 2009) is utilized for such purpose. The derived spatial correlogram of noise, $\rho_{\mathbf{\theta}}(h)$, decreases rapidly from a correlation level between nearby voxels, ρ_{0+}, towards an asymptotic correlation, ρ_{∞}. A critical distance h_{∞}^{ε} can be determined beyond which the correlogram is almost equal to the asymptote, with a tolerance of ε. The parameterization of the rational-quadratic model using $\left(\rho_{0+}, \rho_{\infty}, h_{\infty}^{\varepsilon}\right)$ is given as in (Bellec et al., 2006; Wang & Xia, 2009).

Spatial Multiple Correlations in Noise. The spatial multiple correlations of the noise consider the correlations between any voxel X and a combination of multiple seeds $S_1, S_2, \cdots S_P$. Suppose the distances between the voxel X and the seeds $S_1, S_2, \cdots S_P$ are respectively $h_1, h_2, \cdots h_P$, and the distances between any pair-wise seeds are h_{ij} (for S_i and S_j, $h_{ij} = h_{ji}$). The noise spatial correlation matrix for $\left[X, S_1, S_2, \cdots S_P\right]'$ can then be constructed as:

$$\mathbf{\Lambda}_{spa} = \begin{bmatrix} 1 & \rho_{\mathbf{\theta}}(h_1) & \cdots & \rho_{\mathbf{\theta}}(h_P) \\ \rho_{\mathbf{\theta}}(h_1) & 1 & & \rho_{\mathbf{\theta}}(h_{1P}) \\ \vdots & \vdots & \ddots & \vdots \\ \rho_{\mathbf{\theta}}(h_P) & \rho_{\mathbf{\theta}}(h_{P1}) & \cdots & 1 \end{bmatrix} = \begin{bmatrix} 1 & \boldsymbol{\rho}_S' \\ \boldsymbol{\rho}_S & \mathbf{\Lambda}_{SS} \end{bmatrix}$$

where $\rho_{\mathbf{\theta}}(h)$ is the correlogram estimated above. Let σ_X^2 and $\sigma_{S_p}^2$ respectively denote the noise variance for voxel X, and seed $S_p, p = 1, 2, \cdots P$. Then the corresponding variance-covariance matrix, $\mathbf{\Sigma}_{spa}$, is:

$$\mathbf{\Sigma}_{spa} = \begin{bmatrix} \sigma_X^2 & \rho_{\mathbf{\theta}}(h_1)\cdot\sigma_X\cdot\sigma_{S_1} & \cdots & \rho_{\mathbf{\theta}}(h_P)\cdot\sigma_X\cdot\sigma_{S_P} \\ \rho_{\mathbf{\theta}}(h_1)\cdot\sigma_{S_1}\cdot\sigma_X & \sigma_{S_1}^2 & \cdots & \rho_{\mathbf{\theta}}(h_{1P})\cdot\sigma_{S_1}\cdot\sigma_{S_P} \\ \vdots & \vdots & \ddots & \vdots \\ \rho_{\mathbf{\theta}}(h_P)\cdot\sigma_{S_P}\cdot\sigma_X & \rho_{\mathbf{\theta}}(h_{P1})\cdot\sigma_{S_P}\cdot\sigma_{S_1} & \cdots & \sigma_{S_P}^2 \end{bmatrix} = \begin{bmatrix} \sigma_X^2 & \boldsymbol{\sigma}_{XS}' \\ \boldsymbol{\sigma}_{XS} & \mathbf{\Sigma}_{SS} \end{bmatrix}.$$

The spatial multiple correlation coefficient of the noise between any voxel X and the seeds $\left[S_1, S_2, \cdots S_P\right]'$ is computed as: $R_{spa} = \sqrt{\frac{\boldsymbol{\sigma}_{XS}' \boldsymbol{\Sigma}_{SS}^{-1} \boldsymbol{\sigma}_{XS}}{\sigma_X^2}}$, and can be re-formulated to:

$$R_{spa} = \sqrt{\boldsymbol{\rho}_S' \cdot \boldsymbol{\Lambda}_{SS}^{-1} \cdot \boldsymbol{\rho}_S} \tag{7}$$

Identifying Functional Connectivity of Brain The factors Given the estimation of multiple correlations in noise, we use hypothesis testing to search for significant correlations between any voxel and the seed regions that are statistically unlikely to be due to noise.

Statistical Hypothesis Testing. We would like to test whether the temporal multiple correlation $\hat{R}_{tem}$ is likely to be found only by chance from the noise correlation. The hypothesis is:

$$H_0 : R_{tem} = R_{spa} \text{ vs. } H_1 : R_{tem} > R_{spa} .$$

Under the null hypothesis that the temporal multiple correlation, $\hat{R}_{tem}$, arises from a population whose multiple correlation equals the spatial multiple correlation of the noise, R_{spa}, the following quantity is a non-central F (Anderson, 2003) (pp. 153-154):

$$F = \frac{\hat{R}_{tem}^2}{1 - \hat{R}_{tem}^2} \cdot \frac{T-1-P}{P} \tag{8}$$

Here, the degrees of freedom are P and $T-1-P$, and the noncentrality parameter incorporating our re-formulated R_{spa} in Eq. (7) is $\frac{(T-1)\boldsymbol{\rho}_S' \boldsymbol{\Lambda}_{SS}^{-1} \boldsymbol{\Psi} \hat{\boldsymbol{\Sigma}}_{SS} \boldsymbol{\Psi} \boldsymbol{\Lambda}_{SS}^{-1} \boldsymbol{\rho}_S}{1 - \boldsymbol{\rho}_S' \cdot \boldsymbol{\Lambda}_{SS}^{-1} \cdot \boldsymbol{\rho}_S}$, where we condition on the seeds' time series, and $\boldsymbol{\Psi}$ is a $P \times P$ diagonal matrix with diagonal element $1/\sigma_{S_p}$, for $p = 1,2,\ldots,P$. In this way, the p-value for each voxel can be calculated from this noncentral F distribution. A voxel shall be included in the functional connectivity network if the corresponding p-value is smaller than a pre-chosen type I error α (note: $\alpha = 0.05$ is used in this connectivity work). It can also be shown that under the null hypothesis of the population multiple correlation, R_{spa}, is zero (i.e. our hypothesis becomes: $H_0 : R_{tem} = 0$ vs. $H_1 : R_{tem} > 0$), the F in Eq. (8) is a central F (Anderson, 2003) (pp. 149-150), with P and $T-1-P$ degrees of freedom. In fact, this is equivalent to multiple correlation analysis of multi-seed functional connectivity but without taking the spatial correlations of the noise into consideration.

Effective Degrees of Freedom for Temporal Autocorrelation. A departure from the temporally i.i.d. (independent and identically distributed) assumption due to the temporal autocorrelation will result in a decrease in the degrees of freedom in the above hypothesis testing. To correct such possible bias, we estimate the effective degrees of freedom T_{eff}. This can be achieved through the context of the general linear model (Worsley & Friston, 1995). Note that the T_{eff} estimated this way assumes voxelwise spatial independence, which can be considered as an upper-bound estimation of our effective degrees of freedom. We approximate the effective degrees of freedom as T_{eff}, and use the estimated T_{eff} to replace the T-1 in the F statistic's calculation in Eq. (8).

Multiple Testing using Non-central F Random Field. We need to perform numerous tests equal to the total number of voxels over the brain area. In order to correct this multiple testing problem, different strategies can be potentially applied, such as Bonferroni correction, cluster-size thresholding, random field theory or false discovery rate control (Huettel et al., 2004; Benjamini & Hochbert, 1995; Logan & Rowe, 2004; Nicholos & Holmes, 2001; Zhou & Wang, 2008). The Random field theory (RFT) correction on the *t*-field, Hotelling's T^2 field, χ^2 field, central *F* field, and the correlation field has been developed by Worsley and colleagues (Cao & Worsley, 1999; Worsley, 1994). RFT estimates the number of independent statistical tests based upon the spatial correlation, or smoothness, of the experimental data. With even small to moderate amounts of smoothness in the data, the number of resels (resolution elements) will be much less than the original number of voxels. From the number of resels, one can estimate how many clusters of activity should be found by chance at a given statistical threshold. This number is known as the Euler characteristic of the data. RFT correction is less conservative than the Bonferroni correction. In this work, we use the non-central *F* RFT to correct the multiple comparison problems (Wang & Xia, 2009; Hayasaka et al., 2007).

3.2 Functional connectivity using partial multiple correlations

Estimating Temporal Partial Multiple Correlations The temporal partial multiple correlation coefficient considers the fMRI time series correlation between a given voxel X and a combination of seed regions $S_1, S_2, \cdots S_P$ conditioned on fixed stimuli (experimental paradigms or reference functions, i.e. the convolution functions of the hemodynamic response with the 0-1 boxcar stimulus functions in the case of the block-design experiments), $V_1, V_2, \cdots V_N$. Its estimation is based on the matrix:

$$\begin{bmatrix} \hat{\text{var}}_X & \hat{\text{cov}}_{X,S_1} & \cdots & \hat{\text{cov}}_{X,S_P} & \hat{\text{cov}}_{X,V_1} & \cdots & \hat{\text{cov}}_{X,V_N} \\ \hat{\text{cov}}_{S_1,X} & \hat{\text{var}}_{S_1} & & \hat{\text{cov}}_{S_1,S_P} & \hat{\text{cov}}_{S_1,V_1} & \cdots & \hat{\text{cov}}_{S_1,V_N} \\ \vdots & \vdots & \vdots & \vdots & \vdots & \vdots & \vdots \\ \hat{\text{cov}}_{S_P,X} & \hat{\text{cov}}_{S_P,S_1} & \cdots & \hat{\text{var}}_{S_P} & \hat{\text{cov}}_{S_P,V_1} & \cdots & \hat{\text{cov}}_{S_P,V_N} \\ \hat{\text{cov}}_{V_1,X} & \hat{\text{cov}}_{V_1,S_1} & \cdots & \hat{\text{cov}}_{V_1,S_P} & \text{var}_{V_1} & \cdots & \text{cov}_{V_1,V_N} \\ \vdots & \vdots & \vdots & \vdots & \vdots & \vdots & \vdots \\ \hat{\text{cov}}_{V_N,X} & \hat{\text{cov}}_{V_N,S_1} & \cdots & \hat{\text{cov}}_{V_N,S_P} & \text{cov}_{V_N,V_1} & \cdots & \text{var}_{V_N} \end{bmatrix} = \begin{bmatrix} \hat{\text{var}}_X & \hat{\textbf{cov}}_{XS}' & \hat{\textbf{cov}}_{XV}' \\ \hat{\textbf{cov}}_{XS} & \hat{\boldsymbol{\Sigma}}_{SS} & \hat{\boldsymbol{\Sigma}}_{SV}' \\ \hat{\textbf{cov}}_{XV} & \hat{\boldsymbol{\Sigma}}_{SV} & \boldsymbol{\Sigma}_{VV} \end{bmatrix} = \begin{bmatrix} \hat{\boldsymbol{\Sigma}}_{\{XS\}\{XS\}} & \hat{\boldsymbol{\Sigma}}_{\{XS\}V}' \\ \hat{\boldsymbol{\Sigma}}_{\{XS\}V} & \boldsymbol{\Sigma}_{VV} \end{bmatrix},$$

where var_{V_n} is the time series variances of the stimulus V_n $(n = 1, 2, \cdots N)$; cov_{X,V_n} is the covariance between voxel X and V_n, and cov_{S_p,V_n} is the covariance between the seed S_p and V_n. Their estimation can be achieved through time series and reference function samples of size *T*, though here they are not technically variances and covariances because the V_n are fixed stimuli. With the assumption that the conditional distribution $(X, S_1, \cdots, S_P | V_1 = v_1, V_2 = v_2, \cdots V_N = v_N)'$ is a multi-normal distribution (Anderson, 2008), its variance-covariance matrix can be calculated as:

$$\hat{\boldsymbol{\Sigma}}^*_{tem} = \hat{\boldsymbol{\Sigma}}_{\{XS\}\{XS\}} - \hat{\boldsymbol{\Sigma}}_{\{XS\}V}' \cdot \boldsymbol{\Sigma}_{VV}^{-1} \cdot \hat{\boldsymbol{\Sigma}}_{\{XS\}V} \cdot$$

Let the components of $\hat{\mathbf{\Sigma}}^*_{tem}$ be divided into four groups, $\begin{bmatrix} \hat{\text{var}}^*_X & \hat{\mathbf{cov}}^{*\prime}_{XS} \\ \hat{\mathbf{cov}}^*_{XS} & \hat{\mathbf{\Sigma}}^*_{SS} \end{bmatrix}$, where $\hat{\text{var}}^*_X$ and $\hat{\mathbf{\Sigma}}^*_{SS}$ are variances of voxel X and the seeds holding the reference functions (stimuli) fixed, $\hat{\mathbf{cov}}^*_{XS}$ is their corresponding covariance under the same condition. The temporal partial multiple correlation is:

$$\hat{R}_{tem \bullet \mathbf{V}} = \sqrt{\frac{\hat{\mathbf{cov}}^{*\prime}_{XS} \cdot \hat{\mathbf{\Sigma}}^{*\,-1}_{SS} \cdot \hat{\mathbf{cov}}^*_{XS}}{\hat{\text{var}}^*_X}}$$

Estimating Spatial Partial Multiple Correlations in Noise In Section 3.1, we estimate the voxel-based spatial correlograph of noise using the median of Pearson's linear correlation, i.e. marginal correlation. Here, we take the similar approach but replace the marginal correlation with partial correlation because the stimuli are now considered to be fixed, i.e., $\hat{\rho}^*(h) = median\left\{r_{ij\cdot\mathbf{V}},\ \left(X_i, X_j\right) \in D_h\right\}$,, where $r_{ij\cdot\mathbf{V}}$ is the partial correlation coefficient between voxels X_i and X_j holding $V_1, V_2, \cdots V_N$ fixed. Let the variance-covariance matrix of $\left(X_i, X_j, V_1, \cdots, V_N\right)'$ be $\begin{bmatrix} \hat{\mathbf{\Sigma}}_{XX} & \hat{\mathbf{\Sigma}}_{XV} \\ \hat{\mathbf{\Sigma}}_{XV} & \mathbf{\Sigma}_{VV} \end{bmatrix}'$. $\left(X_i, X_j \middle| V_1 = v_1, V_2 = v_2, \cdots V_N = v_N\right)'$ is assumed to be multi-normal; its variance-covariance matrix is calculated as:

$$\hat{\mathbf{\Sigma}}_{X\cdot V} = \hat{\mathbf{\Sigma}}_{XX} - \hat{\mathbf{\Sigma}}_{XV}' \cdot \mathbf{\Sigma}^{-1}_{VV} \cdot \hat{\mathbf{\Sigma}}_{VX} = \begin{bmatrix} \hat{\sigma}^2_{i\cdot\mathbf{V}} & \hat{\sigma}'_{ij\cdot\mathbf{V}} \\ \hat{\sigma}_{ij\cdot\mathbf{V}} & \hat{\sigma}^2_{j\cdot\mathbf{V}} \end{bmatrix}.$$

The partial correlation coefficient is thus given by (Anderson, 2008):

$$r_{ij\cdot\mathbf{V}} = \frac{\sigma_{ij\cdot\mathbf{V}}}{\sigma_{i\cdot\mathbf{V}} \cdot \sigma_{j\cdot\mathbf{V}}}.$$

The noise spatial partial correlation matrix for $\left[X, S_1, S_2, \cdots S_P\right]'$ holding $V_1, V_2, \cdots V_N$ fixed can be constructed as:

$$\mathbf{\Lambda}^*_{spa} = \begin{bmatrix} 1 & \rho^*_\theta(h_1) & \cdots & \rho^*_\theta(h_P) \\ \rho^*_\theta(h_1) & 1 & & \rho^*_\theta(h_{1P}) \\ \vdots & \vdots & \ddots & \vdots \\ \rho^*_\theta(h_P) & \rho^*_\theta(h_{P1}) & \cdots & 1 \end{bmatrix} = \begin{bmatrix} 1 & \boldsymbol{\rho}^{*\prime}_S \\ \boldsymbol{\rho}^*_S & \mathbf{\Lambda}^*_{SS} \end{bmatrix}$$

where $\rho^*_\theta(h)$ is the correlogram. Let $\sigma^*_{S_p}$ denote the residual standard deviation of the noise for seed S_p, $p = 1, 2, \cdots P$, holding $V_1, V_2, \cdots V_N$ fixed (see Appendix in [Wang & Xia, 2009] for its estimation). The spatial partial multiple correlation coefficient of the noise between any voxel X and the seeds $\left[S_1, S_2, \cdots S_P\right]$ holding the stimuli fixed is computed as:

$$R_{spa \cdot \mathbf{V}} = \sqrt{\boldsymbol{\rho}_\mathbf{S}^{*\prime} \cdot \boldsymbol{\Lambda}_{\mathbf{SS}}^{*-1} \cdot \boldsymbol{\rho}_\mathbf{S}^{*}} .$$

Identifying Conditional Functional Connectivity of Brain We would like to test whether the temporal partial multiple correlation $\hat{R}_{tem \cdot \mathbf{V}}$ is likely to be found only by change from the noise correlation. The hypothesis is:

$$H_0 : R_{tem.\mathbf{V}} = R_{spa \cdot \mathbf{V}} \text{ vs. } H_1 : R_{tem.\mathbf{V}} > R_{spa \cdot \mathbf{V}} .$$

Here, we can show that the following quantity is a non-central F:

$$\frac{\hat{R}_{tem.\mathbf{V}}^2}{1 - \hat{R}_{tem.\mathbf{V}}^2} \cdot \frac{(T-1) - N - P}{P} \tag{9}$$

with the degrees of freedom P and $T-1-N-P$, and the noncentrality parameter $\frac{(T-1)\boldsymbol{\rho}_\mathbf{S}^{*\prime} \boldsymbol{\Lambda}_{\mathbf{SS}}^{*-1\prime} \boldsymbol{\Psi}^* \hat{\boldsymbol{\Sigma}}_{\mathbf{SS}}^* \boldsymbol{\Psi}^* \boldsymbol{\Lambda}_{\mathbf{SS}}^{*-1} \boldsymbol{\rho}_\mathbf{S}^*}{1 - \boldsymbol{\rho}_\mathbf{S}^{*\prime} \boldsymbol{\Lambda}_{\mathbf{SS}}^{*-1} \boldsymbol{\rho}_\mathbf{S}^*}$, where we condition on the seeds' time series; $\boldsymbol{\psi}^*$ is a $P \times P$ diagonal matrix with diagonal element $1/\sigma_{S_p}^*$, for $p = 1, 2, \cdots P$. Note that the temporal autocorrelation can be handled in a similar way as in the multiple correlation case by computing the associated effective degrees of freedom; the multiple testing correction is similarly based on non-central F random field theory (see Section 3.1 for details).

Similar to the multiple correlation case, under the null hypothesis of the population partial multiple correlation, $R_{spa \cdot \mathbf{V}}$, is zero (i.e. our hypothesis becomes: $H_0 : R_{tem.\mathbf{V}} = 0$ vs. $H_1 : R_{tem.\mathbf{V}} > 0$), the F in Eq. (9) is a central F, with P and $T-1-N-P$ degrees of freedom. This is then equivalent to partial multiple correlation analysis of multi-seed functional connectivity but without taking the spatial partial correlations of the noise into consideration.

3.3 Experiments on real fMRI data

The real fMRI data (single-subject) was obtained from the SPM data site (*http://www.fil.ion.ucl.ac.uk/spm/data/attention*) with the detailed description in (Buchel & Friston, 1997). The subject was scanned during four runs, each lasting 5 min 22 s. One hundred image volumes were acquired and the first ten was discarded in each run. Each condition lasted 32.2 s, giving 10 multislice volumes per condition. The fMRI data size was $53 \times 63 \times 46 \times 360$. Four conditions – 'fixation', 'attention', 'no attention', and 'stationary' – were used. Electrophysiological and neuroimaging studies have shown that attention to visual motion can increase the responsiveness of the motion-selective cortical area V5 and some other areas, and an occipito-parieto-frontal network is involved in the visual pathway modulation by attention. The structural model for the dorsal visual pathway includes primary visual cortex (V1), visual cortical area MT (V5), posterior parietal cortex (PP), and modulatory interaction term involving dorsolateral prefrontal cortex (PFC). The activation regions were identified by categorical comparisons using the SPM5 software package, contrasting "attention" and "no attention" and contrasting "no attention" and "stationary". Here we examine the functional interactions by using the different seed regions: V1, or V5 or both V1 and V5, and by using different methods.

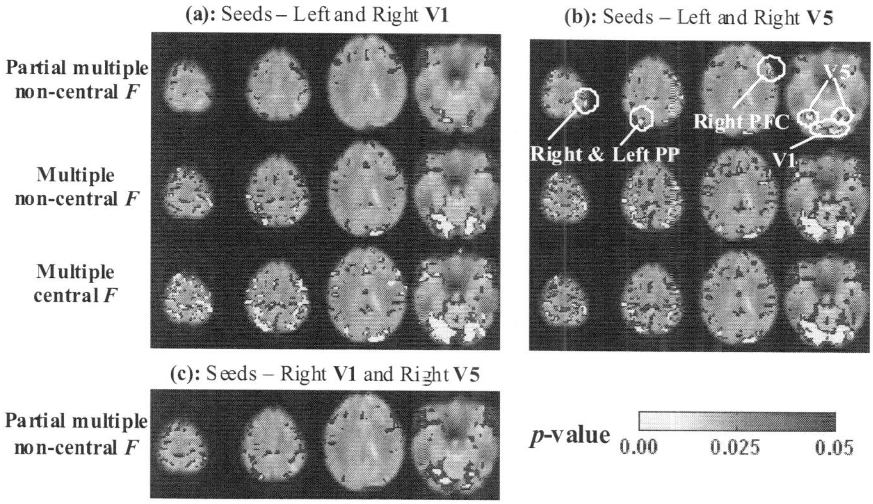

Fig. 4. Comparison and results of functional interaction maps for the real fMRI data.

Partial Correlation Effects - Multiple vs. Partial Multiple Correlations From Fig. 4 (a) and (b), we can see that using multiple correlation (2nd row), both stimulus-locked and task-induced networks are identified, with all the dorsal visual pathway involved regions shown as highly significant (yellow). However, using partial multiple correlation (1st row), since the stimulus-locked effects are accounted for, the network regions and their sizes are considerably reduced. Specifically: i) with V1 as seed regions (Fig. 4(a), 1st row), mainly the low level visual network is identified as highly significant implying task-induced coupling among the visual areas, such as V1 to V5; ii) withV5 as seed regions (Fig. 4(b), 1st row), the two PP and the right PFC regions are still shown as highly significant, suggesting the involved task-induced coupling of attention to motion modulation, after taking account of the stimulus-locked effects.

Effects of Multiple Seeds - Comparison using Both V1 and V5 as Seeds The partial multiple correlation results using V1 or V5 (Fig. 4 (a) and (b), 1st row) as seed regions have been illustrated in the above. With a combination of a V1 and a V5 as seed regions (Fig. 4(c)), using partial multiple correlation, we can not only detect the highly significant low level visual network regions (as in Fig. 4 (a) and (b), 1st row, last slice), but also identify the highly significant attention to motion modulation PP areas (as in Fig. 4(b), 1st row; also compare to Fig. 4(a), 1st row), achieving the combined effects of multiple seed regions involving both V1 and V5. Note that since only one V5 is used here, the region sizes and significance levels for the PP and right PFC are not as large as the ones using both V5 regions in Fig. 4(b) (1st row).

Effects of Spatial Noise - Comparison of Non-central and Central *F*-tests The results without taking the spatial noise correlations into consideration (central *F*-test) are shown in Fig. 4 (a) and (b), 3rd row, with many unjustified areas identified as functionally correlated with the V1 and/or V5 seed regions due to the spatial structured noise in the fMRI data.

4. Conclusions

A new statistical surface morphometry analysis method is presented and developed by using our moments-based permutation tests where the permutation distributions are accurately approximated through Pearson distributions for considerably reduced computation cost. The proposed hybrid strategy takes advantage of nonparametric permutation tests and parametric Pearson distribution approximation to achieve both accuracy/flexibility and efficiency. In addition, hybrid permutation schemes for both the conventional and bioequivalence tests are provided. Compared with the classical hypothesis tests, bioequivalence tests can screen out the non-notable differences and accurately locate the practical or physical significances. In real applications, either the standard or the bioequivalence hypothesis tests can be chosen, depending on the specific problems, i.e. whether the statistical and practical significance differences are negligible or not.

This chapter also presents a novel and general statistical framework for sensitive and reproducible estimation of brain networks from fMRI based on multiple and partial multiple correlation analyses and multiple seed regions, with the standard single-seed region analysis as the degenerate and a special case. Compared with using only a single seed, using multiple seeds can not only lead to more robust estimation of functional connectivity, but also more sensitive identification of functional co-activation networks or regions to multiple seeds that may not be detected in the single-seed method. The use of the partial multiple correlation has the interesting features of providing a convenient summary of conditional independences and hence of being more closely related to the direct functional interactions (i.e. effective connectivity) of the brain than marginal correlation.

The statistical and computational data analysis methods presented in this chapter can lead to precise and efficient recovery of structure and function of the human brain. The discovery of relationship between brain structure and function through combination of different modalities (e.g. sMRI and fMRI) will be a future direction, which may provide a unique perspective (Jiang et al., 2008) and thus further enhance our understanding of the complex system of the human brain.

5. Acknowledgments

This work was supported in part by the National Institute of Health under grant 1K25AG033725-01 from the National Institute of Aging awarded to Dr. Wang; Email: <ymw@illinois.edu>.

6. References

Anderson, T. W. (2003). *An Introduction to Multivariate Statistical Analysis*. 3rd edition, John Wiley and Sons Inc., New Jersey.

Ashburner, J. & Friston, K. J. (2000). Voxel-based morphometry: The methods. *Neuroimage*, 11: 805-821.

Bellec, P.; Perlbarg, V.; Jbabdi, S.; Pelegrini-Issac, M.; Anton, J.; Doyon, J. & Benali, H. (2006). Identification of large-scale networks in the brain using fMRI. *Neuroimage*, 29: 1231-1243.

Benjamini, Y. & Hochberg, Y. (1995). Controlling the false discovery rate: a practical and powerful approach to multiple testing. *Journal of the Royal Statistical Society*, 57: 289-300.

Benjamini, Y.; Krieger, A. M. & Yekutieli, D. (2006). Adaptive linear step-up false discovery rate controlling procedures. *Biometrika*. *93*: 491-507.

Brechbühler, C.; Gerig, G. & Kübler, O. (1995). Parametrization of closed surfaces for 3-D shape description. *Computer Vision, Graphics, and Image Processing*, 61: 154–170.

Brown, L. D.; Hwang, J. T. G. & Munk, A. (1997). An unbiased test for the bioequivalence problem. Ann. Stat. 25: 2345-2367.

Buchel, C. & Friston, K. J. (1997). Modulation of connectivity in visual pathways by attention: Cortical inferences evaluated with structural equation modeling and fMRI. *Cerebral Cortex*, 7: 768-778.

Buckner, R. L.; Head, D.; Parker, J.; Fotenos, A. F.; Marcus, D.; Morris, J. C. & Snyder, A. Z. (2004). A unified approach for morphometric and functional data analysis in young, old, and demented adults using automated atlas-based head size normalization: reliability and validation against manual measurement of total intracranial volume. *Neuroimage*, 23: 724-738.

Calhoun, V. D.; Adali, T.; Pearison, G. D. & Pekar, J. J. (2001). Spatial and temporal independent component analysis of functional MRI data containing a pair of task-related waveforms. *Human Brain Mapping*, 13: 43-53.

Cao, J. & Worsley, K. J. (1999). The geometry of correlation fields with an application to functional connectivity of the brain. *Annals of Applied Probability*, 9: 1021-1057.

Chung, M. K.; Worsley, K. J.; Paus, T.; Cherif, C.; Collins, D. L.; Giedd, J. N.; Rapoport, J. L. & Evans, A. C. (2001). A unified statistical approach to deformation-based morphometry. *Neuroimage*, 14: 595-606.

Cressie, N. (1993). *Statistics for Spatial Data*. John Wiley and Sons, New York.

Cordes, D.; Haughton, V.; Carew, J. D.; Arfanakis, K. & Maravilla, K. (2002). Hierarchical clustering to measure connectivity in fMRI resting-state data. *Magnetic Resonance Imaging*, 20: 305–317.

Davatzikos, C.; Gene, A.; Xu, D. & Resnick, S. M. (2001). Voxel-based morphometry using the RAVENS maps: Methods and validation using simulated longitudinal atrophy. *Neuroimage*, 14: 1361-1369.

Friston, K. J.; Frith, C. D.; Liddle, P. F. & Frackowiak, R. S. J. (1993). Functional connectivity: The principal-component analysis of large (PET) data sets. *Journal of Cerebral Blood Flow & Metabolism*, 13: 5-14.

Hahn, J. & Shapiro, S. S. (1967). *Statistical Models in Engineering*. John Wiley. New York.

Hayasaka, S.; Peiffer, A. M.; Hugenschmidt, C. E. & Laurienti, P. (2007). Power and sample size calculation for neuroimaging studies by non-central random field theory. *Neuroimage*, 37: 721-730.

Horwitz, B. (2003). The elusive concept of brain connectivity. *Neuroimage*, 19: 466-470.

Hubert, L. (1987). *Assignment Methods in Combinatorial Data Analysis*, Marcel Dekker, Inc.

Huettel, S. A. ; Song, A. W. & McCarthy, G. (2004). *Functional Magnetic Resonance Imaging*. Sinauer Associates, Inc. Publisher.

Jack, C. R.; Petersen, R. C.; O'Brien, P. C. & Tangalos, E. G. (1997). MR-based hippocampal volumetry in the diagnosis of Alzheimer's disease. *Neurology*, 42: 183-188.

Jiang, T.; Liu, Y.; Shi, F.; Shu, N.; Liu, B.; Jiang J. & Zhou, Y. (2008). Multimodal magnetic resonance imaging for brain disorders: Advances and perspectives. *Brain Imaging and Behavior*, 2: 249-257.

Lindquist, M. A. (2008). The statisticsl analysis of fMRI data. *Statistical Science*, 23: 439-464.

Logan, B. R. & Rowe, D. B. (2004). An evaluation of thresholding techniques in fMRI analysis," *Neuroimage*, 22: 95-108.

Marrelec, G.; Krainik, A.; Duffau, H.; Pelegrini-Issac, M.; Lehericy, S.; Doyon, J. & Benali, H. (2006). Partial correlation for functional brain interactivity investigation in functional MRI. *Neuroimage*, 32: 228-237.

Martijn, P.; van den Heuvel, P. & Hulshoff Pol, H. E. (2010). Exploring the brain network: A review on resting-state fMRI functional connectivity. *European Neuropsychopharmacology*, 20: 519-534.

McIntosh, A. R. & Lobaugh, N. J. (2004). Partial least squares analysis of neuroimaging data: Applications and advances. *Neuroimage*, 23: S250-S263.

Nichols, T. E. & Holmes, A. P. (2001). Nonparametric permutation tests for functional neuroimaging: A primer with examples. *Human Brain Mapping*, 15: 1–25.

Ogawa, S.; Lee, T. M.; Nayak, A. S. & Glynn, P. (1990). Oxygenation-sensitive contrast in magnetic resonance imaging of rodent brain of high magnetic fields. *Magnetic Resonance in Medicine*, 14: 68-78.

Pantazis, D., Leahy, R. M.; Nichols, T. E. & Styner, M. (2004). Statistical surface-based morphometry using a non-parametric approach. *IEEE International Symposium on Biomedical Imaging*, pp. 1283-1286.

Shen, L.; Saykin, A.; McHugh, T.; West, J.; Rabin, L.; Wishart, H.; Chung, M. & Makedon, F. (2005). Morphometric analysis of 3D surfaces: Application to hippocampal shape in mild cognitive impairment. *6th Int. Conf. on Computer Vision, Pattern Recognition and Image Processing in conjunction with 8th Joint Conference on Information Sciences*, pp. 699-702.

Styner, M.; Lieberman, J. A.; McClure, R. K.; Weinberger, D. R.; Jones, D. W. & Gerig, G. (2005). Morphometric analysis of lateral ventricles in schizophrenia and healthy controls regarding genetic and disease-specific factors. *Proc. Natl. Acad. Sci. U. S. A.*, 102: 4872-4877.

Styner, M.; Oguz, I.; Xu, S.; Brechbuehler, C.; Pantazis, D.; Levitt, J. J.; Shenton, M. E. & Gerig, G. (2006). Framework for the statistical shape analysis of brain structures using SPHARM-PDM, *Open Science Workshop at MICCAI 2006 Insight Journal*.

Symms, M.; Jager, H. R.; Schmierer, K. & Yoursry, T. A. (2004). A review of structural magnetic resonance neuroimaging. *Journal of Neurology, Neurosurgery & Psychiatry*, 75: 1235-1244.

Sun, F. T.; Miller, L. M. & D'Esposito, M. (2004). Measuring interregional functional connectivity using coherence and partial coherence analyses of fMRI data. *Neuroimage*, 21: 647-658.

Thompson, P. M.; Hayashi, K. M.; de Zubicaray, G. I.; Janke, A. L.; Rose, S. E.; Semple, J.; Hong, M. S.; Herman, D. H.; Gravano, D.; Doddrell, D. M. & Toga, A. W. (2004). Mapping hippocampal and ventricular change in Alzheimer disease. *Neuroimage*, 22: 1754-1766.

Wang, L.; Swank, J. S.; Glick, I. E.; Gado, M. H.; Miller, M. I.; Morris, J. C. & Csernansky, J. G. (2003). Changes in hippocampal volume and shape across time distinguish dementia of the Alzheimer type from healthy aging. *Neuroimage*, 20: 667-682.

Wang, Y. M. (2005). Modeling and nonlinear analysis in fMRI via statistical learning. In: *Advanced Image Processing in Magnetic Resonance Imaging*, Marcel Dekker International Publisher, L. Landini, V. Positano, and M. F. Santarelli, Eds., pp. 565-586.

Wang, Y. M.; Schultz, R. T.; Constable, R. T. & Staib, L. H. (2003). Nonlinear estimation and modeling of fMRI data using spatio-temporal support vector regression. In: *Proceedings of the 18th International Conference on Information Processing in Medical Imaging*, Lecture Notes in Computer Science, vol. 2732, pp. 647-659.

Wang, Y. & Staib, L. H. (2000). Boundary finding with prior shape and smoothness models. *IEEE Trans. on Pattern Analysis and Machine Intelligence*, 22: 738-743.

Wang, Y. M. & Xia, J. (2009). Unified framework for robust estimation of brain networks from fMRI using temporal and spatial correlation analyses. *IEEE Transactions on Medical Imaging*, 28: 1296-1307.

Woolrich, M.; Jenkinson, M.; Brady, M. & Smith, S. M. (2004). Fully Bayesian spatio-temporal modeling of fMRI data. *IEEE Transactions on Medical Imaging*, 23:213-230.

Worsley, K. J. (1994). Local maxima and the expected Euler characteristic of excursion sets of χ^2, *F* and *t* fields. *Advances in Applied Probability*, 26: 13-42.

Worsley, K. J. & Friston, K. J. (1995). Analysis of fMRI time-series revisited - again. *Neuroimage*, 2: 173-181.

Worsley, K. J.; Chen, J-I; Lerch, J. & Evans, A. C. (2005). Comparing connectivity via thresholding correlations and SVD. *Philosophical Transactions of the Royal Society*, 360: 913-920.

Zhou, C. & Wang, Y. M. (2008). Hybrid permutation test with application to surface shape analysis. *Statistica Sinica*, 18(4): 1553-1568.

Zhou, C.; Wang, H. & Wang, Y. M. (2009). Efficient Moments-based Permutation Tests. *Advances in Neural Information Processing Systems*, 22: 2277-2285.

Part 4

Cell Therapy and Tissue Engineering

9

Cell Therapy and Tissular Engineering to Regenerate Articular Cartilage

Silvia Mª Díaz Prado[1,2], Isaac Fuentes Boquete[1,2] and Francisco J Blanco[2,3]
[1]*Department of Medicine. INIBIC-University of A Coruña*
[2]*CIBER-BBN-Cellular Theraphy Area*
[3]*INIBIC-Hospital Universitario A Coruña*
Spain

1. Introduction

Osteoarthritis (OA) is a degenerative joint disease characterized by deterioration in the integrity of hyaline cartilage and subchondral bone (Ishiguro et al., 2002). OA is the most common articular pathology and the most frequent cause of disability. Genetic, metabolic and physical factors interact in the pathogenesis of OA producing cartilage damage. The incidence of OA is directly related to age and is expected to increase along with the median age of the population (Brooks, 2002).

The capacity for the self-repair of articular cartilage is very limited, mainly because it is an avascular tissue (Mankin, 1982; Resinger et al., 2004; Fuentes-Boquete et al., 2008). Consequently, progenitor cells in blood and marrow cannot enter the damaged region to influence or contribute to the reparative process (Steinert et al., 2007).

There are a lack of reliable techniques and methods to stimulate growth of new tissue to treat degenerative diseases and trauma (Wong et al., 2005).

Modalities of cellular therapy to repair focal articular cartilage defects include the implantation of cells with chondrogenic capacity (Koga et al., 2008) and creating access to the bone-marrow. Of the numerous treatments available nowadays, no technique has yet been able to consistently regenerate normal hyaline cartilage. Current treatments generate a fibrocartilaginous tissue that is different from hyaline articular cartilage. To avoid the need for prosthetic replacement, different cell treatments have been developed with the aim of forming a repair tissue with structural, biochemical, and functional characteristics equivalent to those of natural articular cartilage (Fuentes-Boquete et al.. 2007). This review summarizes the options for treatment of articular cartilage defects from both the experimental and clinical perspective (Fig. 1).

2. Perforation of the subchondral bone

This treatment is one of the most popular marrow-stimulating techniques based on the principle of inducing invasion of mesenchymal progenitor cells from the underlying subchondral bone to the lesion site, in order to initiate cartilage repair (Pelttari et al., 2009). This minimally invasive procedure has a low cost and is currently being used as the first treatment in patients not treated of cartilage defects. When the defect affecting the cartilage penetrates to the bone and bone marrow spaces (osteochondral injury), mesenchymal cells from the bone marrow migrate with the hemorrhage and remain in the blood clot filling the defect, and are differentiated into articular chondrocytes thus been responsible for the repair of the defect (Fig. 2) (Shapiro et al., 1993). The opening of subchondral vascular spaces is utilized for several surgical strategies, such as arthroscopic abrasion (Friedman et al., 1984), subchondral drilling (Muller & Kohn, 1999), spongialization (Ficat et al., 1979) and microfracture (which produces the best results) (Steadman et al., 1999). In most cases, bone is formed in the bony defect and fibrocartilaginous tissue is formed in the chondral lesion (Johnson, 1986; Buckwalter & Mankin, 1998). In the case of large osteochondral defects, the ability to spontaneously repair the damage is negligible. On the contrary, if the chondral defect is small, articular cartilage can be completely repaired in full. The critical size of the lesion so that it will self-repair remains unknown.

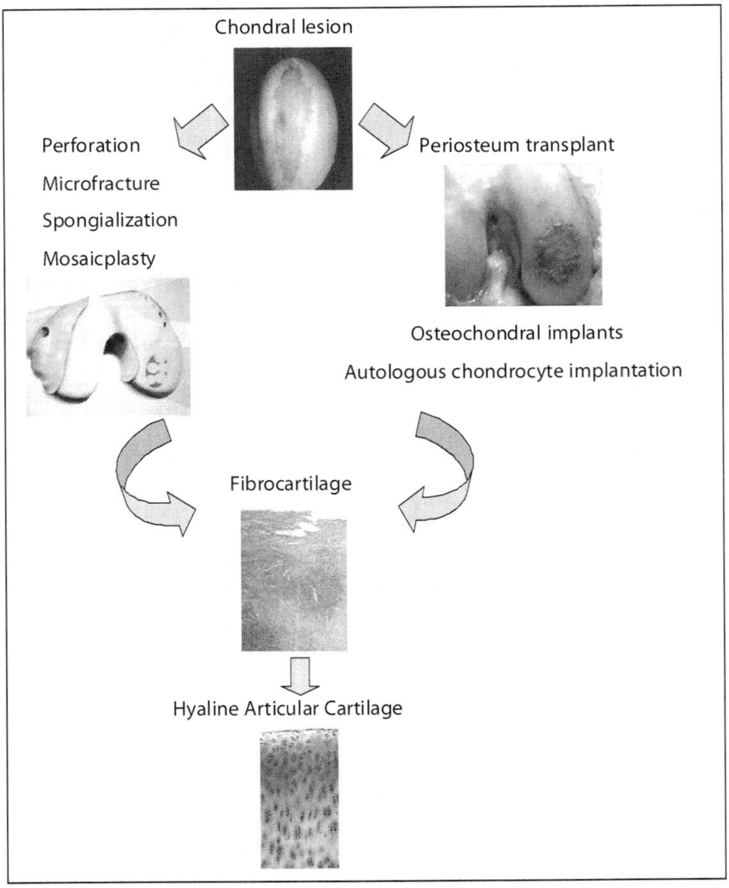

Fig. 1. Different treatments of articular cartilage defects.

The outcome of these procedures is highly variable and frequently results in repair tissue composed of fibrocartilage with some limitations in quality and duration as compared to native hyaline cartilage (Pelttari et al., 2009). Experimental studies in rabbits (Metsaranta et al., 1996; Menche et al., 1996) and dogs (Altman et al., 1992) have shown that the repair tissue generated by these processes is fibrocartilaginous in nature, differing from hyaline articular cartilage in biochemical composition, structural organization, durability and biomechanical properties, and degenerates over time (Shapiro et al., 1993; Menche et al., 1996). In addition, the newly formed subchondral bone is thicker than the native subchondral bone (Qiu et al., 2003). The co-expression of types I and II collagens in repair tissue does not occur until one year following subchondral penetration (Furukawa et al., 1980). Clinical results, to some degree, contradict the findings relating to the quality of the repair tissue. For example, the treatment of knee osteochondral defects by microfracture has provided good clinical results after two years (Knutsen et al., 2004). This longevity, however, seems to be age-dependent, with the most persistent repair cartilage in patients under the age of 40 (Kreuz et al., 2006a). Although the initiation of a degenerative process for tissue repair has been described at 18 months after microfracture (Kreuz et al., 2006b), and 7 to 17 years after microfracture, improvement in articular function and pain relief were preserved (Steadman et al., 2003).

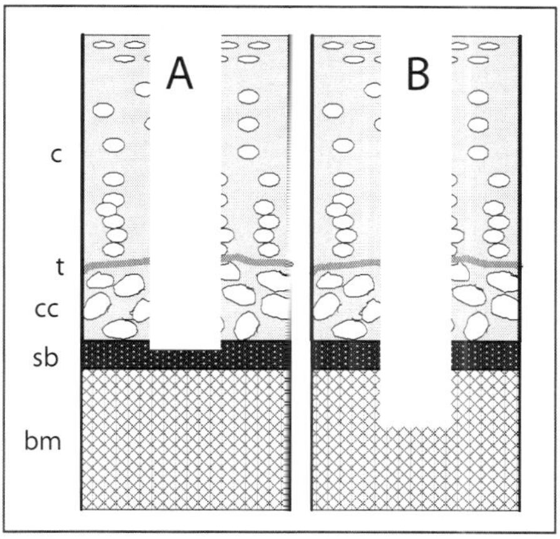

Fig. 2. Types of articular cartilage defects. In a partial defect the lesion includes cartilage tissue and part of the subchondral bone [A]. In a deep defect the lesion extends to the bone marrow [B]. C, uncalcified articular cartilage; t, tidemark; cc, calcified articular cartilage; sb, subchondral bone; bm, bone marrow.

3. Implants of periosteum and perichondrium

Tissue grafts have potential benefits since they allow the introduction of a new cell population embedded in an organic matrix, and reduces the development of fibrous adhesions between the articular surfaces before forming a new articular surface.

Periosteum and perichondrium contain mesenchymal stem cells (MSCs) that are capable of chondrogenesis (O´Driscoll et al., 2001; Duynstee et al., 2002). In particular, periosteum

consists of a fibrous outer layer, containing fibroblasts; and an inner layer or cambium, in direct contact with the bone, of higher cellular density, which contains MSCs.
Experimental studies in rabbits, indicated that the grafts of periosteum and perichondrium produce an incomplete filling of the chondral defect, and showed no significant differences between the two grafts in the quality of the repair tissue (Carranza-Bencano et al., 1999). In contrast, in a horse model, it was observed that chondrogenesis was more frequent and of greater magnitude in the grafts of periosteum than in perichondrium (Vachon et al., 1989). In both cases, these membrane implants forms a fibrocartilaginous repair tissue that does not seem to mature over time (Dounchis et al., 2000; Trzeciak et al., 2006). However, the clinical effects of a perichondrium implant are similar those of subchondral perforation. At 10 years following either procedure there were no significant differences observed between their outcomes (Bouwmeester et al., 2002). However, the graft of perichondrium requires an additional intervention.
With age, decreases the chondrogenic potential of periosteum, decreasing the ability of MSCs to proliferate and differentiate into chondrocytes (O´Driscoll et al., 2001). This procedure has confirmed the improvement of joint function and pain relief (Korkala & Kuokkanen, 1995). The periosteum has the advantage of being readily available for transplantation. However, the technique of obtaining and management of periosteum is a critical step and determining the chondrogenic potential; if the cambium layer is not preserved, the procedure fails (O´Driscoll & Fitzsimmons, 2000).
At present, there is no sufficient evidence to justify the use periosteum and perichondrium implants in the treatment of chondral defects.

4. Osteoperiosteal implants

The cylinder of bone graft covered with periosteum has been used for the treatment of osteochondral defects. Although it has been reported that its clinical application produces improved joint function and pain relief (Korkala & Kuokkanen, 1995), studies in animals show a neosynthesized tissue with fibrous features (van Susante et al., 2003). When the graft is accompanied by chondrogenic inductors it acquires a fibrocartilaginous appearance (Jung et al., 2005). Also, bleeding from bone marrow spaces from the injury probably interferes with the repair action of the periosteum germ layer. In fact, in a rabbit model of osteoperiosteal implant it was found that nearly 67% of repair tissue cells were derived mainly from the bone marrow (Zarnett & Salter, 1989).
Osteochondral grafts have the advantage of providing matrix and viable chondrocytes that maintain this matrix (Czitrom et al., 1990; Schachar et al., 1992; Ohlendorf et al., 1996). In addition, it is possible to retrieve the subchondral bone and the contour of the joint of patients with osteochondral defects or articular incongruity. The articular cartilage transplantation as part of an osteochondral graft provides the decrease in joint pain (Beaver et al., 1992), perhaps by the replacement of the innervated area of the subchondral bone by a graft without innervation.

5. Mosaicplasty

Autologous mosaicplasty is considered to be a promising alternative for treatment of small to medium-sized focal chondral and osteochondral defects (Bartha et al., 2006). This technique involves the translocation of osteochondral cylinders, or plugs, from a low-weight-bearing normal site to a high-weight-bearing diseased site. The injured area is completely covered by means of the combination of different sizes of cylinders (Szerb et al., 2005). The donor sites spontaneously repair with mesenchymal stromal cells from the bone marrow to promote a new fibrocartilaginous tissue.

This procedure, which clinical application started in 1992 (Hangody & Karpati, 1994; Hangody et al., 2001) is considered a promising alternative for the treatment of chondral and osteochondral defects of small and medium-size load in synovial joints (Bartha et al., 2006). However, it is limited by several factors. The ideal diameter of the defect should range between 1 and 4 cm^2. In addition, clinical experience shows that age is a limiting factor, it is recommended to apply this technique only for patients under 50 years. Contraindications to the use of mosaicplasty include infection, tumor and rheumatoid arthritis (Szerb et al., 2005).

Arthroscopic evaluations at 5 (Chow et al., 2004) and 10 years (Hangody & Fules, 2003) after osteochondral cylinder implantation showed survival of the transplanted articular cartilage, congruency between opposing (treated and untreated) joint surfaces and fibrocartilaginous repair of the donor sites. However, if the osteochondral cylinders protrude above the surface, joint problems can arise. At 4 months post-surgery, patients with protruding cylinders experienced a "catching sensation" and some of these patients reported joint pain. Arthroscopic examinations of these cases revealed fissures in the osteochondral cylinders and fibrillation around the recipient site (Nakagawa et al., 2007).

The use of autologous mosaicplasty is limited by the defect size, which determines the number of osteochondral cylinders required. Thus, in large defects the best option is osteochondral allogenic transplantation. In addition, the implanted tissue comes from an area of low load, showing a thin thickness, a different histological structure and, therefore, a lower functional capacity for dealing with charge absorption.

The articular cartilage produced by this technique exhibits topographical variations in morphological, biochemical and physical properties (Xia et al., 2002; Rogers et al., 2006). Because the implanted tissue is harvested from a low-weight-bearing area, the cartilage is thinner and differs in histological structure from cartilage from high weight-bearing areas (Fragonas et al., 1998; Gomez et al., 2000).

6. Osteoarticular allotransplantation

Due to the avascular nature of chondrocytes and the fact that they are encapsulated in the extracellular matrix (ECM), articular cartilage is considered a privileged immunological tissue (Langer & Gross, 1974). Thus, the allogenic transplant may be the solution for problems arising from the autologous mosaicplasty (avoiding injury to the low load zone of cartilage, can produce a large number of osteochondral cylinders and these can come from the same load area). In fact, osteochondral allograft in knee has shown a good integration and provides a functional improvement at 2 years (McCulloch et al., 2007), showing a 85% of implant survival after more than 10 years after intervention (Gross et al., 2005).

7. Autologous chondrocyte implantation

A cell-based therapeutic alternative offering more effective repair of focal articular cartilage defects is autologous chondrocyte implantation (ACI) which was developed in a rabbit experimental model (Grande et al., 1987 & 1989). The first clinical application of this method was performed by the group of Brittberg (Brittberg et al., 1994), which also demonstrated the successful repair of articular cartilage in rabbits transplanted with autologous chondrocytes (Brittberg et al., 1996). Currently the autologous chondrocyte implantation is a safe and effective therapeutic alternative to repair focal articular cartilage lesions (Pérez-Cachafeiro et al., 2010; Brittberg et al., 1994; Richardson et al., 1999; Peterson et al., 2000; Roberts et al., 2001). This procedure is also used for patients with osteochondritis dissecans (Peterson et al., 2002), but not for osteoarthritis joints. Because the results of this technique are highly age-dependent, the use of this procedure is recommended for patients younger than 55 years of age. The technique involves obtaining, by arthroscopy, articular cartilage explants from low-weight-bearing areas. Chondrocytes are then isolated and expanded *in vitro* to obtain a sufficient number of cells (approximately 10-12x10^6 cells) to introduce into the defect site, where they are expected to synthesize new cartilaginous matrix. In a second surgical intervention, the periosteum of the patient is removed from the proximal extremity and sutured to the edge of the cartilage injury, guiding the cambium layer towards de defect. This will close the defect cavity to retain the suspension of chondrocytes. Then, chondrocytes of the patient are resuspended in a liquid medium and injected into the cavity. A recent study assessed the efficacy and safety of ACI in 111 patients and demonstrated good clinical results in about 70%of the cases after 3 to 5 years (Pérez-Cachafeiro et al., 2010). Sometimes these autologous articular chondrocytes are introduced into the defect site as a cell suspension or in association with a supportive matrix (matrix-assisted ACI, MACI) (Pelttari et al., 2009). MACI uses a cell-seeded collagen matrix for treatment of cartilage defects. A prospective clinical investigation carried out in 38 patients with localized cartilage defects for a period of up to 5 years after surgery, showed that MACI represents a viable alternative for treatment of local cartilage defects of the knee (Behrens et al., 2006).

The outcome of these chondrocyte-based techniques is generally quite good (Minas, 2001; Peterson et al., 2000) but in many cases results in the formation of non-hyaline cartilage repair tissue with inferior mechanical properties and limited durability (Pelttari et al., 2009). ACI has several technical limitations: *a)* obtaining cartilage explants requires an additional surgical intervention, adding to the articular cartilage damage that increases the osteoarthritic process (Marcacci et al., 2002); *b) in vitro* chondrocyte proliferation must be limited because the capacity to produce stable cartilage *in vivo* is gradually reduced when cell divisions are increased (Dell´Accio et al., 2001); *c)* aging reduces the cellular density of the cartilage, which impacts chondrocyte proliferation capacity *in vitro* (Menche et al., 1998) and the chondrogenic potential of the periosteum (O´Driscoll & Fitzsimmons, 2001), *d)* cell culture procedures take too long (3 to 6 weeks) and increase the risk of contamination, *e)* risk of leakage of transplanted chondrocytes from the cartilage defects, *f)* the effects of gravity causing the chondrocytes to sink to the dependent side of the defect, resulting in an unequal distribution of cells that hampers the homogenous regeneration of the cartilage (Díaz-Prado et al., 2010c; Sohn et al., 2002), *g)* not the least the reacquisition of phenotypes of dedifferentiated chondrocytes in a monolayer culture (Kimura et al., 1984; Benya & Shaffer, 1982) and *h)* hypertrophy of tissue (Steinwachs & Kreuz, 2007; Haddo et al., 2004). The use of periosteum membrane poses constraints and the need for wide surgical incision, hypertrophy of the periosteum peripheral implant and its potential for ectopic calcification. As an alternative it has been proposed the use of a membrane collagen type I/III (Haddo et al., 2004; Krishnan et al., 2006; Robertson et al., 2007). The use of both kinds of membranes shows no significant differences in the clinical assessment, although arthroscopic analysis

showed that after implantation of periosteum a substantial number of patients required a cleanup of the peripheral hypertrophy (Gooding et al., 2006).
In 1997, the American Society FDA (Food and Drug Administration) approved the cellular technology that uses autologous chondrocytes to repair articular cartilage lesions in the knee. This was the first type of cellular technology that was regulated by the industry for use in human transplantation (Brittberg et al., 2001).
The first article about ACI in humans appeared in 1994 (Brittberg et al., 1994). Clinical and arthroscopic evaluations of femoral implants showed good results after 2 years and the histological study of biopsies of the new tissue showed a similar appearance to hyaline cartilage in 11 of 15 cases of femoral implant. From this first approach further studies, based on clinical or arthroscopic evaluations, have demonstrated the durability of the implant. Thereby, after 5-11 years of treatment showed good or excellent clinical results in 51 of the 61 patients (Peterson et al., 2002). Histological analysis of the *de novo* formed tissue revealed some heterogeneity in the quality of the repair tissue. Of the 41 biopsies obtained one year following implantation, 10% consisted of hyaline cartilage; 24% consisted of a mixture of hyaline cartilage and fibrocartilage; 61% were entirely fibrocartilage and 5% consisted only of fibrous tissue (Tins et al., 2005).
Other studies at one year after implantation have shown that fibrocartilaginous morphology regions and hyaline morphology regions coexist in the same biopsy; both types having proteoglycans and type II collagen (Richardson et al., 1999; Roberts et al., 2001). Furthermore, aggrecanase activity was higher than metalloprotease activities in the fibrocartilaginous regions although both enzymes were found (Roberts et al., 2001). The expression of type IIA and IIB collagen mRNA was also detected (Briggs et al., 2003). These mRNA expressions seem be characteristic of the prechondrocytic state (type IIA) and differentiated chondrocytes (type IIB) (Nah et al., 2001). These results suggest that ACI induces the regeneration of articular cartilage, probably by the turnover and remodelling from an initial fibrocartilaginous matrix using enzymatic degradation and synthesis of type II collagen (Roberts et al., 2001). It is believed that this process continues for more than 24 months following the implantation (Peterson et al., 2000, Bentley et al., 2003) and takes place in three specific stages: cell proliferation (the first 6 weeks), transition (7 to 26 weeks) and remodeling (beyond 27 weeks) (Minas & Peterson, 1997).

8. Allotransplantation and xenotransplantation of chondrocytes

Other therapeutic alternatives are allotransplantation (Wakitani et al., 1989; Rahfoth et al., 1998; Schreiber et al., 1999) and xenotransplantation of chondrocytes (Fuentes-Boquete et al., 2004, Ramallal et al., 2004), that elude the damage added to the joint during autotransplantation to obtain isolated chondrocytes. Allotransplantation is constrained by the necessity for compatible donors and limitations on storage of cartilage or chondrocytes because cryopreservation reduces survival and proliferation of chondrocytes (Rendal-Vázquez et al., 2001). Xenotransplantation may resolve some of these problems, but this therapeutic alternative has rarely been investigated. The immune barrier is an important objection to the use of both of these therapeutic procedures, although its application in articular cartilage presents fewer difficulties than in other tissues. Even though isolated chondrocytes result in immunogenic reaction, alloimplantation of chondrocytes encapsulated in their ECM (Schreiber et al., 1999) or embedded in collagen gel (Wakitani et al., 1989) or agarose (Rahfoth et al., 1998) resulted in few or no rejection reactions. Notably, xenotransplantation *in vivo* of cultured pig chondrocytes into rabbit chondral defects closed with periosteal membrane no signs of infiltration by immune cells (Ramallal et al., 2004).

9. Mesenchymal stem cells transplantation

Within the bone marrow stroma, a subset of non-hematopoietic cells referred to as MSCs exists. These cells can be isolated by adherence to plastic, expanded *ex vivo* and induced, both *in vitro* or *in vivo*, to terminally differentiate into multiple mesoderm-type lineages, including osteocytes, chondrocytes, adipocytes, tenocytes, myotubes, astrocytes and hematopoietic-supporting stroma (Barlow et al., 2008; Minguell et al., 2000; Caplan, 1991) and also into cell types of ectodermal (e.g., neurons) and endodermal (e.g., hepatocytes) origin (Pasquinelli et al., 2007). Furthermore, MSCs from different tissue sources can have biologic distinctions. For example, MSCs derived from bone marrow show a higher potential for osteogenic differentiation (Muraglia et al., 2000), while MSCs of synovial origin show a greater tendency toward chondrogenic differentiation (Djouad et al., 2005). Under identical culture conditions for differentiation, MSCs isolated from the synovial membrane show more chondrogenic potential than those derived from bone marrow, periosteum, skeletal muscle or adipose tissue (Sakaguchi et al., 2005). Studies of cartilage injury repair in animal models using MSCs embedded in collagen gel (Wakitani et al., 1989) or injected into defects closed with periosteal membrane (Im et al., 2001) indicate that MSCs can differentiate *in vivo* into a number of cell types in different biologic environments.

This procedure uses cells isolated from small tissue samples, proliferated in culture, to obtain the appropriate number for clinical applications. They can be implanted in the donor patient, obviating rejection problems. MSCs may be a tool for tissue repair that has the advantage of avoiding the problem of immunological rejection of the allotransplant and the ethical conflict of using embryonic stem cells. The recent use of autologous or allogenic stem cells has been suggested as an alternative therapeutic approach for treatment of cartilage defects (Jung et al., 2009). MSCs have the capability to self-renew and are responsible for repair and repopulation of damaged tissues in the adult (Hombach-Klonisch et al., 2008). For these reasons MSCs are a promising cell resource for tissue engineering and cell-based therapies (Pittenger, 2008). The interest in MSCs and their possible application in cell therapy have resulted in a better understanding of the basic biology of these cells. Due to the low number of MSCs that can be isolated from a tissue sample, culture expansion is necessary to obtain adequate cell numbers for clinical purposes and for the analysis of molecular mechanisms. However, the number of mitotic divisions of MSCs in culture must be limited because MSCs age during *in vitro* culture, causing a reduction in their proliferative capacity (Banfi et al., 2000; Bonab et al., 2006) and gradual loss of the potential for multiple differentiation (Banfi et al., 2000; Izadpanah et al., 2006). The conservation of phenotype and differentiation capacity of MSCs are proportional to telomerization (Abdallah et al., 2005). Telomeres are normally shortened in successive cell divisions, however, in embryonic stem cells the telomere length is restored by telomerase enzyme activity. On the other hand, MSCs lack (Zimmermann et al., 2003) adequate levels of telomerase activity to achieve telomeric restoration (Izadpanah et al., 2006; Parsch et al., 2004; Yanada et al., 2006). Patient age also influences the characteristics of MSCs because their proliferative capacity is reduced by aging (Stenderup et al., 2003).

Three criteria define all types of stem cells: self-renewal, multipotency and the ability to reconstitute a tissue *in vivo*. According to a recent proposal of the International Society for Cellular Therapy (Dominici et al., 2006), MSCs are multipotent nonhematopoietic progenitors located within the stroma of the bone marrow and other organs that are phenotypically characterized by the expression of several markers (e.g., CD73, CD90, and CD105) and the lack of expression of CD14 or CD11b, CD19 or CD79α, CD34, CD45 and HLA-DR surface molecules (Mrugala et al., 2009; Kastrinaki et al., 2008). Because there is no specific marker for MSCs, the principal criteria for identification are adherence to the plastic of the tissue culture flask, fibroblast-like morphology (Prockop, 1997), the prolonged capacity for proliferation in supportive media and the capacity to differentiate *in vitro* into cells of mesodermal origin (chondrocytes, adipocytes, osteoblasts). Furthermore, characteristics of MSCs are the absence of expression of typical hematopoietic antigens like CD34 and CD45, and the expression of surface markers like Stro-1, CD44, CD73, CD90, CD105 and CD166 (Pittenger et al., 1999).

Human MSCs, which are probably responsible for normal tissue renewal, as well as for response to injury (Tsai et al., 2007), have been isolated from several tissues, including bone marrow (Kastrinaki et al., 2008; Yoo et al., 1998), periosteum (Nakahara et al., 1990), perichondrium (Dounchis et al., 1997), synovial membrane (De Bari et al., 2001; Fickert et al., 2003), articular cartilage (Alsalameh et al., 2004); connective tissue of dermis and skeletal muscle (Young et al., 2001), peripheral blood (Villaron et al., 2004; Kuznetsov et al., 2001; Zvaifler et al., 2000), adipose tissue (Zuk et al., 2001 & 2002), lung (In´t Anker et al., 2003), liver (Le Blanc et al., 2005), amniotic fluid (You et al., 2008; Steigman & Fauza, 2007; Fauza, 2004), placenta (Barlow et al., 2008, Steigman & Fauza, 2007; Fauza, 2004: Matikainen & Laine, 2005), amniotic membrane (Díaz-Prado et al., 2010a & 2010b; Alviano et al., 2007), umbilical cord (Baksh et al., 2007) and umbilical cord blood (Mareschi et al., 2001). Although bone marrow is the usual source of MSCs, umbilical cord blood is emerging as an important reservoir for stem cells capable of differentiation into many cell types and possessing the advantages of immune status and relatively unshortened telomere length (McGuckin et al., 2005). Some countries have private and public stem cell banks from umbilical cord blood (UCB) for transplant programs or personal use (Samuel et al., 2008). Multipotent MSCs are a promising cell resource for tissue engineering and cell-based therapeutics because of their ability to self-renew and differentiate into specific functional cell types (Tsai et al., 2007). The list of tissues with the potential for tissue engineering is increasing because of recent progress in stem cell biology (Bianco & Robey, 2001).

In vitro (Pittenger et al., 1999; Majumdar et al., 1998; Muraglia et al., 2000) and in vivo (Gronthos et al., 2003) studies of clonally-derived MSCs demonstrated that the MSC population consists of subsets that have different expression of markers and different capacities for cellular differentiation. To improve the number of MSCs isolated from a tissue it is frequent to use a pre-plating technique that minimizes the number of contaminating fibroblasts in the culture (Richler & Yaffe, 1970). Also, MSCs show phenotypic and functional differences depending on their tissue of origin. For example, MSCs from bone marrow and synovial membrane have been differentiated by their gene expression profiles (Djouad et al., 2005).

Several studies have recently reported the migration of intraarticularly injected MSCs to the site of a cartilage injury to repair chondral defects. In a caprine model for osteoarthritis in which OA is induced by the complete excision of the medial meniscus and resection of the anterior cruciate ligament, the intraarticular injection of MSCs produced meniscus repair after 6 weeks; however, there was no evidence of cartilage or ligament repair (Murphy et al., 2003). This suggests that the injected MSCs migrated to the injured meniscus, but not the

damaged cartilage. The intraarticular injection of MSCs into rat knees, however, showed mobilization of these cells towards all injured tissues, including articular cartilage; the MSCs contributed to tissue regeneration (Nishimori et al., 2006; Agung et al., 2006).
In osteoarthritic knees, MSCs embedded in collagen gel were implanted into chondral defects and closed with periosteal membrane. After 42 weeks, arthroscopic and histological results were better than in osteoarthritic patients without implants, although there was no statistically significant improvement in clinical results (Wakitani et al., 2002). The use of MSCs to treat chondral lesions clinically has not been established, in part because the stages of chondrogenic differentiation of MSCs are not sufficiently defined. In addition, there are currently no protocols that ensure direct differentiation to the desired phenotype; the plasticity of the cells differentiated from MSCs can lead to undesirable phenotypic alterations (De Bari et al., 2004; Pelttari et al., 2006).

10. Scaffolds

The clinical outcome of the techniques described above underline the need of increase the quality of the synthesized repair tissue. To overcome some of the limitations of ACI, cell delivery supports can be used for cell transplantation. Recent research efforts have focused on tissue engineering as a promising approach for cartilage regeneration and repair (Kuo et al., 2006). Tissue engineering is a technique by which a living tissue can be reconstructed by associating the cells with biomaterials that provide a scaffold on which they can proliferate three-dimensionally, under physiological conditions (Iwasa et al., 2009). A biomaterial is any pharmacologically inert compound designed to be implanted or incorporated into the living system. Therefore cartilage tissue engineering is critically dependent on the selection of appropriate cells (differentiated or MSCs), suitable scaffolds for cell delivery and biological stimulation with chondrogenically bioactive molecules (Kuo et al., 2006). The transplantation of chondrocytes seeded on natural and synthetic scaffolds has been used for cartilage tissue engineering (Kuo et al., 2006). Regeneration of a hyaline-like repair tissue could be obtained after the implantation of a pre-engineering, functional cartilage tissue, instead of the delivery of a chondrocyte implantation (Pelttari et al., 2009). A major prerequisite for choosing a scaffold is the property of not producing toxic, injurious, carcinogenic, or immunological responses (either inflammation or rejection) in living tissue (Niknejad et al., 2008). New tissue regeneration should occur as the scaffold degrades, so the new tissue assumes the shape and size of the original scaffold. Design criteria for scaffolds include suitable mechanical strength and surface chemistry, ability to be processed in different shapes and sizes, and the ability to regulate cellular activities such as differentiation and proliferation (Kuo et al., 2006). Moreover, requirements for the biomaterials used as a scaffold include controlled biocompatibility, structurally and mechanically stable, permeability (allowing the exchange of nutrients and metabolites), suitable ligands for implanted cell attachment, must support the loading of an appropriate cell source to allow successful infiltration and attachment with appropriate bioactive molecules in order to promote cellular differentiation and maturation. Also, they must present readily integration with native cartilage, biodegradation into non-toxic products that can be replaced by host cells, initial stability and provide an excellent environment for cell and tissue growth and differentiation crucial to maintain cell function and development of new tissue. Scaffolds must also provide a stable temporary structure while cells seeded within the biodegradable matrix synthesize a new and natural tissue (Frenkel & Di Cesare, 2004). Other important factors in the design of a scaffold are pore size, porosity, adaptive shape, mechanical integrity, the ability to be retained at the implantation site and cost efficiency.

A number of scaffolds have been developed and investigated, in vitro and in vivo, for potential use in tissue engineering and in particular for in vitro regeneration of cartilage tissues (Vinatier et al., 2009). Carries have been marketed and various tissue-engineering techniques have been developed using chondrocytes seeded on biological matrices (Iwasa et al., 2009). For cartilage tissue engineering, scaffolding has been fabricated from both natural and synthetic polymers (Tuli et al., 2003), such as fibrous structures, porous sponges, woven or non-woven meshes and hydrogels (Kuo et al., 2006). Natural biomaterials, such as fibrin, collagen, agarose, alginate, hyaluronic acid or chitosan (Eyrich et al., 2007; Cao & Xu, 2008; Mouw et al., 2005; Lisignoli et al., 2006; Nettles et al., 2002) and synthetic biomaterials, such as poly-lactic glycolic acid (PLGA) (Han et al., 2008) and a polymeric nanofiber (Janjanin et al., 2008), are used alone or in different combinations to make scaffolds. Collagen and hyaluronan-based matrices are among the most popular natural scaffolds in clinical use nowadays, since they contain natural components of the hyaline cartilage. On the contrary, there is no clinical experience using scaffolds such as alginate, agarose and chitosan (Iwasa et al., 2009). Within each kind of biomaterial (natural and synthetic) there are many types of biomaterials that are being studied, with controversial results. The human amniotic membrane (HAM) is considered to be an important potential source for scaffolding material (Niknejad et al., 2008). The HAM possesses clinical considerable advantages that are not shared by other natural or synthetic polymers. On the other hand, HAM has abundant natural cartilage components, which are important in the regulation and maintenance of normal chondrocyte metabolism (Jin et al., 2007); this suggests that the HAM is an excellent candidate for use as native scaffold for cartilage tissue engineering (Niknejad et al., 2008). Amnion allografts are widely applied in ophthalmology, plastic surgery, dermatology, and gynecology (Tejwani et al., 2007; Santos et al., 2005; Rinastiti et al., 2006; Meller et al., 2000; Morton & Dewhurst, 1986). A recent study demonstrated the potential use of the HAM as a scaffold to support human chondrocyte proliferation in cell therapy to repair human OA cartilage (Díaz-Prado et al., 2010c).

Experimental studies in animals with synthetic biomaterials showed disappointing results, since after 8 weeks of implantation, all animals suffered ulceration and loss of cartilage (Oka et al., 1997). The problem that arises with artificial biomaterials is that the implant is not interwoven with adjacent bone, leading to degradation of the recovered surface after only 2 or 3 months (Oka et al., 1997). In a study in rabbits with a biomaterial composed of collagen in which chondrocytes were seeded, a good proliferation and cell phenotype maintenance were shown; therefore good repair results were observed (Frenkel et., 1997). One of the major limitations of the use of matrices is the size of the lesion (Nixon et al., 1993, Sams & Nixon, 1995, Sams et al., 1995). Despite the diffusion of new tissue-engineering techniques and the number of scaffolds that have been investigated, the ideal matrix material has not been identified. However, the clinical use of these materials is currently limited, mainly due to the risk of disease transmission and immunoreaction (Iwasa et al., 2009).

Mechanical and biological properties of biomaterials significantly influence chondrogenesis and the long-term maintenance of the structural integrity of the neo-formed tissue. The three-dimensional nature of the scaffolds promotes maintenance of rounded cell morphology and the elevated expression of glycosaminoglycans and type II collagen (Nettles et al., 2002; Gong et al., 2008). Other advantage is that cell delivery supports may act as barrier to the invasion of the graft by fibroblasts, which may otherwise induce fibrous repair (Frenkel et al., 1997). Indeed, the presence of ECM around cells was reported to increase donor cell retention at the repair site and possibly protect the cells from environmental factors such as inflammatory molecules (Pelttari et al., 2009). The tissue-engineering methods with scaffolds including the arthroscopy technique are less invasive because there is no need to harvest periosteum (Iwasa et al., 2009). Other benefits of this methodology are: reduce surgical time, morbidity, and risk of periosteal hypertrophy and postsurgical adhesions substantially (Iwasa et al., 2009). However, scaffolding biomaterials have differing influences on the metabolism of host cells and, consequently, the quality of the tissue-engineered cartilage (Mouw et al., 2005, Jeon et al., 2007). For example, the use of chitosan, compared to PLGA, for cartilage tissue engineering produces a superior maintenance of structural integrity because the expression of type II collagen protein and mRNA became weaker over time in the PLGA group (Jeon et al., 2007). Scaffolds using hyaluronic acid are also being used with excellent clinical and histological results (Giannini et al., 2008).

11. Gene therapy

The introduction of genetic products into the field of tissue damage repair can enhance the process of articular cartilage restoration. The most obvious would be growth factors, proteinase inhibitors and cytokine antagonists. The gene therapy process involves the determination of the appropriate gene and cell type (chondrocytes, chondrogenic cells and cells of the synovial membrane) for the gene transfer, as well as the determination of the optimal vector to incorporate the cDNA (Trippel et al., 2004). Different anabolic factors, such as members of the TGF-β3 (tumor growth factor beta 3), IGF (insulin growth factor), FGF (fibroblastic growth factor), and HGF (hepatocyte growth factor) superfamily, could induce chondrogenesis and the synthesis of ECM components, while anti-inflammatory molecules, such as interleukins (IL): IL-4, IL-10, Il-1Ra (IL-1 receptor antagonist), and TNFsR (tumor necrosis factor soluble receptor), could act as inhibitors of cartilage degradation (Gelse et al., 2003).

The synovial membrane seems to be useful as a target for chondroprotective therapies (Palmer et al., 2002). The viral transfection *in vivo* with the IL-1Ra gene in rheumatoid arthritis joints reduces the severity of the disease process in animal models (Gouze et al., 2003). Furthermore, this technique makes possible the safe intraarticular expression of the IL-1Ra gene (Evans et al., 2005 & 2001). Chondrocytes and MSCs are the preferred targets for the induction of chondrogenesis. Using animal models, the transplantation *in vivo* of MSCs transfected with BMP-2 (bone morphogenetic protein-2) cDNA produces improved chondral lesion repair with a higher production of proteoglycans and type II collagen compared to controls (Park et al., 2006).

12. Conclusion

Modalities of cellular therapy to repair focal articular cartilage defects include the implantation of cells with chondrogenic capacity and creating access to the bone-marrow. Of the numerous treatments available nowadays, no technique has yet been able to consistently regenerate normal hyaline cartilage. The implantation of autologous chondrocytes and autologous mosaicplasty induces a better quality of articular cartilage whereas the use of stem cell implants is in an early experimental stage at this time. Currently the autologous chondrocyte implantation is the most effective therapeutic alternative to repair focal articular cartilage lesions although this procedure is also used for patients with osteochondritis dissecans but not for osteoarthritis joints. On the other hand the use of tissue-engineered grafts based on scaffolds seems to be as effective as conventional ACI clinically but there are no convincing evidences that scaffold techniques allow the maintenance of the chondrocyte phenotype and the homogeneous distribution of the cells. Therefore it has not verified that the technical and theoretical advantages of scaffold techniques have led to the better clinical and histological results compared with conventional ACI. Further studies would be needed to determine whether articular cartilage repair with scaffolds is the most adequate alternative to ACI.

13. Acknowledgements

This study was supported by grants: Servizo Galego de Saúde, Xunta de Galicia (PS07/84); Cátedra Bioiberica de la Universidade da Coruña; Instituto de Salud Carlos III CIBER BBN CB06-01-0040; Ministerio de Ciencia e Innovacion PLE2009-0144; Fondo de Investigacion Sanitaria-PI 08/2028 with participation of fundus from FEDER (European Community), Silvia Diaz-Prado is beneficiary of an Isidro Parga Pondal contract from Xunta de Galicia, A Coruna, Spain.

14. References

Abdallah BM, Haack-Sorensen M, Burns JS, Elsnab B, Jakob F, Hokland P, Kassem M. (2005). Maintenance of differentiation potential of human bone marrow mesenchymal stem cells immortalized by human telomerase reverse transcriptase gene despite [corrected] extensive proliferation. *Biochem Biophys Res Commun* 326:527-38.

Agung M, Ochi M, Yanada S, Adachi N, Izuta Y, Yamasaki T, Toda K. (2006). Mobilization of bone marrowderived mesenchymal stem cells into the injured tissues after intraarticular injection and their contribution to tissue regeneration. *Knee Surg Sports Traumatol Arthrosc* 14:1307-14.

Alsalameh S, Amin R, Gemba T, Lotz M. (2004). Identification of mesenchymal progenitor cells in normal and osteoarthritic human articular cartilage. *Arthritis Rheum* 50:1522-32.

Altman RD, Kates J, Chun LE, Dean DD, Eyre D. (1992). Preliminary observations of chondral abrasion in a canine model. *Ann Rheum Dis* 51:1056-62.

Alviano F, Fossati V, Marchionni C, Arpinati M, Bonsi L, Franchina M, Lanzoni G, Cantoni S, Cavallini C, Bianchi F, Tazzari PL, Pasquinelli G, Foroni L, Ventura C, Grossi A, Bagnara GP. (2007). Term amniotic membrane is a high throughput source for multipotent mesenchymal stem cells with ability to differentiate into endothelial cells *in vitro*. *BMC Dev Biol* 7:11.

Baksh D, Yao R, Tuan RS. (2007). Comparison of proliferative and multilineage differentiation potential of human mesenchymal stem cells derived from umbilical cord and bone marrow. *Stem Cells* 25:1384-92.

Banfi A, Muraglia A, Dozin B, Mastrogiacomo M, Cancedda R, Quarto R. (2000). Proliferation kinetics and differentiation potential of *ex vivo* expanded human bone marrow stromal cells: Implications for their use in cell therapy. *Exp Hematol* 28:707-15.

Barlow S, Brooke G, Chatterjee K, Price G, Pelekanos R, Rossetti T, Doody M, Venter D, Pain S, Gilshenan K, Atkinson K. (2008). Comparison of human placenta- and bone marrow-derived multipotent mesenchymal stem cells. *Stem Cells Dev* 17:1095-1108.

Bartha L, Vajda A, Duska Z, Rahmeh H, Hangody L. (2006). Autologous osteochondral mosaicplasty grafting. *J Orthop Sports Phys Ther* 36:739-50.

Beaver RJ, Mahomed M, Backstein D, Davis A, Zukor DJ, Gross AE. (1992). Fresh osteochondral allografts for post-traumatic defects in the knee. A survivorship analysis. *J Bone Joint Surg Br* 74:105-10.

Behrens P, Bitter T, Kurz B, Russlies M. (2006). Matrix-associated autologous chondrocyte transplantation/implantation (MACT/MACI)- 5-year follow-up. *Knee* 13:194-202.

Bentley G, Biant LC, Carrington RW, Akmal M, Goldberg A, Williams AM, Skinner JA, Pringle J. (2003). A prospective, randomised comparison of autologous chondrocyte implantation versus mosaicplasty for osteochondral defects in the knee. *J Bone Joint Surg Br* 85:223-30.

Benya PD, Shaffer JD. (1982). Dedifferentiated chondrocytes re-express the differentiated collagen phenotype when cultured in agarose gels. *Cell* 30:215-24.

Bianco P, Robey PG. (2001). Stem cells in tissue engineering. *Nature* 414:118-21.

Bonab MM, Alimoghaddam K, Talebian F, Ghaffari SH, Ghavamzadeh A, Nikbin B. (2006). Aging of mesenchymal stem cell *in vitro*. *BMC Cell Biol* 7:14-20.

Bouwmeester PS, Kuijer R, Homminga GN, Bulstra SK, Geesink RG. (2002). A retrospective analysis of two independent prospective cartilage repair studies: autogenous perichondrial grafting versus subchondral drilling 10 years post-surgery. *J Orthop Res* 20:267-73.

Briggs TW, Mahroof S, David LA, Flannelly J, Pringle J, Bayliss M. (2003). Histological evaluation of chondral defects after autologous chondrocyte implantation of the knee. *J Bone Joint Surg Br* 85:1077-83.

Brittberg M, Lindahl A, Nilsson A, Ohlsson C, Isaksson O, Peterson L. (1994). Treatment of deep cartilage defects in the knee with autologous chondrocyte transplantation. *N Engl J Med* 331:889-95.

Brittberg M, Nilson A, Lindahl A, Ohlsson C, Peterson L. (1996). Rabbit articular cartilage defects treated with autologous cultured chondrocytes. *Clin Orthop Relat Res* (326):270-83.

Brittberg M, Tallhden T, Sjögren-Jansson B, Lindahl A, Peterson L. (2001) Autologous chondrocytes used for articular cartilage repair: an update. *Clin Orthop Relat Res* (391 Suppl):S337-48.

Brooks PM. (2002). Impact of osteoarthritis on individuals and society: how much disability? Social consequences and health economic implications. *Curr Opin Rheumatol* 14:573-7.

Buckwalter JA, Mankin HJ. (1998). Articular cartilage: tissue design and chondrocyte-matrix interactions. *Instr Course Lect* 47: 477-86.

Cao H, Xu SY. (2008). EDC/NHS-crosslinked type II collagen-chondroitin sulfate scaffold: characterization and *in vitro* evaluation. *J Mater Sci Mater Med* 19(2):567-75.

Caplan AI. (1991). Mesenchymal stem cells. *J Orthop Res* 9:641-50.

Carranza-Bencano A, Perez-Tinao M, Ballesteros-Vázquez P, Armas-Padrón JR, Hevia-Alonso A, Martos Crespo F. (1999). Comparative study of the reconstruction of articular cartilage defects with free costal perichondrial grafts and free tibial periosteal grafts: an experimental study on rabbits. *Calcif Tissue Int* 65:402-7.

Chow JC, Hantes ME, Houle JB, Zalavras CG. (2004). Arthroscopic autogenous osteochondral transplantation for treating knee cartilage defects: a 2- to 5-year follow-up study. *Arthroscopy* 20:681-90.

Czitrom AA, Keating S, Gross AE. (1990). The viability of articular cartilage in fresh osteochondral allografts after clinical transplantation. *J Bone Joint Surg Am* 72:574-81.

De Bari C, Dell'Acio F, Tylzanowski P, Luyten FP. (2001). Multipotent mesenchymal stem cells from adult human synovial membrane. *Arthritis Rheum* 44:1928-42.

De Bari C, Dell'Accio F, Luyten FP. (2004). Failure of *in vitro* differentiated mesenchymal stem cells from the synovial membrane to form ectopic stable cartilage *in vivo*. *Arthritis Rheum* 50:142-50.

Dell'Accio F, De Bari C, Luyten FP. (2001). Molecular markers predictive of the capacity of expanded human articular chondrocytes to form stable cartilage *in vivo*. *Arthritis Rheum* 44:1608-19.

Díaz-Prado S, Muíños-López E, Hermida-Gómez T, Rendal-Vázquez ME, Fuentes-Boquete I, de Toro FJ, Blanco FJ. (2010a). Isolation and characterization of mesenchymal stem cells from human amniotic membrane. *Tissue Eng Part C Methods* Aug 1.

Díaz-Prado S, Muíños-López E, Hermida-Gómez T, Rendal-Vázquez ME. Fuentes-Boquete I, de Toro FJ, Blanco FJ. (2010b). Multilineage differentiation potential of cells isolated from the human amniotic membrane. *J Cell Biochem* Jul 21.

Díaz-Prado S, Rendal-Vázquez ME, Muíños López E, Hermida-Gómez T, Rodríguez-Cabarcos M, Fuentes-Boquete I, de Toro FJ, Blanco FJ. (2010c). Potential use of the human amniotic membrane as a scaffold in human articular cartilage repair. *Cell Tissue Bank* 11:183-95.

Djouad F, Bony C, Häupl T, Uzé G, Lahlou N, Louis-Plence P, Apparailly F, Canovas F, Réme T, Sany J, Jorgensen C, Noël D. (2005). Transcriptional profiles discriminate bone marrow-derived and synovium-derived mesenchymal cells. *Arthritis Res Ther* 7:1304-15.

Dominici M, Le Blanc K, Mueller I, Slaper-Cortenbach I, Marini F, Krause D, Deans R, Keating A, Prockop Dj, Horwitz E. (2006). Minimal criteria for defining multipotent mesenchymal stromal cells. The International Society for Cellular Therapy position statement. *Cytotherapy* 8:315-7.

Dounchis JS, Goomer RS, Harwood FL, Khatod M, Coutts RD, Amiel D. (1997). Chondrogenic phenotype of perichondrium-derived chondroprogenitor cells is influenced by transforming growth factor-beta 1. *J Orthop Res* 15:803-7.

Dounchis JS, Bae WC, Chen AC, Sah RL, Coutts RD, Amiel D. (2000). Cartilage repair with autogenic perichondrium cell and polylactic acid grafts. *Clin Orthop Relat Res* (377):248-64.

Duynstee ML, Verwoerd-Verhoef HL, Verwoerd CD, Van Osch GJ. (2002). The dual role of perichondrium in cartilage wound healing. *Plast Reconstr Surg* 110:1073-9.

Evans CH, Robbins PD, Ghivizzani SC, Herndon JH, Wasko MC, Tomaino M, Kang R, Muzzonigro TA, Elder EM, Whiteside TL, Watkins SC. (2001). Transfer and intraarticular expression of the IL-1Ra cDNA in human rheumatoid joints. *Arthritis Res* 3 (Suppl 1):P33.

Evans CH, Robbins PD, Ghivizzani SC, Wasko MC, Tomaino MM, Kang R, Muzzonigro TA, Vogt M, Elder EM, Whiteside TL, Watkins SC, Herndon JH. (2005). Gene transfer to human joints: progress toward a gene therapy of arthritis. *Proc Natl Acad Sci USA* 102:8698-703.

Eyrich D, Brandl F, Appel B, Wiese H, Maier G, Wenzel M, Staudenmaier R, Goepferich A, Blunk T. (2007). Long-term stable fibrin gels for cartilage engineering. *Biomaterials* 28:55-65.

Fauza D. (2004). Amniotic fluid and placental stem cells. *Best Pract Res Clin Obstet Gynaecol* 18:877-91.

Ficat RP, Ficat C, Gedeon P, Toussaint JB. (1979). Spongialization: a new treatment for diseased patellae. *Clin Orthop Rel Res* 144: 74-83.

Fickert S, Fiedler J, Brenner RE. (2003). Identification, quantification and isolation of mesenchymal progenitor cells from osteoarthritic synovium by fluorescence automated cell sorting. *Osteoarthritis Cartilage* 11:790-800.

Fragonas E, Mlynárik V, Jellús V, Micali F, Piras A, Toffanin R, Rizzo R, Vittur F. (1998). Correlation between biochemical composition and magnetic resonance appearance of articular cartilage. *Osteoarthritis Cartilage* 6:24-32.

Frenkel SR, Toolan B, Menche D, Pitman MI, Pachence JM. (1997). Chondrocyte transplantation using a collagen bilayer matrix for cartilage repair. *J Bone Joint Surg Br* 79:831-6.

Frenkel SR, Di Cesare PE. (2004). Scaffolds for articular cartilage repair. *Ann Biomed Eng* 32:26-34.

Friedman MJ, Berasi CC, Fox JM, Del Pizzo W, Snyder SJ, Ferkel RD. (1984). Preliminary results with abrasion arthroplasty in the osteoarthritic knee. *Clin Orthop Rel Res* 182:200-5.

Fuentes-Boquete I, López-Armada MJ, Maneiro E, Fernández-Sueiro JL, Caramés B, Galdo F, de Toro FJ, Blanco FJ. (2004). Pig chondrocyte xenoimplants for human chondral defect repair: an *in vitro* model. *Wound Repair Regen* 12:444-52.

Fuentes-Boquete IM, Arufe Gonda MC, Díaz Prado S, Hermida Gómez T, de Toro Santos FJ, Blanco García FJ. (2007). Tratamiento de lesiones del cartílago articular con terapia celular. *Reumatol Clin* 3 Supl 3:S63-9.

Fuentes-Boquete IM, Arufe Gonda MC, Díaz Prado SM, Hermida Gómez T, de Toro santos FJ, Blanco FJ. (2008). Cell and tissue transplant strategies for joint lesions. *The Open Transplantation Journal* 2:21-8.

Furukawa T, Eyre DR, Koide S, Glimcher MJ. (1980). Biochemical studies on repair cartilage resurfacing experimental defects in the rabbit knee. *J Bone Joint Surg Am* 62:79-89.

Gelse K, von der Mark K, Schneider H. (2003). Cartilage regeneration by gene therapy. *Curr Gene Ther* 3:305-17.

Giannini S, Buda R, Vannini F, Di Caprio F, Grigolo B. (2008). Arthroscopic autologous chondrocyte implantation in osteochondral lesions of the talus: surgical technique and results. *Am J Sports Med* 36:873-80.

Gomez S, Toffanin R, Bernstorff S, Romanello M, Amenitsch H, Rappolt M, Rizzo R, Vittur F. (2000). Collagen fibrils are differently organized in weight-bearing and not-weight-bearing regions of pig articular cartilage. *J Exp Zool* 287:346-52.

Gong Y, Ma Z, Zhou Q, Li J, Gao C, Shen J. (2008) Poly(lactic acid) scaffold fabricated by gelatin particle leaching has good biocompatibility for chondrogenesis. *J Biomater Sci Polym Ed* 19:207-21.

Gooding CR, Bartlett W, Bentley G, Skinner JA, Carrington R, Flanagan A. (2006). A prospective, randomised study comparing two techniques of autologous chondrocyte implantation for osteochondral defects in the knee: Periosteum covered versus type I/III collagen covered. *Knee* 13:203-10.

Gouze E, Pawliuk R, Gouze JN, Pilapil C, Fleet C, Palmer GD, Evans CH, Leboulch P, Ghivizzani SC. (2003). Lentiviral-mediated gene delivery to synovium: potent intra-articular expression with amplification by inflammation. *Mol Ther* 7:460-6.

Grande DA, Singh IJ, Pugh J. (1987). Healing of experimentally produced lesions in articular cartilage following chondrocyte transplantation. *Anat Rec* 218:142-8.

Grande DA, Pitman MI, Peterson L, Menche D, Klein M. (1989). The repair of experimentally produced defects in rabbit articular cartilage by autologous chondrocyte transplantation. *J Orthop Res* 7:208-18.

Gronthos S, Zannettino AC, Hay SJ, Shi S, Graves SE, Kortesidis A, Simmons PJ. (2003). Molecular and cellular characterisation of highly purified stromal stem cells derived from human bone marrow. *J Cell Sci* 116(Pt 9):1827-35.

Gross AE, Shasha N, Aubin P. (2005). Long-term followup of the use of fresh osteochondral allografts for posttraumatic knee defects. *Clin Orthop Relat Res* 435:79-87.

Haddo O, Mahroof S, Higgs D, David L, Pringle J, Bayliss M, Cannon SR, Briggs TW. (2004). The use of chondrogide membrane in autologous chondrocyte implantation. *Knee* 11:51-5.

Han SH, Kim YH, Park MS, Kim IA, Shin JW, Yang WI, Jee KS, Park KD, Ryu GH, Lee JK. (2008). Histological and biomechanical properties of regenerated articular cartilage using chondrogenic bone marrow stromal cells with a PLGA scaffold *in vivo*. *J Biomed Mater Res A* 87:850-61.

Hangody L, Karpati Z. (1994). New possibilities in the management of severe circumscribed cartilage damage in the knee. *Magy Traumatol Ortop Kezseb Plasztikai Seb* 37:237-43.

Hangody L, Feczkó P, Bartha L, Bodó G, Kish G. (2001). Mosaicplasty for the treatment of articular defects of the knee and ankle *Clin Orthop Relat Res* (391 Suppl):S328-6.

Hangody L, Fules P. (2003). Autologous osteochondral mosaicplasty for the treatment of full-thickness defects of weight-bearing joints: ten years of experimental and clinical experience. *J Bone Joint Surg Am* 85-A(Suppl 2):25-32.

Hombach-Klonisch S, Panigrahi S, Rashedi I, Seifert A, Alberti E, Pocar P, Kurpisz M, Schulze-Osthoff K, Mackiewicz A, Los M. (2008). Adult stem cells and their trans-differentiation potential–perspectives and therapeutic applications. *J Mol Med* 86:1301–14.

Im GI, Kim DY, Shin JH, Hyun CW, Cho WH. (2001). Repair of cartilage defect in the rabbit with cultured mesenchymal stem cells from bone marrow. *J Bone Joint Surg Br* 83:289-94.

In't Anker PS, Noort WA, Kruisselbrink AB, Scherjon SA, Beekhuizen W, Willemze R, Kanhai HH, Fibbe WE. (2003). Nonexpanded primary lung and bone marrow-derived mesenchymal cells promote the engraftment of umbilical cord blood-derived CD34(+) cells in NOD/SCID mice. *Exp Hematol* 31:881-9.

Ishiguro N, Kojima T, Poole R. (2002). Mechanism of cartilage destruction in osteoarthritis. *Nagoya J Med Sci* 65:73-84.

Iwasa J, Engebretsen L, Shima Y. (2009). Clinical application of scaffolds for cartilage tissue engineering. *Knee Surg Sports Traumatol Arthrosc* 17:561-77.

Izadpanah R, Trygg C, Patel B, Kriedt C, Dufour J, Gimble JM, Bunnell BA. (2006). Biologic properties of mesenchymal stem cells derived from bone marrow and adipose tissue. *J Cell Biochem* 99:1285-97.

Janjanin S, Li WJ, Morgan MT, Shanti RM, Tuan RS. (2008). Moldshaped, nanofiber scaffold-based cartilage engineering using human mesenchymal stem cells and bioreactor. *J Surg Res* 149:47-56.

Jeon YH, Choi JH, Sung JK, Kim TK, Cho BC, Chung HY. (2007). Different effects of PLGA and chitosan scaffolds on human cartilage tissue engineering. *J Craniofac Surg* 18:1249-58.

Jin CZ, Park SR, Choi BH, Lee KY, Kang CK,m Min BH. (2007). Human amniotic membrane as a delivery matrix for articular cartilage repair. *Tissue Eng* 13:693-702.

Johnson LL. (1986). Arthroscopic abrasion arthroplasty historical and pathologic perspective: present status. *Arthroscopy* 2:54-69.

Jung DI, Ha J, Kang BT, Kim JW, Quan FS, Lee JH, Woo EJ, Park HM. (2009). A comparison of autologous and allogenic bone marrow-derived mesenchymal stem cell transplantation in canine spinal cord injury. *J Neurol Sci* 285:67-77.

Jung M, Gotterbarm T, Gruettgen A, Vilei SB, Breusch S, Richter W. (2005). Molecular characterization of spontaneous and growth factoraugmented chondrogenesis in periosteum-bone tissue transferred into a joint. *Histochem Cell Biol* 123:447-56.

Kastrinaki M-C, Andreakou I, Charbord P, Papadaki HA. (2008). Isolation of human bone marrow mesenchymal stem cells using different membrane markers: comparison of colony/cloning efficiency, differentiation potential, and molecular profile. *Tissue Eng Part C Methods* 14:333-9.

Kimura T, Yasui N, Ohsawa S, Ono K. (1984). Chondrocytes embedded in collagen gels maintain cartilage phenotype during long-term cultures. *Clin Orthop Relat Res* 186:231-9.

Knutsen G, Engebretsen L, Ludvigsen TC, Drogset JO, Grøntvedt T, Solheim E, Strand T, Roberts S, Isaksen V, Johansen O. (2004). Autologous chondrocyte implantation compared with microfracture in the knee. A randomized trial. *J Bone Joint Surg Am* 86-A:455-64.

Koga H, Shimaya M, Muneta T, Nimura A, Morito T, Hayashi M, Suzuki S, Ju YJ, Mochizuki T, Sekiya I. (2008). Local adherent technique for transplanting mesenchymal stem cells as a potential treatment of cartilage defect. *Arthritis Res Ther* 10:R84.

Korkala OL, Kuokkanen HO. (1995). Autoarthroplasty of knee cartilage defects by osteoperiosteal grafts. *Arch Orthop Trauma Surg* 114:253-6.

Kreuz PC, Erggelet C, Steinwachs MR, Krause SJ, Lahm A, Niemeyer P, Ghanem N, Uhl M, Südkamp N. (2006a). Is microfracture of chondral defects in the knee associated wih different results in patients aged 40 years or younger? *Arthroscopy* 22:1180-6.

Kreuz PC, Steinwachs MR, Erggelet C, Krause SJ, Konrad G, Uhl M, Südkamp N. (2006b). Results after microfracture of full-thickness chondral defects in different compartments in the knee. *Osteoarthritis Cartilage* 14:1119-25.

Krishnan SP, Skinner JA, Carrington RW, Flanagan AM, Briggs TW, Bentley G. (2006). Collagen-covered autologous chondrocyte implantation for osteochondritis dissecans of the knee: two- to seven-year results. *J Bone Joint Surg Br* 88:203-5.

Kuo CK, Li WJ, Mauck RL, Tuan RS. (2006). Cartilage tissue engineering: its potential and uses. *Curr Opin Rheumatol* 18:64-73.

Kuznetsov SA, Mankani MH, Gronthos S, Satomura K, Bianco P, Robey PG. (2001). Circulating skeletal stem cells. *J Cell Biol* 153:1133-40.

Langer F, Gross AE. (1974). Immunogenicity of allograft articular cartilage. *J Bone Joint Surg Am* 56:297-327.

Le Blanc K, Götherström C, Ringdén O, Hassan M, McMahon R, Horwitz E, Anneren G, Axelsson O, Nunn J, Ewald U, Nordén Lindeberg S, Jansson M, Dalton A, Aström E, Westgren M. (2005). Fetal mesenchymal stem-cell engraftment in bone after in utero transplantation in a patient with severe osteogenesis imperfecta. *Transplantation* 79:1607-14.

Lisignoli G, Cristino S, Piacentini A, Zini N, Noël D, Jorgensen C, Facchini A. (2006). Chondrogenic differentiation of murine and human mesenchymal stromal cells in a hyaluronic acid scaffold: differences in gene expression and cell morphology. *J Biomed Mater Res A* 77:497-506.

Majumdar MK, Thiede MA, Mosca JD, Moorman M, Gerson SL. (1998). Phenotypic and functional comparison of cultures of marrow-derived mesenchymal stem cells (MSCs) and stromal cells. *J Cell Physiol* 176:57-66.

Mankin HJ. (1982). The response of articular cartilage to mechanical injury. *J Bone Joint Surg Am* 64:460-6.

Marcacci M, Zaffagnini S, Kon E, Visani A, Iacono F, Loreti I. (2002). Arthroscopic autologous chondrocyte transplantation: technical note. *Knee Surg Sports Traumatol Arthrosc* 10:154-9.

Mareschi K, Biasin E, Piacibello W, Aglietta M, Madon E, Fagioli F. (2001). Isolation of human mesenchymal stem cells: bone marrow versus umbilical cord blood. *Haematologica* 86:1099-100.

Matikainen T, Laine J. (2005). Placenta-an alternative source of stem cells. *Toxicol Appl Pharmacol* 207 (2 Suppl):544-9.

McCulloch PC, Kang RW, Sobhy MH, Hayden JK, Cole BJ. (2007). Prospective evaluation of prolonged fresh osteochondral allograft transplantation of the femoral condyle: minimum 2-year follow-up. *Am J Sports Med* 35:411-20.

McGuckin CP, Forraz N, Baradez MO, Navran S, Zhao J, Urban R, Tilton R, Denner L. (2005). Production of stem cells with embryonic characteristics from human umbilical cord blood. *Cell Prolif* 38:245-55.

Meller D, Pires RT, Mack RJ, Figueiredo F, Heiligenhaus A, Park WC, Prabhasawat P, John T, McLeod SD, Steuhl KP, Tseng SC. (2000). Amniotic membrane transplantation for acute chemical or thermal burns. *Ophthalmology* 107:980-9.

Menche DS, Frenkel SR, Blair B, Watnik NF, Toolan BC, Yaghoubian RS, Pitman MI. (1996). A comparison of abrasion burr arthroplasty and subchondral drilling in the treatment of fullthickness cartilage lesions in the rabbit. *Arthroscopy* 12:280-6.

Menche DS, Vangsness CT Jr, Pitman M, Gross AE, Peterson L. (1998). The treatment of isolated articular cartilage lesions in the young individual. *Instr Course Lect* 47:505-15.

Metsaranta M, Kujala UM, Pelliniemi L, Osterman H, Aho H, Vuorio E. (1996). Evidence for insufficient chondrocytic differentiation during repair of full-thickness defects of articular cartilage. *Matrix Biol* 15:39-47.

Minas T, Peterson L. (1997). Chondrocyte transplantation. *Oper Tech Orthop* 7:323-33.

Minas T. (2001). Autologous chondrocyte implantation for focal chondral defects of the knee. *Clin Orthop Relat Res* 391:S349-61.

Minguell JJ, Conget P, Erices A. (2000). Biology and clinical utilization of mesenchymal progenitor cells. *Braz J Med Biol Res* 33:881-7.

Morton KE, Dewhurst CJ (1986). Human amnion in the treatment of vaginal malformations. Br J Obstet & Gynaecol 93:50-4.

Mouw JK, Case ND, Guldberg RE, Plaas AH, Levenston ME. (2005). Variations in matrix composition and GAG fine structure among scaffolds for cartilage tissue engineering. *Osteoarthritis Cartilage* 13:828-36.

Mrugala D, Dossat N, Ringe J, Delorme B, Coffy A, Bony C, Charbord P, Häupl T, Daures J-P, Noël D, Jorgensen C. (2009). Gene expression profile of multipotent mesenchymal stromal cells: identification of pathways common to TGFβ3/BMP2-induced chondrogenesis. *Cloning Stem Cells* 11:61-76.

Muller B, Kohn D. (1999). Indication for and performance of articular cartilage drilling using the Pridie method. *Orthopade* 28:4-10.

Muraglia A, Cancedda R, Quarto R. (2000). Clonal mesenchymal progenitors from human bone marrow differentiate *in vitro* according to a hierarchical model. *J Cell Sci* 113:1161-6.

Murphy JM, Fink DJ, Hunziker EB, Barry FP. (2003). Stem cell therapy in a caprine model of osteoarthritis. *Arthritis Rheum* 48:3464-74.

Nah HD, Swoboda B, Birk DE, Kirsch T. (2001). Type IIA procollagen: expression in developing chicken limb cartilage and human osteoarthritic articular cartilage. *Dev Dyn* 220:307-22.

Nakagawa Y, Suzuki T, Kuroki H, Kobayashi M, Okamoto Y, Nakamura T. (2007). The effect of surface incongruity of grafted plugs in osteochondral grafting: a report of five cases. *Knee Surg Sports Traumatol Arthrosc* 15:591-6.

Nakahara H, Bruder SP, Haynesworth SE, Holecek JJ, Baber MA, Goldberg VM, Caplan AI. (1990). Bone and cartilage formation in diffusion chambers by subcultured cells derived from the periosteum. *Bone* 11:181-8.

Nettles DL, Elder SH, Gilbert JA. (2002). Potential use of chitosan as a cell scaffold material for cartilage tissue engineering. *Tissue Eng* 8:1009-16.

Niknejad H, Peirovi H, Jorjani M, Ahmadiani A, Ghanavi J, Seifalian AM. (2008). Properties of the amniotic membrane for potential use in tissue engineering. *Eur Cell Mater* 15:88-99.

Nishimori M, Deie M, Kanaya A, Exham H, Adachi N, Ochi M. (2006). Repair of chronic osteochondral defects in the rat. A bone marrowstimulating procedure enhanced by cultured allogenic bone marrow mesenchymal stromal cells. *J Bone Joint Surg Br* 88:1236-44.

Nixon AJ, Sams AE, Lust G, Grande D, Mohammed HO. (1993). Temporal matrix synthesis and histological features of a chondrocyte-laden porous collagen cartilage analogue. Am J Vet Res 54:349-56.

O´Driscoll SW, Fitzsimmons JS. (2000). The importance of procedure specific training in harvesting periosteum for chondrogenesis. *Clin Orthop Relat Res* (380):269-78.

O'Driscoll SW, Fitzsimmons JS. (2001). The role of periosteum in cartilage repair. *Clin Orthop Rel Res* 391:S190-207.

O'Driscoll SW, Saris DB, Ito Y, Fitzimmons JS. (2001). The chondrogenic potential of periosteum decreases with age. *J Orthop Res* 19:95-103.

Ohlendorf C, Tomford WW, Mankin HJ. (1996). Chondrocyte survival in cryopreserved osteochondral articular cartilage. *J Orthop Res* 14: 413-6.

Oka M, Chang YS, Nakamura T, Ushio K, Toguchida J, Gu HO. (1997). Synthetic osteochondral replacement of the femoral articular surface. J Bone Joint Surg Br 79:1003-7.

Palmer G, Pascher A, Gouze E, Gouze JN, Betz O, Spector M, Robbins PD, Evans CH, Ghivizzani SC. (2002). Development of gene-based therapies for cartilage repair. *Crit Rev Eukaryot Gene Expr* 12:259-73.

Park J, Gelse K, Frank S, von der Mark K, Aigner T, Schneider H. (2006). Transgene-activated mesenchymal cells for articular cartilage repair: a comparison of primary bone marrow-, perichondrium/periosteum- and fat-derived cells. *J Gene Med* 8:112-25.

Parsch D, Fellenberg J, Brummendorf TH, Eschlbeck AM, Richter W. (2004). Telomere length and telomerase activity during expansion and differentiation of human mesenchymal stem cells and chondrocytes. *J Mol Med* 82:49-55.

Pasquinelli G, Tazzari P, Ricci F, Vaselli C, Buzzi M, Conte R. (2007). Ultrastructural characteristics of human mesenchymal stromal (stem) cells derived from bone marrow and term placenta. *Ultrastruc Pathol* 31:23-31.

Pelttari K, Winter A, Steck E, Goetzke K, Hennig T, Ochs BG, Aigner T, Richter W. (2006). Premature induction of hypertrophy during *in vitro* chondrogenesis of human mesenchymal stem cells correlates with calcification and vascular invasion after ectopic transplantation in SCID mice. *Arthritis Rheum* 54:3254-66.

Pelttari K, Wixmerten A, Martin I. (2009). Do we really need cartilage tissue engineering? *Swiss Med Wkly* 139:602-9.

Pérez-Cachafeiro S, Ruano-Raviña A, Couceiro-Follente J, Benedí-Alcaine JA, Nebot-Sanchis I, Casquete-Román C, Bello-Prats S, Couceiro-Sánchez G, Blanco FJ. (2010). Spanish experience in sutologous chondrocyte implantation. *Open Orthop* 4:14-21.

Peterson L, Minas T, Brittberg M, Nilsson A, Sjogren-Jansson E, Lindahl A. (2000). Two- to 9-year outcome after autologous chondrocyte transplantation of the knee. *Clin Orthop Relat Res* 374:212-34.

Peterson L, Brittberg M, Kiviranta I, Akerlund EL, Lindahl A. (2002). Autologous chondrocyte transplantation. Biomechanics and long-term durability. *Am J Sports Med* 30:2-12.

Pittenger MF, Mackay AM, Beck SC, Jaiswal RK, Douglas R, Mosca JD, Moorman MA, Simonetti DW, Craig S, Marshak DR. (1999). Multilineage potential of adult human mesenchymal stem cells. *Science* 284:143-7.

Pittenger MF. (2008). Mesenchymal stem cells from adult bone marrow. *Methods Mol Biol* 449:27–44.

Prockop DJ. (1997). Marrow stromal cells as stem cells for nonhematopoietic tissues. *Science* 276:71-4.

Qiu YS, Shahgaldi BF, Revell WJ, Heatley FW. (2003). Observations of subchondral plate advancement during osteochondral repair: a histomorphometric and mechanical study in the rabbit femoral condyle. *Osteoarthritis Cartilage* 11:810-20.

Rahfoth B, Weisser J, Sternkopf F, Aigner T, von der Mark K, Brauer R. (1998). Transplantation of allograft chondrocytes embedded in agarose gel into cartilage defects of rabbits. *Osteoarthritis Cartilage* 6:50-65.

Ramallal M, Maneiro E, López E, Fuentes-Boquete I, López-Armada MJ, Fernández-Sueiro JL, Galdo F, de Toro FJ, Blanco FJ. (2004). Xeno-implantation of pig chondrocytes into rabbit to treat localized articular cartilage defects: an animal model. *Wound Repair Regen* 12:337-45.

Rendal-Vázquez ME, Maneiro-Pampín E, Rodríguez-Cabarcos M, Fernández-Mallo O, López de Ullibarri I, Andión-Núñez C, Blanco FJ. (2001). Effect of cryopreservation on human articular chondrocyte viability, proliferation, and collagen expression. *Cryobiology* 42:2-10.

Resinger C, Vécsei V, Marlovits S. (2004). Therapeutic options in the treatment of cartilage defects. Techniques and indications. *Radiologe* 44:756-62.

Richardson JB, Caterson B, Evans EH, Ashton BA, Roberts S. (1999). Repair of human articular cartilage after implantation of autologous chondrocytes. *J Bone Joint Surg Br* 81:1064-8.

Richler C, Yaffe D. (1970). The in vitro cultivation and differentiation capacities of myogenic cell lines. *Dev Bio;* 23:1-22.

Rinastiti M, Harijadi, Santoso AL, Sosroseno W. (2006). Histological evaluation of rabbit gingival wound healing transplanted with human amniotic membrane. *Int J Oral Maxillofac Surg* 35:247-51.

Roberts S, Hollander AP, Caterson B, Menage J, Richardson JB. (2001). Matrix turnover in human cartilage repair tissue in autologous chondrocyte implantation. *Arthritis Rheum* 44:2586-98.

Robertson WB, Fick D, Wood DJ, Linklater JM, Zheng MH, Ackland TR. (2007). MRI and clinical evaluation of collagen-covered autologous chondrocyte implantation (CACI) at two years. *Knee* 14:117-27.

Rogers BA, Murphy CL, Cannon SR, Briggs TW. (2006). Topographical variation in glycosaminoglycan content in human articular cartilage. *J Bone Joint Surg Br* 88:1670-4.

Sakaguchi Y, Sekiya I, Yagishita K, Muneta T. (2005). Comparison of human stem cells derived from various mesenchymal tissues: superiority of synovium as a cell source. *Arthritis Rheum* 52:2521-9.

Sams AE, Minor RR, Wootton JA, Mohammed H, Nixon AJ. (1995). Local and remote matrix responses to chondrocyte-laden collagen scaffold implantation in extensive articular cartilage defects. Osteoarthritis Cartilage 3:61-70.

Sams AE, Nixon AJ. (1995). Chondrocyte-laden collagen scaffolds for resurfacing extensive articular cartilage defects. Osteoarthritis Cartilage 3:47-59.

Samuel GN, Kerridge IH, O'Brien TA. (2008). Umbilical cord blood banking: public good or private benefit? *Med J Aust* 188:533-5.

Santos MS, Gomes JAP, Hofling-Lima AL, Rizzo LV, Romano AC, Belfort R Jr. (2005). Survival analysis of conjuctival limbal grafts and amniotic membrane transplantation in eyes with total limbal stem cell deficiency. *Am J Ophthalmol* 140:223-30.

Schachar N, McAllister D, Stevenson M, Novak K, McGann L. (1992). Metabolic and biochemical status of articular cartilage following cryopreservation and transplantation: a rabbit model. *J Orthop Res* 10:603-9.

Schreiber RE, Ilten-Kirby BM, Dunkelman NS, Symons KT, Rekettye LM, Willoughby J, Ratcliffe A. (1999). Repair of osteochondral defects with allogeneic tissue engineered cartilage implants. *Clin Orthop Rel Res* 367S:382-95.

Shapiro F, Koide S, Glimcher MJ. (1993). Cell origin and differentiation in the repair of full-thickness defects of articular cartilage. *J Bone Joint Surg Am* 75:532-53.

Sohn DH, Lottman LM, Lum LY, Kim SG, Pedowitz RA, Coutts RD, Sah RL. (2002). Effect of gravity on localization of chondrocytes implanted in cartilage defects. *Clin Orthop Relat Res* 394:254-62.

Steadman JR, Rodkey WG, Briggs KK, Rodrigo JJ. (1999). The microfracture technic in the management of complete cartilage defects in the knee joint. *Orthopade* 28:26-32.

Steadman JR, Briggs KK, Rodrigo JJ, Kocher MS, Gill TJ, Rodkey WG. (2003). Outcomes of microfracture for traumatic chondral defects of the knee: average 11-year follow-up. *Arthroscopy* 19:477-84.

Teigman SA, Fauza DO. (2007). Isolation of mesenchymal stem cells from amniotic fluid and placenta. *Curr Protoc Stem Cell Biol*; Chapter 1:Unit 1E.2.

Steinert AF, Ghivizzani SC, Rethwilm A, Tuan RS, Evans CH, Nöth U. (2007). Major biological obstacles for persistent cell-based regeneration of articular cartilage. *Arthritis Res Ther* 9:213.

Steinwachs M, Kreuz PC. (2007). Autologous chondrocyte implantation in chondral defects of the knee with a type I/III collagen membrane: a prospective study with a 3-year follow-up. *Arthroscopy* 23:381-7.

Stenderup K, Justesen J, Clausen C, Kassem M. (2003). Aging is associated with decreased maximal life span and accelerated senescence of bone marrow stromal cells. *Bone* 33:919-26.

Szerb I, Hangody L, Duska Z, Kaposi NP. (2005). Mosaicplasty: long-term follow-up. *Bull Hosp Jt Dis* 63:54-62.

Tejwani S, Kolari RS, Sangwan VS, Rao GN. (2007). Role of amniotic membrane graft for ocular chemical and thermal injuries. *Cornea* 26:21-6.

Tins BJ, McCall IW, Takahashi T, Cassar-Pullicino V, Roberts S, Ashton B, Richardson J. (2005). Autologous chondrocyte implantation in knee joint: MR imaging and histologic features at 1-year follow-up. *Radiology* 234:501-8.

Trippel SB, Ghivizzani SC, Nixon AJ. (2004). Gene-based approaches for the repair of articular cartilage. *Gene Ther* 11:351-9.

Trzeciak T, Kruczynski J, Jaroszewski J, Lubiatowski P. (2006). Evaluation of cartilage reconstruction by means of autologous chondrocyte versus periosteal graft transplantation: an animal study. *Transplant Proc* 38:305-11.

Tsai MS, Hwang SM, Chen KD, Lee YS, Hsu LW, Chang YJ, Wang CN, Feng HH, Chang YL, Chao AS, Chang SD, Lee KD, Wang TH, Wang HS, Soong YK. (2007). Functional network analysis on the transcriptomes of mesenchymal stem cells derived from amniotic fluid, amniotic membrane, cord blood, and bone marrow. *Stem Cells* 25:2511-23.

Tuli R, Li WJ, Tuan RS. (2003). Current state of cartilage tissue engineering. *Arthritis Res Ther* 5:235-8.

Vachon A, McIlwraith CW, Trotter GW, Norrdin RW, Powers BE. (1989). Neochondrogenesis in free intra-articular, periosteal, and perichondrial autografts in horses. *Am J Vet Res* 50:1787-94.

Van Susante JL, Wymenga AB, Buma P. (2003). Potential healing benefit of an osteoperiosteal bone plug from the proximal tibia on a mosaicplasty donor-site defect in the knee. An experimental study in the goat. *Arch Orthop Trauma Surg* 123:466-70.

Villaron EM, Almeida J, Lopez-Holgado N, Alcoceba M, Sánchez-Abarca LI, Sanchez-Guijo FM, Alberca M, Pérez-Simon JA, San Miguel JF, Del Cañizo MC. (2004). Mesenchymal stem cells are present in peripheral blood and can engraft after allogenic haematopoietic stem cell transplantation. *Haematologica* 89:1421-7.

Vinatier C, Mrugale D, Jorgensen C, Guicheux J, Noel D. (2009). Cartilage engineering: a crucial combination of cells, biomaterials and biofactors. *Trends Biotechnol* 27:307-14.

Wakitani S, Kimura T, Hirooka A, Ochi T, Yoneda M, Yasui N, Owaki H, Ono K. (1989). Repair of rabbit articular surfaces with allograft chondrocytes embedded in collagen gel. *J Bone Joint Surg Br* 71:74-80.

Wakitani S, Imoto K, Yamamoto T, Saito M, Murata N, Yoneda M. (2002). Human autologous culture expanded bone marrow mesenchymal cell transplantation for repair of cartilage defects in osteoarthritic knees. *Osteoarthritis Cartilage* 10:199-206.

Wong BJ, Pandhoh N, Truong MT, Diaz S, Chao K, Hou S, Gardiner D. (2005). Identification of chondrocyte proliferation following laser irradiation, thermal injury, and mechanical trauma. *Lasers Surg Med* 37:89-96.

Xia Y, Moody JB, Alhadlaq H, Burton-Wurster N, Lust G. (2002). Characteristics of topographical heterogeneity of articular cartilage over the joint surface of a humeral head. *Osteoarthritis Cartilage* 10:370-80.

Yamada S, Ochi M, Kojima K, Sharman P, Yasunaga Y, Hiyama E. (2006). Possibility of selection of chondrogenic progenitor cells by telomere length in FGF-2-expanded mesenchymal stromal cells. *Cell Prolif* 39:575-84.

Yoo JU, Barthel TS, Nishimura K, Solchaga L, Caplan AI, Goldberg VM, Johnstone B. (1998). The chondrogenic potential of human bone-marrow-derived mesenchymal progenitor cells. *J Bone Joint Surg Am* 80:1745-57.

You Q, Cai L, Zheng J, Tong X, Zhang D, Zhang Y. (2008). Isolation of human mesenchymal stem cells from third-trimester amniotic fluid. *Int J Gynaecol Obstet* 103:149-52.

Young HE, Steele TA, Bray RA, Hudson J, Floyd JA, Hawkins K, Thomas K, Austin T, Edwards C, Cuzzourt J, Duenzl M, Lucas PA, Black AC Jr. (2001). Human reserve pluripotent mesenchymal stem cells are present in the connective tissues of skeletal muscle and dermis derived from fetal, adult, and geriatric donors. *Anat Rec* 264:51-62.

Zarnett R, Salter RB. (1989). Periosteal neochondrogenesis for biologically resurfacing joints: its cellular origin. *Can J Surg* 32:171-4.

Zimmermann S, Voss M, Kaiser S, Kapp U, Waller CF, Martens UM. (2003). Lack of telomerase activity in human mesenchymal stem cells. *Leukemia* 17:1146-9.

Zuk PA, Zhu M, Mizuno H, Huang J, Futrell JW, Katz AJ, Benhaim P, Lorenz HP, Hedrik MH. (2001). Multilineage cells from human adipose tissue: implications for cell-based therapies. *Tisse Eng* 7:211-28.

Zuk PA, Zhu M, Ashjian P, De Ugarte DA, Huang JI, Mizuno H, Alfonso ZC, Fraser JK, Benhaim P, Hedrick MH. (2002). Human adipose tissue is a source of multipotent stem cells. *Mol Biol Cell* 13:4279-95.

Zvaifler NJ, Marinova-Mutafchieva L, Adams G, Edwards CJ, Moss J, Burger JA, Maini RN. (2000). Mesenchymal precursor cells in the blood of normal individuals. *Arthritis Res* 2:477-88.

10

In Vivo Gene Transfer in the Female Bovine: Potential Applications for Biomedical Research in Reproductive Sciences

Miguel A. Velazquez[1] and Wilfried A. Kues[2]
[1]*School of Agricultural Sciences, Autonomous University of Campeche,*
[2]*Friedrich-Loeffler-Institute, Institute of Farm Animal Genetics,*
[1]*Mexico*
[2]*Germany*

1. Introduction

"We still share genes around, and the resemblance of the enzymes of grasses to those of whales is a family resemblance" (Lewis Thomas, The lives of a cell, 1974).

Gene transfer technology is an invaluable research tool to study gene function and its regulation. *In vitro* transfer of exogenous nucleic acids into mammalian cells has been of pivotal importance for the characterization of gene functions (Hampton & Kinnaird, 2010). Likewise, *in vivo* transfer of functionally active foreign genes into target mammalian somatic tissues or organs has played a critical role in the development of effective gene therapy strategies (Yang, 1992) that has escalated into clinical application for the therapeutic treatment of inherited and acquired diseases (Mountain, 2000). In addition, the genetic engineering of model organisms became possible (Niemann & Kues, 2003). Most of the gene transfer research has been conducted on several non-reproductive topics including blood diseases (Nienhuis, 2008), neurological dysfunctions (Manfredsson & Mandel, 2010), cancer (Pei et al., 2010), lung diseases (Geiger et al., 2010), bone healing (Evans, 2010), skin diseases (Long et al., 2009) and heart failure (Poller et al., 2010). To a lesser extent gene transfer research in gynecological diseases (Raki et al., 2006; Hassan et al., 2009) and reproductive medicine (Stribley et al., 2002; Daftary & Taylor, 2003; Yoshimura et al., 2010) has been undertaken using the mouse as model species. Although the mouse model possesses several advantages (*e.g.* short generation interval, large litter size), some large animals (*e.g.* non-human primates, dogs, pigs, sheep, cattle and horses) are considered relevant model species in biomedical research. For instance, pig and sheep species have been used as models for cardiovascular disease (Ishii et al., 2006), wound repair (Graham et al., 2000), respiratory disease (Scheerlinck et al., 2008), cancer (Du et al., 2007), diabetes (Dyson et al., 2006), ophthalmological disorders (Klassen et al., 2008) and neurological dysfunctions (Kragh et al., 2009). The physiology, organ size, genome organization, life span and pathology of farm animal species reflect the human situation much better than rodent models (Casal & Haskins 2006; Habermann et al., 2007; Jacobsen et al., 2010; Muschler et al., 2010).

Implementation of *in vivo* gene transfer technology in relevant large animal models is pivotal to elucidate molecular pathways involved in reproductive processes such as ovarian follicular development, fertilization, and early embryo development. This research will allow the generation of safer and more efficient strategies in human reproductive medicine for infertility treatment and contraception.

A large animal model for gene transfer studies in reproduction should resemble human reproductive features as close as possible. In this regard, the bovine model is increasingly accepted as an alternative model species to generate conceptual models of relevance for human reproduction (Adams & Pierson, 1995; Ménézo & Hérubel, 2002; Baumann et al., 2007; Velazquez, 2008). Both species are monovulatory and displayed similarities regarding ovarian folliculogenesis, gene expression profile during early embryogenesis, and gestation length period (Campbell et al., 2003; Adjaye et al., 2007; Mihm & Evans, 2008; Kues et al., 2008; Xie et al., 2010). Furthermore, several gynaecological procedures are performed virtually in the same fashion as in women (Velazquez et al., 2009b). The aim of this chapter is to highlight the methods than could potentially be applied for *in vivo* gene delivering in the reproductive tract of female bovine species in order to address topics of reproductive relevance for both humans and cattle.

2. Basics of gene transfer technology

2.1 Gene transfer

Broadly speaking, gene transfer technology involves the transfer of exogenous nucleic acids (deoxyribonucleic acid [DNA] or ribonucleic acid [RNA]) into target cells either to produce a biologically active protein or to inhibit protein synthesis. The classic concept of gene transfer involves the insertion of DNA encoding the desire gene as complementary DNA (cDNA) into the nucleus of target cells, followed by transcription into messenger RNA, which is then exported to the cytoplasm and translated into its encoding protein (Grigsby & Leong, 2010). The introduced cDNA may restore a lost gene function, interfere with gene's function or initiate a new function (Stribley et al., 2002). However, progress in gene transfer technology now allows the deliver of large fragments of genomic DNA containing the whole locus of the desired gene (Lufino et al., 2008). Furthermore, with the increasing understanding of the non-coding DNA functions the use of non-coding regulatory RNAs is becoming an important tool for gene transfer technology (Poller et al., 2010). Several RNA-based technologies have been used to down-regulate gene expression in loss-of-function studies including small interfering RNA (siRNA), short hairpin RNA (shRNA) and micro RNA (miRNA) (Guo et al., 2010; Khurana et al., 2010; Poller et al., 2010). Although RNA interference (RNAi) technology (via siRNAs and shRNAs) is only used for gene silencing, miRNA interventions can also be applied for up-regulation of protein expression (Poller et al., 2010). Gene transfer can be targeted to either somatic (somatic gene transfer) or germ-line (*i.e.* oocyte, spermatozoa, and preimplantation embryos) cells (Stribley et al., 2002).

2.2 Gene therapy

Gene transfer studies using *in vitro* cellular assays have been critical to unravel basic features of gene function (Hampton & Kinnaird, 2010). However, gene transfer technology has been put forward for clinical use as a therapeutic tool (*i.e.* gene therapy) (Mountain, 2000). Gene transfer for therapeutic purposes can be aimed at correcting a genetic defect in target cells (*i.e.* correcting gene therapy) or to destroy target cells using a cytotoxic pathway (*i.e.* cytotoxic gene therapy) (Stribley et al., 2002). Gene therapy can be carried out either *ex vivo* or *in vivo* (Yang, 1992; Stribley et al., 2002; Gardlík et al., 2005). The *ex vivo* approach involves the *in vitro* transfer of exogenous genetic material into cells followed by the *in vivo* delivery of the genetically modified cell into the target tissue (Yang, 1992; Stribley et al., 2002; Gardlík et al., 2005). *In vivo* gene therapy makes reference to the direct transfer of nucleic acids into target cells (Yang, 1992; Stribley et al., 2002; Gardlík et al., 2005).

2.3 *In vivo* gene delivery

The delivery of nucleic acids to the nuclei of target cells requires the use of carrier vehicles called vectors. After systemic or topical administration, the vector carrying the transgene has to cross the plasma membrane and move through the cytosol before delivering the transgene into the nucleus target cell (Ziello et al., 2010). In order to achieve efficient gene transfer the vector has to avoid degradation from components in the extracellular matrix (*e.g.* exonucleases) and the cytoplasm (*e.g.* endonucleases) and effectively release the transgene for nuclear uptake and transcriptional processing (Escoffre et al., 2010; Parra-Guillén et al., 2010). Gene transfer vectors can be classified into viral and non-viral (Table 1) (Niidome & Huang, 2002; Niemann & Kues, 2003; Gardlík et al., 2005; Young et al., 2006; Vassaux et al., 2006; Lufino et al., 2008; Al-Dosari & Gao, 2009; Tros de Ilarduya et al., 2010).

Viral vectors	Non-viral vectors
Retrovirus/Lentivirus	Naked plasmid DNA
Adenovirus	Lipoplexes
Adeno-associated virus	Polyplexes
Herpes simplex virus	Inorganic nanoparticles
Alphavirus	Artificial chromosomes
Poxvirus	Peptides
Vaccinia virus	Bacteria
Simian virus 40	Minicircle DNA
Moloney murine leukemia virus	Transposon

Table 1. Common viral and non-viral vectors used for gene transfer technology

Viral vector-mediated gene transfer is based on the innate capacity of viruses to infect cells. Recombinant viruses without the ability to replicate have to be synthesized in order to avoid infectious diseases in the host. This requires the deletion of essential genes for viral replication and the insertion of the gene of interest into the viral genome (Kay et al., 2001). Viral vectors enter target cells via receptor-mediated endocytosis (Ziello et al., 2010). Following endocytosis viral vectors are released from endosomes and travel along the microtubules towards the nucleus where they deliver the transgene through nuclear pores (Fig. 1) (Dinh et al., 2005; Yea et al., 2007). However, other viral vectors (*e.g.* retroviruses) deliver the transgene in the nucleus during mitotic-nuclear-envelope breakdown (Kay et al., 2001) or do not depend on microtubule-mediated transport. Instead, they do not escape endosomes soon after cellular uptake and reach the nucleus in a diffuse motion where they are released from late endosomes or lysosomes (Dinh et al., 2005; Akita et al., 2010).

The majority of non-viral vectors rely on plasmid DNA as the primary carrier of the transgene (Schleef & Blaesen, 2009; Escoffre et al., 2010). Injection of naked plasmid DNA is the simplest gene delivery system, but transgene expression (*i.e.* transfection) is usually low due to its rapid degradation after delivery, especially under systemic administration (Parra-Guillén et al., 2010). This problem has been addressed with the use of chemical vectors, which act as protective complexes (*i.e.* DNA-complexes) that facilitate cellular uptake and intracellular delivery (Tros de llarduya et al., 2010). It has been suggested that DNA complexes can enter the cytosol by fusion with the plasma membrane, but most of the experimental evidence indicates that the main entrance route of non-viral DNA-complexes currently used in gene transfer research is receptor-mediated endocytosis (Medina-Kauwe et al., 2005; Khalil et al., 2006; Ziello et al., 2010). Nevertheless, within a vector line, the origin of the vector could determine its cellular uptake pathway. Accordingly, chemically derived gold nanoparticles enter the cytoplasm using an endocytic pathway, but gold nanoparticles produced by laser ablation can enter cultured bovine immortalized cells by passive diffusion (Taylor et al., 2010).

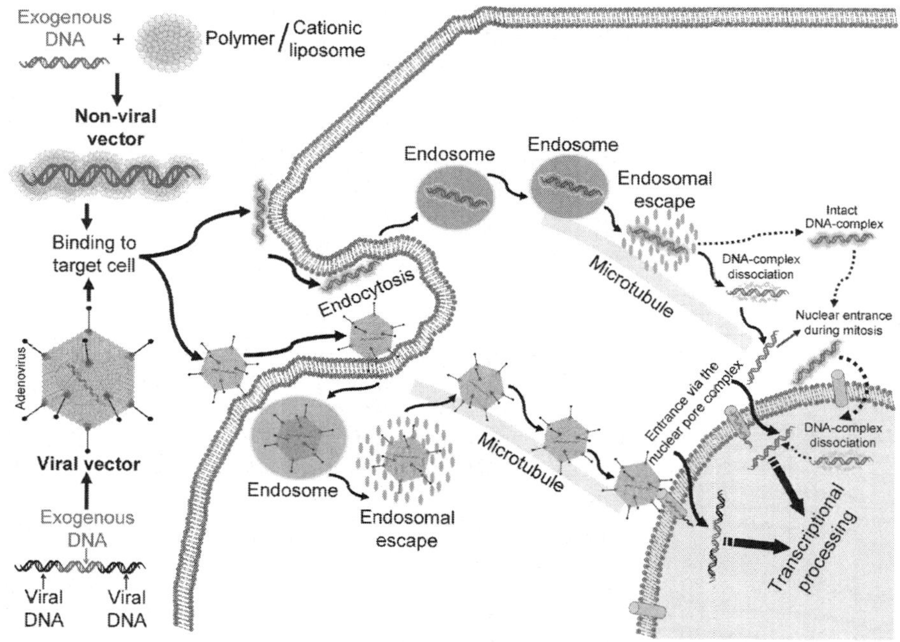

Fig. 1. General pathway of vector cellular uptake via receptor-mediated endocytosis followed by microtubule-mediated transport in viral (*e.g.* adenovirus) and non-viral (*e.g.* polyplexes and lipoplexes) gene delivery systems. Non-viral DNA-complex dissociation can occur in the cytosol or in the nucleus, after nuclear entry of the DNA-complex during mitosis, when the nuclear envelope disassembles. Dissociated exogenous DNA can enter the nucleus either through the nuclear pore complex or during mitosis.

The most accepted model of cellular uptake of non-viral vectors is based in polyplexes (*i.e.* polymer-based transfection agents) and lipoplexes (*i.e.* cationic liposome-based transfection agents). Following endosomal entrapment non-viral vectors undergo microtubule-facilitated trafficking and accumulate within close proximity to the nucleus (Fig. 1) (Vaughan & Dean, 2006; Doyle & Chan, 2007). The site of release of the transgene seems to depend on the type of non-viral DNA-complex. Endosomal release of polyplexes in the cytoplasm can occur without release of DNA from the polymer and the polyplexes may enter the nucleus intact, where they subsequently release the transgene (Cohen et al., 2009). Polyplexes are released from the endosome by a proton-sponge mechanism in which the polyplex exacerbates proton accumulation in the endosome, resulting in passive chloride influx followed by osmotic swelling and endosomal rupture (Medina-Kauwe et al., 2005; Midoux et al., 2009). It has been hypothesized that the nuclear entry of polyplexes takes place at the time of nuclear membrane breakage during mitosis (O'Rorke et al., 2010), but there is evidence that nuclear proteins, such as nucleolin, can incorporate non-viral vectors into the nucleus in an endocytosis-independent manner (Chen et al., 2008b).

Nevertheless, it has been demonstrated that some polyplexes can release their DNA cargo before entering the nucleus via ion exchange with RNA present in the cytoplasm (Huth et al., 2006). Presumably, DNA release from polyplexes in the nucleus could be caused by ion exchange with chromosomal DNA (Schaffer et al., 2000) or by polymerases through stripping of histone proteins during DNA replication (Thomas & Klibanov, 2003a). Release of DNA from polyplexes is affected by polymer degree of deacetylation (DDA) and molecular weight (MW), as high DDA and MW reduced DNA dissociation, whereas intermediate values of these polymer characteristics are associated with efficient DNA dissociation rate (Thibault et al., 2010).

Experimental evidence has shown that lipoplexes are more likely to release the DNA in the cytosol during endosomal escape (Pollard et al., 1998; Cohen et al., 2009). Current evidence indicates that liposomes fuse with endosomal membranes leading to a neutralization of cationic lipids in the lipoplexes by anionic membrane lipids. This process causes endosome destabilization and displaces the DNA from the cationic lipids into the cytoplasm (Tarahovsky et al., 2004; Medina-Kauwe et al., 2005; Caracciolo et al., 2007). Recent evidence suggests that the capacity of lipoplexes to escape the endosome is strongly influenced by its formulation. For instance, multicomponent lipoplexes (*i.e.* incorporation of three to six lipid species simultaneously) displayed an enhanced ability to destabilized endosomes compared to binary complexes (Caracciolo et al., 2009).

Due to their significant size, DNA constructs are unable to cross the nuclear membrane by passive diffusion (Lukacs et al., 2000). Investigations on the mechanism of nuclear translocation of plasmid DNA have documented that nuclear uptake of exogenous DNA occurred during mitosis, when the nuclear envelope breaks down and the permeability barrier to the nucleus is lost (Mortimer et al., 1999; Brunner et al., 2000; Cohen et al., 2009). However, this cytoplasmic to nuclear translocation mechanism does not operate in differentiated non-dividing cells (Dean et al., 2005, Khalil et al., 2006). The other documented form of entry of foreign DNA into the nucleus is through the nuclear pore complex, mediated by nuclear localization signals (NLSs) (Dowty et al., 1995; Dean, 1997; Boulikas, 1998; Dean et al., 2005). Alternatively, non-viral vectors can release the transgene into the nucleus after fusion with the nuclear membrane (Kamiya et al., 2002).

There are several physical methods that can increase the efficiency of vector delivery (Table 2) (Russ & Wagner, 2007; Al-Dosari & Gao, 2009; Escoffre et al., 2010; Wells, 2010). These physical techniques can be applied alone or in combination, and are mainly used in *in vitro* settings (Escoffre et al., 2010). Nonetheless, some of these physical methods (*e.g.* electroporation and ultrasound) have shown to work efficiently under *in vivo* conditions, enhancing nucleic acid delivery at a specific location (Huber & Pfisterer, 2000; Saito & Nakatsuji, 2001; Sato et al., 2003; Brown et al., 2004). Although the precise mechanisms by

Method	Putative Mechanism
Needle injection	Physical damage caused by needle insertion generates pores in the cell membrane
Jet injection	High-speed ultrafine stream generates pores in the cell membrane
Electroporation	Electrical field pulses generate pores in the cell membrane
ltrasound	Ultrasonic waves induce pores in the cell membrane by acoustic cavitation
Hydrodynamic injection	The high pressure of a rapid injection of a large volume of vector solution generates cell membrane pores
Laser irradiation	A short exposure to a laser beam generates cell membrane pores
Photochemical internalization	Illumination induces photochemical damage and rupture of endosomal membranes
Plasma	Ion deposition on the cell surface by direct current plasma induces membrane permeability
Hyperthermia	Cells lose their cytoskeletal structure and contract, causing widening of intercellular gap junctions
Gene gun	Heavy metal macroparticles are impacted at high velocity allowing direct penetration through the plasma membrane into the cytoplasm and even the nucleus
Magnetofection	Magnetic forces accelerate accumulation of vectors (superparamagnetic nanoparticles) on the cell surface followed by endocytosis

Table 2. Physical methods for gene delivery

which these physical methods operate are not totally understood, most of them allow direct entrance of vectors into the cytosol by generating a transient membrane permeabilization, avoiding in this way the endocytic pathway (Escoffre et al., 2010; Wells, 2010).

Alternative strategies to improve transgene delivery include the use of the hybrid vectors. For instance, coating of adenovirus with polymers or liposomes allows the production of "stealth" viruses that can avoid recognition by the host's antibodies and permits targeting of desired receptors following linkage of ligands to the chemical coating (Han et al., 2010; Kim et al., 2010; Zhong et al., 2010). Other hybrid vector combinations include polymer-artificial chromosome (Magin-Lachmann et al., 2004); polymer-gold nanoparticle (Thomas & Klibanov, 2003b); liposome-peptide-artificial chromosome (White et al., 2003); polymer-peptide (Huang et al., 2010), liposome-polymer (Schäfer et al. ,2010) and viral vector combinations such as adenovirus-Epstein-Barr virus (Gardlík et al., 2005).

The general consensus is that viral gene deliver systems achieve stable *in vivo* transgene expression more efficiently than non-viral systems (Gardlík et al., 2005; Hassam et al., 2009; Escoffre et al., 2010; Grigsby & Leong, 2010). The lower efficiency of non-viral vectors seems not to be associated with their capacity to reach the vicinity of the nucleus, but with their ability to cross the nuclear envelope (Dean et al., 2005). Accordingly, Hama et al. (2006)

reported lower efficient transgene expression with lipoplexes than with adenoviral vectors, which was attributed to differences in nuclear transcription efficiency rather than to differences in intracellular trafficking. Nevertheless, advances with artificial chromosomes and transposons could offer an efficient *in vivo* non-viral gene delivery system (Lufino et al., 2008; Wilson & George, 2010). Non-viral vectors offer appealing advantages over viral vectors including higher insert capacity for DNA cargo size, low host immunogenicity, easy manufacturing and potential for repeated administration (Niidome & Huang, 2002; Al-Dosari & Gao, 2009; Grigsby & Leong, 2010).

2.4 Transgene expression

Once in the nucleus, expression vectors (*i.e.* expression cassette in a viral or non-viral vector) may integrate into the host genome or remain as extrachromosomal genetic elements (*i.e.* episomal vector) (Lufino et al., 2008). Nuclear uptake of the expression vector can result in either permanent or transient transgene expression (Ehrhardt et al., 2008; Lufino et al., 2008; Voigt et al., 2008; Romano et al., 2009). Although some viruses can provide transient expression (*e.g.* adenovirus, vaccinia virus), most of the viral gene transfer systems result in permanent transgene expression (*e.g.* retrovirus, adeno-associated virus) due to their capacity to achieve chromosomal integration (Young et al., 2006). Nevertheless, some integrating viruses are prone to epigenetic silencing and provide a transient burst of transgene expression. Lentiviruses have been known to escape epigenetic silencing and are currently the viral vector with most faithful expression (Park, 2009). In contrast, with the exception of transposons (Hackett et al., 2005; Wilson & George, 2010) non-viral vectors so far investigated do not integrate into the host genome (Gardlík et al., 2005). Non-integrated plasmid vectors from non-viral vectors usually produce a transient transgene expression (Gardlík et al., 2005), except when they are combined with viral replicons, which facilitates extrachromosomal replication, the presence of the vector as a stable episome and high efficiency of transfer (Gardlík et al., 2005). Furthermore, advances in extrachromosomal vector technology have allowed the creation of high capacity non-viral episomal vectors with the ability to achieve stable transgene expression (Lufino et al., 2008).

When an expression vector is not integrated into the host genome of dividing cells the extrachromosomally expression vector may not be segregated to all daughter cells during cellular division (Fig. 2) (Ehrhardt et al., 2008; Lufino et al., 2008). This transgene dilution due to a reduction in the number of copies of extrachromosomal DNA in each cell cycle is partially responsible for the transient levels of gene expression (Gardlík et al., 2005). When stable chromosomal integration takes place, the transgene will be inherited to both daughter cells after each cell cycle (Fig. 2). Chromosomal integration of viral vectors and transposons is usually random, which bring the risk of disrupting host gene expression (*i.e.* insertational mutagenesis) (Baum et al., 2006; Hackett et al., 2007). Activation of host cell oncogenes and inactivation of tumor suppressors are among the genetic consequences of insertational mutagenesis (Baum et al., 2006; Hackett et al., 2007). However, whereas retro- and lentiviruses preferentially integrate into promoter and exonic regions of transcribed genes, most transposons integrate into intergenic regions (Yant et al., 2005; Hackett et al., 2005). Thus, transposons represent probably the safest method currently available for genetic engineering (Grabundzija et al., 2010; Kues et al., 2010).

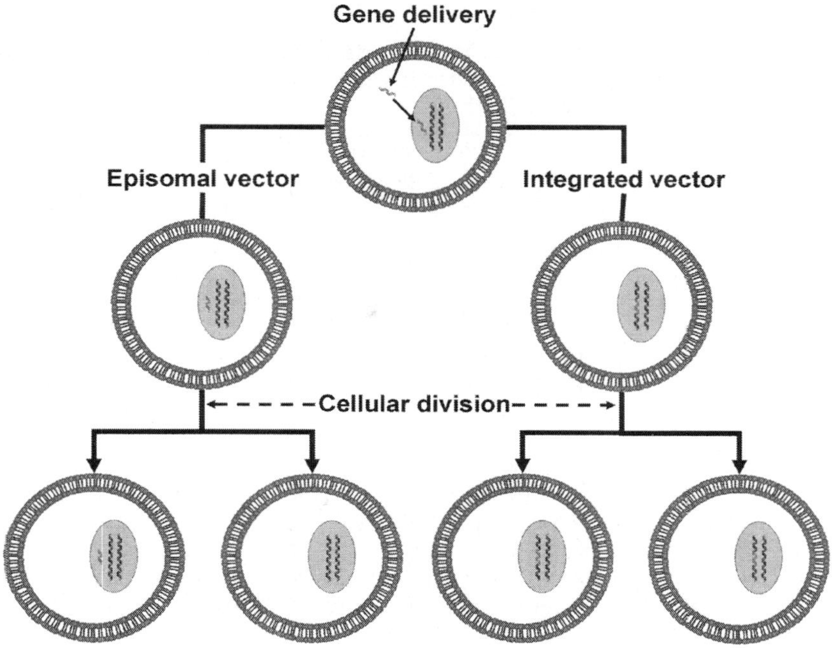

Fig. 2. Transgene segregation in extrachromosomal positioning (episomal) or chromosomal integration of expression vectors after gene delivery.

Regardless of the expression vector position in the nucleus (*i.e.* episomal or chromosomal), transcriptional activity is not always efficient, which can result in ectopic, weak or even undetectable transgene expression (Giraldo & Montoliu, 2001). Possible causes of transgene expression variability include differences in the number of integrations, transgene inactivation, or different genome integration sites of the vector. Transgene expression critically depends on the number of plasmids entering the nucleus (James & Giorgio, 2000; Glover et al., 2010), which not only depends on the ability of vectors to deliver intact DNA but also on the type of cell, as some cells translocate plasmid DNA from the cytoplasm to the nucleus more efficiently than others (James & Giorgio, 2000). However, high copy numbers of the transgene can increase methylation pattern of the promoter and thereby inducing transgene silencing (Garrick et al., 1998). In addition to promoter hypermethylation, transgene silencing may also involve chromatin modifications such as chromatin condensation caused by histone tail deacetylation and histone code switch (He et al., 2005). In some cases formation of repressive heterochromatin on the plasmid DNA backbone without methylation of the promoter can also cause transcriptional silencing of the transgene (Chen et al., 2008a). Moreover, integration into a transcriptionally inactive region of DNA, such as constitutive heterochromatin, will also result in transgene inactivation (Hackett et al., 2007). It is common to observe the transferred gene undergoing a brief period of expression followed by a decline to undetectable levels even though the vector DNA concentration remains constant in cells (Bestor, 2000).

3. Current gene transfer models in bovine species

Current uses of gene transfer models in bovine species include the production of transgenic cattle via germ-line gene transfer to produce valuable proteins in milk and serum of cattle for therapeutic purposes in humans (Table 3).

Protein	Possible therapeutic application	Reference
Human lactoferrin	Infectious complications	Krimpenfort et al., 1991
Human α-lactalbumin	Phenylketonuria	Eyestone et al., 1998
Human serum albumin	Blood volume restoration	Behboodi et al., 2001
Human bile salt-stimulated lipase	Pancreatic insufficiency	Chen et al., 2002
Human immunoglobulin	Immuno-related diseases	Kuroiwa et a., 2002
Human growth hormone	Growth-related disorders	Salamone et al 2006
Human myelin basic protein	Multiple sclerosis	Al-Ghobashy et al., 2009

Table 3. Examples of human proteins produced in transgenic cattle and their possible therapeutic application

Other applications of bovine transgenesis include the production of recombinant antibodies for tumor cell killing therapy (Grosse-Hovest et al., 2004) and the creation of cattle resistant to diseases (*e.g.* mastitis) (Wall et al. ,2005) or with enhanced milk composition (*e.g.* higher levels of casein) (Brophy et al., 2003).

Methodologies to produce transgenic cattle include microinjection of exogenous DNA into the pronuclei of zygotes, sperm-mediated gene transfer (via intracytoplasmic injection), injection (in the perivitelline space) of oocytes with viral vectors, and somatic cell nuclear transfer (SCNT) (Niemann & Kues, 2003; Velazquez, 2008). Currently the most common method to produce transgenic bovine offspring is SCNT. This approach involves the *in vitro* transfer of the foreign DNA into somatic cells followed by the insertion of positive transgenic cells into enucleated oocytes which develop to the blastocyst stage and are subsequently transferred to recipients (Fig. 3).

The use of *in vivo* gene therapy has been reported in a neonatal bovine model of citrullinemia (Lee et al., 1999), a urea-cycle disorder causing hyperammonemia due to the lack of argininosuccinate synthetase (ASS) (Marquis-Nicholson et al., 2010). In this study, two calves diagnosed with citrullinemia were supplemented with arginine and sodium benzoate from 24 hrs after birth onwards to avoid death. At day 10 after birth a single application of a viral vector carrying human ASS cDNA into the external jugular vein caused selective transduction of hepatocytes and resulted in decreased levels of glutamine (an indication of *de novo* synthesis of urea), which lasted until day 18 posttreatment. Since the treatment just restored ASS activity in liver and not in the kidneys, arginine therapy had to be continued. This partial enzymatic correction was lost 3 weeks after vector application (Lee et al., 1999).

In a different *in vivo* gene transfer model, Brown et al. (2004) injected a single dose of plasmid DNA carrying cDNA for growth hormone-releasing hormone (GHRH) in the trapezius muscle of dairy heifers followed by electroporation. Treated animals displayed an increase in haemoglobin, red blood cells, peripheral blood mono-nuclear cells and insulin-like growth factor-1 (IGF-1) compared to control animals at 300 days posttreatment. These physiological effects were observed without effect on concentrations of glucose and insulin.

The treatment was associated with increased body condition score, reduced hoof pathology and decreased mortality (Brown et al., 2004). The same group tested this gene delivery system during heat stress in pregnant heifers (Brown et al., 2009). They reported that calves from treated cows showed lower mortality and a significant improvement of survival from birth to 260 days, along with increased daily weight gain. In dams, milk production and prolactin concentrations were increased. Furthermore, the second pregnancy rate was improved in cows receiving the plasmid-based GHRH (Brown et al., 2009).

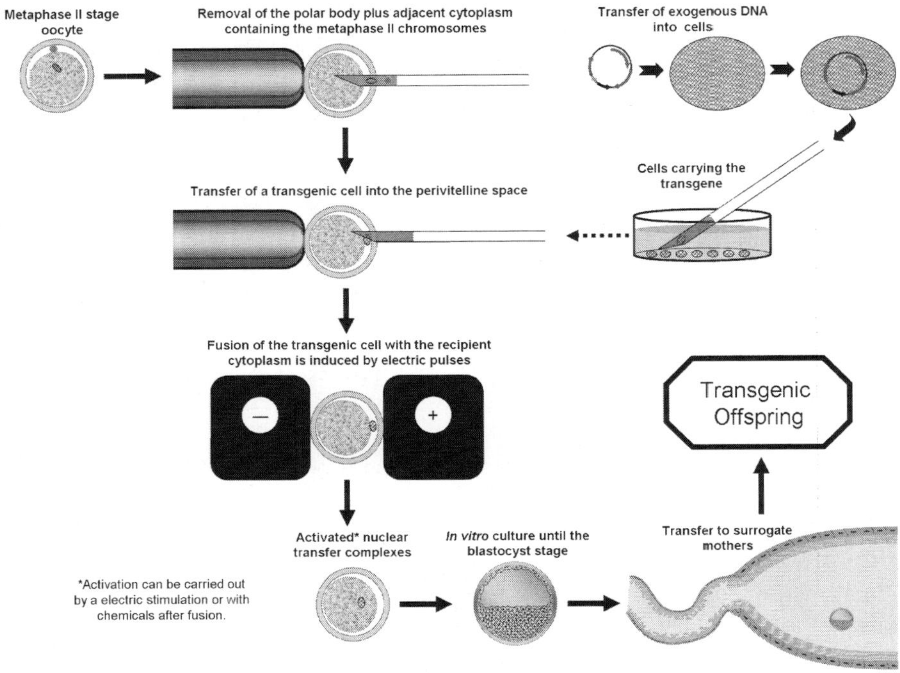

Fig. 3. Main steps in the production of transgenic bovine offspring using conventional somatic cell nuclear transfer.

Previous research has shown that growth hormone and IGF-1 play a significant role on ovarian follicular development and preimplantation embryo development (Kaiser et al., 2001; Sirotkin, 2005; Velazquez et al., 2009b). It will be interesting to test whether the plasmid-based GHRH treatment could serve as therapy to increase the superovulatory response of low responder animals (De Roover et al., 2005) or to increase pregnancy rates in cows with infertility problems (Thatcher et al., 2006).

Bovine models with RNA interference (RNAi) technology have been also implemented in loss-of-function studies to address gene function on ovarian follicular development and development of oocytes and preimplantation embryos (Table 4). Although the effects of gene knockdown on embryo development have been analyzed mostly *in vitro*, approaches using *in vivo* embryo culture have been reported (Tesfaye et al., 2010).

Gene	RNAi	Parameter analyzed	Reference
Cyclin B1	dsRNA	Oocyte maturation	Paradis et al., 2005
C-mos	dsRNA	Oocyte maturation	Nganvongpanit et al., 2006
Oct-4	dsRNA	Embryo development	Nganvongpanit et al., 2006
JY-1	siRNA	Embryo development	Bettegowda et al., 2007
p66Shc	shRNA	Embryo development	Favetta et al., 2007
Survivin	dsRNA	Embryo development	Park et al., 2007
Connexin 43	dsRNA	Embryo development	Tesfaye et al., 2007
E-cadherin	dsRNA	Embryo development	Tesfaye et al., 2007
FIBP	siRNA	Ovarian steroidogenesis	Forde et al., 2008
Betaglycan	siRNA	Ovarian steroidogenesis	Forde et al., 2008
Follistatin	siRNA	Embryo development	Lee et al. ,2009
KPNA7	siRNA	Embryo development	Tejomurtula et al., 2009
CENPF	dsRNA	Embryo development	Toralová et al., 2009
KRT18	dsRNA	Embryo development	Goossens et al., 2010
BIRC6	ds/shRNA	Embryo development	Salilew-Wondim et al., 2010
MSX1	ds/siRNA	Embryo development	Tesfaye et al., 2010

Table 4. Examples of use of RNAi in bovine models. dsRNA=double-stranded RNA, siRNA=small interfering RNA, shRNA=short hairpin RNA.

4. Methods for *in vivo* gene delivery in the reproductive tract of female bovine species

4.1 *In vivo* gene delivery to the ovaries

Since its first reported use as a tool to aspirate bovine oocytes *in vivo* (Pieterse et al., 1988), ovarian transvaginal ultrasonography (OTU) has been used in ovum-pick programs for the *in vitro* production of bovine preimplantation embryos world-wide for commercial purposes (van Wagtendonk-de Leeuw, 2006). Bovine OTU is performed in virtually the same way as in humans, with the advantage that the bovine ovary can be fixed to the probe more precisely via rectal palpation. OTU is considered a non-invasive technique that has played a pivotal role in the elucidation of mechanism involved in the control of follicular growth and developmental capacity of the oocyte in both humans(Revelli et al., 2009) and cattle (Beg & Ginther 2006; Leroy et al., 2008). This has been mainly accomplished with the analysis of aspirated oocytes and ovarian follicular fluid samples. Other possible *in vivo* procedures with OTU include injections in individual follicles (Beg & Ginther 2006), ovarian stroma (Oropeza et al., 2004) and corpus luteum (CL) (Yamashita et al., 2008). Ovarian biopsies can also be performed with OTU for the collection of CL (Kot et al., 1999) and ovarian cortical samples (Aerts et al., 2005). Moreover, OTU allows the *in vivo* transfer of oocytes from one ovarian follicle to another (*i.e.* interfollicular oocyte transfer) (Bergfelt et al., 1998).

Bovine OTU could afford the possibility of *in vivo* delivering of vectors directly to the ovaries without the necessity of surgical procedures. The feasibility of this model is partially supported by the transient transfection of murine ovarian cells achieved after direct *in vivo* intraovarian (IOI) injection of circle plasmid DNA followed by electroporation (Sato et al., 2003). Likewise, production of transgenic mice expressing green fluorescent protein has been achieved after direct IOI of plasmid DNA without subsequent electroporation (Yang et al., 2007). The necessity of surgical exposure of ovaries in these murine models hinders the opportunity for repeated administration of vectors producing transient transgene expression. This could be easily circumvented with the bovine model as intraovarian injections could be carried out at least twice per week (Velazquez et al., 2009a). Advances in ultrasound-triggered targeted gene delivery vehicles such as echogenic liposomes (Smith et al., 2010) could provide an efficient OTU *in vivo* vector delivery system in cattle. Following gene delivery, integration of the transgene could be analyzed in primordial and preantral follicles (Aerts et al., 2005), oocytes from antral follicles (Zaraza et al., 2010) and granulosa cells (Wells et al., 1999) with minimal discomfort for the carrier animal. Furthermore, since sheep ovaries can be imaged *in situ* (*i.e.* ovaries are exteriorized through a mid-ventral laparotomy) with fibered confocal fluorescence microscopy (Al-Gubory, 2005), the possibility of analyzing *in vivo* transgene integration with fluorescent reporter genes such as green fluorescent protein (Zizzi et al., 2010) is plausible (Fig. 4).

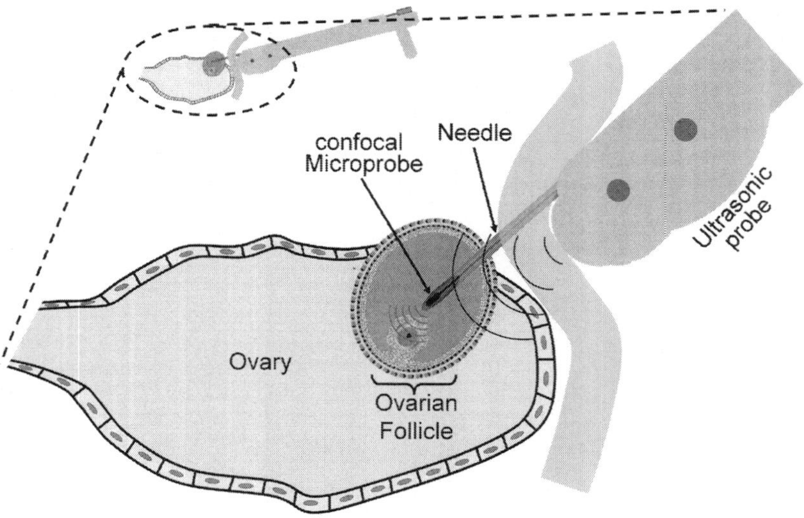

Fig. 4. Hypothetical *in vivo* monitoring of ovarian transgene integration with fluorescent reporter genes using fibered confocal fluorescence microscopy in cattle.

Since human and cattle ovaries are similar in size (Kagawa et al., 2009), the bovine OTU model could be useful to investigate the effect of silencing or overexpressing oocyte-specific genes known to be expressed also in humans such as bone morphogenetic protein 15 (BMP15) and growth differentiation factor 9 (GDF9) (Simpson, 2008). Experiments with these genes in a bovine OTU model aimed at controlling granulosa cell proliferation and follicle-stimulating hormone (FSH) responsiveness (Shimasaki et al., 2003) could substantially contribute to the development of therapeutic strategies for conditions such as premature ovarian failure (Simpson, 2008) or ovarian hyperstimulation syndrome (Mikkelsen, 2005). This latter disorder could be also addressed in the bovine OTU model with gain- or loss-of-function studies with anti-müllerian hormone in superovulated cows, as in both species anti-müllerian hormone is associated with the number of antral follicles responding to ovarian superstimulation (Broer et al., 2010; Monniaux et al., 2010).

The bovine OTU model will be an important tool for *in vivo* silencing of candidate genes involved in the regulation of cattle dominant follicle selection recently identified by genomic approaches (Mihm & Evans, 2008). Monitoring of ovarian follicular development with transrectal ultrasonography is a routine procedure in the cattle industry that was the based for the characterization of the follicular wave pattern in women (Baerwald, 2009). Data generated with the bovine model could provide valuable information for humans, especially when using modified cow models (*i.e.* FSH-suppressed cows during the follicular phase) that mimic the time of follicular recruitment and development of the dominant follicle in a highly analogous manner to women (Campbell et al., 2003).

4.2 In vivo gene delivery to the oviduct

In vivo transfection of oviductal epithelium has been reported in rodents via deposition of naked plasmid DNA or lipoplexes in the lumen of the infundibulum (Relloso & Esponda, 1998; 2000; Rios et al., 2002). Access to the fallopian tubes in this laboratory animal model requires invasive surgery. In cattle, a minimal invasive technique based on transvaginal endoscopy has been developed that allows *in vivo* access to the oviducts (Besenfelder et al., 2001). This endoscopy-mediated transvaginal access to the fallopian tubes has made possible the *in vivo* recovery and transfer of embryos from the zygote to the 8-16 cell stage in standing cows without the necessity of general anaesthesia (Besenfelder et al., 2010). The use of this transvaginal endoscopic procedure was pivotal for the generation of gene expression profiles of *in vivo* preimplantation embryos (Kues et al., 2008). The importance of using this technique to recover early stages embryos relies in the fact that postmortem recovery of *in vivo*-produced embryos can alter embryo gene expression (Knijn et al., 2005). This is especially relevant when studying the effects of gene silencing on preimplantation embryo development *in vivo* (Tesfaye et al. 2010).

With this technique it will be possible to infuse vectors into the lumen of the oviduct repeatedly (Besenfelder et al., 2008) and the efficiency of transfection could be improved with the combined use of transrectal ultrasonography, as ultrasound application can improve *in vivo* vector cellular uptake in the reproductive tract (Maruyama et al., 2004). Transgene integration in the oviductal epithelium with fluorescent reporter genes could be also monitored *in vivo* with flexible fibered confocal fluorescence microscopy microprobes. This is supported by the used of this technology to carry out *in vivo* imaging of fluorochrome-labelled ram spermatozoa to analyze *in situ* sperm motility in the ewe genital tract after surgical positioning of the microprobe (Druart et al., 2009). With the endoscopic approach the positioning of the confocal microprobe into lumen of the oviducts may be feasible (Fig. 5).

Silencing (or overexpression) of genes in the oviduct thought to play similar roles in oviductal biology in humans and cattle (identified during comparison of data from microarray analysis from the two species [Bauersachs et al., 2004]), could provide clues for the development of therapies for human contraception and for the formulation of enhanced embryo culture medium. Suggested candidate genes of bovine embryo developmental competence (El-sayed et al., 2006) could be tested. This may be achieved with an *ex vivo* approach of embryo gene silencing such as the one developed by Tesfaye et. al. (2010). Data from the bovine model could be useful for humans, as global transcription profiles during the maternal-zygotic transition are similar in both species (Xie et al. 2010). The model could be particularly relevant for genes showing high homology between the two species such as HMGN3a and SMARCAL I, which are known to play a critical role in chromatin remodelling during early embryo development (Uzun et al., 2009).

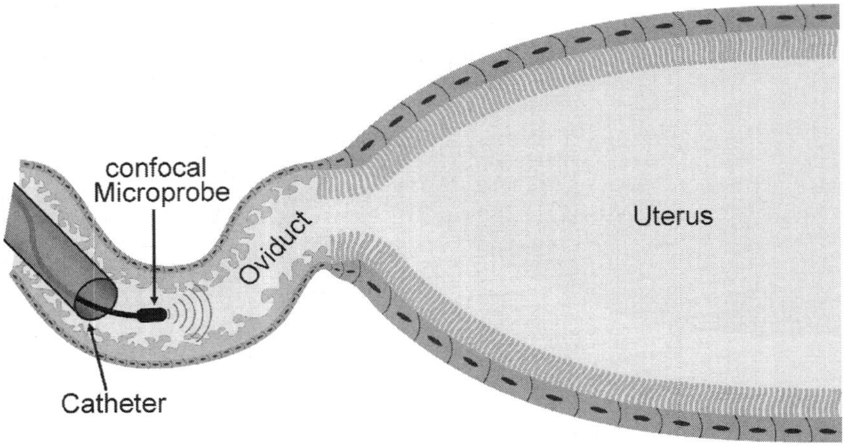

Fig. 5. Hypothetical *in vivo* monitoring of oviductal transgene integration with fluorescent reporter genes using fibered confocal fluorescence microscopy in cattle.

4.3 In vivo gene delivery to the uterus

Non-invasive access to the uterus is a standard procedure broadly used for artificial insemination (AI) and embryo transfer in cattle herds (Velazquez, 2008) that could be applied for repeated *in vivo* gene transfer in the bovine uterus. Uterine *in vivo* gene transfer has been demonstrated in mice (Charnock-Jones et al., 1997; Kimura et al., 2005; Rodde et al., 2008) and rabbits (Laurema et al., 2007). However, accurate access to the lumen of uterus in small animals requires invasive surgical procedures (Ngô-Muller & Muneoka, 2010). As with ovaries and oviducts, transrectal ultrasonography could improve vector cellular uptake via sonoporation (Maruyama et al., 2004). *In vivo* transgene tracking in the uterus with fibered confocal fluorescence microscopy, as previously reported in transgenic rabbits (Al-Gubory and Houdebine, 2006), could be performed in a non-invasive way with transcervical endoscopy (Fig. 6). Transcervical endoscopy is a fairly established technique in cattle used to evaluate uterine involution and its association with uterine diseases (Mordak et al., 2007; Madoz et al., 2010). In addition, confocal laser endomicroscopy technology is already available (Buchner et al., 2010).

Genes with possible roles in uterine biology in humans and cattle, identified during comparison of data from microarray analysis from the two species (Bauersachs et al., 2008), could be silenced (or overexpressed) in order to develop therapies for human contraception and for the formulation of enhanced embryo culture medium. The development of models of uterine cancer in superovulated cows (Velazquez et al. 2009b), will be particularly relevant to test the therapeutic usefulness of tumor suppressor induction (*e.g.* TP53) or silencing of growth factor receptors (*e.g.* IGF-1R). Testing (*i.e.* silencing or overexpression) of candidate genes of bovine embryo developmental competence (El-sayed et al., 2006) can be carried out with the use of embryo transfer, a technique well established in the cattle industry (Velazquez, 2008). Information generated with the bovine embryo transfer model could be useful to human assisted reproduction, as gene expression profiles in blastocysts of both species are to a large extent identical (Adjaye et al., 2007).

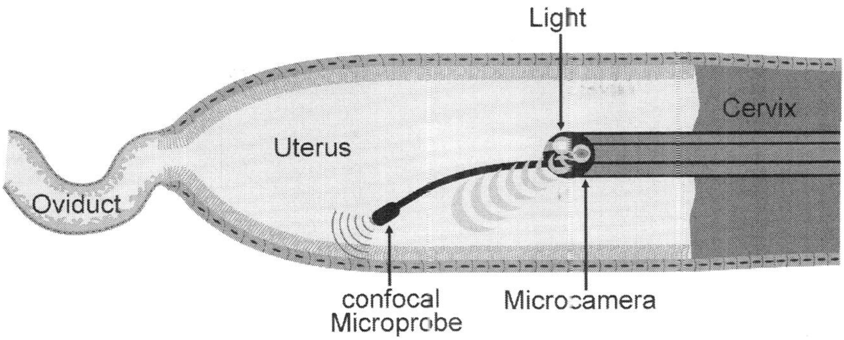

Fig. 6. Hypothetical *in vivo* monitoring of uterine transgene integration with fluorescent reporter genes using fibered confocal fluorescence microscopy in cattle.

5. Animal welfare considerations

All of the techniques mentioned above require special training and should be carried out by professionals that have proper understanding of bovine physiology and anatomy. In the hands of professionals this techniques are safe and cause minimal disturbance to the animal. Nervous cows or those sensitive to rectal palpation (*i.e.* excessive rectal bleeding during exploratory palpation) should be indentified to avoid unnecessary suffering. Environmental enrichment (*e.g.* music or visual effects) should be implemented whenever possible to provide comfort to the animal during the procedure. Health status should be monitored closely after gene delivery to identify and treat ill animals. Euthanasia must be implemented immediately when required.

6. Conclusions

The female bovine could provide a useful model for *in vivo* gene transfer in the reproductive tract. The bovine model may not only offer easiness in the delivering of transgenes in reproductive tract, but also long-term monitoring. This chapter has provided just a handful of the possible scenarios that could be addressed in the bovine model with relevance for human reproductive medicine. The strong similarities in some reproductive characteristics between the two species open the possibility of using the female bovine as a pre-clinical model in reproductive sciences. It is interesting to note that procedures with proved capacity to increase the superovulatory response of cows (*i.e.* aspiration of the dominant follicle) (Bungartz & Niemann, 1994) developed more than a decade ago, are just recently being proposed for application in women as a means to increase the efficiency of assisted reproduction (Bianchi et al. 2010). Perhaps it is time for human reproductive scientists to pay close attention to reproductive large animal models.

7. References

Adams, G.P. & Pierson, R.A. (1995). Bovine model for study of ovarian follicular dynamics in humans. *Theriogenology* 43:113-120.

Adjaye, J., Herwig, R., Brink, T.C., Herrmann, D., Greber, B., Sudheer, S., Groth, D., Carnwath, J.W., Lehrach, H., Niemann, H. (2007). Conserved molecular portraits of bovine and human blastocysts as a consequence of the transition from maternal to embryonic control of gene expression. *Physiological Genomics* 31:315-327.

Aerts, J.M.J., Oste, M. & Bols, P.E.J. (2005). Development and practical applications of a method for repeated transvaginal, ultrasound-guided biopsy collection of the bovine ovary. *Theriogenology* 64:947-957.

Akita, H., Enoto, K., Masuda, T., Mizuguchi, H., Tani, T. & Harashima, H. (2010). Particle tracking of intracellular trafficking of octaarginine-modified liposomes: a comparative study with adenovirus. *Molecular Therapy* 18:955-964.

Al-Dosari, M.S. & Gao, X. (2009). Nonviral gene delivery: Principle, limitations, and recent progress. *The American Association of Pharmaceutical Scientists Journal* 11:671-681.

Al-Ghobashy, M.A., Williams, M.A., Brophy, B. Laible, G. & Harding, D.R. (2009). On-line casein micelle disruption for downstream purification of recombinant human myelin basic protein produced in the milk of transgenic cows. *Journal of Chromatography B, Analytical Technologies in the Biomedical and Life Sciences* 877:1667-1677.

Al-Gubory, K.H. (2005). Fibered confocal fluorescence microscopy for imaging apoptotic DNA fragmentation at the single-cell level in vivo. *Experimental Cell Research* 310:474-481.

Al-Gubory, K.H. & Houdebine, L.-M. (2006). In vivo imaging of green fluorescent protein-expressing cells in transgenic animals using fibred confocal fluorescence microscopy. *European Journal of Cell Biology* 85:837-845.

Baerwald, A.R. (2009). Human antral folliculogenesis: what we have learned from the bovine and equine models. *Animal Reproduction* 6:20-29.

Bauersachs, S., Mitko, K., Ulbrich, S.E., Blum, H. & Wolf, E. (2008). Transcriptome studies of bovine endometrium reveal molecular profiles characteristic for specific stages of estrous cycle and early pregnancy. *Experimental and Clinical Endocrinology & Diabetes* 116:371-384.

Bauersachs, S., Rehfeld, S., Ulbrich, S.E. Mallok, S., Prelle, K., Wenigerkind, H., Einspanier, R., Blum, H. & Wolf, E. (2004). Monitoring gene expression changes in bovine oviduct epithelial cells during the oestrous cycle. Journal of Molecular Endocrinology 32:449-466.

Baum, C., Kustikova, O., Modlich, U., Li, X. & Fehse, B. (2006). Mutagenesis and oncogenesis by chromosomal insertion of gene transfer vectors. *Human Gene Therapy* 17:253-263.

Baumann, C.G., Morris, D.G., Sreenan, J.M. & Leese, H.J. (2007). The quiet embryo hypothesis: molecular characteristics favoring viability. *Molecular Reproduction and Development* 74:1345-1353.

Beg, M.A. & Ginther, O.J. (2006). Follicle selection in cattle and horses: role of intrafollicular factors. *Reproduction* 132:365-377.

Behboodi, E., Groen, W., Destrempes, M.M., Williams, J.L., Ohlrichs, C., Gavin, W.G., Broek, D.M., Ziomek, C.A., Faber, D.C., Meade, H.M. & Echelard, Y. (2001). Transgenic production from in vivo-derived embryos: effect on calf birth weight and sex ratio. *Molecular Reproduction and Development* 60:27-37.

Bergfelt, D.R., Brogliatti, G.M. & Adams, G.P. (1998). Gamete recovery and follicular transfer (GRAFT) using transvaginal ultrasonography. *Theriogenology* 50:15-25.

Besenfelder, U. Havlicek, V. Kuzmany, A. & Brem, G. (2010). Endoscopic approaches to manage in vitro and in vivo embryo development: use of the bovine oviduct. *Theriogenology* 73:768-776.

Besenfelder, U., Havlicek, V. Moesslacher, G., Gilles, M., Tesfaye, D., Griese, J., Hoelker, M., Hyttel, P.M., Laurincik, J., Brem, G. & Schellander, K. (2008). Endoscopic recovery of early preimplantation bovine embryos: effect of hormonal stimulation, embryo kinetics and repeated collection. *Reproduction in Domestic Animals* 43:566-572.

Besenfelder, U. Havlicek, V. Mösslacher, G. & Brem G. (2001). Collection of tubal stage bovine embryos by means of endoscopy. A technique report. *Theriogenology* 55:837-845.

Bestor, TH. (2000). Gene silencing as a threat to the success of gene therapy. *Journal of Clinical Investigation* 105:409-411.

Bettegowda, A., Yao, J., Sen, A., Li, Q., Lee, K.B., Kobayashi, Y., Patel, O.V., Coussens, P.M., Ireland, J.J. & Smith, G.W. (2007). JY-1, an oocyte-specific gene, regulates granulosa cell function and early embryonic development in cattle. *Proceedings of the National Academy of Sciences of the United States of America* 104:17602-17607.

Bianchi, P., Serafini, P., da Rocha, A.M., Hassun, P., da Motta, E., Baruselli, P. & Baracat, E. (2010). Follicular waves in the human ovary: a new physiological paradigm for novel ovarian stimulation protocols *Reproductive Sciences*, in press, pISSN:1933-7191, eISSN:1933-7205, doi:10.1177/1933719110366483

Boulikas, T. (1998). Nucleocytoplasmic trafficking: implications for the nuclear import of plasmid DNA during gene therapy. *Gene Therapy and Molecular Biology* 1:713-740.

Broer, S.L., Dólleman, M., Opmeer, B.C., Fauser, B.C., Mol, B.W. & Broekmans, F.J. (2010). AMH and AFC as predictors of excessive response in controlled ovarian hyperstimulation: a meta analysis. *Human Reproduction Update*, in press, pISSN:1355-4786, eISSN:1460-2369, doi:10.1093/humupd/dmq034

Brophy, B., Smolenski, G., Wheeler, T., Wells, D., L'Huillier P. & Laible, G. (2003). Cloned transgenic cattle produce milk with higher levels of β-casein and κ-casein. *Nature Biotechnology* 21:157-162.

Brown, P.A., Bodles-Brakhop, A.M. & Draghia-Akli, R. (2008). Effects of plasmid growth hormone-releasing hormone treatment. *DNA and Cell Biology* 27:629-635.

Brown, P.A., Davis, W.C. & Draghia-Akli, R. (2004). Immune-enhancing effects of growth hormone-releasing hormone delivered by plasmid injection and electroporation. *Molecular Therapy* 10:644-651.

Brunner, S., Sauer, T., Carotta, S., Cotten, M., Saltik, M. & Wagner, E. (2000). Cell cycle dependence of gene transfer by lipoplex, polyplex and recombinant adenovirus. *Gene Therapy* 7:401-407.

Buchner, A.M. ,Shahid, M.W. Heckman, M.G. Krishna, M., Ghabril, M., Hasan, M., Crook, J.E., Gomez, V., Raimondo, M., Woodward, T., Wolfsen, H.C. & Wallace, M.B. (2010). Comparison of probe-based confocal laser endomicroscopy with virtual chromoendoscopy for classification of colon polyps. *Gastroenterology* 138:834-842.

Bungartz, L. & Niemann, H. (1994). Assessment of the presence of a dominant follicle and selection of dairy cows suitable for superovulation by a single ultrasound examination. *Journal of Reproduction and Fertility* 101:583-591.

Campbell, B.K., Souza, C., Gong, J., Webb, R., Kendall, N., Masters, P., Robinson, G., Mitchell, A., Telfer, E.E. & Baird, D.T (2003). Domestic ruminants as models for the elucidation of the mechanisms controlling ovarian follicle development in humans. *Reproduction* 61(Supplement):429-443.

Caracciolo, G., Caminiti, R., Digman, M.A., Gratton, E. & Sanchez, S. (2009). Efficient escape from endosomes determines the superior efficiency of multicomponent lipoplexes. *Journal of Physical Chemistry B* 113:4995-4997.

Caracciolo, G., Pozzi, D., Amenitsch, H. & Caminiti, R. (2007). Interaction of lipoplexes with anionic lipids resulting in DNA release is a two-stage process. *Langmuir* 23:8713-8717.

Casal, M. & Haskins, M. (2006). Large animal models and gene therapy. *European Journal of Human Genetics* 14:266-272.

Charnock-Jones, D.S., Sharkey, A.M., Jaggers, D.C., Yoo, H.J., Heap, R.B. & Smith, S.K. (1997). In-vivo gene transfer to the uterine endometrium. *Human Reproduction* 12:17-20.

Chen, Z.-Y., Riu, E., He, C.-Y., Xu, H. & Kay, M.A. (2008a). Silencing of episomal transgene expression in liver by plasmid bacterial backbone DNA is independent of CpG methylation. *Molecular Therapy* 16:548-556.

Chen, X., Kube, D.M. Cooper, M. J. & Davis, P.B. (2008b). Cell surface nucleolin serves as receptor for DNA nanoparticles composed of pegylated polylysine and DNA. *Molecular Therapy* 16:333-342.

Chen, S.-H., Vaught, T.D., Monahan, J.A., Boone, J., Emslie, E., Jobst, P.M., Lamborn, A.E., Schnieke, A., Robertson, L., Colman, A., Dai, Y., Polejaeva, I.A. & Ayares, D.L. (2002). Efficient production of transgenic cloned calves using preimplantation screening. *Biology of Reproduction* 67:1488-1492.

Cohen, R.N., van der Aa, M.A.E.M., Macaraeg, N., Lee, A.P. & Szoka, F.C.Jr. (2009). Quantification of plasmid DNA copies in the nucleus after lipoplex and polyplex transfection. *Journal of Controlled Release* 135:166-174.

Daftary, G.S. & Taylor, M.D. (2003). Reproductive tract gene transfer. *Fertility and Sterility* 80:475-484.

De Roover, R., Bols, P.E.J., Genicot, G. & Hanzen, Ch. (2005). Characteristics of low, medium and high responders following FSH stimulation prior to ultrasound-guided transvaginal oocyte retrieval in cows. *Theriogenology* 63:1902-1913.

Dean, D.A. (1997). Import of plasmid DNA into the nucleus is sequence specific. *Experimental Cell Research* 230:293-302.

Dean, D.A., Strong, D.D. & Zimmer, W.E. (2005). Nuclear entry of nonviral vectors. *Gene Therapy* 12:881-890.

Dinh, A.T., Theofanous, T., Mitragotri, S. (2005). A model for intracellular trafficking of Adenoviral vectors. *Biophysical Journal* 89:1574-1588.

Dowty, M.E. ,Williams, P., Zhang, G., Hagstrom, J.E. & Wolff, J.A. (1995). Plasmid DNA entry into postmitotic nuclei of primary rat myotubes. *Proceedings of the National Academy of Sciences of the United States of America* 92:4572-4576.

Doyle, S.R. & Chan, C.K. (2007). Differential intracellular distribution of DNA complexed with polyethylenimine (PEI) and PEI-polyarginine PTD influences exogenous gene expression within live COS-7 cells. *Genetic Vaccines and Therapy* 5:11

Druart, X., Cognié, J., Baril, G., Clément, F., Dacheux, J.-L. & Gatti, J.-L. (2009). In vivo imaging of in situ motility of fresh and liquid stored ram spermatozoa in the ewe genital tract. *Reproduction* 138:45-53.

Du, Z.Q., Vincent-Naulleau, S., Gilbert, H., Vignoles, F., Créchet, F., Shimogiri, T., Yasue, H., Leplat, J.J., Bouet, S., Gruand, J., Horak, V., Milan, D., Le Roy, P., Geffrotin, C. (2007). Detection of novel quantitative trait loci for cutaneous melanoma by genom-wide scan in the MeLiM swine model. *International Journal of Cancer* 120:303-320.

Dyson, M., Allososh, M., Vuichetich, J.P., Mokelke, E.A. & Sturek, M. (2006). Components of metabolic syndrome and coronary artery disease in female Ossabaw swine fed excess atherogenic diet. *Comparative Medicine* 56:35-45.

Ehrhardt, A., Haase, R., Schepers, A., Deutsch, M.J., Lipps, H J. & Baiker. A. (2008). Episomal vectors for gene therapy. *Current Gene Therapy* 8:147-161.

El-Sayed, A. Hoelker, M., Rings, F. Salilew, D. Jennen, D., Tholen, E. Sirard, M.-A., Schellander, K. Tesfaye, D. (2006). Large-scale transcriptional analysis of bovine embryo biopsies in relation to pregnancy success after transfer to recipients. *Physiological Genomics* 28:84-96.

Escoffre, J.-M., Teissié, J. & Rols M.-P. (2010). Gene transfer: how can the biological barriers be overcome? *Journal of Membrane Biology* 236:61-74.

Evans, C.H. (2010). Gene therapy for bone healing. *Expert Review in Molecular Medicine* 12:e18.

Eyestone, W.H., Gowallis, M., Monohan, J., Sink, T., Ball, S.F. & Cooper, J.D. (1998). Production of transgenic cattle expressing human α-lactalbumin in milk. *Theriogenology* 49:386[abstract].

Favetta, L.A., Madam, P., Mastromonaco, G.F., St John, E.J., King, W.A. & Betts, D.H. (2007). The oxidative stress adaptor p66Shc is required for permanent embryo arrest in vitro. *BMC Developmental Biology* 7:132.

Forde, N., Mihn, M., Canty, M.J., Zielak, A.E., Baker, P.J., Park, S., Lonergan, P., Smith, G.W., Coussens, P.M., Ireland, J.J. & Evans, A.C. (2008). Differential expression of signal transduction factors in ovarian follicle development: a functional role for betaglycan and FIBP in granulosa cells in cattle. *Physiological Genomics* 33:193-204.

Gardlík, R., Pálffy, R., Hodosy, J., Lukács, J., Turňa, J. & Celec P. (2005). Vectors and delivery systems in gene therapy. *Medical Science Monitor* 11:RA110-121.

Garrick, D., Fiering, S., Martin, D.I.K. & Whitelaw E. (1998) Repeat-induced gene silencing in mammals. *Nature Genetics* 18:56-59.

Geiger, J., Aneja, M.K. & Rudolph, C. (2010). Vectors for pulmonary gene therapy. *International Journal of Pharmaceutics* 390:84-88.

Giraldo, P. & Montoliu, L. (2001). Size matters: use of YACs, BACs and PACs in transgenic animals. *Transgenic Research* 10:83-103.

Glover, D.J., Leyton, D.L., Moseley, G.W. & Jans, D.A. (2010). The efficiency of nuclear plasmid DNA delivery is a critical determinant of transgene expression at the single cell level. *Journal of Gene Medicine* 12:77-85.

Goossens, K., Tesfaye, D., Rings, F., Schellander, K., Hölker, M, Van Poucke, M., Van Zeveren, A., Lemahieu, I., Van Soom, A. & Peelman, L.J. (2010). Supression of keratin 18 gene expression in bovine blastocysts by RNA interference. *Reproduction Fertility and Development* 22:395-404.

Grabundzija, I., Irgang, M., Mátés, L., Belay, E., Matrai, J., Gogol-Döring, A., Kawakami, K. Chen, W., Ruiz, P., Chuah, M.K., VandenDriessche T., Izsvák, Z. & Ivics, Z. (2010). Comparative analysis of transposable element vector systems in human cells. *Molecular Therapy* 18:1200-1209.

Graham, J.S., Reid, F.M., Smith, J.R., Stotts, R.R., Tucker, E.S., Shumaker, S.M., Niemuth, N.A. & Janny, S.J. (2000). A cutaneous full-thickness liquid sulfur mustard burn model in weanling swine: clinical pathology and urinary excretion of thiodiglycol. *Journal of Applied Toxicology* 20 (Suppl. 1):S161-S172.

Grigsby, C.L. & Leong, K.W. (2010). Balancing protection and release of DNA: tools to address a bottleneck of non-viral gene delivery. *Journal of the Royal Society Interface* 7(Suppl. 1):S67-S82.

Grosse-Hovest, L., Müller, S., Minoia, R., Wolf, E., Zakhartchenko, V., Wenigerkind, H., Lassnig, C., Besenfelder, U., Müller, M., Lytton, S.D., Jung, G. & Brem, G. (2004). Cloned transgenic farm animals produce a bispecific antibody for T-cell mediated tumor cell killing. *Proceedings of the National Academy of Sciences of the United States of America* 101:6858-6863.

Guo, J., Fisher, K.A., Darcy, R., Cryan, J.F. & O'Driscoll, C. (2010). Therapeutic targeting in the silent era: advances in non-viral siRNA delivery. *Molecular Biosystems* 6:1143-1161.

Habermann, F.A., Wuensch, A., Sinowatz, F., Wolf, E. (2007). Reporter genes for embryogenesis research in livestock species. *Theriogenology* 68(Suppl.1):S116-S124.

Hackett, C.S., Geurts, A.M. & Hackett, P.B. (2007). Predicting preferential DNA vector insertion sites: implications for functional genomics and gene therapy. *Genome Biology* 8(Suppl. 1):S12

Hackett, P.B., Ekker, S.C., Largaespada, D.A. & McIvor, R.S. (2005). Sleeping beauty transposons-mediated gene therapy for prolonged expression. *Advances in Genetics* 54:189-232.

Hama, S., Akita, H., Ito, R., Mizuguchi, H., Hayakawa, T. & Harashima, H. (2006). Quantitative comparison of intracellular trafficking and nuclear transcription between adenoviral and lipoplex systems. *Molecular Therapy* 13:786-794.

Hampton, S.L. & Kinnaird, A.I. (2010). Genetic interventions in mammalian cells; applications and uses in high-throughput screening and drug discovery. *Cell Biology and Toxicology* 26:43-55.

Han, J., Zhao, D., Zhong, Z., Zhang, Z., Gong, T., Sun, X. (2010). Combination of adenovirus and cross-linked low molecular weight PEI improves efficiency of gene transduction. *Nanotechnology* 21:105106

Hassan, M.H., Othman, E.E., Hornung, E. & Al-Hendy, A. (2009). Gene therapy in benign genecological diseases. *Advanced Drug Delivery Reviews* 61:822-835.

He, J., Yang, Q. & Chang, L.-J. (2005). Dynamic DNA methylation and histone modifications contribute to lentiviral transgene silencing in murine embryonic carcinoma cells. *Journal of Virology* 79:13497-13508.

Huang, H., Yu, H., Tang, G., Wang, Q. & Li, J. (2010). Low molecular weight polyethylenimine cross-linked by 2-hydroxypropil-gamma-cyclodextrin coupled to peptide targeting HER2 as a gene dleivery vector. *Biomaterials* 31:1830-1838.

Huber, P.E. & Pfisterer, P. (2000). In vitro and in vivo transfection of plasmid DNA in the Dunning prostate tumor R3327-AT1 is enhanced by focused ultrasound. *Gene Therapy* 7:1516-1525.

Huth, S. Hoffmann, F., Von Gersdorff, K., Laner, A., Reinhard, D., Rosenecker, J. & Rudolph C. (2006). Interaction of polyamine gene vectors with RNA leads to the dissociation of plasmid DNA-carrier complexes. *Journal of Gene Medicine* 8:1416-1424.

Ishii, A., Viñuela, F., Murayama, Y., Yuki, I., Nien, Y.L., Yeh, D.T. & Vinters, H.V. (2006). Swine model of carotid artery atherosclerosis: experimental induction by surgical partial ligation and dietary hypercholesterolemia. *American Journal of Neuroradiology* 27:1893-1899.

Jacobsen, J.C., Bawden, C.S., Rudiger, S.R. ,McLaughlan, C.J., Reid, S.J., Waldvogel, H.J., MacDonald, M.E., Gusella, J.F., Walker, S.K., Kelly, J.M., Webb, G.C., Faull, R.L., Rees, M.I., Snell, R.G. (2010). An ovine transgenic Huntington's disease model. *Human Molecular Genetics* 19:1873-1882.

James, M.B. & Giorgio, T.D. (2000). Nuclear-associated plasmid, but not cell-associated plasmid, is correlated with transgene expression in cultured mammalian cells. *Molecular Therapy* 1:339-346.

Kagawa, N., Silber, S. & Kuwayama, M. (2009). Successful vitrification of bovine and human ovarian tissue. *Reproductive Biomedicine Online* 18:568-577.

Kaiser, G.G., Sinowatz, F. & Palma, G.A. (2001). Effects of growth hormone on female reproductive organs. *Anatomia, Histologia, Embryologia* 30:265-271.

Kamiya, H., Fujimura, Y., Matsuoka, I. & Harashima, H. (2002). Visualization of intracellular trafficking of exogenous DNA delivered by cationic liposomes. *Biochemical and Biophysical Research Communications* 298:591-597.

Kay, M.A., Glorioso, J.C. & Naldini, L. (2001). Viral vectors for gene therapy: the art of turning ingectious agents into vehicles of therapeutics. *Nature Medicine* 7:33-40.

Khalil, I.A., Kogure, K., Akita, H. & Harashima, H. (2006). Uptake pathways and subsequent intracellular trafficking in nonviral gene delivery. *Pharmacological Reviews* 58:32-45.

Khurana, B., Goyal, A.K., Budhiraja, A. Arora, D. & Vyas, S.P. (2010). siRNA delivery using nanocarriers - an efficient tool for gene silencing. *Current Gene Therapy* 10:139-155.

Klassen, H., Warfvinge, K., Schwartz, P.H., Kiilgaard, J.F., Shamie, N., Jiang, C., Samuel, M., Scherfig, E., Prather, R.S. & Young, M.J. (2008). Isolation of progenitor cells from GFP-transgenic pigs and transplantation to the retina of allorecipients. *Cloning and Stem Cells* 10:391-402.

Kim, P.H., Kim, T.I., Yockman, J.W., Kim, S.W. & Yun, C.O. (2010). The effect of surface modification of adenovirus with an arginine-grafted bioreducible polymer on transduction efficiency and immunogenicity in cancer gene therapy. *Biomaterials* 31:1865-1874.

Kimura, T., Nakamura, H., Koyama, S., Ogita, K., Tabata, C., Tsutsui, T., Shimoya, K., Koyama, M., Kaneda, Y. & Murata, Y. (2005). In vivo gene transfer into the mouse uterus: a powerful tool for investigating implantation physiology. *Journal of Reproductive Immunology* 67:13-20.

Kot, K., Anderson, L.E., Tsai, S.J., Wiltbank, M.C. & Ginther, O.J. (1999). Transvaginal, ultrasound-guided biopsy of the corpus luteum in cattle. *Theriogenology* 52:987-993.

Knijn, H.M., Wrenzycki, C., Hendriksen, P.J.M., Vos, P.L.A.M., Zeinstra, E.C., van der Weijden, G.C., Niemann, H. & Dielemann, S.J. (2005). *In vitro* and *in vivo* culture effects on mRNA expression of genes involved in metabolism and apoptosis in bovine embryos. *Reproduction Fertility and Development* 17:775-784.

Kragh, P.M., Nielsen, A.L., Li, J., Du, Y., Lin, L., Schmidt, M., Bøgh, I.B., Holm, I.E., Jakobsen, J.E., Johansen, M.G., Purup, S., Bolund, L., Vajta, G. & Jørgensen, A.L. (2009). Hemizygous minipigs produced by random gene insertion and handmade cloning express the Alzheimer´s disease-causing dominant mutation APPsw. *Transgenic Research* 18:545-558.

Krimpenfort, P., Rademakers, A., Eyestone, W., van der Schans A., van den Broek S., Kooiman, P., Kootwijk, E., Platenburg G., Pieper, F, Strijker, R., de Boer, H. (1991). Generation of transgenic dairy cattle using 'in vitro' embryo production. *Bio/Technology* 9:844-847.

Kues, W.A., Garrels, W., Mates, L., Holler, S., Niemann, H., Iszvak, Z., Ivics, Z. (2010). Production of transgenic pigs by the Sleeping Beauty transposon system. *Transgenic Research* 19:336[abstract].

Kues, W.A., Sudheer, S., Herrmann, D., Carnwath, J.W., Havlicek, V., Besenfelder, U., Lehrach, H., Adjaye, J. & Niemann, H. (2008). Genome-wide expression profiling reveals distinct clusters of transcriptional regulation during bovine preimplantation development in vivo. *Proceedings of the National Academy of Sciences of the United States of America* 105:19768-19773.

Kuroiwa, Y., Kasinathan, P., Choi, Y.J., Naeem, R., Tomizuka, K., Sullivan, E.J., Knott, J.G., Duteau, A., Goldsby, R.A., Osborne, B.A., Ishida, I. & Robl, J.M. (2002). Cloned transchromosomic calves producing human immunoglobulin. *Nature Biotechnology* 20:889-894.

Laurema, A., Lumme, S., Heinonen, S.E., Heinonen, S. & Ylä-Herttuala, S. (2007). Transduction patterns and efficiencies in rabbit uterine tissues after intraluminal uterine adenovirus administration vary with the reproductive cycle. *Acta Obstetricia et Gynecologica Scandinavica* 86:1035-1040.

Lee, B., Dennis, J.A., Healy, P.J., Mull, B., Pastore, L., Yu, H., Aguilar-Cordova, E., O'Brien, W., Reeds, P. & Beaudet, A.L. (1999). Hepatocyte gene therapy in a large animal: A neonatal bovine model of citrullinemia. *Proceedings of the National Academy of Sciences of the United States of America* 96:3981-3986.

Lee, K.B., Bettegowda, A., Wee, G., Ireland, J.J. & Smith, G.W. (2009). Molecular determinants of oocyte competence: potential functional role for maternal (oocyte-derived) follistatin in promoting bovine early embryogenesis. *Endocrinology* 150:2463-2471.

Leroy, JLMR, Vanholder, T., Van Knegsel, A.T.M., Garcia-Ispierto, I., Bols, P.E.J. (2008). Nutrient prioritization in dairy cows early postpartum: mismazch between metabolism and fertility? *Reproduction in Domestic Animals* 43(Suppl. 2):96-103.

Long, H.A., McMillan, J.R., Qiao, H., Akiyama, M. & Shimizu, H. (2009). Current advances in gene therapy for the treatment of genodermatoses. *Current Gene Therapy* 9:487-494.

Lufino, M.M.P., Edser, P.A.H. & Wade-Martins, R. (2008). Advances in high-capacity extrachromosomal vector technology: Episomal maintenance, vector delivery, and transgene expression. *Molecular Therapy* 16:1525-1538.

Lukacs, G.L., Haggie, P., Seksek, O., Lechardeur, D., Freedman, N. & Verkman, G.L. (2000). Size-dependent DNA mobility in cytoplasm and nucleus. *Journal of Biological Chemistry* 275:1625-1629.

Madoz, LV., De la Sota, R.L., Suzuki, K., Heuwieser, W. & Drillich, M. (2010). Use of hysteroscopy for the diagnosis of postpartum clinical endometritis in dairy cows. *Veterinary Record* 167:142-143.

Magin-Lachmann, C., Kotzamanis, G., D'Aiuto, L., Cooke, H., Huxley, C. & Wagner, E. (2004). In vitro and in vivo delivery of intact BAC DNA – comparison of different methods. *Journal of Gene Medicine* 6:195-209.

Manfredsson, F.P. & Mandel, R.J. (2010). Development of gene therapy for neurological disorders. *Discovery Medicine* 9:204-211.

Marquis-Nicholson, R., Glamuzina, E., Proser, D., Wilson, C. & Love, D.R. (2010). Citrullinemia type I: molecular screening of the ASS1 gene by exonic sequencing and targeted mutation analysis. *Genetics and Molecular Research* 9:1483-1489.

Maruyama, T., Nagashima, T. Masuda, H., Asada, H., Uchida, H. & Yoshimura, Y. (2004). Female reproductive tract gene transfer by microbubble-enhanced sonoporation. *Fertility and Sterility* 82(Suppl. 2):S2-S3[abstract].

Medina-Kauwe, L.K., Xie, K. & Hamm-Alvarez, S. (2005). Intracellular trafficking of nonviral vectors. *Gene Therapy* 12:1734-1751.

Ménézo, Y.J. & Hérubel, F. (2002). Mouse and bovine models for human IVF. *Reproductive Biomedicine Online* 4:170-175.

Midoux, P., Pichon, C., Yaouanc, J.J. & Jaffrès P.-A. (2009). Chemical vectors for gene delivery: a current review on polymers, peptides and lipids containing histidine or imidazole as nucleic acids carriers. *British Journal of Pharmacology* 157:166-178.

Mihm, M & Evans, A.C.O. (2008). Mechanism for dominant follicle selection in monovulatory species: a comparison of morphological, endocrine and intraovarian events in cows, mares and women. *Reproduction in Domestic Animals* 43 (Suppl. 2):48-56.

Mikkelsen, A.L. (2005). Strategies in human in-vitro maturation and their clinical outcome. *Reproductive Biomedicine Online* 10:593-599.

Mordak, R., Kubiak, K., Jankowski, M. & Nicpoń, J. (2007). Hysteroscopy in cows-picture of postparturient metritis. *Electronic Journal of Polish Agricultural Universities* 10(4):#32.

Mortimer, I., Tam, P., MacLachlan I., Graham, R.W., Saravolac, E.G. & Joshi, P.B. (1999). Cationic lipid-mediated transfection of cells in culture requires mitotic activity. *Gene Therapy* 6:403-411.

Monniaux, D., Barbey, S., Rico, C. Fabre, S. Gallard, Y. & Larroque, H. (2010). Anti-Müllerian hormone: a predictive marker of embryo production in cattle? *Reproduction Fertility and Development* 22:1083-1091.

Mountain, A. (2000). Gene theraphy: the first decade. *Trends in Biotechnology* 18:119-128.

Muschler, G.F., Raut, V.P., Patterson, T.E., Wenke, J.C. & Hollinger, J.O. (2010). The design and use of animal models for translational research in bone tissue engineering and regenerative medicine. *Tissue Engineering Part B, Reviews* 16:123-145.

Nganvongpanit, K., Müller, H., Rings, F., Hoelker, M., Jennen, D., Tholen, E., Havlicek, V., Besenfelder, U., Schellander, K. & Tesfaye D. (2006). Selective degradation of maternal and embryonic transcripts in in vitro produced bovine oocytes and embryos using sequence specific double-stranded RNA. *Reproduction* 131:861-874.

Ngô-Muller, V. & Muneoka, K. (2010). In utero and exo utero surgery on rodent embryos. *Methods in Enzymology* 476:205-226.

Niemann, H. & Kues, W.A. (2003). Application of transgenesis in livestock for agriculture and biomedicine. *Animal Reproduction Science* 79:291-317.

Nienhuis, A.W. (2008). Development of gene therapy for blood disorders. *Blood* 111:4431-4444.

Niidome, T & Huang, L. (2002). Gene therapy progress and prospects: nonviral vectors. *Gene Therapy* 9:1647-1652.

Oropeza, A., Wrenzycki, C., Herrmann, D., Hadeler, K.-G. & Niemann, H. (2004). Improvement of the developmental capacity of oocytes from prepubertal cattle by intraovarian insulin-like growth factor-1 application. *Biology of Reproduction* 70:1634-1643.

O'Rorke, S., Keeney, M. & Pandit, A. (2010). Non-viral lipoplexes: Scaffold mediated delivery for gene therapy. *Progress in Polymer Science* 35:441-458.

Paradis, F., Vigneault, C., Robert, C. & Sirard, M.A. (2005). RNA interference as a tool to study gene function in bovine oocytes. *Molecular Reproduction and Development* 70:111-121.

Park, F. (2009). Lentiviral vectors: are they the future of animal transgenesis? *Physiological Genomics* 31:159-173.

Park, S.Y., Kim, E.Y., Jeon, K., Cui, X.S. Lee, W.D., Kim, N.H., Park, S.P. & Lim, J.H. (2007). Survivin acts as anti-apoptotic factor during the development of bovine pre-implantation embryos. *Molecular Reproduction and Development* 74:582-590.

Parra-Guillén, Z.P., González-Aseguinolaza, G., Berraondo, P. & Trocóniz, I.F. (2010). Gene therapy: a pharmacokinetic/pharmacodynamic modelling overview. *Pharmaceutical Research* 27:1487-1497.

Pei, D.S., Di, J.H., Chen, F.F. & Zheng, J.N. (2010). Oncolytic-adenovirus-expressed RNA interference for cancer therapy. *Expert Opinion in Biological Therapy* 10:1331-1341.

Pieterse, M.C., Kappen, K.A., Kruip, Th.A.M., Taverne, M.A.M. (1988). Aspiration of bovine oocytes during transvaginal ultrasound scanning of the ovaries. *Theriogenology* 30:751-762.

Pollard, H., Remy, J.S., Loussouarn, G., Demolombe, S., Behr, J.P. & Escande, D. (1998). Polyethylenimine but not cationic lipids promotes transgene delivery to the nucleus in mammalian cells. *Journal of Biochemical Chemistry* 273:7507-7511.

Poller, W., Hajjar, R., Schultheiss, H.-P. & Fechner, H. (2010). Cardiac-targeted delivery of regulatory RNA molecules and genes for the treatment of heart failure. *Cardiovascular Research* 86:353-364.

Raki, M., Rein, D.T., Kanerva, A. & Hemminki, A. (2006). Gene transfer approaches for Gynecological disease. *Molecular Therapy* 14:154-163.

Relloso, M. & Esponda, P. (1998). In vivo gene transfer to the mouse oviduct epithelium. *Fertility and Sterility* 70:366-368.

Relloso, M. & Esponda, P. (2000). In-vivo transfection of the female reproductive tract epithelium. *Molecular Human Reproduction* 6:1099-1105.

Revelli, A., Delle Piane, L., Casano, S., Molinari, E., Massobrio, M. & Rinaudo, P. (2009). Follicular fluid content and oocyte quality: from single biochemical markers to metabolomics. *Reproductive Biology and Endocrinology* 7:40.

Rios, M., Venegas, A. & Croxatto, H.B. (2002). In vivo expression of β-galactosidase by rat oviduct exposed to naked DNA or messenger RNA. *Biological Research* 35:333-338.

Rodde, N., Munaut, C., Prince, S., Olivier, F., Bellemin, A.L. Chaouat, G. & Sandra, O. (2008). In vivo gene delivery of the murine uterus: what and why? *American Journal of Reproductive Immunology* 60:87[abstract].

Romano, G., Marino, I.R., Pentimalli, F., Adamo, V. & Giordano, A. (2009). Insertional mutagenesis and development of malignancies induced by integrating gene delivery systems: implications for the design of safer gene-based interventions in patients. *Drug News & Perspectives* 22:185-196.

Russ, V. & Wagner, E. (2007). Cell and tissue targeting of nucleic acids for cancer gene therapy. *Pharmaceutical Research* 24:1047-1057.

Saito, T. & Nakatsuji, N. (2001). Efficient gene transfer into the embryonic mouse brain using in vivo electroporation. *Developmental Biology* 240:237-246.

Salamone, D., Barañao, L., Santos, C., Bussmann, L., Artuso, J., Werning, C., Prync, A., Carbonetto, C., Dabsys, S., Munar, C., Salaberry, R., Berra, G., Berra, I., Fernández, N., Papouchado, M., Foti, M., Judewicz, N., Mujica, I., Muñoz, L., Fenández Alvarez, S., González, E., Zimmermann, J., Criscuolo, M. & Melo, C. (2006). High level expression of bioactive recombinant human growth hormone in the milk of a cloned transgenic cow. *Journal of Biotechnology* 124:469-472.

Salilew-Wondim, D., Hölker, M., Rings, F., Phatsara, C., Mohammadi-Sangcheshmeh, A., Tholen, E., Schellander, K. & Tesfaye, D. (2010). Depletion of BIRC6 leads to retarded bovine early embryonic development and blastocyst formation in vitro. *Reproduction Fertility and Development* 22:564-579.

Sato, M., Tanigawa, M., Kikuchi, N., Nakamura, S. & Kimura, M. (2003). Efficient gene delivery into murine ovarian cells by intraovarian injection of plasmid DNA and subsequent in vivo electroporation. *Genesis* 35:169-174.

Schaffer, D.V., Fidelman, N.A., Dan, N. & Lauffenburger, D.A. (2000). Vector unpacking as a potential barrier for receptor-mediated polyplex gene delivery. *Biotechnology and Bioengineering* 67:598-606.

Scheerlinck., J.-P.Y., Snibson, K.J., Bowles, V.M. & Sutton, P. (2008). Biomedical applications of sheep models: from asthma to vaccines. *Trends in Biotechnology* 26:259-266.

Schäfer, J., Höbel, S., Bakowsky, U. & Aigner, A. (2010). Liposome-polyethylenimine complexes for enhanced DNA and siRNA delivery. *Biomaterials* 31:6892-6900.

Schleef, M. & Blaesen, M. (2009). Production of plasmid DNA as a pharmaceutical. In: *Methods in Molecular Biology, Gene Therapy of Cancer,* Wolgang Walther and Ulrike S. Stein (eds), Humana Press, 542:471-495.

Shimasaki, S., Moore, R.K., Erickson, G.F. & Otsuka, F. (2003). The role of bone morphogenetic proteins in ovarian function. *Reproduction* 61(Supplement):323-337.

Simpson, J.L. (2008). Genetic and phenotypic heterogeneity in ovarian failure: overview of selected candidate genes. *Annals of the New York Academy of Sciences*. 1135:146-154.

Sirotkin, A.V. (2005). Control of reproductive processes by growth hormone: extra- and intracellular mechanisms. *Veterinary Journal* 170:307-317.

Smith, D.A., Vaidya, S.S., Kopechek, J.A., Huang, S.L., Klegerman, M.E., McPherson, D.D. & Holland, C.K. (2010). Ultrasound-triggered release of recombinant tissue-type plasminogen activator from echogenic liposomes. *Ultrasound in Medicine & Biology* 36:145-157.

Stribley, J.M., Rehman, K.S., Niu, H. & Christman, G.M. (2002). Gene therapy and reproductive medicine. *Fertility and Sterility* 77:645-657.

Tarahovsky, Y.S., Koynova, R., MacDonald, R.C. (2004). DNA release from lipoplexes by anionic lipids: correlation with lipid mesomorphism, interfacial curvature, and membrane fusion. *Biophysical Journal* 87:1054-1064.

Taylor, U., Sabine, K., Petersen, S., Kues, W., Barcikowski, S. & Rath, D. (2010). Nonendosomal cellular uptake of ligand-free positively charged gold nanoparticles. *Cytometry Part A* 77A:439-446.

Tejomurtula, J., Lee, K.B., Tripurani, S.K., Smith, G.W. & Yao, J. (2009). Role of importin alpha8, a new member of the importin alpha family of nuclear transport proteins, in early embryonic development in cattle. *Biology of Reproduction* 81:333-342.

Tesfaye, D., Lonergan, P., Hoelker, M., Rings, F. Nganvongpanit, K., Havlicek, V., Besenfelder, U., Jennen, D., Tholen, E., Schellander, K. (2007). Suppresion of connexin 43 and E-cadherin transcripts in in vitro derived bovine embryos following culture in vitro or in vivo in the homologous bovine oviduct. *Molecular Reproduction and Development* 74:978-988.

Tesfaye, D., Regassa, A. ,Rings, F. ,Ghanem, N., Phatsara, C., Tholen, E., Herwig, R., Un, C. Schellander, K. & Hoelker, M. (2010). Suppresion of the transcription factor MSX1 gene delays bovine preimplantation embryo development in vitro. *Reproduction* 139:857-870.

Thatcher, W.W., Bilby, T.R., Bartolome, J.A. Silvestre, F., Staples, C.R. & Santos, J.E. (2006). Strategies for improving fertility in the modern dairy cow. *Theriogenology* 65:30-44.

Thibault, M., Nimesh, S., Lavertu, M. & Buschmann, MD. (2010). Intracellular trafficking and decondensation kinetics of chitosan-pDNA polyplexes. *Molecular Therapy*, in press. pISSN:1525-0016, eISSN:1525-0024, doi:10.1038/mt.2010.143

Thomas, M. & Klibanov, A.M. (2003a). Non-viral gene therapy: polycation-mediated DNA delivery. *Applied Microbiology and Biotechnology* 62:27-34.

Thomas, M. & Klibanov, M. (2003b). Conjugation to gold nanoparticles enhances polyethylenimines´s transfer of plasmid DNA into mammalian cells. *Proceedings of the National Academy of Sciences of the United States of America* 100:9138-9143.

Toralová, T., Susor, A., Nemcová, L., Kepková, K. & Kanka, J. (2009). Silencing CENPF in bovine preimplantation embryos induces arrest at 8-cell stage. *Reproduction* 138:783-791.

Tros de Ilarduya, C., Sun, Y. & Düzgüneş, N. (2010). Gene delivery by lipoplexes and polyplexes. *European Journal of Pharmaceutical Sciences* 40:159-170.

Uzun, A., Rodriguez-Osorio, N., Kaya, A., Wang, H., Parrish, J.J., Ilyin, V.A. & Memili, E. (2009). Functional genomics of HMGN3a and SMARCAL I in early mammalian embryogenesis. *BMC Genomics* 10:183.

van Wagtendonk-de Leeuw, AM. (2006). Ovum pick up and in vitro production in the bovine after use in several generations: a 2005 status. *Theriogenology* 65:914-25.

Vassaux, G., Nitcheu, J. Jezzard, S. & Lemoine, N.R. (2006). Bacterial gene therapy strategies. *Journal of Pathology* 208:290-298.

Vaughan, E.E. & Dean, D.A. (2006). Intracellular trafficking of plasmids during transfection is mediated by microtubules. *Molecular Therapy* 13:422-428.

Velazquez, M.A. (2008). Assisted reproductive technologies in cattle: application in livestock production, biomedical research and conservation biology. *Annual Review of Biomedical Sciences* 10:36-62.

Velazquez, M.A., Hadeler, K.G., Beckers, J.F., Remy, B., Niemann, H. (2009a). Effects of intraovarian application of insulin-like growth factor-1 (IGF-1) on the superovulatory response of dairy cattle. *Reproduction in Domestic Animals* 44(Suppl. 1):38[abstract].

Velazquez, M.A., Zaraza, J., Oropeza, A., Webb, A. & Niemann, H. (2009b). The role of IGF1 in the in vivo production of bovine embryos from superovulated donors. *Reproduction* 137:161-180.

Voigt, K. Izsvák, Z. & Ivics, Z. (2008). Targeted gene insertion for molecular medicine. *Journal of Molecular Medicine* 86:1205-1219.

Wall, R.J., Powell, A.M., Paape, M.J., Kerr, D.E., Bannerman, D.D., Pursel, V.G., Wells, K.D., Talbot, N. & Hawk, H.W. (2005). Genetically enhanced cows resist intramammary Staphylococcus *aureus* infection. *Nature Biotechnology* 23:445-451.

Wells, D.J. (2010). Electroporation and ultrasound enhanced non-viral gene delivery in vitro and in vivo. *Cell Biology and Toxicology* 26:21-28.

Wells, D.N., Misica, P.M. & Tervit, H.R. (1999). Production of cloned calves following nuclear transfer with cultured adult mural granulosa cells. *Biology of Reproduction* 60:996-1005.

White, R.E., Wade-Martins, R., Hart, S.L., Frampton, J., Huey, B., Desai-Mehta, A., Cerosaletti, K.M., Concannon, P. & James, M.R. (2003). Functional delivery of large genomic DNA to human cells with a peptide-lipid vector. *Journal of Gene Medicine* 5:883-892.

Wilson, M.H. & George, A.L. Jr. (2010). Designing and testing chimeric zinc finger transposases. *Methods in Molecular Biology* 649:353-363

Xie, D., Chen, C.-C., Ptaszek, L.M., Xiao, S., Cao, X., Fang, F., Ng, H.H., Lewin, H.A., Cowan C. & Zhong, S. (2010). Rewirable gene regulatory networks in the preimplantation embryonic development of three mammalian species. *Genome Research* 20:804-815.

Yamashita, H. Kamada, D., Shirasuna, K., Matsui, M., Shimizu, T., Kida, K., Berisha, B., Schams, D. & Miyamoto, A. (2008). Effect of local neutralization of basic fibroblast growth factor or vascular endothelial growth factor by a specific antibody on the development of the corpus luteum in the cows. *Molecular Reproduction and Development* 75:1449-1456.

Yang, N.-S. (1992). Gene transfer into mammalian somatic cells *in vivo*. *Critical Reviews in Biotechnology* 12:335-356.

Yang, S.-Y., Wang, J.-G., Cui, H.-X., Sun, S.-G , Li, Q., Gu, L., Hong, Y., Liu, P.P. & Liu, W-Q. (2007). Efficient generation of transgenic mice by direct intraovarian injection of plasmid DNA. *Biochemical and Biophysical Research Communications* 358:266-271.

Yant, S.R., Wu, X., Huang, Y., Garrison, B., Burgess, S.M. & Kay, M.A. (2005). High-resolution genome-wide mapping of transposon integration in mammals. *Molecular and Cellular Biology* 25:2085-2094.

Yea, C., Dembowy, J., Pacione, L. & Brown, M. (2007). Microtubule-mediated and microtubule-independent transport of adenovirus type 5 in HEK293 cells. *Journal of Virology* 81:6899-6908.

Yoshimura, N., Kato, R., Chancellor, M.B., Nelson, J.B. & Glorioso, J.C. (2010). Gene therapy as future treatment of erectile dysfunction. *Expert Opinion in Biological Therapy* 10:1305-1314.

Young, L.S., Searle, P.F., Onion, D. & Mautner, V. (2006). Viral gene therapy strategies: from basic science to clinical application. *Journal of Pathology* 208:299-318.

Zaraza, J., Oropeza, A., Velazquez, M.A., Korsawe, K., Herrmann, D. Carnwath, J.W. & Niemann, H. (2010). Developmental competence and mRNA expression of preimplantation in vitro-produced embryos from prepubertal and postpubertal cattle and their relationship with apoptosis after intraovarian administration of IGF-1. *Theriogenology* 74:75-89.

Zhong, Z., Shi, S., Han, J., Zhang, Z. & Sun, X. (2010). Anionic liposomes increase the efficiency of adenovirus-mediated gene transfer to coxsackie-adenovirus receptor deficient cells. *Molecular Pharmaceutics* 7:105-115.

Ziello, J. E., Huang, Y. & Jovin, IS. (2010). Cellular endocytosis and gene delivery. *Molecular Medicine* 16:222-229.

Zizzi, A., Minardi, D., Ciavattini, A., Giantomassi, F., Montironi, R., Muzzonigro, G., Di Primio, R. & Lucarini, G. (2010). Green fluorescent protein as indicator of nonviral transient transfection efficiency in endometrial and testicular biopsies. *Microscopy Research and Technique* 73:229-233.

11

Nanocarriers for Cytosolic Drug and Gene Delivery in Cancer Therapy

Srinath Palakurthi, Venkata K. Yellepeddi and Ajay Kumar
Irma Lerma Rangel College of Pharmacy, Texas A&M Health Science Center
USA

1. Introduction

In this burgeoning era of personalized medicine we have witnessed a humongous increase in novel therapeutics encompassing wide range of modalities including small molecule drugs which can elicit their action upon encountering certain cellular component, protein macromolecules interfering cellular signaling pathways and nucleotide and DNA based therapies which alter protein/gene expression (Gonzalez-Angulo et al., 2010). The major factor which underscores the success of these novel therapeutic modalities is their propensity to reach the target site of action. Undoubtedly, the ultimate target for all these therapeutic modalities according to traditional paradigm is the cell. But there is a need for change in this paradigm since many of these modalities are targeted towards very specific subcellular organelles. Even though the major subcellular target even today is nucleus, there is growing body of evidence that other organelles also have role in many diseases (Davis et al., 2007). Targeting therapeutics to subcellular organelles would positively improve treatment in a myriad of diseases of metabolic, genetic and oncologic nature. Oncology is perhaps the most demanding area for organelle specific targeting since the standard therapy for oncology involves random interaction with cellular components and is harbinger of potential problems like toxicity and immunogenicity (Fulda et al., 2010; Galluzzi et al., 2008). Subcellular organelles in eukaryotic cells comprise of a complex organization of distinct membrane-bound compartments and these form the cellular basis of human physiology. These subcellular organelles by virtue of highly specialized metabolic functions interact with each other to uphold various cellular functions. Organelle biogenesis regulated by transcriptional networks modulating expression of genes encoding organellar proteins results in inheritance and proliferation of subcellular organelles such as nucleus, mitochondria, endoplasmic reticulum, peroxisomes and lysosomes (Hill et al., 1995; Nunnari et al., 1996; Warren et al., 1996). The recent developments in molecular and cellular biology opened up new vistas in the development of metabolic disorders due to disruption of organelle biogenesis. The disorders pertaining to organelles are not limited to genetic and metabolic origin. They are also involved in metabolic disturbances occurred during diseases due to infections, intoxications and drug treatments (Dhaunsi, 2005). The subcellular organelles are involved in wide array of diseases known to human nature like myopathy, obesity, type 2 diabetes, Zellweger syndrome, cancer etc., and these diseases are explained in detail further in the review. Thus, appropriate targeting of subcellular organelles not only provides direct amelioration of genetic and metabolic disorders but also aid in cure for diseases whose causes underlie subcellularly.

The approach of using nanocarriers for subcellular delivery of drugs, macromolecules and DNA therapeutics is proved to be more effective. This is because inherent physiochemical properties of the carriers such as size, shape and molecular weight are bestowed upon the molecule it is carrying. There is huge body of evidence reported in literature where nanocarriers were able to passively and actively target tumor vasculature and tumor cells (Magadala, 2008; Sawant, 2006; Soman, 2009; Torchilin, 2007: Yang, 2010). Now the major task ahead is to tailor these nanocarriers to cater the needs of subcellular targeting. This can be achieved by developing nanocarriers either by virtue of their inherent predilection toward a cellular compartment, or by attaching subcellular targeting ligands to direct nanocarriers to organelle of interest. For example, dequalinium (DQA)-based liposome like vesicles DQAsomes have inherent capability to target mitochondria for DNA and small molecule drugs (D'Souza et al., 2005; D'Souza et al., 2003; Weissig et al., 2001; Weissig et al., 2000). The examples of targeting using ligand involve use of folic acid, low density lipoprotein, mannose-6-phosphate, transferrin, riboflavin, ICAM-1 antibody etc.,(D'Souza et al., 2009). This ability to control the intracellular trafficking and fate of nanocarriers is by far the most important advantage of using nanocarriers for organelle targeting.

The major challenge posed for subcellular trafficking of nanocarriers is the constitution of the cell interior. This cell interior is very different from an aqueous buffer and it contains many large molecules mainly proteins, nucleic acids and complex sugars. The high concentration of these molecules (up to 400 grams per liter) causing the 'macromolecular crowding' is an important barrier for intracellular trafficking of nanocarriers (Ellis et al., 2003). The complex array of microtubules, actin, and intermediate filaments organized into a mesh resembling lattice also influence the diffusion of solutes inside cell. The other factors that might perpetuate hindrance of diffusion of nanocarriers are fluid phase viscosity, binding to cytosolic components and collisional interactions due to macromolecular crowding (Garner et al., 1994). Hence, it is important to consider these factors while designing nanocarriers for subcellular targeting.

Traditionally, the interactions of nanocarriers with cells and intracellular organelles were considered to be strongly influenced by size. But recent advances in microscopy and particle fabrication techniques has led us to understand the interdependent role of size, shape and surface chemistry on cellular internalization and intracellular trafficking (Geng et al., 2007). Once internalized into the cell, the most important determinant of successful delivery of therapeutics is the intracellular fate of endosomal content. The intracellular fate of the nanocarriers can be controlled depending on endocytic pathway. For example clathrin dependent endocytosis results in lysosomal degradation whereas clathrin independent internalization results in endosomal accumulation and sorting to a nondegradative path. The major aim of subcellular targeted delivery system is to avoid lysosomal trafficking so as to protect the drug or biomolecule from enzymatic degradation (Bareford et al., 2007). As cellular uptake and fate can be controlled by endocytic mechanism, the subcellular distribution can be directed by presence of additional peptide sequences that direct the nanocarrier to a desired subcellular site.

Concept of targeting chemotherapeutic drugs to malignant tissue by identifying certain overexpressed receptors and proteins has been investigated in great detail. The concept of targeting to cancer can be studied by dividing the therapeutics into two classes. The first one being the category where drug itself is capable to act specifically on mechanisms unique to malignant cells. For example, imatinib inhibits Bcr-Abl tyrosine kinase which is overexpressed in chronic myelogenous leukemia and trastuzumab binds and inhibits HER2/neu receptor which is overexpressed in breast cancers (Droogendijk et al., 2006; Hudis, 2007). The second category is utilization of structural moieties such as ligands and antibodies which will be attached to the drug to direct it toward certain features unique to cancer cells. For example, folate is a very good ligand to target cancer cells as folate receptors are over expressed in many cancers and anti-CD22 antibody epratuzumab was conjugated with ^{90}Yttrium for specific diagnosis of B cell lymphoma (Allen, 2002). However, the selectivity to the certain tissue or cell is not sufficient to produce the desired therapeutic effect if the drug is not accumulated at appropriate subcellular target organelle. There also exists other complications such as, efflux of drug after internalization by efflux pumps such as p-glycoprotein (P-gp) and multidrug resistance associated protein (MRP). Thus, subcellular targeting of cancer therapeutics is of prime importance since drugs are designed to act against specific subcellular targets. For example, certain DNA therapeutics are expressed only after they reach nucleus and certain drugs intended for tumor regression by reducing endoplasmic reticulum stress response have to act at endoplasmic reticulum (Nori et al., 2005).

The present review is an attempt to elucidate the importance of nanocarriers in subcellular targeting. The scope for subcellular targeting lies in understanding diseases affected due to malfunctioning of organelles. It is also very important to understand the challenges posed by intracellular environment for effective transport of nanocarriers. The recent targeting strategies employed to target each subcellular organelle is explained in detail. Thus, a comprehensive understanding of role of the nanocarriers in subcellular targeting and their application in amelioration of diseases like cancer is provided to the reader through this review.

2. Cellular organelles and related disorders

Subcellular organelles are responsible for cellular metabolic state which in turn is responsible for maintaining physiologic functions of tissue. Important subcellular organelles like mitochondria, peroxisomes, lysosomes, endoplasmic reticulum and cytoskeleton carry out important functions like production of energy, sorting of proteins, supporting and providing shape to the cell. A defect in any of the components of the network of organelles leads to a serious pathological state. A better understanding of diseases of organelles is of paramount importance in developing efficient targeting strategies. The list of cellular organelle related disorders is tabulated as Table-1 at the end of this section.

Mitochondria, the powerhouse of eukaryotic cells plays a key role in energy metabolism in many tissues. The defects in mitochondrial functions such as respiratory coupling, reactive oxygen species production (ROS), enzymatic activity (fatty acid oxidation), and mitochondrial content and size may result in metabolic disorders such as aging, insulin resistance and type 2 diabetes. Most important diseases of mitochondria arise due to mitochondrial DNA (mtDNA) deletions which cause the formation of mutant mtDNA. Examples of these diseases include Kearns-Sayre syndrome and Pearson syndrome which can be fatal in infancy or early childhood (Johannsen et al., 2009). Mitochondria also regulates cellular life cycle through release of *cytochrome c* which is an important stimulator of apoptosis thus indicating its role in cancer. It was also proved that mitochondrial oxidative and phosphorylation capacity and mitochondrial content are decreased with age thus showing importance of mitochondria in aging. Mitochondrial dysfunction was also implicated in insulin resistance and type 2 diabetes. Recent reports suggest that `metabolic overload' of muscle mitochondria is a key player in insulin resistance (Koves et al., 2008). Another important mitochondrial dysfunction is increased damage by ROS, which in turn results in cancer and neurodegenerative diseases (de Moura et al., 2010).

Impaired ribosome biogenesis and function due to genetic abnormalities result in a class of diseases called ribosomopathies. These ribosomopathies result in distinct clinical phenotypes most often involving bone marrow failure and craniofacial or other skeletal defects. The ribosomopathies are generally congenital syndromes due to mutations of genes encoding ribosomal proteins. The first discovered ribosomopathy was Diamond-Blackfan anemia (DBA) which is due to mutation in *RPS19* gene. DBA is a rare congenital bone marrow failure syndrome with a striking erythroid effect (Draptchinskaia et al., 1999). The other congenital syndromes linked to defective ribosome biogenesis are Schwachman-Diamond syndrome (SDS), X-linked dyskeratosis congenital (DKC), cartilage hair hypoplasia (CHH), and Treacher Collins syndrome (TCS). All of these ribosomopathies except TCS were reported to pose risk to cancers like osteosarcoma and acute myeloid leukemia (Narla et al., 2010).

Endosomes and lysosomes envisage important functions within cells including antigen presentation, innate immunity, autophagy, signal transduction, cell division, and neurotransmission. The cellular function will be compromised if undegraded substrates accumulate in endosomes and lysosomes due to lysosomal dysfunction. Lysosomal storage disorders constitute a group of genetic diseases involving dysfunction of lysosomal hydrolases resulting in impaired substrate degradation. Lysosomal diseases are manifested by enlarged lysosomes which contain partially degraded material due to 1) glycosaminoglycan, lipid or protein degradation defects, 2) transport across lysosomal membrane or 3) endosome-lysosome trafficking. The first discovered diseases of lysosomes are related to lipidoses and mucopolysaccharidoses. They include diseases like Tay-Sach disease, Gaucher disease, Fabry disease, Niemann-Pick disease, Hurler syndrome. However, much of the initial concept for the lysosomes and its dysfunction came from the studies of Pompe disease characterized by cardiomegaly, cardio respiratory failure, hepatomegaly and progressive muscle weakness (Parkinson-Lawrence et al., 2010).

Peroxisomes are single membrane bound organelles which contain more than 50 different proteins, mainly enzymes essential for various metabolic processes, which include hydrogen peroxide based respiration, β-oxidation of very long chain fatty acids, bile acid synthesis and plasmalogen biosynthesis. There exists several genetic disorders associated with peroxisomal system and are divided into two categories. The first category is related to peroxisome biogenesis and second is the single protein defects in which a single metabolic function is different. The examples of first category are heterogeneous group of autosomal recessive disorders including Zellweger syndrome, neonatal adrenoleukodystrophy, infantile Refsum disease and rhizomelic chondrodysplasia punctata. The examples of second category are X-linked adrenoleukodystrophy, hyperoxaluria type I and thiolase deficiency (Gartner, 2000).

The endoplasmic reticulum (ER) apart from playing an important role in many cellular functions is also involved in protein folding and trafficking. The important manifestation of failure of the ER's adaptive capacity is activation of unfolded protein response (UPR), which in turn affects various inflammatory and stress signaling pathways. UPR is closely integrated with inflammation, stress signaling and JNK activation. These pathways play a

critical role in chronic metabolic diseases such as obesity, insulin resistance, and type 2 diabetes. It was also reported that chronic ER stress and activation of the UPR may also result in oxidative stress, causing a toxic accumulation of ROS within the cell (Hotamisligil, 2010). Mice were subjected to obesity-induced stress and then treated chemical chaperones phenyl butyric acid and tauro-ursodeoxycholic acid. After treatment the stress was relieved and also there was observed an increase in insulin sensitivity and reduction in fatty liver disease in those obese mice, showing the link between ER induced stress and metabolic disorders. (Ozcan et al., 2004). A small molecule Salubrinal was reported to protect cells against ER stress induced cell death *in vitro* and *in vivo*. Salubrinal prevents the dephosphorylation of eIF2α (Boyce et al., 2005). ER stress associated disorders also include various neurodegenerative disorders. Recently, various neurological disorders including Alzheimer's disease, Parkinson's disease, Amyotrophic lateral sclerosis have shown disruption of ER homoeostasis and up-regulation of UPR. Another recent ER related neurodegenerative disorder which was reported recently was `seipinopathy', which is a motor neuron disease related to protein seipin. This protein seipin activates the UPR and induces ER stress-mediated cell death (Ito et al., 2009). Thus, targeting ER would be an attractive approach to ameliorate inflammatory and chronic metabolic disorders.
The Golgi complex is an important organelle within the secretory system of the cell. Its organization is maintained by proteinaceous matrix, cytoskeletal components and inositol phospholipids. It carries out two important tasks, one being sorting of secretory cargo to various destinations in cell and other being modification of protein during its way to plasma membrane. Certain pathological conditions, pharmacological agents and over expression of golgi-associated proteins cause profound morphological changes of golgi apparatus. These morphological changes were shown by neuronal golgi apparatus in many neurodegenerative disorders like Alzheimer's disease, amyotrophic lateral sclerosis, Creutzfeldt-Jacob disease, multiple system atrophy, Parkinson's disease, spinocerebelar ataxia type 2 and Niemann-Pick type C (Fan et al., 2008). Protein glycosylation is another important function of Golgi apparatus. A defective glycosylation process by golgi network would result in disorders like congenital disorders of glycosylation and also cause acquired glycosylation defects associated with epidemic diseases such as cancer and diabetes (Ungar, 2009).

3. Role of nanocarriers in cytosolic delivery

During past decade numerous efforts were made to efficiently direct the polymeric and/or nanoparticulate carriers to the organelle of choice. Most of those efforts were successful in delivering small molecule drugs (S. R. Yang et al., 2006), proteins (Bale et al., 2010) and nucleic acids (Jensen et al., 2003) to specific organelle inside cell. The major advantage of use of nanocarriers in cytosolic delivery arises from their characteristic properties like nanosize (1-100 nm), ability to carry high drug/gene payload, feasibility to modify the surface functionality for active targeting, ability to utilize its surface charge for passive targeting. The arsenal of nanocarriers investigated for organelle specific targeting includes inorganic and organic materials. The major units of this arsenal are liposomes (Fattal et al., 2004), micelles (Bontha et al., 2006), quantum dots (QDs)(Hoshino et al., 2004), polymeric nanoparticles (Nori et al., 2003; Yessine et al., 2004), gold nanoparticles (Bergen et al., 2006), magnetic nanoparticles (Xu et al., 2008), dendrimers (Samuelson et al., 2009), carbon nanotubes (Z. Yang et al., 2010).

Cellular Organelle	Disease	Defective gene/Function	Clinical Features	Ref
Mitochondria	Leigh's syndrome	*mtDNA* deletion	Ataxia, seizures, hypotonia, lactic acidosis	(Corona et al., 2002)
	Type 2 diabetes	GLUT4 Translocation	Insulin resistance	(Johannsen et al., 2009)
	Progressive external ophthalmoplegia	*mtDNA* deletion	Developmental delay, lactic acidosis	(Holt et al., 1988)
Endoplasmic reticulum (ER)	Obesity	ER stress-induced autophagy	Increased body mass index	(Hotamisligil, 2010)
	Seipinopathies	*Seipin/BSCL2*	Spastic paraplegia, muscle weakness	(Ito et al., 2009)
Lysosomes	Pompe disease	Lysosomal glycogen hydrolysis	Cardiomegaly, hepatomegaly, Progressive muscle weakness	(Parkinson-Lawrence et al., 2010)
	Gaucher disease	Lipid degradation in macrophages	Hepatosplenomegaly, Osteonecrosis, neurodegeneration	
	Fabry disease	Glycosphingolipid hydrolysis	Growth restriction, Cardio-respiratory problems, Lipid accumulation	
Peroxisomes	Zellweger syndrome	*PEX* gene	Abnormal facial appearance	(Gartner, 2000)
	X-linked adrenoleukodystrophy	*ALD* gene	Progressive neurodegenration	
Ribosomes	Diamond-Blackfan anemia	*RPS19, RPS24, RPS17, RPL35A*	Macrocytic anemia, Short stature, craniofacial defects	(Narla et al., 2010)
	Shwachman-Diamond syndrome	*SBDS*	Neutropenia/infections, Pancreatic insufficiency, Short stature	
Golgi Apparatus	Alzheimer's disease	Dysregulation of Ca^{2+} signalling	Cerebral deposition of amyloid plaques	(Fan et al., 2008)
	Amyotrophic Lateral Sclerosis	Dysregulation of Ca^{2+} signalling	Progressive degeneration of cortical and spinal motoneurons	
Nucleus	Primary biliary cirrhosis	Antibodies against nucleoporins	Cirrhosis of liver with destroyed bile ducts	(Cronshaw et al., 2004)
	Triple A syndrome	*AAAS* gene	Hypoglycemia, achalasia, alacrima	

Table 1. Cellular organelle related disorders with specific genes involved and their clinical sysmptoms

Nanocarriers are internalized into the cell by a process called endocytosis. After the carriers have been successfully endocytosed, depending on the intended target, these carriers are directed to respective organelles of cell by means of specialized mechanisms. There exists a wide plethora of enodocytic mechanisms depending on the physicochemical property of the internalizing nanocarriers. Heterogeneity in mechanisms of endocytosis can be utilized to efficiently translocate the cargo to specific cellular organelles and are subjected to required interactions during their journey towards the target (Maxfield et al., 2004). Process of endocytosis can be broadly classified into two categories, one is phagocytosis that involves uptake of large particles, and the other is pinocytosis which involves uptake of fluid and solutes. Phagocytosis is observed mainly in specialized mammalian cells such as macrophages whereas pinocytosis is observed in all cells. Pinocytosis is underscored by four major mechanisms macropinocytosis, clathrin-mediated endocytosis, caveolae-mediated endocytosis, and clathrin- and caveolae-independent endocytosis. The endocytic route which is of most interest in targeting of nanocarriers is clathrin-mediated endocytosis because it engages mainly receptor-ligand complexes (Conner et al., 2003). Upon ligand-receptor binding, certain adaptor proteins like adaptor protein 2 are engaged which interact with clathrin triskelion to trigger the formation of clathrin-coated pits. A small GTPase dynamin cuts the invaginated pits and release them into the cytoplasm as vesicles. Thus, the endocytosed cargo after being delivered into endosomes is then recycled, sorted for degradation or delivered to the golgi complex (Schmid, 1997). Some of the examples of receptors which are exploited for targeting drugs intracellularly are folate receptors, transferrin receptors and LDL receptors for tumor targeting, gene delivery and brain targeting respectively. There also exist other routes that are non-clathrin-mediated which involve internalization of many proteins, lipids, viruses and toxins. These are referred to as caveolae/raft-mediated endocytosis and cholesterol plays a crucial role in these mechanisms and role of dynamin is seen in some cargo (Rajendran et al., 2010). The other clathrin independent route of cellular internalization which involves internalization of glycophosphatidyl-inositol (GPI)-anchored proteins is GEEC (glycophosphatidyl-inositol (GPI)-anchored protein-enriched early endosomal compartment) pathway. The salient features of this pathway are that it is dynamin independent and bypasses the step of early endosome sorting by using long invaginations from the surface. Nanocarriers are thus directed towards their intracellular compartment using one of the above mentioned mechanisms and in some cases there exists interplay between the mechanisms also.

The strategies employed for targeting nanocarriers to organelles include making the nanocarriers pH responsive and thus rendering them endosmolytic (e.g Poly(methacrylic acid), PEG-Dendrimer), use of fusogenic peptides (e.g, GALA and KALA), use of cell penetrating peptides (e.g Tat, Antennapedia, Tp10), use of small molecule targeting sequences like triphenylphosphonium, attachment of nuclear localization sequence and making nanocarriers which have intrinsic endosmolytic escape capacity. However, each of these targeting strategies will be discussed in detail when dealing with individual organelle targeting.

4. Challenges posed by intracellular environment

The intracellular environment is very different from routine biochemical assay environment. Two complex fluids occupy a large portion of cellular interior, the cytoplasm and nucleoplasm. The cytoplasm is comprised of organelles which are dispersed, macromolecules and the cytoskeletal network and chromosomal DNA constitutes nucleoplasm. This constitution of cytoplasm and nucleoplasm confer to their respective properties. Both cytoplasm and nucleoplasm thus, show a considerable degree of macromolecular crowding (Minton, 2006). It is very important to understand the spatial aspects of intracellular environment to obtain an appropriate description of cell's behavior. This would help in better design of nanocarriers for organelle targeting.

The very high total concentration of proteins, nucleic acids and complex sugars inside cell give rise to 'macromolecular crowding', which has energetic consequences which affect cellular functions like diffusion of proteins within cytosol. The important effects of macromolecular crowding can be formation of protein aggregates such as amyloid deposits and reduction in the diffusion rate of the diffusing particle. A new technique called cryoelectron tomography provided a direct evidence of crowded state of cell interior. The pictures showed a high density of actin filaments and ribosomes confirming that cytoplasm consists of huge compacts of macromolecules rather than freely diffusing and colloiding macromolecules (Medalia et al., 2002). Nanocarriers depict macromolecules because of their size, shape and surface functionality thus it is quite imperative that nanocarriers should be able to overcome this entire gamut of macromolecular crowding inside cell for efficient targeting.

The complex environment of intracellular milieu is mainly attributed by factors like immobile barriers, molecular crowding and binding interactions. These factors hinder the intracellular diffusion. The effect of immobile barriers and crowding agents on translational mobility was assessed using multi-photon fluorescence correlation spectroscopy. The immobile barriers were mimicked by using silica-based nanostructures and macromolecular crowding agents were mimicked by high molecular mass dextrans. The data suggested that when tagged molecules like dextran-tetramethylrhodamine or eGFP-CaM are placed in heterogeneous environments as described above, there exist various mechanisms of diffusion. The first one being characterized as Fickian diffusion which is normal but slowed diffusion due to crowding. In some data it was also observed that molecules have a less hindered mobility due to relative size between tracer molecule and dimensions of crowding agents. In other data the molecule showed a subdiffusive like behavior and hindered mobility and it is explained by the idea that molecules can be trapped in either mobile or immobile cages (Sanabria et al., 2007).

There exists a pH gradient across many biological membranes. The pH gradient play important role in cellular functioning like modulating bilayer asymmetry, loading of vesicles with molecules bearing charge like amino acid, peptide, protein, controlling of fusion process and maintaining degradative functions in acidic organelles. It was observed that vesicles with a pH gradient across their membrane have different electrophoretic mobilities and is due to pH associated changes in surface density (Hope et al., 1989). Using capillary electrophoresis with laser induced fluorescence detection it was shown that pH gradient across liposomal membrane induce electrophoretic mobility shifts based on capacity theory. Moreover, it was also proved that mobilities of acidic organelles are in congruency with predictions based on liposomal models (Chen et al., 2007).

The major determinants of cytoplasmic rheology are fluid-phase viscosity and translational diffusion coefficient. For smaller solutes the collisions with intracellular components was determined to be the principal diffusive barrier which hindered translational diffusion (Kao et al., 1993). Seksek et al have reported that macromolecule size solutes (FITC-dextrans and Ficoll) when microinjected into fibroblasts and epithelial cells, the translational diffusion slowed three- to four folds in cytoplasm and nucleus compared with water and the degree of slowing did not depend on molecular size up to at least 300 A° gyration radius (Seksek et al., 1997). The mobility of DNA in cytoplasm after it is released from a nanocarrier is a very important aspect to assess the efficacy of gene delivery using nanocarriers. Mobility of DNA in cytoplasm is also assessed by the same parameter described above which is translational diffusion. Fluorescein-labeled double stranded DNA fragments of increasing sizes (in base pairs (bp): 21, 100, 250, 500, 1000, 2000, 3000, 6000) were microinjected into cytoplasm and nucleus of HeLa cell and their diffusion was measured using photobleaching. Results indicated that the translational diffusion of smaller DNA fragments was not greatly impeded but the larger DNA fragments showed little or no diffusion especially for DNAs > 2000 bp. Such a slowing of DNA mobility is largely due to a combination of collisional interactions and macromolecular crowding effects. Interestingly, in nucleus DNA fragments of all sizes showed no mobility and this immobilization was attributed to extensive DNA binding to nuclear components like histones (Lukacs et al., 2000).

In an attempt to establish the exact mechanism involved in this reduced mobility with increase in DNA size, the diffusion studies were performed in presence of crowded solutions containing predominantly actin filaments. The results indicated that actin mesh rather than cytoplasmic crowding is the major barrier for cellular diffusion of large DNA. This result was consolidated by fact that when actin filaments were disrupted using cytochalasin D (5 μM) the size dependent reduction in mobility was not seen (Dauty et al., 2004). Thus, cytoskeletal barrier is an important limiting factor for non-viral gene delivery vectors. However, some viruses such as SV40 antigen overcome this barrier by activating tyrosine kinase-induced signaling cascades which dissociates the filamentous actin.

5. Effect of size and shape of nanoparticles in subcellular trafficking

Particle size of the nanocarriers have played a pivotal role in undermining many useful characteristics of the nanocarriers like enhanced permeation and retention (EPR) effect, cellular internalization and cellular trafficking. For example, to efficiently utilize the EPR effect the nanocarrier must fall in between a size range of 10 nm to 100 nm. If the nanocarrier is smaller than 10nm they will be rapidly cleared by kidneys and larger carriers are cleared by reticuloendothelial system. Particle sizes of nanocarrier also influence some of the very important characteristics such as degradation and clearance. It was reported that degradation of particles is size-dependent and degradation products formed within the particle can diffuse freely to the surface if they are from smaller particles (Dunne et al., 2000; Panyam et al., 2003). Particle size more importantly dictates the endocytic mechanism which will be engaged to internalize the nanocarrier. Large particles 2-3 μm are internalized by phagocytosis by macrophages. Internalization of considerably smaller particles >1 μm is facilitated by macropinocytosis, much smaller nanosacle range particles are internalized by caveolar-mediated (~60 nm), clathrin-mediated (~120 nm) and clathrin-independent and caveolin-independent endocytosis (~90 nm) processes (Petros et al., 2010). However, it is not just the particle size that governs the properties of the nanocarriers, particle shape also have a strong impact on the carrier performance.

The impact of particle shape was poorly understood earlier, perhaps due to lack of appropriate fabrication techniques. Recently, many fabrication techniques for synthesis of conventional non-spherical particles were reported in literature. The fabrication methods generally use techniques such as lithography, microfluidics, film-stretching, non-wetting molding and photopolymerization. Many times, these techniques will be used in combination. By virtue of these fabrication methods particles of various morphologies like disks, toroids, ellipsoids form a variety of polymers such as poly(ethyleneglycol), poly styrene, poly vinyl alcohol, poly lactide-co-glycolide, poly(methylmethacrylate) etc, were synthesized and their properties were evaluated. Non-wetting molding and film-stretching methods produced a variety of two and three dimensional shapes in diameters of nanoscale (Champion et al., 2007).

Polystyrene particles of various shapes and sizes were prepared and their phagocytosis was studied in alveolar macrophages(Champion et al., 2006). The polystyrene particles were fabricated into six different shapes encompassing various shape characteristics such as aspect ratio, size, concavity and curvature. The geometric shapes of particles fabricated are spheres (radius 1.0-12.5 μm), oblate ellipsoids (major axis 4μm, aspect ratio 4), prolate ellipsoids (major axis 2-6 μm, aspect ratio 1.3-3), elliptical disks (EDs) (major axis 3-14 μm, aspect ratio 2-4, thickness 400-1,000 nm), rectangular disks (major axis 4-8 μm, aspect ratio 1.5-4.5), and UFO shaped particles (sphere radius 1.5μm, ring radius 4μm). These poly styrene particles were investigated in their nonopsonized and IgG-opsonized forms. It was reported that particle shape at the contact, not the size, dictates whether cells will proceed with phagocytosis or merely spread on the particle size. However, particle size was shown to affect the completion of phagocytosis especially when volume of particle is greater than macrophage volume. The interesting observation of this study was that except for spheres point of initial contact of particle with cell was major determinant in internalization. It was reported that internalization did not occur when cells initial point of contact was concave region whilst, attachment to dome or ring regions proceeded internalization process. The mechanism of internalization as elucidated by formation of actin cup was also influenced by point of initial contact and was in accordance with observations reported above (Champion et al., 2006). The following Figure 1 depicts the influence of point of initial contact on internalization of particles.

The influence of particle shape on *in vivo* circulation and its extravasation through microvasculature was also investigated in rodents using filamentous micelles (Geng et al., 2007). Cylindrically shaped filamentous micelles called filomicelles were fabricated using hydrophilic polyethyleneglycol (PEG) and hydrophobic polycaprolactone (biodegradable) or polyethylene (nonbiodgeradable). These stable filomicelles were fluorescently labeled and then compared with spherical micelles for transport and trafficking after intravenous injection into mice. Filomicelles have shown to exist in circulation for upto one week and filomicelles with longer initial lengths showed increased circulation times. It was also shown that these filomicelles enter cells under static conditions but under conditions of constant flow due to hydrodynamic shear cylindrical filomicelles are pulled off from phagocytes as they come into contact. It was also reported that when a chemotherapeutic agent Paclitaxel was loaded into these filomicelles, they shrunk tumors with longer filomicelles being more effective at a given dose (Geng et al., 2007).

A novel top-down lithographic fabrication method called PRINT (Particle Replication In Non-wetting Templates) was used to prepare micro and nanoparticles from cationic, cross linked poly (ethyleneglycol) hydrogels. These particles were then investigated for the interdependent effect of size, shape and surface charge (zeta potential) on cellular internalization by human cervical carcinoma epithelial (HeLa) cells. Using this technology three different types of particles were fabricated, a micrometer-sized series of cubic-shape

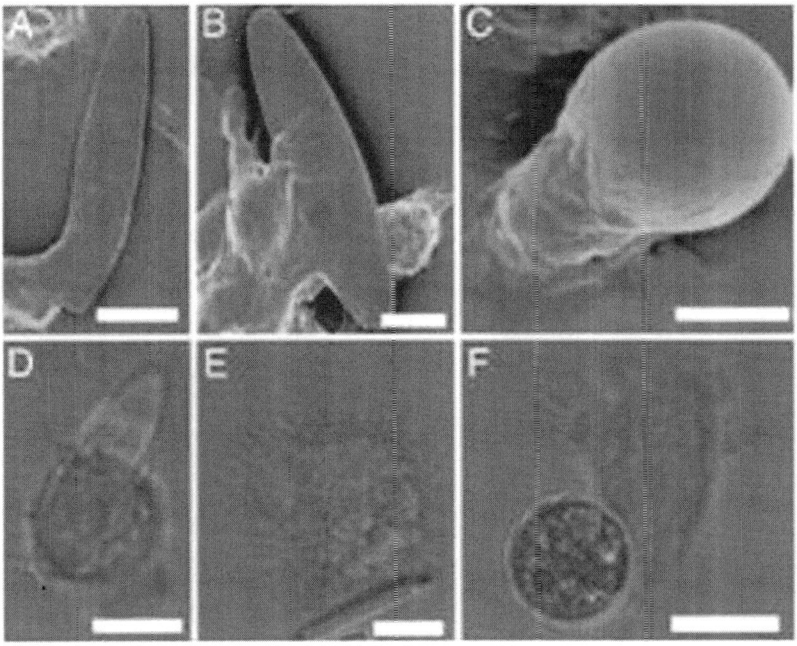

Fig. 1. Scanning electron micrographs (A-C) and actin staining (D-F) depicting the influence of initial point of contact on phagocytosis. In figures A-C cells and particles were colored brown and purple, respectively. (A) The elliptical disk (ED) which was opsonized can be seen to be engulfed by the cell. (Scale bar: 10μm). (B) The flat side of the particle (ED) attached by the cell. (C) A spherical particle with approximately half of its surface was covered by the cell membrane. Figures D-F depict the overlays of bright and fluorescent images after fixing and staining actin cells with rhodamine phalloidin. (D) At the leading edge of membrane new actin polymerization enables membrane to progress over an opsonized ED and formation of actin ring can be seen. (E) No actin cup or ring is visible when cell is attached to the flat side of the opsonized ED. (F) Formation of actin cup at the end of the sphere as internalization begins after attachment. (Scale bars in D-F: 10μm.) Numbers of cells observed for each orientation of each particle were not less than five. Figure was obtained with permission from reference by (Champion et al., 2006) © The National Academy of Sciences of the USA.

particles, micrometer-sized cylindrical particles with same heights but different diameters and finally a cylindrical-shape nanoparticle series. A very important observation of this work was that particles upto 3 μm sizes were internalized by the nonphagocytic HeLa cells. This contradicts the current dogma that upper limit of the size of any nanoparticle to be internalized into cells by means of nonspecific endocytosis is 150 nm. It was reported that of all shapes, rod like cylindrical nanoparticles with high aspect ratio (ratio of height to diameter) were internalized ~4 times faster than low-aspect ratio particles, and cylindrical particles with varying size and volume have shown varying degrees of internalization. It

was also shown that 84% of positively charged nanoparticles were internalized in comparison with <5% of identically shaped negatively charged indicating the importance of surface chemistry in cellular internalization (Gratton et al., 2008).
Similarly, Huang et al fabricated mesoporous silica nanoparticles with various shapes and aspect ratios and their cellular internalization was studied. The three shapes fabricated were spheres, short and long rods each with similar diameter but with different aspect ratios (ARs, 1, 2, and 4). The results indicated that particles with larger aspect ratios were internalized at faster rates and to a greater extent. It was also reported that long rod-shaped particles disrupted the cell cytoskeleton, where as spherical and short rod shaped particles did not. Finally, the long rod-shaped nanoparticles reduced the cell viability to a greater extent when compared to short-rods and spheres (Huang et al., 2010).

6. Intracellular fate of nanocarriers and factors affecting the intracellular fate

Nanocarriers are used profusely for many biomedical applications like drug delivery, gene delivery, imaging, targeted chemotherapy etc. Thus, it is of great importance to understand the intricate complex processes that regulate the intracellular fate of nanocarriers as they govern major properties of nanocarriers like biocompatibility, targeting efficiency etc.,. The traditional paradigm of intracellular fate of nanocarriers suggest that after cellular internalization, nanoparticles gets entrapped in endosomes which later fuse with acidic lysosomes and results in degradation of its contents (Watson et al., 2005). However, in recent years nanocarriers are designed in a way to protect its contents from lysosomal degradation. The strategies involve use of targeting ligands to directly target the organelle of interest, make nanocarriers pH sensitive thus making them endosmolytic or using alternative endocytic mechanisms which evade lysosomal degradation. Thus, intracellular fate of nanocarriers has become highly subjective and varies depending on physical and chemical characteristics of the nanocarrier.
The poly(lactide)-co-glycolide (PLGA) nanoparticles (NPs) were shown to follow a typical endocytosis-exocytosis route. The NPs initially encounter endosomes followed by retrieval or escape from the compartment and then interact with exocytic organelles of the cell like endoplasmic reticulum, golgi apparatus and secretory vesicles. PLGA NPs avoid lysosomes and are capable to bypass intracellular digestive compartment (Cartiera et al., 2009), Whereas, polystyrene NPs once internalized were not contained in endosomes or lysosomes but were found to localize within mitochondria of cell lines. It was also reported that polystyrene NPs were accumulated within bile canaliculi suggesting that NPs can be eliminated within bile. In another study where intracellular fate of a Tat-conjugated quantum dots were investigated, the results have shown that Tat peptide was digested in lysosomes by enzymes leaving the Tat-detached quantum dots in lysosomes for excretion (Xiong et al., 2010).
Liposomes are another important class of nanocarriers whose intracellular fate has been investigated. Tat-peptide conjugated liposomes were fluorescently labeled using Rhodamine-phosphatidylethanolamine (Rh-PE) and their intracellular fate was investigated using epi-fluorescence and differential interference contrast microscopy. The results have shown a typical time dependent pattern of distribution of liposomes inside the cell. The localization of intact liposomes within cytoplasm was observed after 1 hr. The liposomes after 2 and 4 hr were seen clustered in perinuclear region and at 9 hr the degradation of liposomes was observed. Finally, after 24 hr no liposome was seen inside cell (Torchilin, 2005).

7. Current approaches and strategies for optimal organelle targeting

7.A NUCLEUS

Nucleus is perhaps the most important cellular organelle which needs efficient targeting because it is the ultimate target for treatment for genetic diseases. Gene therapy which underscores the use of therapeutic DNA usually fails due to lack of transfection of DNA into nucleus. Thus it is very important to develop strategies that improve targeting of DNA molecules directly to nucleus. The prime barrier for a DNA or any molecule whose intended site of action is nucleus is the nuclear envelope. Both active and passive transport in and out of nucleus takes place via nuclear pore complexes (NPCs) embedded in nuclear envelope. The NPC structurally can be divided into three components, a central domain and a nuclear and cytoplasmic ring constructed from 50 different nucleoporin proteins. The central domain forms a aqueous channel through the nuclear envelope of ~9 nm in diameter. Passive diffusion is the mechanism underlying translocation of small molecules. Whereas, molecules >45 kDa must possess a nuclear localizing signal (NLS) which are recognized by importin family proteins which in turn mediate the nuclear transport (Poon et al., 2005).

In order to efficiently deliver the cargo into the nucleus we have to overcome two major impediments. One is the passage through cytoplasm and other is translocation via nuclear membrane. The common consideration in both these constraints is the size of the cargo. As described in previous sections, cytoplasm is a highly crowded environment containing organelles, macromolecules and cytoskeleton forming a `cytoplasmic sieve'. Large molecules thus diffuse slowly in cytoplasm, in comparison with their diffusion in water. To overcome this impediment a successful strategy was provided by taking example of trafficking of herpes simplex virus (HSV). HSV utilizes the microtubule cytoskeleton motor proteins dynein and kinesins for nuclear transport (Dohner et al., 2005). The transport of 125 nm HSV caspid to nucleus clearly demonstrates that by utilizing the cytoskeleton we can efficiently diffuse large molecules through cytoplasm to nucleus. In order to counteract the second barrier which is presented by NPC, the cargo should be packaged to a size/structure below ~40 -60 nm and a NLS has to be attached (Pante et al., 2002). Thus, it is imperative to consider these two barriers in designing strategies to deliver macromolecules like DNA to nucleus.

The most important strategy to target nucleus is by using DNA binding proteins. Most DNA binding proteins are inherently equipped with NLS to enable them to efficiently translocate into the nucleus to perform necessary functions. GAL4, a yeast transcription factor whose N-terminal 147 residues contain a DNA binding domain and the first 74 amino acids of this domain function as NLS. Thus, it was reported that enhanced GAL4-mediated gene delivery was achieved when a large SV40 T antigen was linked to the complex. This addition resulted in switching of nuclear import from an importin β-mediated to an importin α/β-mediated pathway(Chan et al., 2001). Nuclear factor κ B (NF κB) also has a NLS through which it internalizes into nucleus via a importin dependent fashion. The NFκB protein p50 which have NLS was shown not only to enhance the nuclear transport of DNA but also enhanced the migration of DNA towards nucleus from cytoplasm through microtubules (Mesika et al., 2005).

There has been an increase in considerable amount of interest in recent years in active targeting to nucleus. This stemmed from the rise of non-viral gene therapy to deliver large molecules of DNA to the nucleus. Initially, active targeting involved co-administration of NLS peptide after microinjection of DNA, but with this strategy, there remains a question whether NLS and DNA remain bound in endosome or cytoplasm, or even after binding of NLS to importin. Thus coupling of NLS peptides to DNA emerged as a more attractive approach for nuclear targeting. But this strategy was not highly efficient as increase in gene expression was limited to 2 to 5 fold only (Pouton et al., 2007). An alternative to this strategy would be attaching a polypeptide or protein containing an NLS to the DNA by using covalent coupling, reversible interaction or streptavidin-biotin binding technology. This strategy of attaching a NLS as a part of protein or polypeptide would make NLS more likely to be presented with appropriate tertiary structure to impinge strong binding to the importin or relevant nuclear transport protein involved (Pouton et al., 2007). NLS-streptavidin was coupled to DNA molecules with a single biotinylated nucleotide end and microinjected into cells or administered to digitonin-permeabilised cells to investigate uptake of DNA by nucleus. This study reported that NLS-mediated transport delivered the DNA into nucleus, but there exists a size limitation of approximately 1 kb DNA.

Another strategy which is still in its infancy is the use of multifunctional fusion proteins which are equipped with a DNA binding domain and nuclear import moiety which allows efficient delivery and trafficking of DNA to the nucleus. A recombinant fusion protein was constructed based on multidomain structure of the bacterial pseudomonas exotoxin A. The protein consists of ErbB-2 specific antibody which imparts target cell specificity, the exotoxin A translocation domain executes endosomal escape and a DNA binding domain from yeast GAL4 enable sequence-specific high affinity binding to DNA. Transient expression of the luciferase gene was observed and correlates with the amount of carrier protein in the complex and when carrier protein was truncated lacking either cell recognition domain or translocation domain resulted in failure of DNA transfer (Fominaya et al., 1996).

7.B Mitochondria

Mitochondria are distinct cellular organelles which occupy a major volume of animal cell cytoplasm. Mitochondria are also called as power plants of the cell because they provide the bulk of cellular ATP. Mitochondria structurally are composed of two membranes and are primarily composed of phospholipid bilayers with proteins embedded in them. Because of presence of two membranes there exists two aqueous spaces, the inner one being called the matrix space and the one between the membranes is called the intermembrane space. The outer membrane consists of channel-forming protein called voltage-dependent anion channel (VDAC) and limits the passage of molecules to intermembrane space to a MW of 5000 Da or less. Proteins and other large molecules use a unique protein import apparatus to cross the outer membrane. The inner membrane has a composition distinct from outer membrane, it is more proteinaceous and contains an unusual phospholipid, cardiolipin. The major function of mitochondria, the ATP synthesis occurs in matrix thus inner membrane is then major barrier which governs the transport of molecules in and out of matrix. Inner membrane is thus embedded with many transporters which allow specific compounds with a specific ligand to reach matrix space. One of those transporters is the ATP/ADP carrier which transfers ATP out from matrix space while simultaneously allowing ADP to cross inner membrane (Mukhopadhyay et al., 2007).

Mitochondrial proteins synthesized in cytosolic ribosomes are translocated into mitochondria by receptor-translocator complexes present in inner and outer membranes, which are TIM (translocator inner membrane) and TOM (translocator outer membrane) respectively. An *N*-terminal leader sequence of protein is recognized by the TIM and TOM complexes and thus enables protein to be translocated into mitochondria. Apart from their central role in energy metabolism and bioenergetics, mitochondria are also involved in regulation of apoptotic cell death, calcium metabolism, cardio protection and free radical formation (Biasutto et al., 2010). Thus, targeting mitochondria would benefit in alleviating many pathological conditions whose causes underlie in mitochondrial functioning.

The initial attempts to target mitochondria involved use of hydrophobic molecules which take the advantage of the hydrophobic nature of the membrane and diffuse across the membrane. The first compound showing that property was triphenyl phosphonium ion (Jauslin et al., 2003). We can either attach functional groups to the phosphorous atom or the phenyl rings can be modified to attach drugs and thus carried into the matrix space and released there. The important advantage of triphenyl phosphonium (TPP) or a methyl derivative of TPP is that without requiring a receptor they can penetrate into mitochondria due to their hydrophobicity and delocalized positive charge (Jauslin et al., 2003). TPP has been proved useful in targeting antioxidants to mitochondria which protect oxidative damage (Adlam et al., 2005; Sheu et al., 2006). Polymer based targeting of mitochondria was also investigated by attaching TPP covalently to HPMA copolymer. Results have indicated that TPP was able to transport electrically neutral and very low molecular weight conjugates (Callahan et al., 2006). A more recent study involved targeting of cyclosporin A to mitochondria using TPP. The results have shown that this conjugate amplified CsA activity, which is to abolish cell necrosis which in turn is due to deprivation of oxygen and glucose (Malouitre et al., 2009). TPP was also used to target peptide nucleic acid to mitochondria for treatment of mtDNA diseases (Muratovska et al., 2001). Dequalinium (DQA) is another dicationic amphiphilic compound which has the potential to localize exclusively in mitochondria. Another advantage of DQA is that it has shown to form liposome like aggregates in water called DQAsomes which can also bind plasmid DNA. Weissig et al have demonstrated that DQAsomes complexed with plasmid DNA can transport and release nucleic acid into mitochondria after interacting with mitochondrial membrane (D'Souza et al., 2003).

Mitochondrial proteins encoded in nucleus carry targeting signal that allow delivery into mitochondria through translocases, TIM and TOM. Peptides representing those signal sequences termed as mitochiondrial-targeted peptides are used to target mitochondria. Yamamoto and co-workers attached mitochondrial targeting peptide to *n*-trioctlyphosphine oxide (TOPO)-capped quantum dots and this conjugate exhibited a strong mitochondrial localization in contrast to quantum dots covered with a control peptide (Hoshino et al., 2004). In another attempt to internalize peptide nucleic acid into isolated mitochondria, a presequence of cytochrome *c* oxidase subunit VIII was used (Chinnery et al., 1999). These peptides thus provide a promising approach for targeting small molecules and nucleic acids to mitochondria.

Mitochondrial targeting also witnessed some reports where without any targeting sequence or lipophilic cation, molecules were localized in mitochondria. Block copolymer micelles that were made of poly(caprolactone)-b-poly(ethylene oxide) were unexpectedly localized into mitochondria suggesting these micelles have a important role in mitochondrial targeting (Savic et al., 2003).

There are many strategies used to target mitochondria in the pretext of cancer. Cardiolipin a mitochiondrial inner membrane phospholipid is important component for efficient functioning of various carriers, protein import apparatus and for respiratory chain. Cardiolipin also plays an important role in apoptosis as it is an essential collaborator for caspase-8, t-Bid and Bax thus indicating an avenue for mitochondrial targeting which can promote or prevent apoptosis. Mitochondrial channels like VDAC (porin), Shaker-type K^+ have been shown to play a role in apoptosis. Thus, these channels can be attacked to promote apoptosis in cancer cells. Certain mitochondriotropic polyphenols having antioxidant activity were used to counteract the production of reactive oxygen species. Antioxidants quercetin and resveratrol were shown to preferentially accumulate in mitochondria when conjugated with TPP (Biasutto et al., 2010).

7.C Endoplasmic Reticulum

Endoplasmic reticulum (ER) is an important intracellular organelle involved in expression and control of functional proteins required for the cellular communication and activity. ER is characterized by extensive membrane surfaces in cell extending from the nuclear envelope to cell periphery. ER embedded with ribosomes is known as rough ER and it's continuity with smooth membranes that provide surfaces for vesicle formation at ER exit sites. ER is involved in many key activities of the cell including biosynthesis of lipids, assembly and folding of proteins, homeostasis and control of Ca^{2+} signaling. Protein assembly and folding by the ER is the most important function which affects many essential biological activities. Improper handling of protein in ER leads to development of a myriad of unrelated diseases affecting different organs like heart, thyroid, kidney etc. (Aridor et al., 1999). The protein assembly and folding are controlled by two execution pathways. In one pathway, proteins are directed towards proteasome degradation from a folding pathway and in other folded and assembled proteins are transported to golgi complex by virtue of activity of cytosolic protein complex, the COPII coat.

Dysfunctional processing of proteins by ER can lead to either loss or gain of essential cellular functions. Loss of function of protein is the basis of many ER derived diseases and arise due to mutations that hinder protein folding which eventually lead to retention and degradation in ER. One such example is the loss of cystic fibrosis transmembrane conductance regulator (CFTR) function due to mutation of protein leading to lung fibrosis (Rowe et al., 2005). Inhibition of degradation of mutant protein leading to accumulation and aggregation of protein is the underlying cause of gain of function related ER processing diseases. This leads to generation of signals by transmembrane receptors in ER and can lead to induction of inflammatory response and can culminate in cellular apoptotic response leading to degenerative disease. A mutated protein α 1-antitrypsin which regulates elastase activity when not efficiently degraded gets accumulated in ER and lead to propagation of inflammatory response. This inflammatory response results in liver injury along with normal manifestation of lung emphysema (Hidvegi et al., 2005).

Unfolded protein response (UPR) is an extensive adaptive response that initially upregulates cellular biosynthetic activities in response to signals generated from the ER. Chronic UPR activation leads to apoptotic cell death and UPR is observed in many neurodegenerative diseases.

Stabilization of protein folding is the prime target to alleviate a variety of ER derived diseases. When protein kinetics of ΔF508 mutant of CFTR were modulated at reduced temperatures (27°C) the protein efficiently folds and egresses from the ER (French et al., 1996). Chemical chaperones can also be used to support protein folding without direct binding to mutant proteins. One important class of chemical chaperones is presented by osmolytes. These osmolytes like glycerol, trimethylamine-*N*-oxide or deuterated water

increase the hydration layer of folding intermediates in the ER. The other classes of chemical chaperones include dimethyl sulfoxide, 4-phenyl butyrate (4-PBA). 4-PBA an FDA approved drug for urea cycle disorders was also found to be effective in reducing UPR in cells and animal models. Thus, these chemical chaperones can be utilized to target certain proteins to ER. Another approach for targeting protein in ER is using hydrophobic ligands capable to enter cells and stabilize protein function. Glibenclamide a sulfonylurea, binds to the sulfonylurea receptor protein SUR1 and rescues the ER-retained mutated SUR1 to support delivery and expression of Kir6.2 which otherwise lead to development of congenital hyperinsulinism (Yan et al., 2006).
The above strategies can be applied to efficiently target endoplasmic reticulum to alleviate ER derived disease due to improper processing of proteins.

7.D Endosomes / lysosomes

Endocytosis is the primary route of uptake of many small drugs and macromolecular therapeutics. Especially, the receptor mediated endocytosis is probably the most efficient one for specific uptake of therapeutics. The receptor mediated endocytosis usually begins with uptake of molecule at plasma membrane by binding to cell surface receptors at clathrin coated pits. This complex then in the form of clathrin coated vesicles called endosomes, enters the cell. These early endosomes then mature into late endosomes and then fuse with and release their contents into lysosomes, where the contents are degraded. So targeting of endosomes and lysosomes has to be studied together since the entry of molecules into these organelles in interconnected. Moreover, even though targeting of therapeutics to endosomal uptake pathway enhances the intracellular concentration of molecules up to 1000 fold it is not devoid of demerits (Breunig et al., 2008) Since the end point of the therapeutics like peptides, proteins, DNAzymes is either nucleus or any other organelles, these molecules have to be released in cytosol intact. But unfortunately acidic pH and degradative enzymes in lysosomes degrade those molecules and render them ineffective. Thus, targeting endosomes/lysosomes have to be studied in two contrasting parts. In one part we discuss strategies to enhance intracellular uptake of therapeutics mediated by receptor mediated endocytosis which explains direct targeting to endo-/lysosomes. The other part involves strategies applied for escape of molecules from endo-/lysosomes so that therapeutics are not degraded and delivered intact into cytosol for further action into other organelles.

7.D.1 Targeting endosomes / lysosomes

Apart from being the channel for degradation and recycling of molecules and receptors at cell surface, endosomal system is also an essential site of signal transduction. So, targeting endosomes or endosomal signaling pathway has very important therapeutic effects. For example, endosomal ECE-1 (endothelin-converting enzyme 1) is important target for diseases involving inflammation and pain, an ECE-1 inhibitor exhibited an anti-inflammatory effect thus proving the potential of targeting endosomal signaling pathway (Cattaruzza et al., 2009). The other important way of targeting endosomes involves use of cell surface receptors like folate, transferrin, and low density lipoprotein (LDL) receptors. Several anti cancer drugs like doxorubicin, cisplatin, chlorambucil, mitomycin, gemcitabine and DNAzymes were efficiently targeted to tumor cells through transferrin receptors (Breunig et al., 2008).

Lysosomes apart from serving as acidic organelles involved in degradation of extracellular molecules, are also responsible for turnover of intracellular cytosolic molecules and organelles by a process known as autophagy. In this process lysosomal enzymes are secreted by rough endoplasmic reticulum and reach lysosomes via mannose-6-phosphate receptors. The deficiency of lysosomal enzymes can lead to accumulation of missing enzyme's substrate and eventually leads to metabolic disorders called lysosomal storage diseases like pompe's disease, gaucher's disease, fabry's disease and hurler-Scheie syndrome (Pastores et al., 2005). Thus, targeting of degradative enzymes to lysosomes would result in reversing of those disease conditions. For example, enzyme replacement therapy with agalsidase alpha which is an exogenous source of α-galactosidase A is proved to be effective in treatment of Fabry's disease (Mehta et al., 2010).

7.D.2 Endo-/lysosomal escape strategies

The important strategy for endo-/lysosomal escape of protein and nucleotide therapeutics is to use pH responsive carriers. These pH responsive carriers utilize the low pH of endosomes to release the therapeutics into the cytoplasm. Several approaches have been proposed to achieve this task like use of fusogenic peptides, use of pH sensitive polymers use of cell penetrating peptides or photochemical internalization which involve rupture of endosomal membrane loaded with photosensitizing molecules.

The fusogenic peptides at pH 7 assume a random coil structure and when encounters acidic pH, a conformational transition takes place which enables their interaction with phospholipid membrane resulting in pore formation or lysis or membrane fusion. These peptides can be of natural origin like N-terminus of hemagglutinin subunit HA-2 of influenza virus or synthetic like WEAALAEALAEALAEHLAEALAEALEALAA(GALA), orWEAKLAKALAKALAKHLAKALAKALKACEA (KALA). Intracellular delivery of many therapeutics including oligonucleotides, peptides or plasmid DNA was enhanced when these peptides were incorporated into delivery systems. When a siRNA to silence suppressor of cytokine signaling 1 (SOCS1) gene was loaded in an octaarginine (R8) modified lipid envelope type nanoparticles (R8-MEND) with a fusogenic peptide GALA, successful endosomal escape was achieved. The results have shown that siRNA loaded R8/GALA- MEND nanoparticles efficiently suppress endogenous gene expression (Akita et al., 2010).

Many cationic polymers have an intrinsic endosmolytic activity which results in swelling and rupture of endosomes due to proton sponge effect. Cationic polymers such as polyethyleneimine (PEI) can result in endosomal escape and subsequent release of DNA into cytoplasm by two mechanisms. One involves proton sponge effect where PEI buffers endosomal environment resulting in osmotic swelling of vesicle and subsequent burst of endosome which leads to release of DNA into cytoplasm (Behr, 1994). Other involves direct interaction of PEI with endosomal membrane creating holes in the membrane (Bieber et al., 2002). In another attempt, hydrophobic groups were attached to dendrimers by an acid-sensitive acetal linkage and thus in acidic conditions the complex will lose its hydrophobic molecules making it hydrophilic and thus destabilizing the micelle and allow escape of drug doxorubicin (Gillies et al., 2005).

Inspite of the advantages offered by above strategies for delivery of therapeutics into cytosol a direct targeting strategy to cytosol, would be of prime importance. In order to achieve this objective, a novel approach using "cell penetrating peptides" (CPPs) or "protein transduction domains" (PTDs) has been described. These peptides are tethered either directly to the therapeutic molecules or to the delivery system and then transported through cellular membrane. The cell penetrating peptides involve either chimeric CPPs like transportan and MPG or synthetic CPPs like oligoarginine and model amphipathic peptides (MAP). The protein transduction domains reported are penetratin and Tat peptide (Said Hassane et al., 2010). CPPs were successful in transporting many therapeutics and carriers such as proteins, DNA, antibodies and liposomes, nanoparticles into the mammalian cells (Gupta et al., 2005).

7.E GOLGI APPARATUS

Camillo Golgi more than 100 years ago first described the Golgi apparatus as 'internal reticular apparatus'. Golgi apparatus is central organelle of the cell secretory pathway and interacts with ER on both sides of the stack. It is comprised of a flattened stacks of cisternae arranged into a ribbon that are punctuated by openings of various sizes through which tubules project and vesicles move. Golgi apparatus mainly contains enzymes involved in processes like phosphorylation, acylation, glycosylation, methylation and sulphation which are post translational modification processes of newly synthesized proteins. The trans golgi network (TGN) is where cargo is sorted before it is sent to various organelles inside the cell and for secretion outside the cell (Marsh et al., 2002). Transport of cargo through golgi is bidirectional, one is anterograde (that is forward transport of cargo) and other is retrograde (transport of molecules backward within the golgi, and from the golgi to ER) and is mediated by vesicles, tubules or the process of cisternal progression/maturation. Both the anterograde and retrograde transport processes are mediated by coatomer protein complex I (COPI) dependent mechanism of vesicular transport (Marsh et al., 2002). The retrograde trafficking pathway gained importance since it involves delivery of drugs and macromolecules from endosomes to Golgi apparatus and to ER thus bypassing the acidic and hydrolytic environment of the lysosome.

The retrograde transport route was mainly reported to be exploited by toxins like shiga toxin and shiga like toxin to reach ER where they translocate into cytosol to exert their toxic effect. Movement of this toxin to ER is considered to follow a COPI independent process involving Rab6 which normally operates in cycling of enzymes from golgi apparatus to ER. Shiga toxin has two subunits A and B. Targeting property of the Shiga toxin resides in the B subunit of the toxin and subunit A involves in cell death. The B subunit binds to the cell surface glycosphingolipid, globotriaosylceramide or Gb_3 and internalizes the toxin in a receptor mediated endocytosis process. Gb_3 is also shown to be expressed in antigen presenting cells such as dendritic cells and some B cells. The unique retrograde trafficking pathway of shiga toxin combined with the expression of Gb_3 provides us with a strategy to deliver antigens to the MHC class I pathway of APC using shiga toxin as vector. It was also shown that expression of Gb_3 was enhanced in various cancers such as ovarian carcinoma, lymphoma, breast cancer cells, astrocytoma cells, malignant meningiomas, colon cancer and testicular cancer. Thus, shiga toxin can also be used to target the cancerous tissues for diagnostic as well as therapeutic purposes. Finally, since the B subunits of the shiga toxin can be produced as a polypeptide it can be used to target drugs, genes or proteins (antigens) for treatment and diagnosis of cancer and for delivery of antigens to MHC class I pathway (Tarrago-Trani et al., 2007).

7.F PEROXISOMES

Peroxisomes initially described as "microbodies" are single membrane bound organelles found in cytoplasm that encompass large variety of functions in all eukaryotic cells (Platta et al., 2007). Peroxisomes are multifunctional organelles responsible for a wide variety of biochemical and metabolic processes. Peroxisomes house biosynthetic pathways for bile acids, docosahexanenoic acids and ether phospholipids. By virtue of α- and β-oxidation reactions peroxisomes, degrade variety of fatty acids including 3-methyl-branched fatty acids, eicosanoids, prostaglandins, thromboxanes and leukotrienes. Detoxification of certain xenobiotics such as glyoxylate and hydrogen peroxide were also performed by peroxisomes (Wanders et al., 2006).

Peroxisomal enzymes are encoded by nuclear genes and then transported into lumen of peroxisomes from cytosol. The peroxisomal enzymes destined for matrix are first recognized by a peroxisomal targeting signal (PTS) type 1 or 2 (PTS1 or PTS2). A group of specific protein called peroxins play crucial role in proper formation and trafficking of matrix enzymes. Two peroxin receptors Pex5p and Pex7p recognize the enzyme's PTS1 and PTS2 respectively. These peroxin receptors bind to the cargo in cytosol and transport the complex to peroxisome membrane. The peculiar feature of protein import to peroxisomes which is different from mitochondria is its ability to accommodate fully folded, oligomeric, and co-factor bound proteins by shuttling receptors peroxins. Peroxins Pex 13p and Pex 14p which are membrane associated peroxins initiate the receptor/cargo docking. The translocation is then advanced by formation of RING membrane protein network which forms a larger complex the importomer from peroxins Pex2p, Pex 10p, ad Pex12p (Rosenkranz et al., 2006). Peroxisome membrane proteins are transported to membrane by chaperone peroxin Pex19p and other membrane-associated peroxins Pex3p and Pex16p. Subsequent to release of cargo Pex5p, Pex7p and Pex20p are exported back to cytosol for further transportation (Platta et al., 2007).

Peroxisomal related disorders include peroxisome biogenesis disorders, single enzyme deficiencies, or pathological situations associated with oxidative stress. The peroxisome assembly, protein import and consequent metabolic pathways are severely affected if there are any defects in genes encoding peroxins. Sometimes this might also result in complete loss of peroxisomal function. Thus, it would be of great clinical value if therapeutic proteins can be transported to peroxisomes of above discussed disease conditions.

As mentioned earlier peroxisomes have unique ability of internalizing fully folded and oligomeric proteins. Thus, in many peroxisome related conditions when therapeutic proteins or enzymes are targeted directly to peroxisomes they will alleviate the disease conditions. The most important criteria for a protein to be targeted to peroxisomes is that it should possess PTSs. PTS1 and PTS2 are the two PTSs. PTS1 is the best characterized as a short carboxy terminal sequence specifically recognized by the peroxin Pex5p and PTS2 is a N-terminal sequence recognized and transported by peroxin Pex7p (Miyata et al., 2009).

In order to target proteins which do not possess these targeting signal related sequences can be easily introduced through recombinant DNA molecular biology. For example an SKL sequence can be introduced to make protein accessible to PTS1 receptor Pex5p. One important consideration is that the attached sequence must be accessible and should not be buried inside the protein. To make it accessible spacers such as polyglycine can be introduced (Terlecky et al., 2007).

One classic example of peroxisomal targeting is administration of catalase enzyme in peroxisomal hypocatalasemia. In this condition, hydrogen peroxide and related ROS initiate

a 'peroxisomal deterioration spiral' which affect the peroxisomal import apparatus and hence catalase with weak KANL PTS1 is specifically affected. To overcome this, catalase was engineered such that it contains a high affinity SKL PTS1 and hence, its import into peroxisomes is enhanced. The results have shown that when catalase-SKL along with a cell penetrating peptide Pep-1 delivered into human hypocatalasemic fibroblasts, it reduced cellular hydrogen peroxide levels by 80% (Wood et al., 2006).
The following table summarizes various nuclear import machineries and their substrates present in cellular organelles.

Cellular Organelle	Import Apparatus	Substrates (Examples)	References
Nucleus	Importin α and β	Nuclear localization signals (SV40, GAL4)	(Chan et al., 2001)
Mitochondria	ATP/ADP Carrier	ATP, ADP	(Mukhopadhyay et al., 2007)
	TIM, TOM	Mitochondrial targeting peptide	(Hoshino et al., 2004)
	Mitochondrial membrane	Triphenyl phosphinium, Dequalinium	(Jauslin et al., 2003), (D'Souza et al., 2003)
Endosomes/lysosomes	Folate, transferrin cell surface receptors	Folic acid, Transferrin	(Breunig et al., 2008)
Golgi Apparatus	Coatomer protein complex 1 (COP I)	Shiga toxin	(Tarrago-Trani et al., 2007)
Peroxisomes	Peroxins	Peroxisomal targeting signal	(Miyata et al., 2009)

Table 2. Table of import machineries of various cellular organelles and their respective susbtrates.

8. Conclusions and future perspectives

The strategy of targeting therapeutics like small molecule drugs, proteins, enzymes, siRNA, DNA etc to specific cell population like cancer was proved to be successful. But that itself does not ensure the therapeutic efficiency of the molecule, since the molecule has to reach its intracellular target where it acts. Thus, it is very important to understand the concept of intracellular organelle targeting and intricacies involved therein. In order to establish a pattern for strategies it is first very important to understand how these intracellular organelles communicate with each other and how do they overcome the barriers due to intracellular environment. Next, it is very important to understand how do some natural viruses and other pathogens decode the intracellular processes and evade the organelle of interest and make it defective. When we combine both the strategies, we can definitely provide excellent strategies to target therapeutics of organelle of interest. Improvements in the field of polymer chemistry and molecular biology allowed us to design novel carriers and signaling agents for targeting organelles with superior level of sophistication. Like other fields of biomedical research, targeting to organelles has to evolve from a laboratory experiments to clinical success.

9. References

Adlam, V. J., Harrison, J. C., Porteous, C. M., James, A. M., Smith, R. A., Murphy, M. P., et al. (2005). Targeting an antioxidant to mitochondria decreases cardiac ischemia-reperfusion injury. *FASEB J,* 19. 9. (Jul 2005), 1088-1095.1530-6860.

Akita, H., Kogure, K., Moriguchi, R., Nakamura, Y., Higashi, T., Nakamura, T., et al. (2010). Nanoparticles for ex vivo siRNA delivery to dendritic cells for cancer vaccines: programmed endosomal escape and dissociation. *J Control Release,* 143. 3. (May 10 2010), 311-317.1873-4995.

Allen, T. M. (2002). Ligand-targeted therapeutics in anticancer therapy. *Nat Rev Cancer,* 2. 10. (Oct 2002), 750-763.1474-175.

Aridor, M., & Balch, W. E. (1999). Integration of endoplasmic reticulum signaling in health and disease. *Nat Med,* 5. 7. (Jul 1999), 745-751.1078-8956

Bale, S. S., Kwon, S. J., Shah, D. A., Banerjee, A., Dordick, J. S., & Kane, R. S. (2010). Nanoparticle-mediated cytoplasmic delivery of proteins to target cellular machinery. *ACS Nano,* 4. 3. (Mar 23 2010), 1493-1500.1936-086.

Bareford, L. M., & Swaan, P. W. (2007). Endocytic mechanisms for targeted drug delivery. *Adv Drug Deliv Rev,* 59. 8. (Aug 10 2007), 748-758.0169-409.

Behr, J. P. (1994). Gene transfer with synthetic cationic amphiphiles: prospects for gene therapy. *Bioconjug Chem,* 5. 5. (Sep-Oct 1994), 382-389.1043-1802.

Bergen, J. M., von Recum, H. A., Goodman, T. T., Massey, A. P., & Pun, S. H. (2006). Gold nanoparticles as a versatile platform for optimizing physicochemical parameters for targeted drug delivery. *Macromol Biosci,* 6. 7. (Jul 14 2006), 506-516.1616-5187.

Biasutto, L., Dong, L. F., Zoratti, M., & Neuzil, J. (2010). Mitochondrially targeted anti-cancer agents. *Mitochondrion*(Jul 1 2010).1872-8278.

Bieber, T., Meissner, W., Kostin, S., Niemann, A., & Elsasser, H. P. (2002). Intracellular route and transcriptional competence of polyethylenimine-DNA complexes. *J Control Release,* 82. 2-3. (Aug 21 2002), 441-454.0168-3659.

Bontha, S., Kabanov, A. V., & Bronich, T. K. (2006). Polymer micelles with cross-linked ionic cores for delivery of anticancer drugs. *J Control Release,* 114. 2. (Aug 28 2006), 163-174.0168-3659.

Boyce, M., Bryant, K. F., Jousse, C., Long, K., Harding, H. P., Scheuner, D., et al. (2005). A selective inhibitor of eIF2alpha dephosphorylation protects cells from ER stress. *Science,* 307. 5711. (Feb 11 2005), 935-939.1095-9203.

Breunig, M., Bauer, S., & Goepferich, A. (2008). Polymers and nanoparticles: intelligent tools for intracellular targeting? *Eur J Pharm Biopharm,* 68. 1. (Jan 2008), 112-128.0939-6411.

Callahan, J., & Kopecek, J. (2006). Semitelechelic HPMA copolymers functionalized with triphenylphosphonium as drug carriers for membrane transduction and mitochondrial localization. *Biomacromolecules,* 7. 8. (Aug 2006), 2347-2356.1525-7797.

Cartiera, M. S., Johnson, K. M., Rajendran, V., Caplan, M. J., & Saltzman, W. M. (2009). The uptake and intracellular fate of PLGA nanoparticles in epithelial cells. *Biomaterials,* 30. 14. (May 2009), 2790-2798.1878-5905.

Cattaruzza, F., Cottrell, G. S., Vaksman, N., & Bunnett, N. W. (2009). Endothelin-converting enzyme 1 promotes re-sensitization of neurokinin 1 receptor-dependent neurogenic inflammation. *Br J Pharmacol,* 156. 5. (Mar 2009), 730-739.1476-5381.

Champion, J. A., Katare, Y. K., & Mitragotri, S. (2007). Particle shape: a new design parameter for micro- and nanoscale drug delivery carriers. *J Control Release,* 121. 1-2. (Aug 16 2007), 3-9.1873-4995.

Champion, J. A., & Mitragotri, S. (2006). Role of target geometry in phagocytosis. *Proc Natl Acad Sci U S A,* 103. 13. (Mar 28 2006), 4930-4934.0027-8424.

Chan, C. K., & Jans, D. A. (2001). Enhancement of MSH receptor- and GAL4-mediated gene transfer by switching the nuclear import pathway. *Gene Ther,* 8. 2. (Jan 2001), 166-171.0969-7128.

Chen, Y., & Arriaga, E. A. (2007). Individual electrophoretic mobilities of liposomes and acidic organelles displaying pH gradients across their membranes. *Langmuir,* 23. 10. (May 8 2007), 5584-5590.0743-7463.

Chinnery, P. F., Taylor, R. W., Diekert, K., Lill, R., Turnbull, D. M., & Lightowlers, R. N. (1999). Peptide nucleic acid delivery to human mitochondria. *Gene Ther,* 6. 12. (Dec 1999), 1919-1928.0969-7128.

Conner, S. D., & Schmid, S. L. (2003). Regulated portals of entry into the cell. *Nature,* 422. 6927. (Mar 6 2003), 37-44.0028-0836.

Corona, P., Lamantea, E., Greco, M., Carrara, F., Agostino, A., Guidetti, D., et al. (2002). Novel heteroplasmic mtDNA mutation in a family with heterogeneous clinical presentations. *Ann Neurol,* 51. 1. (Jan 2002), 118-122.0364-5134.

Cronshaw, J. M., & Matunis, M. J. (2004). The nuclear pore complex: disease associations and functional correlations. *Trends Endocrinol Metab,* 15. 1. (Jan-Feb 2004), 34-39.1043-2760.

D'Souza, G. G., Boddapati, S. V., & Weissig, V. (2005). Mitochondrial leader sequence--plasmid DNA conjugates delivered into mammalian cells by DQAsomes co-localize with mitochondria. *Mitochondrion,* 5. 5. (Oct 2005), 352-358.1567-7249.

D'Souza, G. G., Rammohan, R., Cheng, S. M., Torchilin, V. P., & Weissig, V. (2003). DQAsome-mediated delivery of plasmid DNA toward mitochondria in living cells. *J Control Release,* 92. 1-2. (Sep 19 2003), 189-197.0168-3659.

D'Souza, G. G., & Weissig, V. (2009). Subcellular targeting: a new frontier for drug-loaded pharmaceutical nanocarriers and the concept of the magic bullet. *Expert Opin Drug Deliv,* 6. 11. (Nov 2009), 1135-1148.1744-7593.

Dauty, E., & Verkman, A. S. (2004). Molecular crowding reduces to a similar extent the diffusion of small solutes and macromolecules measurement by fluorescence correlation spectroscopy. *J Mol Recognit,* 17. 5. (Sep-Oct 2004), 441-447.0952-3499.

Davis, J. R., Kakar, M., & Lim, C. S. (2007). Controlling protein compartmentalization to overcome disease. *Pharm Res,* 24. 1. (Jan 2007), 17-27.0724-8741.

de Moura, M. B., dos Santos, L. S., & Van Houten, B. (2010). Mitochondrial dysfunction in neurodegenerative diseases and cancer. *Environ Mol Mutagen,* 51. 5. (Jun 2010), 391-405.1098-2280.

Dhaunsi, G. S. (2005). Molecular mechanisms of organelle biogenesis and related metabolic diseases. *Med Princ Pract,* 14 Suppl 1. 2005), 49-57.1011-7571.

Dohner, K., Nagel, C. H., & Sodeik, B. (2005). Viral stop-and-go along microtubules: taking a ride with dynein and kinesins. *Trends Microbiol,* 13. 7. (Jul 2005), 320-327.0966-842.

Draptchinskaia, N., Gustavsson, P., Andersson, B., Pettersson, M., Willig, T. N., Dianzani, I., et al. (1999). The gene encoding ribosomal protein S19 is mutated in Diamond-Blackfan anaemia. *Nat Genet,* 21. 2. (Feb 1999), 169-175.1061-4036.

Droogendijk, H. J., Kluin-Nelemans, H. J., van Doormaal, J. J., Oranje, A. P., van de Loosdrecht, A. A., & van Daele, P. L. (2006). Imatinib mesylate in the treatment of systemic mastocytosis: a phase II trial. *Cancer,* 107. 2. (Jul 15 2006), 345-351.0008-543.

Dunne, M., Corrigan, I., & Ramtoola, Z. (2000). Influence of particle size and dissolution conditions on the degradation properties of polylactide-co-glycolide particles. *Biomaterials,* 21. 16. (Aug 2000), 1659-1668.0142-9612.

Ellis, R. J., & Minton, A. P. (2003). Cell biology: join the crowd. *Nature,* 425. 6953. (Sep 4 2003), 27-28.1476-4687.

Fan, J., Hu, Z., Zeng, L., Lu, W., Tang, X., Zhang, J., et al. (2008). Golgi apparatus and neurodegenerative diseases. *Int J Dev Neurosci,* 26. 6. (Oct 2008), 523-534.0736-5748.

Fattal, E., Couvreur, P., & Dubernet, C. (2004). "Smart" delivery of antisense oligonucleotides by anionic pH-sensitive liposomes. *Adv Drug Deliv Rev,* 56. 7. (Apr 23 2004), 931-946.0169-409.

Fominaya, J., & Wels, W. (1996). Target cell-specific DNA transfer mediated by a chimeric multidomain protein. Novel non-viral gene delivery system. *J Biol Chem,* 271. 18. (May 3 1996), 10560-10568.0021-9258.

French, P. J., van Doorninck, J. H., Peters, R. H., Verbeek, E., Ameen, N. A., Marino, C. R., et al. (1996). A delta F508 mutation in mouse cystic fibrosis transmembrane conductance regulator results in a temperature-sensitive processing defect in vivo. *J Clin Invest,* 98. 6. (Sep 15 1996), 1304-1312.0021-9738.

Fulda, S., Galluzzi, L., & Kroemer, G. (2010). Targeting mitochondria for cancer therapy. *Nat Rev Drug Discov,* 9. 6. (Jun 2010), 447-464.1474-1784.

Galluzzi, L., Morselli, E., Kepp, O., Tajeddine, N., & Kroemer, G. (2008). Targeting p53 to mitochondria for cancer therapy. *Cell Cycle,* 7. 13. (Jul 1 2008), 1949-1955.1551-4005.

Garner, M. M., & Burg, M. B. (1994). Macromolecular crowding and confinement in cells exposed to hypertonicity. *Am J Physiol,* 266. 4 Pt 1. (Apr 1994), C877-892.0002-9513.

Gartner, J. (2000). Disorders related to peroxisomal membranes. *J Inherit Metab Dis,* 23. 3. (May 2000), 264-272.0141-8955.

Geng, Y., Dalhaimer, P., Cai, S., Tsai, R., Tewari, M., Minko, T., et al. (2007). Shape effects of filaments versus spherical particles in flow and drug delivery. *Nat Nanotechnol,* 2. 4. (Apr 2007), 249-255.1748-3395.

Gillies, E. R., & Frechet, J. M. (2005). pH-Responsive copolymer assemblies for controlled release of doxorubicin. *Bioconjug Chem,* 16. 2. (Mar-Apr 2005), 361-368.1043-1802.

Gonzalez-Angulo, A. M., Hennessy, B. T., & Mills, G. B. (2010). Future of personalized medicine in oncology: a systems biology approach. *J Clin Oncol,* 28. 16. (Jun 1 2010), 2777-2783.1527-7755.

Gratton, S. E., Ropp, P. A., Pohlhaus, P. D., Luft, J. C., Madden, V. J., Napier, M. E., et al. (2008). The effect of particle design on cellular internalization pathways. *Proc Natl Acad Sci U S A,* 105. 33. (Aug 19 2008), 11613-11618.1091-6490.

Gupta, B., Levchenko, T. S., & Torchilin, V. P. (2005). Intracellular delivery of large molecules and small particles by cell-penetrating proteins and peptides. *Adv Drug Deliv Rev,* 57. 4. (Feb 28 2005), 637-651.0169-409.

Hidvegi, T., Schmidt, B. Z., Hale, P., & Perlmutter, D. H. (2005). Accumulation of mutant alpha1-antitrypsin Z in the endoplasmic reticulum activates caspases-4 and -12, NFkappaB, and BAP31 but not the unfolded protein response. *J Biol Chem,* 280. 47. (Nov 25 2005), 39002-39015.0021-9258.

Hill, C. S., & Treisman, R. (1995). Transcriptional regulation by extracellular signals: mechanisms and specificity. *Cell,* 80. 2. (Jan 27 1995), 199-211.0092-8674.

Holt, I. J., Harding, A. E., & Morgan-Hughes, J. A. (1988). Deletions of muscle mitochondrial DNA in patients with mitochondrial myopathies. *Nature,* 331. 6158. (Feb 25 1988), 717-719.0028-0836.

Hope, M. J., Redelmeier, T. E., Wong, K. F., Rodrigueza, W., & Cullis, P. R. (1989). Phospholipid asymmetry in large unilamellar vesicles induced by transmembrane pH gradients. *Biochemistry,* 28. 10. (May 16 1989), 4181-4187.0006-2960.

Hoshino, A., Fujioka, K., Oku, T., Nakamura, S., Suga, M., Yamaguchi, Y., et al. (2004). Quantum dots targeted to the assigned organelle in living cells. *Microbiol Immunol,* 48. 12. 2004), 985-994.0385-5600.

Hotamisligil, G. S. (2010). Endoplasmic reticulum stress and the inflammatory basis of metabolic disease. *Cell,* 140. 6. (Mar 19 2010), 900-917.1097-4172.

Huang, X., Teng, X., Chen, D., Tang, F., & He, J. (2010). The effect of the shape of mesoporous silica nanoparticles on cellular uptake and cell function. *Biomaterials,* 31. 3. (Jan 2010), 438-448.1878-5905.

Hudis, C. A. (2007). Trastuzumab--mechanism of action and use in clinical practice. *N Engl J Med,* 357. 1. (Jul 5 2007), 39-51.1533-4406.

Ito, D., & Suzuki, N. (2009). Seipinopathy: a novel endoplasmic reticulum stress-associated disease. *Brain,* 132. Pt 1. (Jan 2009), 8-15.1460-2156.

Jauslin, M. L., Meier, T., Smith, R. A., & Murphy, M. P. (2003). Mitochondria-targeted antioxidants protect Friedreich Ataxia fibroblasts from endogenous oxidative stress more effectively than untargeted antioxidants. *FASEB J,* 17. 13. (Oct 2003), 1972-1974.1530-6860.

Jensen, K. D., Nori, A., Tijerina, M., Kopeckova, P., & Kopecek, J. (2003). Cytoplasmic delivery and nuclear targeting of synthetic macromolecules. *J Control Release,* 87. 1-3. (Feb 21 2003), 89-105.0168-3659.

Johannsen, D. L., & Ravussin, E. (2009). The role of mitochondria in health and disease. *Curr Opin Pharmacol,* 9. 6. (Dec 2009), 780-786.1471-4973.

Kao, H. P., Abney, J. R., & Verkman, A. S. (1993). Determinants of the translational mobility of a small solute in cell cytoplasm. *J Cell Biol,* 120. 1. (Jan 1993), 175-184.0021-9525.

Koves, T. R., Ussher, J. R., Noland, R. C., Slentz, D., Mosedale, M., Ilkayeva, O., et al. (2008). Mitochondrial overload and incomplete fatty acid oxidation contribute to skeletal muscle insulin resistance. *Cell Metab,* 7. 1. (Jan 2008), 45-56.1550-4131.

Lukacs, G. L., Haggie, P., Seksek, O., Lechardeur, D., Freedman, N., & Verkman, A. S. (2000). Size-dependent DNA mobility in cytoplasm and nucleus. *J Biol Chem,* 275. 3. (Jan 21 2000), 1625-1629.0021-9258.

Malouitre, S., Dube, H., Selwood, D., & Crompton, M. (2009). Mitochondrial targeting of cyclosporin A enables selective inhibition of cyclophilin-D and enhanced cytoprotection after glucose and oxygen deprivation. *Biochem J,* 425. 1. (Jan 1 2009), 137-148.1470-8728.

Marsh, B. J., & Howell, K. E. (2002). The mammalian Golgi--complex debates. *Nat Rev Mol Cell Biol,* 3. 10. (Oct 2002), 789-795.1471-0072.

Maxfield, F. R., & McGraw, T. E. (2004). Endocytic recycling. *Nat Rev Mol Cell Biol,* 5. 2. (Feb 2004), 121-132.1471-0072.

Medalia, O., Typke, D., Hegerl, R., Angenitzki, M., Sperling, J., & Sperling, R. (2002). Cryoelectron microscopy and cryoelectron tomography of the nuclear pre-mRNA processing machine. *J Struct Biol,* 138. 1-2. (Apr-May 2002), 74-84.1047-8477.

Mehta, A., Beck, M., Eyskens, F., Feliciani, C., Kantola, I., Ramaswami, U., et al. (2010). Fabry disease: a review of current management strategies. *QJM,* 103. 9. (Sep 2010), 641-659.1460-2393.

Mesika, A., Kiss, V., Brumfeld, V., Ghosh, G., & Reich, Z. (2005). Enhanced intracellular mobility and nuclear accumulation of DNA plasmids associated with a karyophilic protein. *Hum Gene Ther,* 16. 2. (Feb 2005), 200-208.1043-0342.

Minton, A. P. (2006). How can biochemical reactions within cells differ from those in test tubes? *J Cell Sci,* 119. Pt 14. (Jul 15 2006), 2863-2869.0021-9533.

Miyata, N., Hosoi, K., Mukai, S., & Fujiki, Y. (2009). In vitro import of peroxisome-targeting signal type 2 (PTS2) receptor Pex7p into peroxisomes. *Biochim Biophys Acta,* 1793. 5. (May 2009), 860-870.0006-3002.

Mukhopadhyay, A., & Weiner, H. (2007). Delivery of drugs and macromolecules to mitochondria. *Adv Drug Deliv Rev,* 59. 8. (Aug 10 2007), 729-738.0169-409.

Muratovska, A., Lightowlers, R. N., Taylor, R. W., Turnbull, D. M., Smith, R. A., Wilce, J. A., et al. (2001). Targeting peptide nucleic acid (PNA) oligomers to mitochondria within cells by conjugation to lipophilic cations: implications for mitochondrial DNA replication, expression and disease. *Nucleic Acids Res,* 29. 9. (May 1 2001), 1852-1863.1362-4962.

Narla, A., & Ebert, B. L. (2010). Ribosomopathies: human disorders of ribosome dysfunction. *Blood,* 115. 16. (Apr 22 2010), 3196-3205.1528-0020.

Nori, A., Jensen, K. D., Tijerina, M., Kopeckova, P., & Kopecek, J. (2003). Tat-conjugated synthetic macromolecules facilitate cytoplasmic drug delivery to human ovarian carcinoma cells. *Bioconjug Chem,* 14. 1. (Jan-Feb 2003), 44-50.1043-1802.

Nori, A., & Kopecek, J. (2005). Intracellular targeting of polymer-bound drugs for cancer chemotherapy. *Adv Drug Deliv Rev,* 57. 4. (Feb 28 2005), 609-636.0169-409.

Nunnari, J., & Walter, P. (1996). Regulation of organelle biogenesis. *Cell,* 84. 3. (Feb 9 1996), 389-394.0092-8674.

Ozcan, U., Cao, Q., Yilmaz, E., Lee, A. H., Iwakoshi, N. N., Ozdelen, E., et al. (2004). Endoplasmic reticulum stress links obesity, insulin action, and type 2 diabetes. *Science,* 306. 5695. (Oct 15 2004), 457-461.1095-9203.

Pante, N., & Kann, M. (2002). Nuclear pore complex is able to transport macromolecules with diameters of about 39 nm. *Mol Biol Cell,* 13. 2. (Feb 2002), 425-434.1059-1524.

Panyam, J., Dali, M. M., Sahoo, S. K., Ma, W., Chakravarthi, S. S., Amidon, G. L., et al. (2003). Polymer degradation and in vitro release of a model protein from poly(D,L-lactide-co-glycolide) nano- and microparticles. *J Control Release,* 92. 1-2. (Sep 19 2003), 173-187.0168-3659.

Parkinson-Lawrence, E. J., Shandala, T., Prodoehl, M., Plew, R., Borlace, G. N., & Brooks, D. A. (2010). Lysosomal storage disease: revealing lysosomal function and physiology. *Physiology (Bethesda),* 25. 2. (Apr 2010), 102-115.1548-9221.

Pastores, G. M., & Barnett, N. L. (2005). Current and emerging therapies for the lysosomal storage disorders. *Expert Opin Emerg Drugs,* 10. 4. (Nov 2005), 891-902.1744-7623.

Petros, R. A., & DeSimone, J. M. (2010). Strategies in the design of nanoparticles for therapeutic applications. *Nat Rev Drug Discov,* 9. 8. (Aug 2010), 615-627.1474-1784.

Platta, H. W., & Erdmann, R. (2007). The peroxisomal protein import machinery. *FEBS Lett,* 581. 15. (Jun 19 2007), 2811-2819.0014-5793.

Poon, I. K., & Jans, D. A. (2005). Regulation of nuclear transport: central role in development and transformation? *Traffic,* 6. 3. (Mar 2005), 173-186.1398-9219.

Pouton, C. W., Wagstaff, K. M., Roth, D. M., Moseley, G. W., & Jans, D. A. (2007). Targeted delivery to the nucleus. *Adv Drug Deliv Rev,* 59. 8. (Aug 10 2007), 698-717.0169-409.

Rajendran, L., Knolker, H. J., & Simons, K. (2010). Subcellular targeting strategies for drug design and delivery. *Nat Rev Drug Discov,* 9. 1. (Jan 2010), 29-42 1474-1784.

Rosenkranz, K., Birschmann, I., Grunau, S., Girzalsky, W., Kunau, W. H., & Erdmann, R. (2006). Functional association of the AAA complex and the peroxisomal importomer. *FEBS J,* 273. 16. (Aug 2006), 3804-3815.1742-464.

Rowe, S. M., Miller, S., & Sorscher, E. J. (2005) Cystic fibrosis. *N Engl J Med,* 352. 19. (May 12 2005), 1992-2001.1533-4406.

Said Hassane, F., Saleh, A. F., Abes, R., Gait, M. J., & Lebleu, B. (2010). Cell penetrating peptides: overview and applications to the delivery of oligonucleotides. *Cell Mol Life Sci,* 67. 5. (Mar 2010), 715-726.1420-9071.

Samuelson, L. E., Dukes, M. J., Hunt, C. R., Casey, J. D., & Bornhop, D. J. (2009). TSPO targeted dendrimer imaging agent: synthesis, characterization, and cellular internalization. *Bioconjug Chem,* 20. 11. (Nov 2009), 2082-2089.1520-4812.

Sanabria, H., Kubota, Y., & Waxham, M. N. (2007). Multiple diffusion mechanisms due to nanostructuring in crowded environments. *Biophys J,* 92. 1. (Jan 1 2007), 313-322.0006-3495.

Savic, R., Luo, L., Eisenberg, A., & Maysinger, D. (2003). Micellar nanocontainers distribute to defined cytoplasmic organelles. *Science,* 300. 5619. (Apr 25 2003), 615-618.1095-9203.

Schmid, S. L. (1997). Clathrin-coated vesicle formation and protein sorting: an integrated process. *Annu Rev Biochem,* 66. 1997), 511-548.0066-4154.

Seksek, O., Biwersi, J., & Verkman, A. S. (1997). Translational diffusion of macromolecule-sized solutes in cytoplasm and nucleus. *J Cell Biol,* 138. 1. (Jul 14 1997), 131-142.0021-9525.

Sheu, S. S., Nauduri, D., & Anders, M. W. (2006). Targeting antioxidants to mitochondria: a new therapeutic direction. *Biochim Biophys Acta,* 1762. 2. (Feb 2006), 256-265.0006-3002.

Tarrago-Trani, M. T., & Storrie, B. (2007). Alternate routes for drug delivery to the cell interior: pathways to the Golgi apparatus and endoplasmic reticulum. *Adv Drug Deliv Rev,* 59. 8. (Aug 10 2007), 782-797.0169-409.

Terlecky, S. R., & Koepke, J. I. (2007). Drug delivery to peroxisomes: employing unique trafficking mechanisms to target protein therapeutics. *Adv Drug Deliv Rev,* 59. 8. (Aug 10 2007), 739-747.0169-409.

Torchilin, V. P. (2005). Fluorescence microscopy to follow the targeting of liposomes and micelles to cells and their intracellular fate. *Adv Drug Deliv Rev,* 57. 1. (Jan 2 2005), 95-109.0169-409.

Ungar, D. (2009). Golgi linked protein glycosylation and associated diseases. *Semin Cell Dev Biol,* 20. 7. (Sep 2009), 762-769.1096-3634.

Wanders, R. J., & Waterham, H. R. (2006). Biochemistry of mammalian peroxisomes revisited. *Annu Rev Biochem,* 75. 2006), 295-332.0066-4154.

Warren, G., & Wickner, W. (1996). Organelle inheritance. *Cell,* 84. 3. (Feb 9 1996), 395-400.0092-8674.

Watson, P., Jones, A. T., & Stephens, D. J. (2005). Intracellular trafficking pathways and drug delivery: fluorescence imaging of living and fixed cells. *Adv Drug Deliv Rev,* 57. 1. (Jan 2 2005), 43-61.0169-409.

Weissig, V., D'Souza, G. G., & Torchilin, V. P. (2001). DQAsome/DNA complexes release DNA upon contact with isolated mouse liver mitochondria. *J Control Release,* 75. 3. (Aug 10 2001), 401-408.0168-3659.

Weissig, V., Lizano, C., & Torchilin, V. P. (2000). Selective DNA release from DQAsome/DNA complexes at mitochondria-like membranes. *Drug Deliv,* 7. 1. (Jan-Mar 2000), 1-5.1071-7544.

Wood, C. S., Koepke, J. I., Teng, H., Boucher, K. K., Katz, S., Chang, P., et al. (2006). Hypocatalasemic fibroblasts accumulate hydrogen peroxide and display age-associated pathologies. *Traffic,* 7. 1. (Jan 2006), 97-107.1398-9219.

Xiong, R., Li, Z., Mi, L., Wang, P. N., Chen, J. Y., Wang, L., et al. (2010). Study on the intracellular fate of Tat peptide-conjugated quantum dots by spectroscopic investigation. *J Fluoresc,* 20. 2. (Mar 2010), 551-556.1573-4994.

Xu, C., Xie, J., Kohler, N., Walsh, E. G., Chin, Y. E., & Sun, S. (2008). Monodisperse magnetite nanoparticles coupled with nuclear localization signal peptide for cell-nucleus targeting. *Chem Asian J,* 3. 3. (Mar 7 2008), 548-552.1861-471.

Yan, F. F., Casey, J., & Shyng, S. L. (2006). Sulfonylureas correct trafficking defects of disease-causing ATP-sensitive potassium channels by binding to the channel complex. *J Biol Chem,* 281. 44. (Nov 3 2006), 33403-33413.0021-9258.

Yang, S. R., Lee, H. J., & Kim, J. D. (2006). Histidine-conjugated poly(amino acid) derivatives for the novel endosomolytic delivery carrier of doxorubicin. *J Control Release,* 114. 1. (Aug 10 2006), 60-68.0168-3659.

Yang, Z., Zhang, Y., Yang, Y., Sun, L., Han, D., Li, H., et al. (2010). Pharmacological and toxicological target organelles and safe use of single-walled carbon nanotubes as drug carriers in treating Alzheimer disease. *Nanomedicine,* 6. 3. (Jun 2010), 427-441.1549-9642.

Yessine, M. A., & Leroux, J. C. (2004). Membrane-destabilizing polyanions: interaction with lipid bilayers and endosomal escape of biomacromolecules. *Adv Drug Deliv Rev,* 56. 7. (Apr 23 2004), 999-1021.0169-409.

Part 5

Biomaterials and Medicines

12

Antimicrobial Peptides: Diversity and Perspectives for Their Biomedical Application

Joel E. López-Meza[1], Alejandra Ochoa-Zarzosa[1]
José A. Aguilar[2] and Pedro D. Loeza-Lara[2]
[1]*Centro Multidisciplinario de Estudios en Biotecnología, CMEB-FMVZ-UMSNH Morelia, Michoacán*
[2]*Genómica Alimentaria, Universidad de La Ciénega del Estado de Michoacán de Ocampo UCM, Sahuayo, Michoacán,*
[1,2]*México*

1. Introduction

For over fifty years, people have used antibiotics to treat illnesses caused by pathogens. However, the excessive and inappropriate use of these antibiotics in clinical treatment of humans and animals has increased pathogen resistance to these compounds, turning them into less effective agents. There has also been an increase in the generation of multidrug-resistant pathogens, primarily bacteria and fungi that resist the effects of most currently available antibiotics (Heuer et al., 2006; Field, 2010).

Until now, the pharmaceutical industry is facing this problem by looking for new antibiotics or modifying existing ones. However, pathogens have proven to have the ability to quickly develop and disseminate resistance mechanisms, which compromises this strategy, becoming it less effective. This clearly shows the need to develop new biomedical treatments with different action mechanisms from those of conventional antibiotics (Parisien et al., 2008).

This problem has led that efforts being made on research and development of new biomedical alternatives, among which antimicrobial peptides (AMPs) are considered one of the most promising options. AMPs are produced by a wide variety of organisms as part of their first line of defense (eukaryotes) or as a competition strategy for nutrients and space (prokaryotes). These molecules are usually short peptides (12-100 amino acid residues); have a positive charge (+2 to +9), although there are also neutral and negatively charged. They are amphipathic and have been isolated from bacteria, plants and animals, including humans; which give us an overview of the enormous structural diversity of these molecules and their different action mechanisms (Murray & Liu, 2008).

The continuous discovery of new AMPs groups in diverse organisms has turned these natural antibiotics into the basic elements of a new generation of potential biomedical treatments against infectious diseases in humans and animals. Besides the above, the broad spectrum of biological activities reported for these molecules suggests a potential benefit in cancer treatment, viral and parasitic infections and in the modulation of the immune system, which reinforces the importance of studying these molecules (Mercado et al., 2005; Schweizer, 2009).

The contents of this chapter shows the importance of AMPs for living organisms, not only from the antimicrobial point of view, but also in bacterial cell communication processes, immune response modulation in animals and plant defense mechanisms. It also emphasizes on AMPs' biological and structural diversity, as well as their various action mechanisms and, finally, their possible biotechnological development for the pharmaceutical industry is discussed.

2. AMPs from Gram positive bacteria and their classification

During their evolution, bacteria have acquired mechanisms that allow them to have success in competition for nutrients and space in their habitat. These mechanisms include from the enhancement of chemotaxis systems to the acquisition of defense systems such as the production of antimicrobial peptides (AMPs), also called bacteriocins (Riley & Wertz, 2002). AMPs are biologically active molecules that have the ability to inhibit the growth of other members of the same specie or members of different bacterial genres (Cotter et al., 2005b).

These molecules are synthesized by the vast majority of bacterial groups; in fact, it has been proposed that 99% of bacteria produce at least one, as they have been found in most examined species, covering Gram positive and Gram negative bacteria and archaea; in addition they are used as an important tool in evolutionary and ecological studies (Klaenhammer, 1988). Also, the successful commercial development of nisin (produced by *Lactococcus lactis*) and the use of molecular biology and genetic engineering tools in recent years have provoked a resurgence in AMPs studies, particularly in relation to their potential biomedical applications (Cotter et al., 2005a, b; Bierbaum & Sahl, 2009; Field et al., 2010).

AMPs from Gram positive bacteria represent a heterogeneous group of chemical molecules; nevertheless only three main categories have been established based on their structural modifications, size, thermostability and action mechanisms (Table 1). Class I (lantibiotics) is constituted by cationic peptides ranging from 19 to 38 amino acid residues, which undergo posttranslational modifications and exert their effect at membrane and cell wall levels. Their posttranslational modifications are diverse; the most important involve dehydration reactions of serine and threonine residues, resulting in the formation of didehydroalanine (Dha) and didehydroaminobutyric acid (Dhb), respectively (Cotter et al., 2005b). The reaction of these amino acids with the thiol group (SH) of a cysteine residue generates a thioether bond producing lanthionine (in the case of Dha) and β-methyl-lanthionine (in the case of Dhb). The formation of these bonds within the peptide generates a series of "globular" structures that are characteristic of lantibiotics. This AMPs class is further divided into subgroups A and B, having nisin as the representative member of subgroup A, while mersacidin, produced by bacteria of the *Bacillus* genus, is a member of subgroup B (Table 1) (McAuliffe et al., 2001; Cotter et al., 2005a).

On the other hand, class II (non lantibiotics) is formed by AMPs constituted by 30 to 60 amino acid residues; they do not contain lanthionine, are thermostable and induce the formation of pores in the membrane of target cells. These peptides in turn are divided into subclasses IIa, IIb, IIc and IId (Table 1). Subclass IIa is the largest and its members posses the amino terminal motif YGNGVXCXXXXVXV (X indicates any amino acid residue) and have one or two disulfide bonds. AMPs from this subclass show specific activity against the bacteria *Listeria monocytogenes* (Ennahar et al., 2000). Leucocin A from *Leuconostoc gelidum* is a representative member of this subclass (Hastings et al., 1991).

Class	Subclass	Representative AMPs	Producing bacteria
I Lantibiotic	I A	Nisin	*Lactococcus lactis*
I Lantibiotic	I B	Mersacidin	*Bacillus* spp.
II Non lantibiotic	IIa	Leucocin A	*Leuconostoc gelidum*
II Non lantibiotic	IIb	Lactococcin G	*L. lactis*
II Non lantibiotic	IIc	AS-48 enterocin	*Enterococcus faecalis*
II Non lantibiotic	IId	Lactococcin A	*L. lactis*
III Proteins		Helveticin J	*L. helveticus*

Table 1. Classification of AMPs found in Gram positive bacteria (Cotter et al., 2005a; Drider et al., 2006)

Subclass IIb comprises AMPs that require the combined action of two peptides in order to have activity; these peptides do not show inhibitory activity on an individual basis. Lactococcin G from *L. lactis* is a representative member of this subclass (Moll et al., 1996). The AMPs that make up subclass IIc posses a cyclic structure as a result of the covalent binding of their carboxyl and amino terminal ends; AS-48 enterocin from *Enterococcus faecalis* is one of the main representatives of this subclass (Sanchez et al., 2003). Subclass IId is formed by a variable group of linear peptides, among which lactococcin A from *L. lactis* is found (Holo et al., 1993). Finally, the class III is formed by proteins with molecular masses higher than 30 kDa, the helveticin J from *L. helveticus*, is an example (Drider et al., 2006).

2.1 Genes involved in AMPs synthesis and expression regulation from Gram positive bacteria

The genes encoding AMPs are organized as operons, which could contain several genes involved in the synthesis and regulation. For example, the enterocin A operon of *Enterococcus faecium* contains the *entA* gene that codifies for pre-enterocin; in addition, this operon contains the genes that codify for the protein involved in the self-protection of the producing strain (*entI*), the AMP synthesis induction gene (*entF*), genes for proteins involved in extracellular transport (*entT, D*), as well as the genes of proteins related to the AMP synthesis regulation (*entK, R*) (Nilsen et al., 1998). In the case of lantibiotics, these have additional genes that codify for AMP modification enzymes (McAuliffe et al., 2001).
AMPs synthesis regulation is mediated by two signal transduction systems constituted by two or three components. Diverse factors activate these systems, which include: the presence of other competing bacteria (Maldonado et al., 2004), temperature or pH stress (Ennahar et al., 2000) and a mechanism of "quorum sensing" (Kuipers et al., 1998). An

interesting example is the three-component system that regulates the synthesis of enterocin A in *E. faecium,* which is regulated by the mechanism of quorum sensing. This system includes: 1) a histidine kinase (HK), located in the cytoplasmic membrane which detects extracellular signals, and 2) a cytoplasmic response regulator (RR) that mediates an adaptive response, which usually is a change in the gene expression and an induction factor (IF), whose presence is detected by the HK protein (Figure 1, stage 1) (Cotter et al., 2005b). In this case, the system is triggered as a result of an IF excess concentration through a slow accumulation during cell growth, the HK detects this concentration and initiates the signaling cascade that activates the transcription of genes involved in enterocin A synthesis (Figure 1, stages 2 and 3) (Ennahar et al., 2000). Other examples of this type of regulation include several class II members such as sakacin P and A from *Lactobacillus sake* (Hühne et al., 1996). Moreover, some examples of regulation mediated by two-component systems include numerous lantibiotics, for example, subtilin from *Bacillus subtilis* and nisin from *L. lactis.* In these systems AMPs have a dual function, as they have antimicrobial activity and also act as a signal molecule by inducing its own synthesis (not shown) (Kleerebezem, 2004).

2.2 AMPs secretion and self-protection mechanisms from Gram positive bacteria

AMPs are synthesized as inactive pre-peptides containing a signal peptide at the N-terminal region (Figure 1, stage 3). This signal keeps the molecule in an inactive form within the producing cell facilitating its interaction with the carrier, and in the case of lantibiotics plays an important role in the pre-peptide recognition by the enzymes that perform posttranslational modifications. The signal peptide may be proteolytically removed during transport of the pre-peptide into the periplasmic space by the same transport proteins (ATP-dependent ABC membrane transporters, which may also contain a proteolytic domain) (Figure 1, stage 4), or by serine-proteases present on the outside of the cell membrane. Thus, the carboxyl terminus is separated from the signal peptide and is released into the extracellular space to produce the biologically active peptide (Figure 1, stage 5) (Ennahar et al., 2000; Cotter et al., 2005b).

AMPs producing bacteria possess proteins that protect them from the action of their own peptides. The exact molecular mechanisms by which these proteins confer protection to the producing bacteria are unknown; however, two protection systems have been proposed, which, in some cases act in the same bacteria (Kleerebezem, 2004). The protection can be provided by a specific protein that sequesters and inactivates the AMP, or that binds to the AMP receptor causing a conformational change in its structure making it inaccessible to the AMP (Figure 1, stage 6) (Venema et al., 1994). The second system is constituted by the ABC transport proteins, which in some cases provide the protection mechanism through the expulsion of the membrane-binding AMPs (Otto et al., 1998).

2.3 AMPs spectrum and action mechanisms from Gram positive bacteria

In general, the antibacterial action spectrum of AMPs of Gram positive bacteria is restricted to this bacterial group. However, there are several molecules with a wide range of action, inhibiting the growth of Gram positive (McAuliffe et al., 2001) and Gram negative bacteria (Motta et al., 2000), human pathogenic fungi (De Lucca & Walsh, 1999) and viruses (Jenssen et al., 2006). Also, AMPs have activity against various eukaryotic cells, such as human and bovine erythrocytes (Datta et al., 2005). With regard to their antimicrobial activity, AMPs possess essential characteristics in order to carry out the activity, regardless of their target

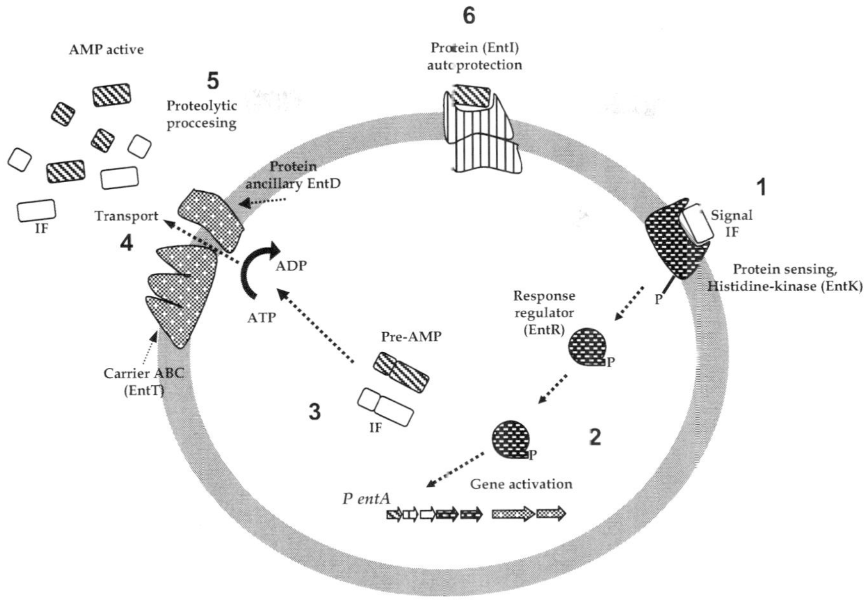

Fig. 1. Regulation of the synthesis of enterocin A from *Enterococcus faecium* (non-lantibiotic). Stage 1, the EntK protein detects the presence of the induction factor (IF) and autophosphorylates. Stages 2 and 3, the phosphate group is transferred to the EntR response regulator, which activates genes involved in the synthesis of the pre-peptide (pre-enterocin A) and of the IF. Stages 4 and 5, the pre-enterocin A and the IF are transported to the outside by the EntT and EntD proteins, and processed by the same system, releasing the active enterocin A and the IF. Stage 6, the EntI protein protects the producing bacteria from the effect of enterocin A (Ennahar et al., 2000; Cotter et al., 2005b)

cell. These include, 1) a net positive charge which favors its interaction with the negatively charged lipopolysaccharide membrane of Gram negative bacteria, or with teichoic and lipoteichoic acids from the wall of Gram positive bacteria; 2) hydrophobicity, required for the insertion of the AMP in the cell membrane; and 3) flexibility, which allows a conformational change from a soluble state to one of membrane interaction. These characteristics vary from molecule to molecule; however, all are important for antimicrobial activity (Jenssen et al., 2006).

It has been shown that the action targets of AMPs studied to date are the cell membrane and wall, as well as some important enzymes for cell metabolism. The action mechanisms include: *i*) pore formation in the cell membrane, causing loss of cell contents, this is the mechanism described for nisin (Enserink, 1999) and lactococcin A from *L. lactis* (Van Belkum et al., 1991); *ii*) cell wall synthesis inhibition, this mechanism has been described for mersacidin, which involves binding to lipid II, the main transporter of peptidoglycan subunits (UDP-Mur -Nac-pentapeptide-GlcNAc) (Brotz et al., 1995); and *iii*) inhibition of the activity of enzymes such as phospholipase A2, which is involved in membrane repair; this is the reported mechanism for cinamicin from *Streptomyces cinnamoneus* (Marki et al., 1991).

Additionally, there have been reports of AMPs that possess a dual action mechanism, such as nisin (Figure 2) (Breukink et al., 1999; Bierbaum & Sahl, 2009). The most accepted model showing the dual action mechanism of nisin proposes that it initially binds to the cell wall by electrostatic attraction, events that are facilitated due to the positive charge of this peptide and negative charges of cell wall components (Figure 2, stage 1). Subsequently, nisin binds to lipid II, the main transporter of peptidoglycan subunits, and uses this molecule to anchor itself to the cell membrane (Figure 2, stage 2). Then, it changes its orientation with respect to the membrane and inserts itself in it; this involves the translocation of its carboxyl terminus through the membrane. Finally, the binding of different peptides in the insertion site leads to the formation of a transmembrane pore that allows the exit of important molecules such as amino acids and ATP, leading the bacteria to a rapid cell death (Figure 2, stage 3) (Wiedemann et al., 2001; Bierbaum & Sahl, 2009).

2.4 AMPs resistance from Gram positive bacteria

Resistance development in pathogenic bacteria that are normally sensitive to AMPs is of great interest because of their possible use in biomedical therapies, as bacterial resistance might limit their use. Within a particular bacterial species there may be naturally resistant members to AMPs or resistance may arise as a result of continuous exposure; which are known as intrinsic and acquired resistance, respectively (Xue et al., 2005).

Most research in this area has focused on specific AMPs such as nisin and class IIa members. In the first case, *L. monocytogenes, L. innocua, Streptococcus pneumoniae* and *S. bovis* resistant mutants have been detected, whose resistance has been correlated to changes in the wall and cell membrane (Gravesen et al., 2002). More specifically the synthesis and incorporation of various structural components to the membrane (Li et al., 2002) and the cell wall (Mantovani & Russell, 2001) have been observed in the mutants, which has favored an increase in positive charges in these cell structures and reduced the antibacterial activity of nisin (which has a net positive charge). Likewise, changes in the fluidity of cell membrane (Verheul et al., 1997) and an increase in the thickness of the cell wall of some mutant bacteria have been observed (Maisnier & Richard, 1996; Murray & Liu, 2008).

The mechanisms of resistance to type II AMPs have been studied in strains of *L. monocytogenes*, essentially towards class IIa peptides, in which the resistance is related to several factors including reduced expression of a permease that acts as a potential receptor (Dalet et al., 2001), as well as changes in membrane fluidity (Vadyvaloo et al., 2002), and in cell surface charges (Vadyvaloo et al., 2004). The importance of studying the resistance lies not only in the possible long term ineffectiveness of AMPs, but also in generating knowledge that could serve as a basis for strategies to improve the therapeutic potential of these antimicrobial molecules, i.e. the development of protein engineering strategies to improve the biological properties of AMPs (Field et al., 2010).

Currently, the existence of natural AMPs variants suggests that there is flexibility in the location of some important amino acid residues for antimicrobial activity, which indicates that it is possible to generate mutants with changes that increase this activity. Thus, additional studies are needed to determine the mechanisms of resistance to AMPs, as well as the frequency with which it occurs (Cotter et al., 2005a).

2.5 Current and potential Gram positive AMPs applications in biomedical therapies

AMPs null toxicity to humans and animals and activity directed towards pathogenic bacteria has allowed investigating their potential applications in biomedical therapies. In particular, the action mechanisms of these peptides and their activity against pathogens

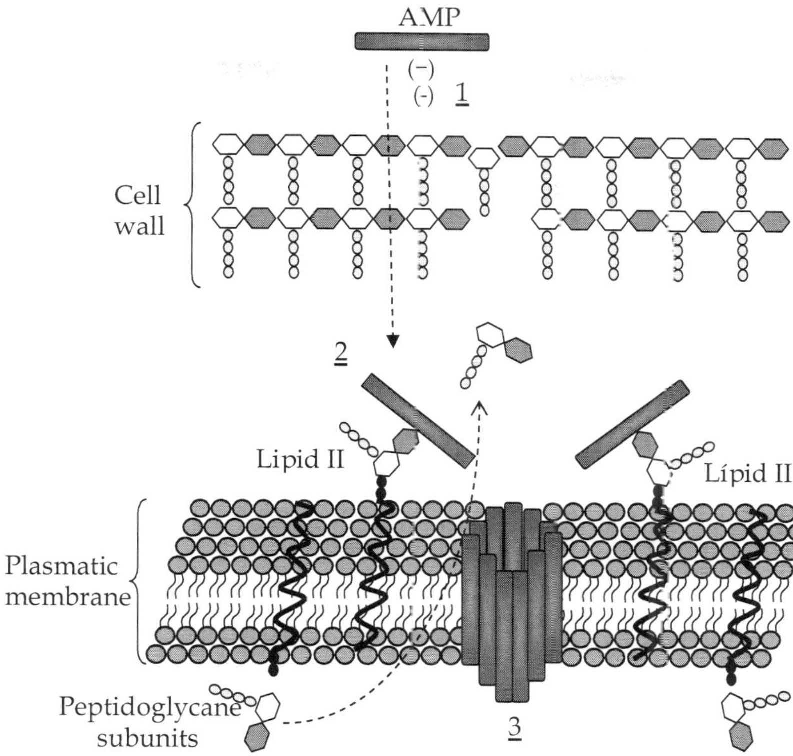

Fig. 2. Model showing the dual action mechanism of nisin from *Lactococcus lactis*. Stage 1, nisin has a net positive charge that increases its interaction with the negative charges of the cell wall components. Stage 2, nisin binds to lipid II, the main transporter of peptidoglycan subunits from the cytoplasm to the cell wall, interfering with its synthesis, leading the bacteria to cell death. Stage 3, in addition, several nisin molecules use lipid II to anchor and insert themselves into the cell membrane and begin the formation of pores, leading the bacteria to a rapid cell death (Wiedemann et al., 2001; Cotter et al., 2005a)

resistant to conventional antibiotic therapy, making them an attractive option as antimicrobial agents (Table 2) (Cotter et al., 2005a, b; Piper et al., 2009). Broad spectrum AMPs or bioengineered AMPs could be used against Gram positive pathogens of humans and animals. For example, lacticin 3147 from *L. lactis* has shown *in vitro* activity against methicillin-resistant *Staphylococcus aureus* (MRSA); vancomycin-resistant enterococci (VRE); vancomycin-intermediate *S. aureus* (VISA); streptococci, *S. pneumoniae, S. pyogenes, S. agalactiae, S. dysgalactiae, S. uberis, S. mutans; Clostridium botulinum* and *Propionibacterium acnes* (Galvin et al., 1999; Piper et al., 2009). In the same way, it has been created two nisin variants by bioengineered (nisin V and nisin T) with enhanced antimicrobial activity against Gram positive pathogens like MRSA, VRE, VISA, *Clostridium difficile, L. monocytogenes* and *B. cereus* (Field et al., 2010).

AMPs and producing strain	Activity	Potential biomedical applications
Nisin *L. lactis*	Inhibits Gram positive and Gram negative bacteria, including *Helicobacter pylori*	Bacterial mastitis, oral hygiene, treatment of methicillin-resistant *Staphylococcus*, enterococcal infections, topical formulations, deodorants and cosmetics, treatment of peptic ulcers and enterocolitis
Epidermin *S. epidermidis*	Inhibits *Propionibacterium acnes*, staphylococci, streptococci	Acne, folliculitis, impetigo
Mersacidin *Bacillus* spp.	Inhibits staphylococci and streptococci strains	Treatment of methicillin-resistant *Staphylococcus aureus* and streptococcal infections
Cinamicin *Streptomyces cinnamoneus*	Phospholipase A2 inhibitor, angiotensin and HSV converting enzyme	Inflammation reduction, blood pressure regulation and viral infection treatment

Table 2. A few Gram positive AMPs examples and their potential biomedical use (Cotter et al., 2005a)

On the other hand, *in vivo* experiments using animal models have shown positive results after using lantibiotics, such as mersacidin and nisin in the treatment of respiratory tract infections caused by *S. aureus* MRSA (Kruszewska et al., 2004; De Kwaadsteniet et al., 2009), and *Streptococcus pneumonia* (Goldstein et al., 1998), in addition to skin care and oral therapies, such as tooth paste for prevention of teeth loss, bad breath and gingivitis (Howell et al., 1993; Arauz et al., 2009). Likewise, nisin has showed that has the potential for treatment of human mastitis (Fernández et al., 2008).

The Oragenics pharmaceutical company has realized extensive preclinical testing on the lantibiotic mutacin MU1140 of *S. mutans,* which has demonstrated activity against wide variety of disease-causing Gram positive bacteria, including MRSA, VRE, *Mycobacterium tuberculosis,* and anthrax. For the complete trials, this company has created the synthetic version MU1140-S, and they expect to conclude the preclinical testing in 2011. Likewise, in New Zealand, the BLIS K12® dietary supplement is sold as an inhibitor of bacteria responsible for bad breath, because it contains a strain of *S. salivarus* that produces salivaricin A2 and B peptides (Tagg, 2004).

In relation to animal disease, several AMPs have been proposed as potential alternatives to bovine mastitis control. Nisin has activity against mastitis pathogens and has been formulated in Wipe Out® and Mast Out®, commercially available products (Ryan et al., 1998; Wu et al., 2007). Also, AMPs produced by *S. aureus, S. epidermidis* and *Streptococcus gallolyticus* have been tested against strains of both *S. aureus* and *Streptococcus* species

isolated from bovine mastitis (Varella et al., 2007; Pieterse et al., 2008). Finally, *B. thuringiensis* AMPs have showed inhibitory action against *S. aureus* isolates from bovine mastitis (Barboza-Corona et al., 2009).
From a non antimicrobial medical perspective, AMPs such as cinamicin may have different biomedical applications, because this peptide inhibits the function of phospholipase A2 and the angiotensin converting enzyme, which are involved in the immune system and in maintaining blood pressure in humans, respectively; so that they could be used in inflammatory processes and in blood pressure regulation (Ernahar et al., 2000) (Table 2). In the same way, nisin has shown contraceptive activity (Gupta et al., 2009) and protector activity in rabbits and mice vaginas in *in vitro* and *in vivo* studies (Reddy et al., 2004).

3. AMPs from Gram negative bacteria and their classification

The term "bacteriocinogenicity" is used to describe the ability of Gram negative bacteria to synthesize and excrete AMPs (Daeschel et al., 1990). These molecules were first detected in *Escherichia coli* and were called colicins. Later, they were found in Gram positive bacteria and have been studied with great interest, especially those produced by lactic acid bacteria, which can be used in food preservation because its activity against Gram negative bacteria, the leading cause of food poisoning (Hardy, 1975; Tagg et al., 1976). Colicin V from *E. coli* and pyocin from *Pseudomonas aeruginosa*, are the two best studied peptides in the Gram negative bacteria group (Table 3) (Jack et al., 1995).
The colicin group has been taken as the representative group of Gram negative AMPs, although there are differences between them. Pyocins are AMPs of high molecular weight synthesized by *P. aeruginosa* strains, which could participate in establishing and protection of bacteria. There are three types of pyocins: R, F and S, which resemble the tails of bacteriophages of the Myoviridae family. Type R pyocins show broad similarities with the fibers of the tails of these phages. Type R pyocins are contractile and not flexible, the F type are flexible, but are not contractile; and the S type are susceptible to proteases (Michel-Briand & Baysse, 2002; Waite & Curtis, 2009).
The colicins are proteins between 29 and 90 kDa, which have binding, transport and specific activity domains, same as those found in pyocins. The secretion of colicins is carried out in cell lysis, which involves their death (Riley & Wertz, 2002; Sano et al., 1993). Other kind of AMPs produced by *E. coli* and other enterobacteria are the microcins, which are a group of circular peptides, from which microcin J25, produced by *E. coli* AY25, has been taken as a model (Craik et al., 2003). Microcins are low molecular weight molecules under 10 kDa, which play an important role in competition for colonization of the gastrointestinal tract. They are generally hydrophobic, highly stable in relation to heat, extreme pH and proteases (Duquesne et al., 2007). Some other Gram negative AMPs are: Serracin P, produced by *Serratia plymithicum* J7; mundticin KS, synthesized by *Enterococcus mundtii*, NFRI 7393 and caratovoricin, produced by *Pectobacterium carotovorum* subsp. *carotovorum* (Jabrane et al., 2002; Kawamoto et al., 2002; Yamada et al., 2008).

3.1 Genes involved in Gram negative AMPs synthesis

The genes required for colicin synthesis are encoded usually in plasmids, and consist of a colicin gene, a gene for immunity and a lysis gene. Most of the genes coding for AMPs in Gram negative bacteria probably derived from recombination of existing AMPs genes. Colicins contains a central domain (50%) involved in the recognition of the target cell receptor; a N-terminal domain (> 25%) responsible for the translocation of the peptide to the

AMPs and producing bacteria	Group	Main features
Colicin *Escherichia coli*	Group A	N-terminal domain rich in glycine (~20-40%)
	Group B	N-terminal domain rich in glycine (~10-20%)
Microcins *E. coli*	Class I	The self-immunity genes are not close to microcin structural gene
	Class IIa	Cluster of four genes encoded in plasmids
	Class IIb	Chromosomally encoded, have a complex transcriptional organization
Pyocins *P. aeruginosa*	Type R	Resemble the fibers of the tails of bacteriophages of the Myoviridae family and are contractile but are not flexible
	Type F	Flexible, but are not contractile peptides
	Type S	Susceptible to proteases

Table 3. Principal groups of Gram negative AMPs

target cell, and the rest of the protein has the lethal and immunity activities. Pyocin genes from *P. aeruginosa* PAO1 strain are found in the chromosome, are present as a group of 16 open reading frames, of which 12 are analogous to bacteriophage genes (Riley & Wertz, 2003; Williams et al., 2008). Microcins are encoded in plasmids or the chromosome; a typical gene clusters include the microcin precursor, the self-immunity factor, the secretion proteins and frequently the post-translational modification enzymes (Duquesne et al., 2007).

3.2 Synthesis and AMPs secretion from Gram negative bacteria

The production of colicins is performed under stress, reason why it is mediated by the SOS regulon (Gillor et al., 2008). The number of cells producing colicin in culture is very small, but the proportion increases when cells are exposed to stressors such as mitomycin and UV light (Jack et al., 1995). Pyocin synthesis in *P. aeruginosa* PAO1 occurs in a similar way. Synthesis starts when the stressor (which could cause damage to DNA) stimulates the expression of the RecA protein, whose main function is the repair of damaged DNA and to degrade the repressor protein (PRTR) to initiate the expression of the *prtN* activator gene; the PrtN protein then activates the expression of genes that codify for pyocins (Waite & Curtis, 2009). Microcins are also synthesized under stress conditions like a pro-microcin that is secreted to the medium after suffering a cut of 15 to 37 amino acid residues to release the active microcin; only the MccC7/C5 AMP from *E. coli* does not undergo this change (Duquesne et al., 2007; Novikova et al., 2007).

3.3 Gram negative AMPs action mechanisms

Colicins generally present three action mechanisms: some of them form pores or ion channels in the membrane, others have nuclease activity (colicin E2 and pyocin S3), others inhibit the synthesis of macromolecules (colicin E3), or as in the case of microcin, the action mode depends upon the organism that it is acting on. Microcin J25 acts on *E. coli* inhibiting RNA polymerase, while on *Salmonella enterica* forms pores in the membrane (Pugsley, 1984; Craik et al., 2003).

AMPs whose action is to form pores in the membrane destroy the organism by altering the membrane permeability, affecting the normal flow of ions like potassium, magnesium, sodium and chloride, as well as inhibiting ATP synthesis through the dissipation of the membrane electric potential and of the pH gradient. Examples of these AMPs are: glycinecin A from *Xanthomonas campestris*; A, E1, K, Ia and Ib colicins from *E. coli*, pyocin S5 from *P. aeruginosa* and xenocin from *Xenorhabdus nematophila* (Pham et al., 2004; Cascales et al., 2007; Singh & Banerjee, 2008; Zhang et al., 2010). Once released, some AMPs are attached to a membrane receptor present in the target cell, afterwards enter to the cell, usually helped by Tol-like proteins, and finally they may have access to intracellular targets (Lazaroni et al., 2002; Singh & Banerjee, 2008).

The AMPs that have nuclease activity enter to the cell and bind to tRNA or rRNA and break it at specific sites, thus inhibiting protein synthesis. Also, several AMPs can degrade nucleic acids without any specificity, for example: colicins E5, D and E7, and pyocins S1, S2, S3, S4 and AP41 (Masaki & Ogawa, 2002; Michel-Briand & Baysse, 2002; Hsia et al., 2005).

In the case of microcins, the facts that have a great diversity of post-translational modifications suggests that also have a great variety of action mechanisms; however, they show the typical nuclease and pore-formation mechanisms, although the latter is related to the production of siderophores. This dual mechanism of siderophore production and pore formation has been found in some microcins such as MccE492, produced by *Klebsiella pneumoniae* RYC492. The mechanism works as follows: the bacteria produces the siderophore to chelate environmental Fe^{3+}, thus preventing its use by other microorganisms; afterwards the siderophore undergoes post-translational modification and creates a glycopeptide capable of forming pores in the membrane of competing bacteria (Thomas et al., 2004; Duquesne et al., 2007; Nolan et al., 2007; Mercado et al., 2008).

3.4 AMPs resistance from Gram negative bacteria

Resistant mechanisms for Gram negative AMPs, different to self-immunity, have been described. It has been found some strains of *E. coli* resistant to others *E. coli* colicins, which have a Tol or Ton mechanisms altered, but is very specific and only works with the specific colicin. These resistant strains have been used to study the Tol and Ton mechanism (Braun et al., 1994). The pyocin resistant strains of *Neisseria gonorrhoeae* and *Haemophilus ducreyi*, have been found to be associated with structural differences in the outer membrane lipooligosaccharides in both species (John et al., 1991; Filiatrault et al., 2001). An *E. coli* K12 microcin resistant has been found, this strain possess a YojI protein which works as microcin J25 efflux pump (Socias et al., 2009). These examples show the variety of mechanisms displayed by bacteria to counteract the AMPs activity.

3.5 Potential Gram negative AMPs applications in biotechnology and biomedical therapies

The consumption of AMPs producing bacteria or the consumption of the purified peptides can be useful in establishing probiotic microorganisms in the gastrointestinal tract of humans and animals, which can lead to health improvements (Gillor et al., 2009). It has been found that in cystic fibrosis patients with an *P. aeruginosa* infection this organism produces pyocins that inhibit the growth of its closest competitors, so it could also be used as a therapeutic agent in these kind of patients and minimize the effects of the infection, that besides rooting out other susceptible. *P. aeruginosa* strains, also has an effect on *Haemophilus*,

Neisseria and *Campylobacter*. Regarding the latter, peritonitis treatment in mice has been successful (Scholl & Martin, 2008; Waite & Curtis, 2009; Williams et al., 2008). In other studies, colicin E1 has shown to inhibit the growth of *E. coli* O157:H7 *in vitro*, and the next step is to try it in meat and in the feeding of cattle to avoid the growth of *E. coli* O157:H7 in the gut (Callaway et al., 2004). The pyocin R-Type is studied as an antibiotic against *E. coli, Salmonella, Yersinia pestis and Pseudomonas* species by AvidBiotics Corp., with the name "Avidocin™ Proteins", but there is not still commercially available.

4. Animal and plant AMPs

As part of the defense mechanisms of multicellular organisms it can be found the production of compounds to eliminate invading microorganisms. Among these AMPs stand out; they are components of the innate immune response in higher eukaryotes. AMPs are mostly small, amphipathic and cationic peptides that possess diverse functions in addition to their antimicrobial properties. Currently, there have been over 1500 different AMPs described (Guaní-Guerra et al., 2010). Because of their great diversity, AMPs classification in higher eukaryotes has been hampered; however, five groups have been established based on their amino acid sequence and structural conformation; whereas in plants 10 families have been classified. Here are some general aspects of AMPs produced by animals and plants, emphasizing their action mechanism and their therapeutic and biomedical properties.

4.1 Animal AMPs

In animals, AMPs are produced at sites that are in constant contact with microorganisms, such as mucosal epithelial cells (respiratory, oral, genitourinary, gastrointestinal, etc.) or skin cells. In the case of insects, they are also produced in the fat body and hemocytes; and in vertebrates are produced and stored in monocytes, neutrophils, and mast cells, which constitute some of the non-oxidative effector mechanisms against potential pathogens. Animal AMPs can be produced constitutively or in response to infection (Brogden, 2005).

4.2 Animal AMPs classification

AMPs diversity is so large that their classification has been held back; however, five main groups are proposed which consist of those found in plants, vertebrates and invertebrates. These are described in Table 4, and the main representatives of the groups mentioned. Briefly, a group comprises anionic peptides including small peptides rich in glutamic and aspartic acid; a second group contains short cationic peptides (<40 residues) which lack cysteines and that in some environments adopt certain α-helical structures; a third group includes cationic peptides rich in various amino acids. There is a fourth group of anionic and cationic AMPs that present several cysteine residues, and therefore form disulfide bonds and stable α-sheets. These include most of the AMPs produced by plants as described below. Finally, there is a fifth group containing anionic and cationic peptides, which are fragments of larger proteins.

4.3 Plant AMPs

Plant AMPs are part of the defense mechanisms of these, they may be expressed constitutively or can be induced in response to a pathogen attack, and although lack of the sophistication of vertebrate adaptive immunity, they offer "fast" protection against pathogens. Compared with the production and action of secondary metabolites, AMPs can

Group	Representative AMPs	Source
Anionic peptides	Dermacidin Maximin H5	Human sweat glands Amphibians
Linear cationic peptides with α-helical structures	Melittin Magainin 2 Cecropin 37 Dermaseptin Cathelicidin LL37	Bee venom Amphibian skin Insects Amphibian skin Humans
Cationic peptides rich in certain amino acid residues	Histatin-5 (histidin rich) PR-39 (proline and arginine rich) Indolicin (triptophan rich)	Human saliva Pig neutrophils Cattle
Anionic and cationic peptides that contain cysteine and form disulfide bonds	Brevinin (1 S-S bond) Protegrin (2 S-S bonds) α and β defensins (3 S-S bonds) Defensins and Thionins (>3 S-S bonds) Drosomycin (>3 S-S bonds)	Amphibians Pigs Mammals (α and β), avians (α) Plants *Drosophila melanogaster*
Cationic and anionic peptides that are fragments of larger proteins	Lactoferricin from lactoferrin	Bovine milk

Table 4. Animal and plants AMPs classification based on amino acid composition, net charge and secondary structure (Epand & Vogel, 1999; Bradshaw, 2003; Brogden, 2005)

be released immediately after the infection is produced; they are expressed by a single gene and therefore require less biomass and energy expenditure (Thomma et al., 2002; Lay & Anderson, 2005). Most of characterized plant AMPs to date have a molecular weight in the range of 2 to 10 kDa; are basic and contain 4, 6, 8 or 12 cysteines that form disulfide bonds, giving them structural and thermodynamic stability (García-Olmedo et al., 2001; Lay & Anderson, 2005)

4.4 Plant AMPs classification

Plant AMPs are classified based on the identity of their amino acid sequence and the number and position of cysteines forming disulfide bonds. So far, 10 families have been described in plants, these are listed in Table 5 (García-Olmedo et al., 2001; Lay & Anderson, 2005). These include lipid transfer peptides (LTPs), thionins, defensins, hevein and knottin like proteins, as well as antimicrobial proteins isolated from *Macadamia integrifolia* (MBP-1) and *Impatiens balsamina* (Ib-AMP). All these AMPs exert their effect at the plasma membrane of the microorganisms that they attack, although their action mechanisms vary depending on the family. The cyclotides are members of a recently discovered peptide family rich in cysteine, commonly found in the *Rubiaceae*, *Violaceae* and *Cucurbitaceae* families; they present antibacterial and antiviral activities, as well as insecticide properties; besides containing a head-tail cyclic backbone and a knotted arrangement of three conserved disulfide bonds (Daly et al., 2009).

Family	Amino acid number	Disulfide bonds	Acitivity vs.
LTPs	90–95	3–4	Bacteria and fungi
Snakins	61–70	6	Bacteria and fungi
Defensins	45–54	4	Bacteria and fungi
Thionins	45–47	3–4	Bacteria and fungi
Hevein-like	43	4	Gram (+) bacteria and fungi
Knottin-like	36–37	3	Gram (+) bacteria and fungi
Shepherins**	28–38	0 (linear)	Bacteria and fungi
MBP-1*	33	2	Bacteria and fungi
Cyclotides	29–31	3	Bacteria, viruses and insects
Ib-AMP*	20	2	Gram (+) bacteria and fungi

Table 5. Plant AMPs families (Lay & Anderson, 2005; García-Olmedo et al., 1998; Daly et al., 2009). * One member family; **two member family, which are derived from a polypeptide precursor

Thionins were the first AMPs whose antimicrobial activity against plant pathogens was demonstrated *in vitro* (García-Olmedo et al., 2001). This class of molecules has been found in various plant tissues, such as the seed endosperm, the stem and roots; they present a three-dimensional structure that can be represented by gamma letter (γ), where the vertical portion consists of a pair of antiparallel α-helices and the short horizontal arm consists of an antiparallel β-sheet (Thevissen et al., 1996). Thionins belong to a small group of basic peptides rich in cysteine that are toxic to bacteria and phytopathogenic fungi (Vignutelli et al., 1998; Zasloff, 2002). It has been suggested that toxicity requires the electrostatic interaction of the thionins with the negative charges of the membrane, causing the formation of pores (Thevissen et al., 1996).

Plant defensins are AMPs with an approximate molecular weight of 5 kDa, they are composed of 45 to 54 amino acids; they are basic and typically have eight cysteines. γ-purotionina (γ-1P) and γ-hordotionina (γ-1H) were the first isolated defensins, which were obtained from wheat and barley grains, respectively. These AMPs have been found in all studied plants, even it is hypothesized that they are ubiquitous in the plant kingdom. They have been isolated from sorghum, pea, tobacco, potato, petunia, beet, radish and several members of the *Brassicaceae* family (García-Olmedo et al., 1998), also from broad beans (*Vicia faba*) (Zhang & Lewis, 1997) and maize (*Zea mays*) (Kushmerick et al., 1998). AMPs have been detected in various tissues, mainly in those that are most exposed to contact with pathogens such as leaf primordia, the cells adjacent to the substomatal cavity, epidermis and stomata; in addition to seeds, leaves, pods, tubers, fruit, roots and bark (García-Olmedo et al., 1998; Lay & Anderson, 2005).

In relation to shepherins, they have been isolated from *Capsella bursa-pastoris*, they are rich in glycine and histidine and show activity against Gram negative bacteria and fungi (Park et al., 2000). The snakins are peptides containing 12 cysteines, 6 disulfide bonds and have been isolated from potato. They present activity against plant pathogenic fungi and bacteria (Berrocal-Lobo et al., 2002).

4.5 Animal and plant AMPs genes

With regard to the genes that codify for animals and plants AMPs, they can be found in one or more copies with a variable intron number. In animals, it has been found that many of the genes that codify for AMPs have κB regulatory sequences, and therefore many of them are activated by NF-κB transcription factors, although it has also been reported that in higher eukaryotes there are other expression regulatory factors, such as the hypoxia-inducible factor (HIF), which regulates the expression of cathelicidins in mammals (Zarember & Malech, 2005; Hölzl et al., 2008), and the activator protein 1 (AP-1) transcription factor that regulates the expression of mammalian defensins (Wehkamp, 2004).

4.6 Animal and plant AMPs posttranslational modifications

Most studied AMPs are the product of larger proteins that contain a signal peptide, a pre-domain and a region corresponding to the mature peptide. The presence, length and relative position of these three regions varies among the different AMPs families, and only the mature peptide is the one that interacts with microorganisms (Lay & Anderson, 2005). They can also show modifications such as glycosylation, circularization, amidation of the ends and amino acid modification including D-amino acids (Boman, 1995; Nissen-Meyer & Nes, 1997).

4.7 Animal and plant AMPs action mechanisms

The nature of AMPs, based on their amino acid composition, charge and size allows them to be easily inserted into the lipid bilayer membranes of microorganisms. The general mechanism by which AMPs damage plasma membranes is considered universal for all described peptides, and is based on electrostatic interactions. In the case of bacteria, the interaction of cationic AMPs with anionic membrane phospholipids (phosphatidylglycerol and cardiolipin), and with the phosphate groups of Gram negative lipopolysaccharide (LPS), as well as the interaction with teichoic acids in Gram positive bacteria, occurs through electrostatic mechanisms, constituting the first step of action. Subsequently, peptides that are in close contact with the bacterial cell must pass through the capsular polysaccharide or teichoic and lipoteichoic acids to interact with the plasma membrane Once the peptides have contacted it they can interact with the lipid bilayer. The second step is the permeabilizaton of the membrane; this mechanism is given by the formation of pores in the membrane due to interactions and arrangements of the AMPs. This leads to cell lysis by osmotic shock (Ogata et al., 1992; Boman, 1995, 2003).

These mechanisms may vary depending on different AMPs types, their concentration and the organism with which they interact. Besides, recently novel action mechanisms have been described that include the synthesis inhibition of nucleic acids, proteins, the cell wall, as well as the activity inhibition of some other enzymes (Bradshaw, 2003; Murray & Liu, 2008). The mechanisms related to cell membrane disruption and to intracellular target interactions are described below.

The AMPs interaction with membranes has been studied mainly in cationic peptides with α-helical structures. Although the interaction mechanism may be different for each type of peptide, their main action involves the instability of the outer membrane, translocating it through the outer bilayer (Bradshaw, 2003; Téllez & Castaño, 2010); these mechanisms are explained in the "barrel-stave", "toroidal pore", "carpet", "molecular electroporation" and perforation of the" lipid raft" models, which are described below.

4.7.1 "Barrel-stave" model

This model proposes that initially, a group of cationic AMPs molecules with α-helical structures interact with each other on the surface of the plasma membrane to form a complex. Subsequently, the peptides are oriented perpendicular to the plane of the membrane allowing the hydrophobic region of the peptide to interact with the hydrophobic region of the bilayer, while the hydrophilic surface of the peptide is oriented inwards, forming a hydrophilic channel that expands along the membrane. In this way, the formed protein complex behaves as a pore inserted into the membrane. The formation of these channels causes alterations in the membrane potential, provokes the output of solutes and eventually results in cell lysis (Zhao et al., 2003) (Figure 3).

4.7.2 "Carpet" model

In this model it is proposed that cationic AMPs bind to the phospholipids in the outer layer of the membrane covering the bilayer as a "carpet", but without inserting themselves in it. At the beginning of the interaction, the peptides orient themselves parallel to the membrane. When the peptide reaches a certain critical concentration, the monomers rotate and reorient towards the hydrophobic core of the membrane causing the formation of micelles and the collapse of the membrane (Shai, 1995). The early stages of the AMP interface with the membrane are based on electrostatic interactions between the peptide positive charges and the negative charges of the membrane phospholipid heads (Shai, 1995, 1999); while pore formation is mainly governed by interactions between the hydrophobic region of the AMP and the hydrophobic center of the bilayer (Papo & Shai, 2003). The peptides that are characterized by having a "carpet"-type action mechanism have a low affinity for zwitterionic lipids in comparison with acidic lipids (Zhao et al., 2003). This model describes the action mechanism of most cationic AMPs, including dermaseptin from the skin of amphibians and insect cecropin. The "carpet" model (Figure 4) may explains the action mechanism of peptides with a size of less than 23 or 24 amino acid residues that do not cross the plasma membrane and whose action mechanism cannot be explained by the "barrel-stave" model (Zhao et al., 2003).

4.7.3 "Toroidal pore" model

The "toroidal pore" model explains the action mechanism of cationic peptides with α-helical structures and from those that form disulfide bonds. Initially, the peptide orients itself parallel to the plane of the plasma membrane and binds to the region of the phospholipid polar heads in a functionally inactive state. When the threshold of a peptide-lipid molar ratio is exceeded (e.g., 1:30 for magainin 2), the peptides are reoriented perpendicular to the plane of the bilayer, and in conjunction with several surrounding lipids they invert themselves towards the interior of the membrane's hydrophobic region. This forms a "dynamic supramolecular peptide-lipid complex", which causes the irreversible rupture of the membrane. The transition between the inactive and active state of the peptide bound to the membrane depends on AMPs concentration and the phospholipid composition of the bilayer (Huang, 2000).

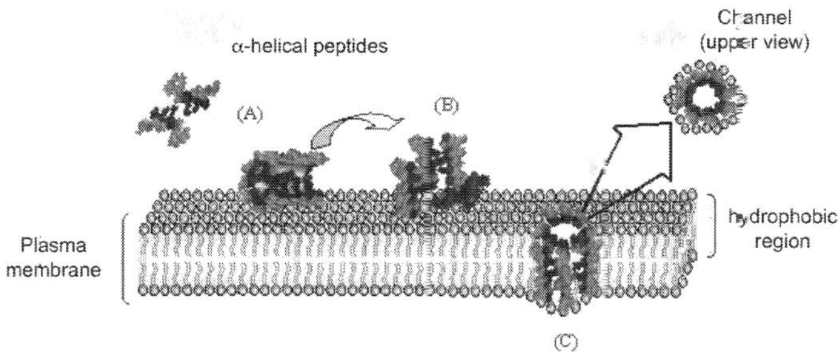

Fig. 3. Schematic representation of the "barrel stave" model explaining the interaction of antimicrobial peptides with bacterial membranes. In a first step (recruitment), the peptide monomers are joined together on the surface of the outer membrane of the bilayer. This process is governed primarily by the interaction of the peptide hydrophilic regions (shown in black), the recruited peptides are oriented parallel to the plane of the bilayer (panel A), when sufficient peptides are recruited (at least three of them) the peptide complex undergoes a perpendicular re-orientation to the plasma membrane (panel B), and finally the complex enters through the hydrophobic region of the bilayer (inset), forming a channel (panel C). Modified from Zhao et al., 2003

According to this model, the pores are formed by rows of lipids interposed to the peptides, which are oriented perpendicularly to the surface of the membrane, allowing the interaction of the hydrophilic regions of the pore with the polar heads of the phospholipids; which causes the lipid heads and the polar face of the α-helix, in the case of cationic peptides, to become oriented towards the pore's interior. As a result, the outside and interior faces of the bilayer become a continuous layer that delimits the interior of the pore. The newly formed pore allows for a coupled lipid and peptide transport across the bilayer with an increase of transmembrane movement of phospholipids ("flip-flop") and the orientation of the peptide monomers towards the interior of the bilayer. This arrangement differs from the classical channel depicted in the "barrel-stave" model (Figure 5); where interactions occur mainly between the hydrophobic face of the pore and the acyl chains of the bilayer's lipid core (Zhao et al., 2003). The magnitude, duration and required concentration for pore formation depends on the peptide, but is generally considered that the multipore state is the most stable structure and is formed when high concentrations of the peptide exist. However, individual pores may have a short lifetime and allow ion diffusion (Matsuzaki et al., 1997).

4.7.4 "Molecular electroporation" model

In this model, cationic AMPs are associated to the bacterial membrane generating an electric potential difference across it. The pore is generated when the potential difference reaches 0.2 V (Murray et al., 2008).

4.7.5 "Lipid raft" perforation model

This model proposes that the binding of an amphipathic AMP causes a mass imbalance and therefore an increase in the curvature of the membrane, which provides sufficient force to it to translocate through itself. Since AMPs self-associate, in this model they would sink into the membrane, generating a transient pore in which the peptides would be in both sides of it

(Murray & Liu, 2008). Moreover, there is growing evidence that indicates that AMPs have intracellular targets in addition to their plasma membrane interactions, because targets have been identified within microbial cells, and also because this mechanism explains why AMPs can enter the microbial cell without affecting its outer structure by passive transport (Nicolas, 2009).

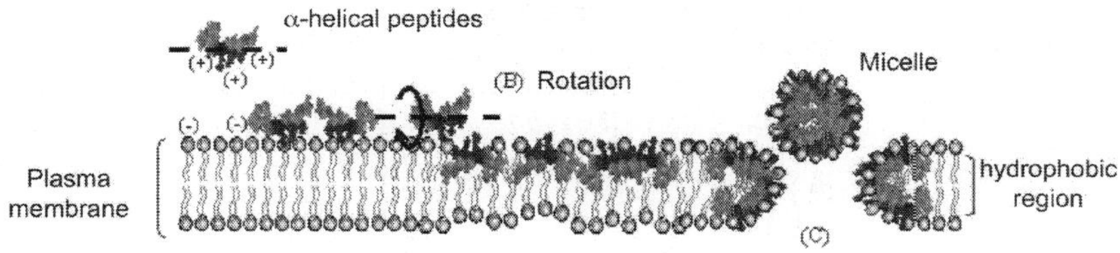

Fig. 4. Schematic representation of the "carpet" model explaining the interaction between antimicrobial peptides and bacterial membranes. This model describes the interaction that occurs between the positive charges of the α-helical cationic peptides and negatively charged polar phospholipid heads, which are oriented towards the outside of the membranes. Bound peptides remain parallel to the outer membrane of the bilayer (panel A), when they reach a critical concentration, the peptides rotate on their axis, causing the phospholipids bound to them to redirect (panel B), this shift produces the collapse of the structure of the plasma membrane and the formation of micelles with a hydrophobic core, forming a pore in the membrane (panel C). Modified from Zhao et al., 2003

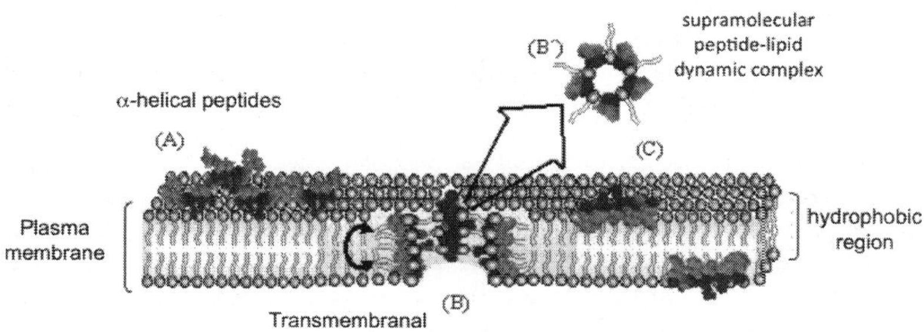

Fig. 5. Schematic representation of the "toroidal pore" model describing the interaction of antimicrobial peptides with bacterial membranes. This model, also known as a "two stage" model, describes the transition of the peptide from an inactive state to an active state. At low concentrations (inactive state), the peptides are oriented parallel to the plane of the bilayer (panel A). When they reaches a critical concentration, the peptide molecules are reoriented perpendicularly penetrating the hydrophobic region of the bilayer (active state) and together with some lipid molecules they adopt a multipore transitional state, known as a supramolecular peptide-lipid dynamic complex (panel B '), this produces the irreversible rupture of the plasma membrane and an increase in the "transmembranal movement" of lipids (two-headed arrow) (panel B). As a result of this increased "transmembranal movement" of lipids an orientation of the peptide molecules towards the inner layer of the bilayer may occur (panel C). Modified from Zhao et al., 2003

Two general mechanisms have been proposed to describe the process by which AMPs enter microbial cells: 1) spontaneous assisted translocation by lipids, and 2) a stereospecific receptor-mediated endocytosis. These internalization mechanisms vary depending on the peptide type and the target cell. In addition, the AMPs amino acid composition plays a crucial role in the internalization, since they are composed mainly of basic amino acids (principally arginine), AMPs can interact in a better way with membrane lipids allowing them to pass inside (Nicolas, 2009).
Once AMPs access the interior of the microbial cells, they interfere in metabolic functions such as: cytoplasm alteration, intracellular content agglutination, signaling pathways modification, regulation of transcription and inhibition of the transcription process, cell wall synthesis, nucleic acid synthesis, protein synthesis or enzyme activity (Brogden, 2005).

4.7.6 Other plant and animal AMPs action mechanisms

It has been reported that some AMPs from plants and insects carry out their effects through specific receptors localized in the membranes of some fungi. Such is the case of plant defensins RsAFP2 and DmAMP1 from *Raphanus sativus* and *Dahlia merckii* respectively, and the insect defensin heliomicin from *Helicthis virescens*; which interact with specific sphingolipids of plant and animal pathogenic fungi (Thevissen et al., 2007).
Many antimicrobial peptides are ineffective in normal mammalian cells. This seems to be related mainly to the lipid composition of target membrane (i.e. fluidity, negative charge density and the presence or absence of cholesterol), and to present a highly negative transmembrane electric potential (Nicolas, 2009). In tumor cells, AMPs interact with the membrane of cancer cells, which contain a small amount of phosphatidylserine giving them a greater negative charge compared to normal cells. In addition, cancer cells contain O-glycosylated mucins that attract serines and threonines from the AMPs. Another possible explanation for the peptide interaction with cancer cells is the high number of microvilli present in them, compared to normal cells, which increases the bonding surface of cancer cell membranes for AMPs (Papo & Shai, 2005).
The action mechanism of AMPs may also vary depending on their concentration, for example, at high concentrations the peptides can "carpet" the plasma membrane quickly generating micelles, causing cell lysis. On the other hand, at low concentrations, AMPs can slowly form pores in the membrane, they can also insert their polar region between phospholipids through the membrane from side to side causing the thinning of it, or they can cross the cell membrane without causing damage and attack or block an intracellular target (Hancock & Rozek, 2002; Brogden, 2005). It has also been shown that some AMPs regulate diverse functions of innate immunity such as neutrophil, mast cell or monocyte chemotaxis; they induce phagocytosis, are involved in tissue repair and angiogenesis, they can show anti-inflammatory properties and in some cases stimulate the production of cytokines and increase vascular permeability (Nicolas, 2009; Téllez & Castaño, 2010; Hölzl, 2008).

4.8 Resistance mechanisms towards animal and plant AMPs

Although AMPs production is an essential component of the plant and animal immunity, microorganisms, particularly bacteria, have developed various resistance mechanisms to them. These include mechanisms against AMP adhesion and insertion, as well as mechanisms that modify membrane permeability. In this sense, some bacteria have developed modifications in the net charge on their surface, changes in membrane proteins, proteolytic enzyme production, removal of AMPs by transporters, etc. (Brogden, 2005).

4.9 Potential application of plant and animal AMPs in biomedical therapies

The potential usefulness of plant and animal AMPs clinical purposes resides in their use as antimicrobial agents, alone or in synergy with existing antibiotics. Similarly they can be employed as immunomodulatory agents or bacterial toxin neutralizers. Because many of them have low toxicity towards normal eukaryotic cells, but not for tumor cells, their use as anticancer drugs has been considered (Schweizer, 2009).

AMPs offer a good alternative for treating infections in relation to conventional antibiotics based on their broad spectrum activity and quick efficiency. However, very few plant and animal AMPs or synthetic derivatives of these have applications in clinical trials (Gordon et al., 2005). This follows the fact that they are susceptible to proteolysis, and that because of their chemical characteristics, their activity depends on the serum concentration of salts, or the pH of the medium in which they occur. For this reason the most promising AMPs in clinical evaluations are the ones that apply topically (Hancock & Sahl, 2006).

However, despite promising AMPs application, there are none currently approved for human use by the Food and Drug Administration (FDA). Only an AMP with topical application has shown efficiency in Phase III trials: AMP MX-226 (Omiganan pentahydrochloride, 1% gel; Migenix Laboratories), a synthetic peptide based on bovine indolicin and developed to prevent infections caused by the use of catheters. AMP synthetic derivatives are based on modifications to their three-dimensional structure and their biochemical properties, in order to show more stability and activity in different environments (Hancock & Sahl, 2006; Marr et al., 2006; Téllez & Castaño, 2010). Additionally, currently the possibility of inducing the endogenous production of AMPs is being considered, such is the case for the administration of sodium butyrate to induce the production of intestinal AMPs for the treatment of infectious or inflammatory diseases (Guaní-Guerra et al., 2010).

In the case of plant biotechnology transgenic plants resistant to diseases and pests have been produced through the introduction of AMPs genes from other plant species or even human defensins have been expressed in experimental models, and a better response to the attack of fungal pathogens has been observed (Aerts et al., 2007). Moreover, through biotechnological approaches, plant defensins and thionins have been expressed in mammalian cells in our working group; which showed activity against bacteria, fungi and tumor cells (Anaya-López et al., 2006; Loeza-Ángeles et al., 2008).

Among the studies that have been done with transgenic animals, those that demonstrate the protection conferred by human lactoferrin expressed in bovine mammary gland, conveying a delayed onset of clinical signs and inflammation caused by intramammary bacteria, stand out (Simojoki et al., 2010). In addition, bovine lactoferricin has been used in aquaculture to produce fish resistant to various infections (Lin et al., 2010).

5. Conclusion

AMPs are structurally diverse molecules, whose characteristics place them as a current and potential alternative to combat infections caused by pathogens resistant to conventional antibiotics. In addition, diverse AMPs have shown biological properties different to antimicrobial activity, which positions them as tools for new biomedical therapies such as the modulation of the immune response, improved conventional antibiotic treatments, development of anticancer and anti-inflammatory therapies, the regulation of blood pressure and other biotechnological developments. Therefore, AMPs benefits in the biomedical area are well known; however, for the therapeutic application to succeed there is a multitude of their effects remains to be studied, as well as their biological and chemical characteristics in order to elucidate their action mechanisms.

6. Acknowledgements

This publication was supported by grants from CONACyT to A.O.Z (83895) and J.E.L.M (101451).

7. References

Aerts, A.; Thevissen, K.; Bresseleers, S.; Sels, J.; Wouters, P.; Cammue, B. & François, I. (2007). *Arabidopsis thaliana* plants expressing human beta-defensin-2 are more resistant to fungal attack: functional homology between plant and human defensins. *Plant & Cell Reports,* Vol. 26, No. 8, 1391-1398, 0721-7714.

Anaya-López, J.; López-Meza, J.; Baizabal-Aguirre, V.; Cano-Camacho, H. & Ochoa-Zarzosa, A. (2006). Fungicidal and cytotoxic activity of a *Capsicum chinense* defensin expressed by endothelial cells. *Biotechnology Letters,* Vol. 28, No. 14, 1101-1108, 0141-5492.

Arauz, L.; Jozala, A.; Mazzola, P. & Vessoni, T. (2009). Nisin biotechnological production and applications: a review. *Trends in Food Science & Technology,* Vol. 20, No. 3-4, 146-154, 0924-2244.

Barboza-Corona, J.; de la Fuente-Salcido, N.; Alva-Murillo, N.; Ochoa-Zarzosa, A. & López-Meza, J. (2009). Activity of bacteriocins synthesized by *Bacillus thuringiensis* against *Staphylococcus aureus* isolates associated to bovine mastitis. *Veterinary Microbiology,* Vol. 138, No. 2, 179-183, 0378-1135.

Berrocal-Lobo, M.; Segura, A.; Moreno, M.; López, M.; García-Olmedo, F. & Molina, A. (2002). Snakin-2, an antimicrobial peptide from potato whose gene is locally induced by wounding and responds to pathogen infection. *Plant physiology,* Vol. 128, No. 3, 951-961, 0032-0889.

Bhunia, A.; Johnson, M.; Ray, B. & Belden, E. (1990). Antigenic property of pediocin AcH produced by *Pediococcus acidilactici* H. *Journal of Applied Microbiology,* Vol. 69, No. 2, 211-215, 1364-5072.

Bierbaum, G. & Sahl, H. (2009). Lantibiotics: mode of action, biosynthesis and bioengineering. *Current Pharmaceutical Biotechnology,* Vol. 10, No. 1, 2-18, 1389-2010.

Boman, H. (1995). Peptide antibiotics and their role in innate immunity. *Annual Review of Immunology,* Vol. 13, 61-92, 0732-0582.

Boman, H. (2003). Antibacterial peptides: basic facts and emerging concepts. *Journal of Internal Medicine,* Vol. 254, No. 3, 197-215, 1365-2796.

Bradshaw, P. (2003). Cationic antimicrobial peptides issues for potential clinical use. *Biodrugs,* Vol. 17, No. 4, 233-240, 1173-8804.

Braun, V.; Pilsl, H. & Grob, P. (1994). Colicins: structure, modes of action, transfer through membranes and evolution. *Archives of Microbiology*, Vol. 161, No. 3, 199-206, 0302-8933.

Breukink, E.; Wiedemann, I.; Van Kraaij, C.; Kuipers, O.; Sahl, H. & Kruijff, B. (1999). Use of the cell wall precursor lipid II by a pore-forming peptide antibiotic. *Science*, Vol. 286, No. 5448, 2361-2364, 0036-8075.

Brogden, K. (2005). Antimicrobial peptides: pore formes or metabolic inhibitors in bacteria? *Nature Reviews Microbiology*, Vol. 3, No. 3, 238-250, 1740-1526.

Brotz, H.; Bierbaum, G.; Markus, A.; Molitor, E. & Sahl, H. (1995). Mode of action of the lantibiotic mersacidin-inhibition of peptidoglycan biosynthesis via a novel mechanism. *Antimicrobial Agents and Chemotherapy*, Vol. 39, No. 3, 714-719, 0066-4804.

Callaway, T.; Stahl, C.; Edrington, T.; Genovese, K.; Lincoln, L.; Anderson, R.; Lonergan, S.; Poole, T.; Harvey, R. & Nisbet, D. (2004). Colicin concentrations inhibit growth of *Escherichia coli* O157:H7 *in vitro*. *Journal of Food Protection*, Vol. 67, No. 11, 2603-2607, 0362-028X.

Cascales, E.; Buchanan, S.; Duché, D.; Kleanthous, C.; Lloubès, R.; Postle, K.; Riley, M.; Slatin, S. & Cavard, D. (2007). Colicin biology. *Microbiology and Molecular Biology Reviews*, Vol. 71, No. 1, 158-229, 1092-2172.

Cotter, P.; Hill, C. & Ross, R. (2005a). Bacterial lantibiotics: strategies to improve therapeutic potential. *Current Protein and Peptides Science*, Vol. 6, No. 1, 61-75, 1389-2037.

Cotter, P.; Hill, C. & Ross, R. (2005b). Bacteriocins: Developing innate immunity for food. *Nature Reviews Microbiology*, Vol. 3, 777-788, 1740-1526.

Craik, D.; Daly, N.; Saska, I.; Trabi, M. & Rosengren K. (2003). Structures of naturally occurring circular proteins from bacteria. *Journal of Bacteriology*, Vol. 185, No. 14, 4011-4021, 0021-9193.

Daeschel, M.; McKenney, M. & McDonald, L. (1990). Bacteriocidal activity of *Lactobacillus plantarum* C-11. *Food Microbiology*, Vol. 7, No. 2, 91-98, 0740-0020.

Dalet, K.; Cenatiempo, Y.; Cossart, P. & Hechard, Y. 2001. A σ^{54}-dependent PTS permease of the mannose family is responsible for sensitivity of *Listeria monocytogenes* to mesentericin Y105. *Microbiology*, Vol. 147, 3263-3269, 1350- 0872.

Daly, N.; Rosengren, J. & Craik, D. (2009). Discovery, structure and biological activities of cyclotides. *Advanced Drug Delivery Reviews*, Vol. 61, No. 11. 918-930. 0169-409X.

Datta, V.; Myskowski, S.; Kwinn, L.; Chiem, D.; Varki, N.; Kansal, R.; Kotb, M. & Nizet, V. (2005). Mutational analysis of the group A streptococcal operon encoding streptolysin S and its virulence role in invasive infection. *Molecular Microbiology*, Vol. 56, No. 3, 681-695, 0950-382X.

De Kwaadsteniet, M.; Doeschate, K. & Dicks, L. (2009). Nisin F in the treatment of respiratory tract infections caused by *Staphylococcus aureus*. *Letters in Applied Microbiology*, Vol. 48, No. 1, 65-70, 0266-8254.

De Lucca, A. & Walsh, T. (1999). Antifungal peptides: Novel therapeutic compounds against emerging pathogens. *Antimicrobial Agents and Chemotherapy*, Vol. 43, No. 1, 24-29, 0066-4804.

Drider, D.; Fimland, G.; Hechard, Y.; McMullen, L. & Prevost, H. (2006). The continuing story of class IIa bacteriocins. *Microbiology and Molecular Biology Reviews*, Vol. 70, No. 2, 564-582, 1092-2172.

Duquesne, S.; Destoumieux-Garzón, D.; Peduzzi, J. & Rebuffat, S. (2007). Microcins, gene-encoded antibacterial peptides from enterobacteria. *Natural Products Report*, Vol. 24, No. 4, 708-734, 0265-0568.

Ennahar, S.; Sashihara, T.; Sonomoto, K. & Ishizaki, A. (2000). Class IIa bacteriocins: biosynthesis, structure and activity. *FEMS Microbiology Reviews*, Vol. 24, No. 1, 85-106, 0168-6445.

Enserink, M. (1999). Promising antibiotic candidate identified. *Science*, Vol. 286, No. 5448, 2245-2247, 0036-8075.

Epand, R. & Vogel, H. (1999). Diversity of antimicrobial peptides and their mechanisms of action. *Biochimica et Biophysica Acta*, Vol. 1462, No. 1-2, 11-28, 0005-2736.

Fernández, L.; Delgado, S.; Herrero, H.; Maldonado, A. & Rodríguez, J. (2008). The bacteriocin nisin, an effective agent for the treatment for staphylococcal mastitis during lactation. *Journal of Human Lactation*, Vol. 24, No. 3, 311-316, 0890-3344.

Field, D.; Quigley, L.; O'Connor, P.; Rea, M.; Daly, K.; Cotter, P.; Hill, C. & Ross, R. (2010). Studies with bioengineered nisin peptides highlight the broad-spectrum potency of nisin V. *Microbial Biotechnology*, Vol. 3, No. 4, 473-486, 1751-7915.

Filiatrault, M.; Munson, R. & Campagnari, A. (2001). Genetic analysis of a pyocin-resistant lipooligosaccharide (LOS) mutant of *Haemophilus ducreyi*: restoration of full-length LOS restores pyocin sensitivity. *Journal of Bacteriology*, Vol. 183, No. 19, 5756-5761, 0021-9193.

Galvin, M.; Hill, C. & Ross, R. (1999). Lacticin 3147 displays activity in buffer against Gram-positive bacterial pathogens which appear insensitive in standard plate assays. *Letters in Applied Microbiology*, Vol. 28, No. 5, 355-358, 0266-8254.

García-Olmedo, F.; Molina, A.; Alamillo, M. & Rodríguez, F. (1998). Plant defense peptides. *Biopolymers*, Vol. 47, No. 6, 479-491, 0006-3525.

García-Olmedo, F.; Rodríguez, P.; Molina, A.; Alamillo, J.; López, E.; Berrocal, M. & Poza, C. (2001). Antibiotic activities of peptides, hydrogen peroxide and peroxynitrite in plant defence. *FEBS Letters*, Vol. 498, No. 2-3, 219-222, 0014-5793.

Gillor, O.; Giladi, I. & Riley, M. (2009). Persistence of colicinogenic *Escherichia coli* in the mouse gastrointestinal tract. *BMC Microbiology*, Vol. 9, 165-171, 1471-2180.

Gillor, O.; Virezen, J. & Riley, M. (2008). The role of SOS boxes in enteric bacteriocin regulation. *Microbiology*, Vol. 154, No. 6, 1783-1792, 1350-0872.

Goldstein, B.; Wei, J.; Greenberg, K. & Novick, R. 1998. Activity of nisin against *Streptococcus pneumoniae, in vitro*, and in a mouse infection model. *Journal of Antimicrobial Chemotherapy*, Vol. 42, No. 2, 277-278, 0305-7453.

Gordon, Y.; Romanowski, E. & Mcdermott, A. (2005). A review of antimicrobial peptides and their therapeutic potential as anti-infective drugs. *Current Eye Research*, Vol. 30, No. 7, 505-515, 0271-3683.

Gravesen, A.; Axelsen, J.; Méndez, D.; Hansen, T. & Knochel, S. (2002). Frequency of bacteriocin resistance development and associated fitness costs in *Listeria monocytogenes*. *Applied and Environmental Microbiology*, Vol. 68, No. 2, 756-764, 0099-2240.

Guaní-Guerra, E.; Santos-Mendoza, T.; Lugo-Reyes, S. & Terán, L. (2010). Antimicrobial peptides: General overview and clinical implications in human health and disease. *Clinical Immunology*, Vol. 135, No. 1, 1-11, 1521-6616.

Gupta, S.; Arahna, C.; Bellare, J. & Reddy, K. (2009). Interaction of contraceptive antimicrobial peptide nisin with target cell membranes: implications for use as vaginal microbiocide. *Contraception*, Vol. 80, No. 3, 299-307, 0010-7824.

Hancock, R. & Rozek, A. (2002). Role of membranes in the activities of antimicrobial cationic peptides. *FEMS Microbiology Letters*, Vol. 206, No. 2, 143-149, 1574-6968.

Hancock, R. & Sahl, H. (2006). Antimicrobial and host-defense peptides as new anti-infective therapeutic strategies. *Nature Biotechnology*, Vol. 24, No. 12, 1551-1557, 1087-0156.

Hardy, K. (1975). Colicinogeny and related phenomena. *Bacteriological Reviews*, Vol. 39, No. 4, 464-515, 0005-3678.

Hastings, J.; Sailer, M.; Johnson, K.; Roy, K.; Vederas, J. & Stiles, M. (1991). Characterization of leucocin A-UAL 187 and cloning of the bacteriocin gene from *Leuconostoc gelidum*. *Journal of Bacteriology*, Vol. 171, No. 23, 7497-7500, 0021-9193.

Heuer, O.; Hammerum, A.; Collignon, P. & Wegener, H. (2006). Human health hazard from antimicrobial-resistant enterococci in animals and food. *Clinical Infectious Diseases*, Vol. 43, No. 7, 911-916, 1058-4838.

Holo, H.; Nilssen, O. & Nes, I. (1991). Lactococcin A, a new bacteriocin from *Lactococcus lactis* subsp. *cremoris* isolation and characterization of the protein and its gene. *Journal of Bacteriology*, Vol. 173, No. 12, 3879-3887, 0021-9193.

Hölzl, M.; Hofer, J.; Steinberger, P.; Pfistershammer, K. & Zlabinger, G. (2008). Host antimicrobial proteins as endogenous immunomodulators. *Immunology Letters*, Vol. 119 No. 1-2, 4-11, 0165-2478.

Howell, T.; Fiorellini, J.; Blackburn, P.; Projan, S.; De la Jarpe, J. & William, R. (1993). The effect of a mouthrinse based on nisin, a bacteriocin, on developing plaque and gingivitis in beagle dogs. *Journal of Clinical Periodontology*, Vol. 20, No. 5, 335-339, 0303-6979.

Hsia, K.; Li, C. & Yuan, H. (2005). Structural and functional insight into sugar-nonespecific nucleases in host defense. *Current Opinion in Structural Biology*, Vol. 15, No. 1, 126-134, 0959-440X.

Huang, H. (2000). Action of antimicrobial peptides: two-state model. *Biochemistry*, Vol. 39, No. 29, 8347-8352, 0006-2960.

Hühne, K.; Axelsson, L.; Holck, A. & Kröckel, L. (1996). Analysis of the sakacin P gene cluster from *Lactobacillus sake* Lb674 and its expression in sakacin-negative *L. sake* strains. *Microbiology*, Vol. 142, 1437-1448, 1350-0872.

Jabrane, A.; Sabri, A.; Compère, P.; Jacques, P.; Vandenberghe, I.; Van Beeumen, J. & Thonart, P. (2002). Characterization of Serracin P, a phage-tail-like bacteriocin, and its activity against *Erwinia amylovora*, the fire blight pathogen. *Applied and Environmental Microbiology*, Vol. 68, No. 11, 5704-5710, 0099-2240.

Jack, R.; Tagg, J. & Ray, B. (1995). Bacteriocins of Gram-positive bacteria. *Microbiology and Molecular Biology Reviews*, Vol. 59, No. 2, 171-200, 1092-2172.

Jenssen, H.; Hamill, P. & Hancock, E. (2006). Peptide antimicrobial agents. *Clinical Microbiology Reviews*, Vol. 19, No. 3, 491-511, 0893-8512.

John, C.; Griffisst, J.; Apicellaq, M.; Mandrelig, R. & Gibson B. (1991). The Structural Basis for Pyocin Resistance in *Neisseria gonorrhoeae* Lipooligosaccharides. *Journal of Biological Chemistry*, Vol. 266, No. 29, 19303-19311, 0021-9258.

Kawamoto, S.; Shima, J.; Sato, R.; Eguchi, T.; Ohmomo, S.; Shibato, J.; Horikoshi, N.; Takeshita, K. & Sameshima, T. (2002). Biochemical and genetic characterization of Mundticin KS, an antilisterial peptide produced by *Enterococcus mundtii* NFRI 7393. *Applied and Environmental Microbiology*, Vol. 68, No. 8, 3830-3840, 0099-2240.

Klaenhammer, T. (1988). Bacteriocins of acid lactic bacteria. *Biochimie*, Vol., 70, No. 3, 337-349, 0300-9084.

Kleerebezem, K. (2004). Quorum sensing control of lantibiotic production; nisin and subtilin autoregulate their own biosynthesis. *Peptides*, Vol. 25, No. 9, 1405-1414, 0196-9781.

Kruszewska, D.; Sahl, H.; Bierbaum, G.; Pag, U.; Hynes, S. & Ljungh, A. (2004). Mersacidin eradicates methicillin-resistant *Staphylococcus aureus* (MRSA) in a mouse rhinitis model. *Journal of Antimicrobial Chemotherapy*, Vol. 54, No. 3, 648-653, 0305-7453.

Kuipers, P.; De Ruyter, P.; Beerthuyzen, M. & De Vos, W. (1998). Quorum sensing-controlled gene expression in lactic acid bacteria. *Journal of Biotechnology*, Vol. 64, No. 1, 15-21, 0168-1656.

Lay, F. & Anderson, M. (2005). Defensins: Components of the innate immune system in plants. *Current Protein and Peptide Science*, Vol. 6, No. 1, 85-101, 1389-2037.

Lazzaroni, J.; Dubuisson, J. & Vianney, A. (2002). The Tol proteins of *Escherichia coli* and their involvement in the translocation of group A colicins. *Biochimie*, Vol. 84, No. 5, 391-397, 0300-9084.

Li, J.; Chikindas, M.; Ludescher, R. & Montville, T. (2002). Temperature-and surfactant-induced membrane modifications that alter *Listeria monocytogenes* nisin sesitivity by different mechanisms. *Applied and Environmental Microbiology*, Vol. 68, No. 12, 5904-5910, 0099-2240.

Lin, C.; Yang, P.; Kao, C.; Huang, H. & Tsai, H. (2010). Transgenic zebrafish eggs containing bactericidal peptide is a novel food supplement enhancing resistance to pathogenic infection of fish. *Fish & Shellfish Immunology*, Vol. 28, No. 3; 419-127, 1050-4648.

Loeza-Ángeles, H.; Sagrero-Cisneros, E.; Lara-Zárate, L.; Villagómez-Gómez, E.; López-Meza, J. & Ochoa-Zarzosa, A. (2008). Expression of thionin Thi2.1 from *Arabidopsis thaliana* in endothelial cells with antibacterial, antifungal and cytotoxic activity. *Biotechnology Letters*, Vol. 30, No. 10, 1713-1719, 0141-5492.

Maisnier, P. & Richard, J. (1996). Cell wall changes in nisin-resistant variants of *Listeria innocua* grow in the presence of high nisin concentrations. *FEMS Microbiology Letters*, Vol. 140, No. 1, 29-35, 0378-1097.

Maldonado, A.; Jiménez, D. & Ruiz, B. (2004). Induction of plantaricin production in *Lactobacillus plantarum* NC8 after coculture with specific Gram positive bacteria is mediated by autoinduction mechanism. *Journal of Bacteriology*, Vol. 186, No. 5, 1556-1564, 0021-9193.

Marki, F.; Hanni, E.; Fredenhagen, A. & Van Oostrum, J. (1991). Mode of action of the lanthionine-containing peptide antibiotics duramycin, duramycin B, duramycin C, and cinnamycin as direct inhibitors of phospholipase A2. *Biochemical Pharmacology*, Vol. 42, No. 10, 2027-2035, 0006-2952.

Marr, A.; Gooderham, W. & Hancock, R. (2006). Antibacterial peptides for therapeutic use: obstacles and realistic outlook. *Current Opinion in Pharmacology*, Vol. 6, No. 5, 468-472, 1471-4892.

Masaki, H. & Ogawa, T. (2002). The modes of action of colicins E5 and D, and related cytotoxic tRNAses. *Biochimie*, Vol. 84, No. 5-6, 433-438, 0300-9084.

Matsuzaki, K.; Sugishita, K.; Haranda, M.; Fuji, N. & Miyajima, K. (1997). Interactions of an antimicrobial peptide, magainin 2, with outer and inner membranes of Gram-negative bacteria. *Biochimica et Biophysica Acta*, Vol. 1327, No. 1, 119-130, 0005-2736.

McAuliffe, O.; Ross, R. & Hill, C. (2001). Lantibiotics: structure, biosynthesis and mode of action. *FEMS Microbiology Reviews*, Vol. 25, No. 3, 285-308, 0168-6445.

Mercado, G.; Tello, M.; Marín, M.; Monasterio, O. & Lagos, R. (2008). The production *in vivo* of microcin E492 with antibacterial activity depends on salmochelin and EntF. *Journal of Bacteriology*, Vol. 190, No. 15, 5464–5471, 0021-9193.

Mercado, L.; Schmitt, P.; Marshall, S. & Arenas, G. (2005). Gill tissues of the mussel *Mytilus edulis chilensis*: A new source for antimicrobial peptides. *Electronic Journal of Biotechnology*, Vol. 8, No. 3, 284-290, 0717-3458.

Michel-Briand, Y. & Baysse, C. (2002). The pyocins of *Pseudomonas aeruginosa*, *Biochimie*, Vol. 84, No. 5-6, 499-510, 0300-9084.

Moll, G.; Ubbink, K.; Hilden, H.; Nissen, M.; Nes, I.; Konings, W. & Driessen, A. (1996). Lactococcin G is a potassium ion-conducting, two-component bacteriocin. *Journal of Bacteriology*, Vol. 178, No. 3, 600-605, 0021-9193.

Montovani, H. & Rusell, J. (2001). Nisin resistance of *Streptococcus bovis*. *Applied and Environmental Microbiology*, Vol. 67, No. 2, 808-813, 0099-2240.

Motta, M.; Lapointe, G.; Lacroix, C. & Lavoine, M. (2000). MICs of mutacin B-Ny266, nisin A, vancomycin and oxacillin against bacterial pathogens. *Antimicrobial Agents and Chemotherapy*, Vol. 44, No. 1, 24-29, 0066-4804.

Murray, R. & Liu, C. (2008). Properties and applications of antimicrobial peptides in biodefense against biological warfare threat agents. *Critical Reviews in Microbiology*, Vol. 34, No. 2, 89-107, 1040-841X.

Nicolas, P. (2009). Multifunctional host defense peptides: intracellular-targeting antimicrobial peptides. *FEBS Journal*, Vol. 276, No. 22, 6483-6496, 1742-464X.

Nilsen, T.; Nes, I. & Holo, H. (1998). An exported inducer peptide regulates bacteriocin production in *Enterococcus faecium* CTC492. *Journal of Bacteriology*, Vol. 180, No. 7, 1848-1854, 0021-9193.

Nissen-Meyer, J. & Nes, I. (1997). Ribosomally synthesized antimicrobial peptides: their function, structure, biogenesis, and mechanism of action. *Archives of Microbiology*, Vol. 167, No. 2-3, 67-77, 0302-8933.

Nolan, E.; Fischbach, M.; Koglin, A. & Walsh, C. (2007). Biosynthetic tailoring of microcin E492m: post-translational modification affords an antibacterial siderophore-peptide conjugate. *Journal of the American Chemical Society*, Vol. 129, No. 46, 14336–14347, 0002-7863.

Novikova, M.; Metlitskaya, A.; Datsenko, K.; Kazakov, T.; Wanner, B. & Severinov, K. (2007). The *Escherichia coli* Yej transporter is required for the uptake of translation inhibitor microcin. *Journal of Bacteriology*, Vol. 189, No. 22, 8361–8365, 0021-9193.

Ogata, K.; Linzer, B.; Zuberi, R.; Ganz, T. & Catanzaro, S. (1992). Activity of defensins of human neutrophilic granulocytes against *Mycobacterium avium* and *Mycobacterium intracellulare*. *Infection and Immunity*, Vol. 60, No. 11, 4720-4725, 0019-9567.

Otto, M.; Peschel, A. & Gotz, F. (1998). Producer self-protection against the lantibiotic epidermin by the ABC transporter EpiFEG of *Staphylococcus epidermidis* Tu3298. *FEMS Microbiology Letters*, Vol. 166, No. 2, 203-211, 0378-1097.

Papo, N. & Shai, Y. (2003). Can we predict biological activity of antimicrobial peptides from their interactions with model phospholipid membranes? *Peptides*, Vol. 24, No. 11, 1693–1703, 0196-978.

Parisien, A.; Allain, B.; Zhang, J.; Mandeville, R. & Lan, C. (2008). Novel alternatives to antibiotics: bacteriophages, bacterial cell wall, hydrolases, and antimicrobial peptides. *Journal of Applied Microbiology*, Vol. 104, No 1, 1-13, 1364-5072.

Park, C.; Park, C.; Hong, S.; Lee, H.; Lee, S. & Kim, C. (2000). Characterization and cDNA cloning of two glycine- and histidine-rich antimicrobial peptides from the roots of shepherd's purse, *Capsella bursa-pastoris*. *Plant Molecular Biology*, Vol. 44, No. 2, 187–197, 0167-4412.

Pham, H.; Riu, K.; Jang, K.; Cho, S. & Cho, M. (2004). Bacterial activity of Glycinecin A, a bacteriocin derived from *Xanthomonas campestris* pv. glycines, on phytopathogenic *Xanthomonas campestris* pv. vesicatoric cells. *Applied and Environmental Microbiology*, Vol. 70, No. 8, 4486-4490, 0099-2240.

Pietersen, R.; Todorov, S. & Dicks, L. (2008). Bacteriocin ST91KM, produced by *Streptococcus gallolyticus* subsp. *macedonicus* ST91KM, is a narrow-spectrum peptide active against bacteria associated with mastitis in dairy cattle. *Canadian Journal of Microbiology*, Vol. 54, No. 7, 525-531, 1480-3275.

Piper, C.; Draper, L.; Cotter, P.; Ross, R. & Hill, C. (2009). A comparison of the activities of lacticin 3147 and nisin against drug-resistant *Staphylococcus aureus* and *Enterococcus* species. *Journal of Antimicrobial Chemoteraphy*, Vol. 64, No. 3, 546-551, 0305-7453.

Pugsley, A. (1984). The ins and outs of colicins. II. Lethal action, immunity and ecological implications. *Microbiological Sciences*, Vol. 1, No. 8, 203-205, 0265-1351.

Reddy, K.; Aranha, C.; Gupta, S. & Yedery, R. (2004). Evaluation of antimicrobial peptide nisin as a safe vaginal contraceptive agent in rabbits: *in vitro* and *in vivo* studies. *Reproduction*, Vol. 128, No. 1, 117-126, 1470-1626.

Riley, R. & Wertz, J. (2002). Bacteriocins: Evolution, ecology and application. *Annual Reviews of Microbiology*, Vol. 56, 117-137, 0066-4227.

Ryan, M.; Meaney, W.; Ross, R. & Hill, C. (1998). Evaluation of lacticin 3147 and a teat seal containing this bacteriocin for inhibition of mastitis pathogens. *Applied and Environmental Microbiology*, Vol. 64, No. 6, 2287-2290, 0099-2240.

Sánchez, B.; Martínez, R.; Gálvez, A.; Valdivia, E.; Maqueda, M.; Cruz, V. & Albert, A. (2003). Structure of bacteriocin AS-48: From soluble state to membrane bound state. *Journal of Molecular Biology*, Vol. 334, No. 3, 541-549, 0022-2836.

Sano, Y.; Kobayashi, M. & Kageyama, M. (1993). Functional domains of S-type pyocins deduced from chimeric molecules. *Journal of Bacteriology*, Vol. 175, No. 19, 6179-6185, 0021-9193.

Scholl, D. & Martin, W. (2008). Antibacterial efficacy or R-Type pyocins towards *Pseudomonas aeruginosa* in a murine peritonitis model. *Antimicrobial Agents and Chemotheraphy*, Vol. 52, No. 5, 1647-1652, 0066-4804.

Schweizer, F. (2009). Cationic amphiphilic peptides with cancer-selective toxicity. *European Journal of Pharmacology*, Vol. 625, No. 1-3, 190-194, 0014-2999.

Shai, Y. (1995). Molecular recognition between membrane-spanning polypeptides. *Trends in Biochemical Sciences*, Vol. 20, No. 11, 460-465, 0968-0004.

Shai, Y. (1999). Mechanism of the binding, insertion and destabilization of phospholipid bilayer membranes by α-helical antimicrobial and cell non-selective membrane-lytic peptides. *Biochimica et Biophysica Acta*, Vol. 1462, No. 1-2, 55-70, 0005-2736.

Simojoki, H.; Hyvönen, P.; Orro, T. & Pyörälä, S. (2010). High concentration of human lactoferrin in milk of rhLf-transgenic cows relieves signs of bovine experimental *Staphylococcus chromogenes* intramammary infection. *Veterinary Immunology and Immunopathology*, Vol. 136, No. 3-4, 265-271, 0165-2427.

Singh, J. & Banerjee, N. (2008). Transcriptional analysis and functional characterization of a gene pair encoding iron-regulated xenocin and immunity proteins of *Xenorhabdus nematophila*. *Journal of Bacteriology*, Vol. 190, No. 11, 3877-3885, 0021-9193.

Socias, S.; Vincent, P. & Salomon, R. (2009). The leucine-responsive regulatory protein, Lrp, modulates microcin J25 intrinsic resistance in *Escherichia coli* by regulating expression of the YojI microcin exporter. *Journal of Bacteriology*, Vol. 191, No. 4, 1343-1348, 0021-9193.

Tagg, J.; Dajani, A. & Wannamaker, L. (1976). Bacteriocins of Gram-positive bacteria. *Bacteriological Reviews*, Vol. 40, No. 3, 722-756, 0005-3678.

Tagg, J. (2004). Prevention of streptococcal pharyngitis by anti-*Streptococcus pyogenes* bacteriocin-like inhibitory substances (BLIS) produced by *Streptococcus salivarus*. *Indian Journal of Medical Research*, Vol. 119, 13-16, 0971-5916.

Téllez, G. & Castaño, J. (2010). Antimicrobial peptides. *Infectio*, Vol. 14, No. 1, 55-67, 0123-9392.

Thevissen, K.; Ghazi, A.; De Samblax, G.; Brownlee, C.; Osborn, R. & Broekaert, W. (1996). Fungal membrane responses induced by plant defensins and thionins. *Journal of Biological Chemistry*, Vol. 271, No. 25, 15018-15025, 0021-9258.

Thevissen, K.; Kristensen, H.; Thomma, B.; Cammue, B. & François, I. (2007). Therapeutic potential of antifungal plant and insect defensins. *Drug Discovery Today*, Vol. 12, No. 21-22, 966-971, 1359-6446.

Thomas, X.; Destoumieux-Garzón, D.; Péduzzi, J.; Alfonso, C.; Blond, A.; Birlirakis, N.; Goulard, C.; Dubost, L.; Thai, R.; Tabet, J. & Rebuffat, S. (2004). Siderophore peptide, a new type of post-translationally modified antibacterial peptide with potent activity. *The Journal of Biological Chemistry*, Vol. 279, No. 27, 28233-28242, 0021-9258.

Thomma, B.; Cammue, B. & Thevissen, K. (2002). Plant defensins. *Planta*, Vol. 216, No. 2, 193-202, 0032-0935.

Vadyvaloo, V.; Arous, S.; Gravesen, A.; Héchard, Y.; Chauchan, H.; Hastings, J. & Rautenbach, M. (2004). Cell-surface alterations in class IIa bacteriocin-resistant *Listeria monocytogenes*. *Microbiology*, Vol. 150, No. 9, 3025-3033, 1350- 0872.

Vadyvaloo, V.; Hastings, J.; Van Der Merwe, M. & Rautenbach, M. (2002). Membranes of class IIa bacteriocin-resistant *Listeria monocytogenes* cells contain increased levels of desaturated and short-acyl-chains phophatidylglycerols. *Applied and Environmental Microbiology*, Vol. 68, No. 11, 5223-5230, 0099-2240.

Van Belkum, M.; Kok, J.; Venema, G.; Holo, H.; Nes, I.; Konings, W. & Abee, T. (1991). The bacteriocin lactococcin A specifically increases permeability of lactococcal cytoplasmic membranes in a voltage-independent, protein-mediated manner. *Journal of Bacteriology*, Vol. 173, No. 24, 7934-7941, 0021-9193.

Varella, M.; Santos, J.; Fagundes, P.; Madureira, D.; Oliveira, S.; Vasconcelos, M. & Freire, C. (2007). Activity of staphylococcal bacteriocins against *Staphylococcus aureus* and *Streptococcus agalactie* involved in bovine mastitis. *Research in Microbiology*, Vol. 158, No.7, 625-630, 0923-2508.

Verheul, A.; Rusell, N.; Van, T.; Rombouts, F. & Abee, T. (1997). Modifications of membrane phospholipids composition in nisin-resistant *Listeria monocytogenes* Scott. *Applied and Environmental Microbiology*, Vol, 63, No. 9, 3451-3457, 0099-2240.

Vignutelli, A.; Wasternack, C.; Apel, K. & Bohlmann, H. (1998). Systemic and local induction of an *Arabidopsis* thionin gene by wounding and pathogens. *Plant Journal*, Vol. 14, No. 3, 285-295, 1365-313X.

Waite, R. & Curtis, M. (2009). *Pseudomonas aeruginosa* PAO1 pyocin production affects population dynamics within mixed-culture biofilms. *Journal of Bacteriology*, Vol. 191, No. 4, 1349-1354, 0021-9193.

Wehkamp, J., Harder, J.; Wehkamp, J.; Wehkamp-von Meissner, B.; Schlee, M.; Enders, C.; Sonnenborn, U.; Nuding, S.; Bengmark, S.; Fellermann, K.; Schröder, J. & Stange, E. (2004). NF-κB- and AP-1-mediated induction of human beta defensin-2 in intestinal epithelial cells by *Escherichia coli* nissle 1917: a novel effect of a probiotic bacterium. *Infection and Immunity*, Vol. 72, No. 10, 5750-5758, 0019-9567.

Wiedemann, I.; Breukink, E.; Van Kraaij, C.; Kuipers, O.; Bierbaum, G.; De Kruijff, B. & Sahl, H. (2001). Specific binding of nisin to the peptidoglycan precursor lipid II combines pore formation and inhibition of cell wall biosynthesis for potent antibiotic activity. *Journal of Biological Chemistry*, Vol. 276, No. 1, 1772-1779, 0021-9258.

Williams, S.; Gebhart, D.; Martin, D. & Scholl, D. (2008). Retargeting R-Type Pyocins to generate novel bactericidal protein complexes. *Applied and Environmental Microbiology*, Vol. 74, No. 12, 3868-3876, 0099-2240.

Wu, J.; Hu, S. & Cao, L. (2007). Therapeutic effect of nisin Z on subclinical mastitis in lactating cows. *Antimicrobial Agents and Chemotherapy*, Vol. 51, No. 9, 3131-3135, 0066-4804.

Xue, J.; Hunter, I.; Steinmetz, T.; Peters, A.; Ray, B. & Miller, K. (2005). Novel Activator of mannose-specific phosphotransferase system permease expression in *Listeria innocua*, identified by screening for pediocin AcH resistance. *Applied and Environmental Microbiology*, Vol. 71, No. 3, 1283-1290, 0099-2240.

Yamada, K.; Kaneko, J.; Kamio, Y. & Itoh, Y. (2008). Binding sequences for RdgB, a DNA damage-responsive transcriptional activator, and temperature-dependent expression of bacteriocin and pectin lyase genes in *Pectobacterium carotovorum* subsp. *carotovorum*. *Applied and Environmental Microbiology*, Vol. 74, No. 19, 6017-6025, 0099-2240.

Zarember, K. & Malech, H. (2005). HIF-1 alpha: a master regulator of innate host defenses? *Journal of Clinical Investigation*, Vol. 115, No. 7, 1702–1704, 0021-9738.

Zasloff, M. (2002). Antimicrobial peptides of multicellular organisms. *Nature*, Vol. 415, No. 6870, 389-395, 0028-0836.

Zhang, Y.; Li, C.; Vankemmelbeke, M.; Bardelang, P.; Paoli, M.; Penfold, C. & James, R. (2010). The crystal structure of the TolB box of colicin A in complex with TolB reveals important differences in the recruitment of the common TolB translocation portal used by group A colicins. *Molecular Microbiology*, Vol. 75, No. 3, 623-636, 0950-382X.

Zhao, H.; Rinaldi, A.; Rufo, A; Bozzi, A; Kinnunen, P. & Di Giulio, A. (2003). Structural and charge requirements for antimicrobial peptide insertion into biological and model membranes. In: Cellular and Molecular Mechanism of Toxin Action. Pore-Forming Peptides and Protein Toxins. Menestrina, G.; Dalla-Serra, M. & Lazarovici, P. (Ed.), 151-177, Taylor & Francis Group, 0-415-29852-0, New York, NY.

Surfactin – Novel Solutions for Global Issues

Gabriela Seydlová, Radomír Čabala and Jaroslava Svobodová
Charles University in Prague
Czech Republic

1. Introduction

The constant demand for new, effective therapeutic agents has triggered intensive research in the field of diverse antimicrobials of natural origin. These compounds are synthesized by all forms of life and have important biomedical and biotechnological properties, and are thus widely considered a potential solution to the growing problem of resistance to conventional antibiotics, fungal infection and life-threatening diseases.

Among these molecules, lipopeptides represent a unique class of bioactive secondary metabolites with increasing scientific, therapeutic and biotechnological interest. The principal representative of the anionic lipopeptide family is surfactin, which is produced by bacterium *Bacillus subtilis*. This most potent known biosurfactant (i.e. surface-active compound of microbial origin), was named surfactin due to its exceptional surface activity. Since its discovery (Arima et al., 1968) and the identification of its molecular structure as a macrolide lipopeptide (Kakinuma et al., 1969) it has been best recognized for its high amhiphilicity and strong tendency for self-aggregation (Ishigami et al., 1995). Due to these characteristics it shows remarkable surface-, interface- and membrane-active properties, resulting in a number of promising biological activities, which are of great relevance in health care and biotechnology. These properties make surfactin a candidate drug for the resolution of a number of global issues in medicine (Banat et al., 2010; Cao et al., 2010), industry (Nitschke & Costa, 2007; Abdel-Mawgoud et al., 2008) and environmental protection (Mulligan, 2009).

2. Structure and physicochemical properties

Surfactin (M.W. 1036 Da), an amphipathic cyclic lipopeptide, is constituted by a heptapeptide (ELLVDLL) with the chiral sequence LLDLLDL interlinked with β-hydroxy fatty acid of the chain lengths 12 to 16 carbon atoms to form a cyclic lactone ring structure (Fig. 1). Hydrophobic amino acid residues are located at positions 2, 3, 4, 6 and 7, while the glutamyl and aspartyl residues, located at positions 1 and 5 respectively, introduce two negative charges to the molecule. Several surfactin isoforms usually coexist in the cell as a mixture of several peptidic variants with a different aliphatic chain length (Hue et al., 2001; Bonmatin et al., 2003; Tang et al., 2007). The pattern of amino acids and β-hydroxy fatty acids in the surfactin molecule depends not only on the producing bacterial strain involved, but also on the type of culture conditions.

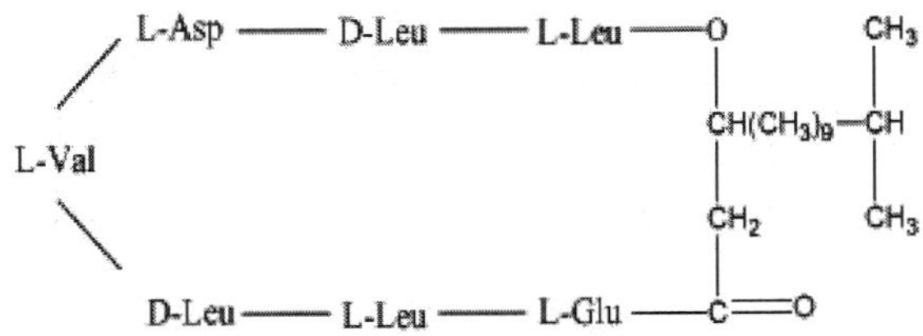

Fig. 1. Primary structure of surfactin

The molecular assembly of surfactin in an aqueous solution and the conformation of the molecules in aggregates condition its physicochemical activities and biological properties. Surfactin adopts a β-turn, forming a β-sheet with a characteristic horse-saddle conformation, which is probably responsible for its broad spectrum of biological activities, even at such low concentrations. The β-turn may be formed by an intramolecular hydrogen bond, whereas the β-sheet may depend on an intermolecular hydrogen bond (Bonmatin et al., 1994; Han et al., 2008; Zou et al., 2010). The two charged side-chains are gathered on the same side and form a "claw", providing a polar head opposite to the hydrophobic domain (Tsan et al., 2007).

The three-dimensional structure of surfactin (Fig. 2) was determined via a high-resolution ^{1}H NMR combined with molecular imaging techniques. On one side of the molecule, residues 2 and 6 face each other in the vicinity of the acidic Glu-1 and Asp-5 side chains, which define a minor polar domain (Bonmatin et al., 1995). On the opposite side, residue 4 faces the connection of the lipidic chain constituting a major hydrophobic domain, which includes the side-chains of residues 3 and 7 to a lesser extent, accounting for its amphiphilic nature and its strong surfactant properties (Tsan et al., 2007). Below the critical micelle concentration (CMC), the lipidic chain should extend freely in solution but it strongly participates in hydrophobic interactions in supramolecular structures such as lipid micelles or oligomers at the air/water interface (Peypoux et al., 1999).

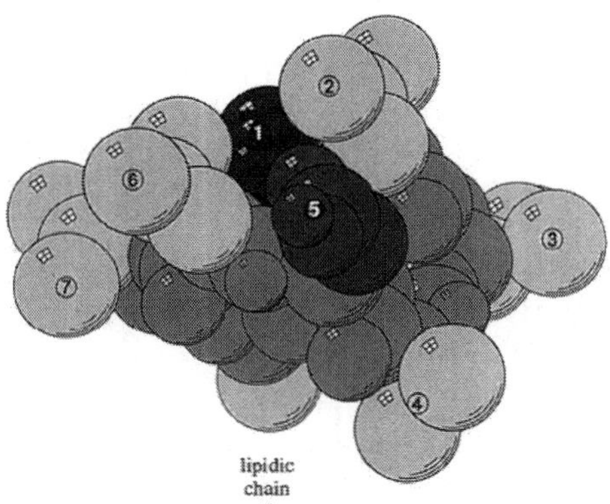

Fig. 2. Three-dimensional structure of surfactin peptide moiety. Backbone atoms are shown in grey. The heavy atoms of amino acid residues (1 to 7) are shown. Pale grey represents hydrophobic residues 2, 3, 4, 6, 7 and the attachment of the lipidic chain. Acidic residues 1 and 5 are in black and dark grey respectively (Peypoux et al., 1999).

Surfactin lowers the surface tension of water from 72 mN.m^{-1} to 27 mN.m^{-1} at a concentration as low as 10 μmol/l (Heerklotz & Seelig, 2001). The critical micelle concentration varies depending on the methods and experimental conditions used, but reaches values of 7.5 - 20 μmol/l (Morikawa et al., 2000; Shen et al., 2010b; Zou et al., 2010), which is about two orders of magnitude smaller than those of most other detergents. Consequently, the consumption of surfactin in practical applications can be lower by several orders when compared with chemical surfactants.

Surfactin has a strong self-assembly ability to form micelles, and these micelles tend to form larger aggregates. Surfactin micelles are inhomogeneous with regard to size distribution with different configurations. The aggregation number of sphere-like micelles is much smaller than that of conventional surfactants, i.e. 11 (Zou et al., 2010) or 20 (Shen et al., 2009). The structure of the micelle is of the core-shell type, with the hydrocarbon chain and the hydrophobic residues forming the core of the micelle (Shen et al., 2009). However, different types of micelles with up to 170 surfactin molecules forming spherical, ellipsoidal and/or cylindrical structures were also found (Heerklotz & Seelig, 2001; Zou et al., 2010).

3. Surfactin-membrane interactions

Recognition of the interaction between surfactin and membrane is an essential prerequisite to understanding its biological activity. Amphiphilic surfactin molecules destabilize the membrane and disturb its integrity (Bernheim & Avigad, 1970). Since this early observation was made, many excellent studies have focused on the description of the surfactin-membrane bilayer system, documenting its exceptional complexity (see parts 3.1., 3.2.). The hypothetical mechanisms of the interactions of surfactin with membrane structures exhibit a complex pattern of effects, such as insertion into lipid bilayers, chelating of mono- and divalent cations, modification of membrane permeability by channel formation or membrane solubilisation by a detergent-like mechanism.

Surfactin penetrates into the lipid membrane through hydrophobic interactions, thus influencing both the order of hydrocarbon chains and the membrane thickness. Upon this primary collision, the peptide cycle then shows conformational changes, which further facilitate the process of interaction (Maget-Dana & Ptak, 1995). Following the incorporation of surfactin into the membrane, the dehydration of the phospholipid polar head groups occurs, perturbing the local lipid packing and strongly compromising bilayer stability, i.e. its barrier properties. A key step for membrane destabilization and leakage is the dimerisation of surfactin into the bilayer. These structural fluctuations may well explain the primary mode of the antibiotic action and the other important biological effects of this lipopeptide (Carrillo et al., 2003).

3.1 Impact of surfactin nature

The extent of perturbation of the phospholipid bilayer correlates with the concentration of surfactin. In a model dimyristoylphosphatidylcholine (DMPC) bilayer system disintegration occurs in three stages. At low concentrations (up to 4 mol%), surfactin penetrates readily into the outer leaflet of the membrane within the head group and part of the adjacent hydrophobic chain region (Shen et al., 2010b). Here it is miscible with the phospholipids, forming mixed micelles. After it reaches a threshold level, the lipopeptide forms domains segregated within the phospholipid bilayer, i.e. pores in the membrane, and the lipid bilayer

is progressively disrupted into sheet-like lamellar membrane fragments due to increasing strains in the membrane caused by further uptake of surfactin molecules (up to 10 mol%). Finally, at a surfactin concentration higher than 10 mol%, thread-like micelles of 6.5 nm in diameter were detected which tended to organize into loops of various sizes (Kell et al., 2007; Boettcher et al., 2010; Liu et al., 2010; Shen et al., 2010a).
Surfactin-membrane interactions can also be described via the quantification of the local surfactin-to-lipid mole ratio within the membrane R_b. This parameter determines the concentration of membrane-bound detergent and the lipid concentration. Membrane leakage starts at $R_b \sim 0.05$ with an aqueous surfactin concentration of 2 µmol/l. The permeabilising activity of surfactin is thus stronger by one order of magnitude than that of detergents such as Triton X-100, which solubilises the membrane at about $R_b \sim 0.6$. At higher concentrations, i.e. $R_b \sim 0.15$, surfactin-rich clusters are formed in the membrane, inducing leaks. Membrane lyses or solubilisation to micelles begin at $R_b \sim 0.22$ and a concentration of 9 µmol/l (Heerklotz and Seelig, 2007). Periodic variations of fluid, surfactin-rich regions and gel lipid-rich domains within the bilayer membrane result in the formation of stable nanoripple structures with intriguing potential in biomedical and biotechnological applications (Brasseur et al., 2007; Kell et al., 2007; Banat et al., 2010).
Membrane penetration by surfactin is facilitated by the presence of cations (Maget-Dana & Ptak, 1995). The Glu-1 and Asp-5 acidic residues form a tailored "claw", which can easily stabilize a surfactin-Ca^{2+} 1:1 complex via an intramolecular bridge (Maget-Dana & Ptak, 1992). This effect of Ca^{2+} ions on the surfactin conformation promotes the deeper insertion of lipopeptide into the membrane (Grau et al., 1999). Surfactin can also drive mono- and divalent cations through an organic barrier, divalent cations being transported with greater efficiency (Thimon et al., 1992). The selective affinity can be correlated with the partial neutralization of the two acidic residues at the air/water interface in the presence of Na^+ or K^+, whereas Ca^{2+} induces a complete neutralization (Maget-Dana & Ptak, 1992). One physiological result of surfactin cation chelation is the inhibition of the cyclic AMP phosphodiesterase activity (Hosono & Suzuki, 1983). The presence of counterions such as Na^+, Li^+, K^+, Mg^{2+} and Ca^{2+} increases the surface activity of surfactin and reduces its CMC. These ions decrease electrostatic repulsions between the surfactin head groups and enhance the formation of micelles (Li et al., 2009a; Li et al., 2009b).
The cyclic nature of the peptide moiety and the number of negative charges, as well as the fatty acid chain length, play a significant role in lipopeptide activity. Variations both in the peptide and lipid moiety of the surfactin molecule can profoundly modulate the structure-function relationship. Within the large hydrophobic domain, position 4 showed a high contribution as the L-Val4/L-Ile4 substitution induced a 2-fold decrease in CMC and a substantial gain in monolayer stability at the air/water interface (Bonmatin et al., 1995). The loss of cyclic nature weakens the degree of surfactin binding. With regards to the effect of the surfactin acyl chain length, the longer the acyl chain, the better its insertion into the lipid bilayer (Razafindralambo et al., 2009). Higher surface activity was observed with a C14 acyl chain, while antiviral properties were stronger when the C15 chain prevailed in surfactin (Bonmatin et al., 2003; Eeman et al., 2006). The membrane activity of surfactin has also been shown to increase with the number of ionic charges of the polar head (Francius et al., 2008).

3.2 Impact of target membrane composition

Several *in vitro* studies have demonstrated the impact of lipid composition on surfactin-membrane interaction and its penetration into the target bilayer; however the mechanism

has so far not been described in detail. Both the polar heads and fatty acid chains play a role in the formation of complexes of surfactin with phospholipids. Surfactin perturbs more strongly membranes containing phospholipids with a shorter chain length (Grau et al., 1999).
These data were also confirmed for the model monolayer system using atomic force microscopy (AFM). This method has become an additional, powerful tool in the investigation of the organization of lipid monolayers and bilayers and the monitoring of their interaction with membrane active peptides, such as surfactin. As the biological activity of surfactin is directly related to its interaction with membranes, understanding the mixing behaviour and domain formation of this molecule within lipid monolayers and bilayers is an important challenge (Deleu et al., 2001; Brasseur et al., 2008).
Polar headgroup composition profoundly affects the interfacial behaviour of surfactin. The miscibility of surfactin with dipalmitoylated (DP) phospholipids decreases in the order phosphatidylcholine > phosphatidylethanolamine > phosphatidylserine (PC>PE>PS). These surfactin-phospholipid interactions are modulated by not only the volume of the phospholipid headgroups (Bouffioux et al., 2007), but also their electrostatic properties and shape (Buchoux et al., 2008). The inverted-cone conformation of surfactin tends to counter-balance the ability of cone-shaped phosphatidylethanolamine molecules to form a hexagonal phase, thereby promoting surfactin stabilization in the membrane. In the case of DPPS, surfactin decreases the electrostatic repulsions between the negative headgroups of DPPS through the large surfactin peptide cycles that result in DPPS-surfactin stability (Grau et al., 1999; Carrillo et al., 2003).
Regarding phospholipid chain lengths, the miscibility between surfactin and phospholipids is higher for shorter chain lengths in the order DMPC (dimyristoyl) > DPPC (dipalmitoyl) > DSPC (distearoylphosphatidylcholine), i.e. 14, 16 and 18 carbon atoms (Bouffioux et al., 2007). On the other hand, the fact that lipid chains are in a fluid or gel phase does not appear to be important, in contrast to other antimicrobial peptides, such as melittin (Buchoux et al., 2008).
There is still some uncertainty regarding the role played by the presence of a negative charge on the phospholipid polar head, which, according to Maget-Dana and Ptak (Maget-Dana & Ptak, 1995) gives rise to electrostatic shielding, preventing the peptide cycle of surfactin from coming close to the phospholipid headgroups. The presence of a net negative charge in the phospholipid monolayer promotes the immiscibility of surfactin into the lipid matrix, therefore favouring surfactin self-assembly. By contrast, this phenomenon is the basis of the pore-forming activity of surfactin in membranes with a significantly high amount of anionic lipids, such as bacterial membranes and some cancer cells (Eeman et al., 2006). A hypothetical model has been proposed for membrane lyses based on charge repulsions between surfactin negative charges and the lipid head group negative charges. This leads to a local increase in membrane curvature and the complete destabilization of the planar membrane, i.e. its direct lyses (Buchoux et al., 2008).
All of the above findings were obtained *in vitro* on model monolayers or bilayers. By contrast, no research deals with the interaction of surfactin with real membrane phospholipids or even intact membranes, where proteins play a crucial role. Our results show subsequent accumulation of cardiolipin (CL) in the *B. subtilis* cytoplasmic membrane during the stationary phase of growth, when surfactin is synthesized. Such an increase in CL, which is regarded as a stress phospholipid stabilizing the membrane bilayer, may therefore support membrane integrity. Additionally, CL bearing two negative charges could prevent the anionic surfactin from coming close to the surface of the membrane bilayer.

However, the putative relation between the surfactin production and the extensive membrane reconstruction would require further analysis (Seydlova & Svobodova, 2008a).

4. Biological and physiological relevance of surfactin

B. subtilis initiates the synthesis of secondary metabolite surfactin through the onset of the stationary growth phase when the culture is becoming short of nutrients and oxygen. Under these famine conditions the cells also activate other survival strategies, such as antibiotic production, sporulation, genetic competence development and the production of extracellular degradative enzymes. Therefore it is reasonable that surfactin or antibiotic synthesis in general provide at least some benefits for the producer, otherwise it would not retain in nature (Stein, 2005).

Lipopeptides are amongst the most frequently produced *B. subtilis* antibiotics. Several possible roles have been proposed for these compounds, such as participation in the acquisition of hydrophobic water-insoluble nutrients and influencing the attachment or detachment of bacteria to and from surfaces (Rosenberg & Ron, 1999). Surfactin is required for raising the fruiting-body-like aerial structures on the surface of *B. subtilis* colonies, where the spores are preferentially developed (Branda et al., 2001). On the other hand, it inhibits the aerial hyphal growth of *Streptomyces coelicolor*, suggesting a possible ecological role (Straight et al., 2006). These properties probably contribute to the survival of *B. subtilis* in its natural habitat.

Surfactin plays a key role in the induction and development of biofilms, i.e. highly structured multicellular communities that adhere to surfaces and constitute the majority of bacteria in most natural ecosystems and are also responsible for many health and industrial problems (Stanley & Lazazzera, 2004). Cells within biofilms are more resistant to biocides and antibiotics; part of this resistance is attributed to the protection provided to the self-produced extracellular matrix, which encases the cells (Lopez et al., 2009b). Swarming, motility in colonies of *B. subtilis* cells, is conditioned by proteins encoded by swrA, swrB, swrC and efp genes (Kearns et al., 2004) and is strictly dependent on the production of surfactin, which reduces surface tension and allows spreading (Kinsinger et al., 2005). Its secretion is stimulated by potassium ions (Kinsinger et al., 2003). Recent improvements in time-of-flight secondary ion mass spectrometry (TOF-SIMS) imaging have enabled the demonstration of surfactin distribution and its precise localization within a swarming colony. Secreted surfactin diffuses freely from the mother colony to the periphery of the swarm and forms a gradient (Debois et al., 2008). This gradient generates surfactant waves, i.e. surface-tension gradients on which the colony spreads outward (Angelini et al., 2009). Laboratory strains such as *B. subtilis* 168, which fail to produce surfactin, do not exhibit swarming motility (Julkowska et al., 2005; Patrick & Kearns, 2009).

Within biofilm, cells differentiate from a predominantly unicellular motile state to a genetically identical mixture of cell types with distinct phenotypes. Cells exhibit specialized functions such as sporulation, matrix production, genetic competence, production of surfactin, cannibalism toxins or exoproteases (Kolter, 2010; Lopez & Kolter, 2010). The formation of these multicellular communities involves extensive intercellular communication via the recognition of and responding to small, secreted, self-generated molecules, i.e. quorum sensing. This also applies to surfactin, which does not trigger multicellularity acting as a surfactant, but rather as autoinducer or a signalling molecule for quorum sensing. It causes potassium leakage across the cytoplasmic membrane, which leads to the activation of protein kinase KinC, affecting the expression of genes involved in the synthesis of the extracellular matrix. This represents a previcusly undescribed quorum-sensing mechanism (Lopez et al., 2009a).

Extracellular surfactin signalling is unidirectional. Surfactin production is triggered in a small subset of cells responding to another signalling molecule ComX, which is synthesized by most cells in the population. Surfactin then acts as a paracrine signal that leads to extracellular matrix production in a different subpopulation of cells, which can then no longer respond to ComX and therefore cannot became surfactin producers (Lopez et al., 2009d). The blockage of signalling molecules caused by the extracellular matrix has been reported in eukaryotes to define the distinct cell fates in morphogenesis. These results indicate that bacteria display attributes of multicellular organisms.

In the same undifferentiated subpopulation of cells, surfactin can trigger not only the production of extracellular matrix but also cannibalism, as a mechanism to delay sporulation. Cannibal cells secrete Skf (sporulation-killing factor) and Sdp (sporulation-delaying factor) toxin systems while at the same time expressing self-resistance to these peptides. The nutrients released from the sensitive siblings promote growths of matrix producers and their DNA can be taken up by competent cells that originate from the fraction of surfactin producers. The coordinated expression of cannibalism and matrix production can result in a fitness advantage in natural habitats by providing both protection and an effective tool to compete for the same resources with neighbouring bacteria (Lopez et al., 2009c).

The developmental pathways controlling sporulation, cannibalism and matrix production are strongly interconnected - they are activated by the same master regulatory protein Spo0A, which can be phosphorylated by the action of different kinases (KinA-E) and presumably therefore different levels of phosphorylation can be reached. Higher levels are necessary to trigger sporulation, whereas lower levels activate matrix production and cannibalism (Fujita et al., 2005).

In our experiments (unpublished data) we determined an interval of sublethal surfactin concentrations that modify the growth of *B. subtilis* 168 that does not produce surfactin. Unexpectedly, two different effects, dependent on surfactin concentration, were discovered that either inhibit or even stimulate the growth of *B. subtilis* 168, the former concentration being higher than the latter. When an exponentially growing *B. subtilis* culture is exposed to exogenously-added surfactin on a nutrient agar plate, the growth stops for a time and is restored with a decreased growth rate in inhibitory concentration, whereas the stimulatory concentration accelerates growth and results in a higher final density of the population. The observations mentioned in the above paragraph led us to speculate that a low concentration of surfactin may induce both matrix production, which protects the cells from the deleterious effect of surfactin, and cannibalism that provides the population with nutrients released from killed siblings. Although this hypothesis has yet to be verified, it is apparent that some optimum surfactin concentration benefits the population as a whole.

5. Potential biomedical applications

The high demand for new chemotherapeutics driven by the increased drug resistance of pathogenes has drawn attention to the use of biosurfactants as new antimicrobial agents (Seydlova & Svobodova, 2008b). Surfactin exhibits a wide range of interactions with target cell membranes and has potential for various medical applications. Besides its antifungal and antibacterial effects (Thimon et al., 1992), surfactin can also inhibit fibrin clot formation

(Arima et al., 1968), inhibits platelet and spleen cytosolic phospholipase A2 (PLA2) (Kim et al., 1998) and exhibits antiviral (Kracht et al., 1999) and antitumor activities (Kameda et al., 1974). Another interesting property of surfactin is that high surfactin concentration affects the aggregation of amyloid β-peptide (Aβ(1-40)) into fibrils, a key pathological process associated with Alzheimer's disease (Han et al., 2008).

Resistance is generally rare against all lipopeptides and the development of a well-defined resistance mechanism has been suggested to be unlikely (Barry et al., 2001). The explanation for this can be found in the complex chemical composition of membranes. The single-component modification of this target structure can hardly cause resistance to surfactin. Therefore, lipopeptide molecules with their unusual structures, which act rapidly on membrane integrity, rather than on other cell targets, are of growing interest in modern medicine and might hold promise for the development of a new generation of antibiotics (Goldberg, 2001).

This is of particular importance at a time when multi-resistant pathogens overcoming the last-resort drugs, including methicillin and vancomycin, pose a growing threat (Singh & Cameotra, 2004). These antibiotics are used not only in the therapy of nosocomial infections caused by enterococci and *Staphylococcus aureus* (Yoneyama & Katsumata, 2006) but also in the therapy of community-acquired methicillin resistant *S. aureus* (caMRSA), which is much more aggressive than its hospital relatives due to having a particular preference for the young and healthy (Hadley, 2004). The recent detection of Enterobacteriaceae with the New Delhi Metallo-β-lactamase (NDM-1) enzyme, which makes bacteria resistant to the main classes of antibiotics used in the treatment of Gram-negative infections, is alarming (Yong et al., 2009). Furthermore, most isolates carried the bla_{NDM-1} gene on plasmids, which are readily transferable (Kumarasamy et al., 2010).

5.1 Antibacterial, anti-inflammatory and antifungal effects

It has long been asserted that the antibacterial properties of anionic antimicrobial peptides are limited due to the repulsive forces between their negative charge and the negatively charged surface of the bacterial surface. Nevertheless, a number of recent studies show inhibitory effects against different bacteria of high medical, environmental or agricultural importance.

Lipopeptide biosurfactants produced by *B. subtilis* R14 (Fernandes et al., 2007) and the marine *Bacillus circulans* (Das et al., 2008) share a lot of surfactin characteristics and were found to be active against multidrug-resistant bacteria such as *Proteus vulgaris, Alcaligenes faecalis, Pseudomonas aeruginosa, Escherichia coli* and methicillin-resistant *Staphylococcus aureus*. The minimal inhibitory (MIC) and minimal bactericidal (MBC) concentrations used were much lower than those of the conventional antibiotics tested in the same time (Das et al., 2008).

The increasing trend to limit the use of chemical food preservatives has generated considerable interest in natural alternatives. It has been observed that a lipopeptide substance containing surfactin is able to damage the surface structure of spores of the recognized food-borne bacterium *B. cereus,* leading to their disruption (Huang et al., 2007). Other results showed that *E. coli* in milk had high sensitivity to a mixture of surfactin with fengycin and can be sterilised by five orders of magnitude even at the temperature of 5.5 °C (Huang et al., 2008). Similar promising observations were made using a combination of surfactin with another lipopeptide iturin to sterilise *Salmonella enteritidis* in meat (Huang et al., 2009). The same antimicrobial peptides were also successful in the antifungal effect against *Penicillium notatum* (Huang et al., 2010). This is of particular relevance in order to ensure food safety.

A culture broth containing surfactin was used to selectively control bloom-forming cyanobacteria, which cause environmental problems due to the production of malodorous compounds and toxins in eutrophic lakes. The surfactin-containing broth inhibited the growth of *Microcystis aeruginosa* and *Anabaena affinis* at a concentration at which chemical surfactants such as Tween 20, Span 80 and Triton X-100 had no effect (Ahn et al., 2003).

Environmentally-friendly solutions are still needed for application in agriculture. It has been found that surfactin and iturin synergistically exhibit an antifungal effect against the fungal pathogen *Colletotrichum gloeosporioides*, causing damage to crops around the world (Kim et al., 2010). These lipopeptides are less toxic and show better reduction and control of phytopathogens than agrochemicals (Souto et al., 2004; Chen et al., 2008; Kim et al., 2010). In another study a mixture of surfactin and iturin disintegrated the cell wall of the gram-negative phytopathogen *Xanthomonas campestris* (Etchegaray et al., 2008). Surfactin was also shown to display antimicrobial activity against *Paenibacillus larvae*, an extremely contagious and dangerous pathogen of honeybees (Sabate et al., 2009).

Surfactin is known to inhibit phospholipase A2, involved in the pathophysiology of inflammatory bowel disease, which is related to ulcerative colitis and Crohn's disease. Oral administration of a natural probiotic *B. subtilis* PB6 secreting surfactin in a rat model with TNBS-induced (trinitrobenzene sulfonic acid) colitis suppressed the colitis, significantly lowering the plasma levels of pro-inflammatory cytokines and significantly increasing anti-inflammatory cytokine (Selvam et al., 2009). Lipopeptide production by probiotic *Bacillus* strains is one of the main mechanisms by which they inhibit the growth of pathogenic microorganisms in the gastrointestinal tract (Hong et al., 2005).

Several recent studies have revealed the impact of surfactin in silencing the inflammatory effect of lipopolysaccharide (LPS) interaction with eukaryotic cells. Compounds that inactivate LPS activity have potential as new anti-inflammatory agents. Surfactin was shown to suppress the interaction of lipid A with LPS-binding protein (LBP) that mediates the transport of LPS to its receptors. Moreover, surfactin did not influence the viability of the eukaryotic cell lines tested (Takahashi et al., 2006). Surfactin also inhibits the LPS-induced expression of inflammatory mediators (IL-1β and iNOS) (Hwang et al., 2005) and reduces the plasma endotoxin, TNF-α and nitric oxide levels in response to septic shock in rats (Hwang et al., 2007). Surfactin downregulates LPS-induced NO production in macrophages by inhibiting the NF-κB transcription factor (Byeon et al., 2008). The surfactin-induced inhibition of NF-κB, MAPK and Akt pathways also leads to the suppression of the surface expression of MHC-II and costimulatory molecules in macrophages, suggesting the impairment of their antigen-presenting function. These results indicate that surfactin is a potent immunosuppressive agent and suggest an important therapeutic implication for transplantation and autoimmune diseases including arthritis, allergies and diabetes (Park & Kim, 2009).

5.2 Anti-mycoplasma effects

Mycoplasmata are the etiological agents of several diseases and also the most significant contaminants of tissue culture cells. Surfactin is already used commercially for the curing of cell cultures and cleansing of biotechnological products of mycoplasma contamination (Boettcher et al., 2010). The treatment of mammalian cells contaminated by mycoplasmata with surfactin improved proliferation rates and led to changes in cell morphology. In addition, the low cytotoxicity of surfactin to mammalian cells permitted the specific inactivation of mycoplasmata without having significantly detrimental effects on the metabolism of cells in the culture (Vollenbroich et al., 1997b). A recent study confirmed the potential of surfactin to kill *Mycoplasma pneumoniae* (MIC 25 μM) independently of target cell concentration, which is a significant advantage over the mode of action of conventional antibiotics. Surfactin has exhibited, in combination with enrofloxacin, a synergistic effect resulting in mycoplasma-killing activity at about two orders of magnitude greater than when entire molecules are used separately (Fassi Fehri et al., 2007). More recently, surfactin was described as inhibiting the expression of proinflammatory cytokines and NO production in macrophages induced by *Mycoplasma hyopneumoniae* (Hwang et al., 2008a). In another study, surfactin showed a strong cidal effect (MIC 62 μM) and in combination with other antibacterials exhibited additive interaction, which could be clinically relevant (Hwang et al., 2008b).

5.3 The role of surfactin in surface colonization by pathogens

Swarming motility and biofilm formation are the key actions in the colonization of a surface by bacteria and increase the likelihood of nosocomial infections associated with various medical appliances, such as central venous catheters, urinary catheters, prosthetic heart valves, voice prostheses and orthopaedic devices. These infections share common characteristics even though the microbial causes and host sites vary greatly (Rodrigues et al., 2006). The most important of these features is that bacteria in biofilms are highly resistant to antibiotics, evade host defenses and withstand traditional antimicrobial chemotherapy, making them difficult to treat effectively (Morikawa, 2006). Moreover, in food-processing environments, the control of microorganisms' adherence to material surfaces is an essential step to meet food safety requirements.

Recent studies have suggested that non-antibiotic molecules naturally produced within bacterial communities, such as surface active biosurfactants, could also interfere with biofilm formation by modulating microbial interaction with interfaces (Banat et al., 2010). Biosurfactants, such as surfactin, have been found to inhibit the adhesion of pathogenic organisms to solid surfaces or infection sites. Surfactin decreases the amount of biofilm formed by *Salmonella typhimurium, Salmonella enterica, Eschericha coli* and *Proteus mirabilis* in polyvinyl chloride wells, as well as vinyl urethral catheters. The precoating of catheters by running the surfactin solution through them prior to inoculation with media was just as effective as the inclusion of surfactin in the growth medium. Given the importance of opportunistic infections with Salmonella species, including the urinary tract of AIDS patients, these results have potential for practical application (Mireles et al., 2001).

Substances containing surfactin have also been shown to possess specific anti-adhesive activity that selectively inhibits the biofilm formation of two pathogenic strains of *S. aureus* and *E. coli* on polystyrene by 97% and 90%, respectively (Rivardo et al., 2009). In another study, Rivardo et al. observed a synergistic interaction between surfactin and silver, acting as effective antibiofilm agents. Negatively charged surfactin increases metal solubility and may therefore facilitate the penetration through the exopolymeric substance that encapsulates biofilm and provides its protection (Rivardo et al., 2010). Moreover it was demonstrated that surfactin increases the efficiency of eradication of different antibiotics against a urinary tract-infective *E. coli* strain (Banat et al., 2010).

The preconditioning of stainless steel and polypropylene surfaces with 0.1% (w/v) surfactin reduces the number of adhered cells of food pathogens *Listeria monocytogenes* and

Enterobacter sakazakii. The absorption of surfactin on polystyrene also reduced the colonization of *Salmonella enteritidis* (Nitschke et al., 2009). Considering that surfactin has an anionic nature, the observed anti-adhesive effect can be due to the electrostatic repulsion between bacteria and the molecules of surfactin adsorbed onto the polystyrene surface (Zeraik & Nitschke, 2010). All in all, these results outline a new potential of surfactin as an anti-adhesive compound that can be explored in the protection of surfaces from microbial contamination.

5.4 Anti-viral activity

Surfactin is active against several viruses, including the Semliki Forest virus, herpes simplex virus (HSV-1 and HSV-2), vesicular stomatitis virus, simian immunodeficiency virus, feline calicivirus and the murine encephalomyocarditis virus. The inactivation of enveloped viruses, especially herpes viruses and retroviruses, is significantly more efficient than that of non-enveloped viruses. This suggests that the antiviral action of surfactin is primarily due to the physicochemical interaction between the membrane active surfactant and the virus lipid membrane (Vollenbroich et al., 1997a). One important factor for virus inactivation is the number of carbon atoms in the acyl chain of surfactin. The capacity for virus inactivation increases with rising fatty acid hydrophobicity. During the inactivation process, surfactin permeates into the lipid bilayer, inducing complete disintegration of the envelope containing the viral proteins involved in virus adsorption, and penetration to the target cells. Its absence accounts for the loss of viral infectivity (Kracht et al., 1999).

Recently, it has also been observed that antimicrobial lipopetides containing surfactin inactivate cell-free viruses of the porcine parvovirus, pseudorabies virus, Newcastle disease virus and bursal disease virus (Huang et al., 2006).

5.5 Antitumor activity

Surfactin has been reported to show antitumor activity against Ehrlich's ascite carcinoma cells (Kameda et al., 1974). A recent study on the effect of surfactin on the proliferation of a human colon carcinoma cell line showed that surfactin strongly blocked cell proliferation. The inhibition of growth by surfactin was due to the induction of apoptosis and cell cycle arrest via the suppression of cell survival regulating signals such as ERK and PI3K/Akt (Kim et al., 2007).

Another study revealed that surfactin inhibits proliferation and induces apoptosis of MCF-7 human breast cancer cells trough a ROS/JNK-mediated mitochondrial/caspase pathway. Surfactin causes the generation of reactive oxygen species (ROS), which induce the sustained activation of survival mediator ERK1/2 and JNK, which are key regulators of stress-induced apoptosis. These results suggest that the action of surfactin is realized via two independent signalling mechanisms (Cao et al., 2010). The induction of apoptotic cell death is a promising emerging strategy for the prevention and treatment of cancer.

5.6 Thrombolytic activity

The plasminogen-plasmin system involved in the dissolution of blood clots forms part of a variety of physiological and pathological processes requiring localized proteolysis. Plasminogen is activated proteolytically using a urokinase-type plasminogen activator (u-PA), which is initially secreted as a zymogen prourokinase (pro-u-PA). Along with activation by u-PA, the plasminogen itself has an activation mechanism involving conformational change. The reciprocal activation of plasminogen and prourokinase is an important mechanism in the initiation and propagation of local fibrinolytic activity. Surfactin at concentrations of 3 – 20 μmol/l enhances the activation of prourokinase as well as the conformational change in the plasminogen, leading to increased fibrinolysis *in vitro* and *in vivo* (Kikuchi & Hasumi, 2002). In a rat pulmonary embolism model, surfactin increased plasma clot lysis when injected in combination with prourokinase (Kikuchi & Hasumi, 2003). Surfactin is also able to prevent platelet aggregation, leading to the inhibition of additional fibrin clot formation, and to enhance fibrinolysis with the facilitated diffusion of fibrinolytic agents (Lim et al., 2005). The anti-platelet activity of surfactin is due not to its detergent effect, but to its action on downstream signalling pathways (Kim et al., 2006). These results suggest a possible use for surfactin in urgent thrombolytic therapy related to pulmonary, myocardial and cerebral disorders. Moreover, surfactin has advantages over other available thrombolytic agents because it has fewer side effects and therefore has potential for long-term use.

5.7 Antiparasitic activity

Vector control is a key point of various strategies aiming at interrupting the transmission of mosquito-borne diseases. The culture supernatant of a surfactin producing *B. subtilis* strain was found to kill the larval and pupal stages of mosquito species *Anopheles stephensi, Culex quinquefasciatus* and *Aedes aegypti*. As few biocontrol agents or insecticides are effective against mosquito pupae, this could be a promising tool for application in control programmes (Geetha et al., 2010).

Surfactin was also reported to act as a Sir2 inhibitor (silent information inhibitor 2). Sir2 belongs to the NAD^+ dependent histone deacetylases, which modulate the acetylation status of histones, regulate transcription, DNA replication and repair and have been implicated in pathogenesis of *Plasmodium falciparum*, causing cerebral malaria. Surfactin functions as a competitive inhibitor of NAD^+ and an uncompetitive inhibitor of acetylated peptide. Surfactin was also found to be a potent inhibitor of intra-erythrocytic growth of *P. falciparum in vitro*, with an IC_{50} value in the low micromolar range (Chakrabarty et al., 2008).

Surfactin can also be used as alternative treatment for nosemosis. When exposed to surfactin, the spores of *Nosema ceranae*, the causative agent of the most frequently parasitic infection in *Apis mellifera*, reveal a significant reduction in infectivity. Moreover, when surfactin is administered *ad libitum* and is introduced into the digestive tract of a bee, it also leads to a substantial reduction in parasitosis development (Porrini et al., 2010).

6. Obstacles and perspectives

In general, biosurfactants produced from microorganisms possess more advantages over their chemical counterparts, such as diversity, biodegradability, lower toxicity, biocompatibility and stability over wide range of pH. Nevertheless, they have not been widely used so far due to their high production costs, caused primarily due to low yields and high recovery expenses that cannot meet the economic needs of industrial production. Similar limitations hinder the exploitation of surfactin potential applications in medicine and industry, as well as environmental protection. Numerous studies have been made on the optimization of surfactin yields at the level of production conditions, hyperproducing mutant construction and downstream processing of the crude product or in seeking surfactin producers in extreme habitats (Das et al., 2008) and the development of novel methods for the rapid screening of producers (das Neves et al., 2009). On the other hand, the relatively low (μmol/l) effective concentration in biological systems could facilitate its use in biomedicine.

However, surfactin also needs to conform to some additional requirements, such as detailed knowledge of the mechanism of interaction with the target cells and possible cytotoxicity effects to the treated macroorganism. Genetic and biochemical engineering approaches to create a tailor-made molecules (Symmank et al., 2002), or surfactin analogues with modified properties represent a possible solution for the future. Surprisingly, almost no research has been focused on the principle of surfactin resistance of the producer, which can not only bring a valuable piece of information for improving yields, but is also crucial for possible medical applications.

6.1 Toxicity

One of the plausible drawbacks of the potential use of surfactin in medical applications is its haemolytic activity, as observed in *in vitro* experiments, which results from surfactin's ability to disturb the integrity of the target cell membranes. The concentration-dependent haemolytic effect of surfactin was described as the concentration of surfactin that bursts 50% of red blood cells (HC_{50}), which is equal to 300 μmol/l (Dufour et al., 2005). On the other hand, surfactin concentrations used in various biomedical studies were far below the threshold, i.e. 30 μmol/l. The lowest surfactin concentration that completely inhibited the growth of mycoplasmata after 48 h (MIC) was 25 μmol/l (Fassi Fehri et al., 2007); 30 μmol/l surfactin treatment displayed significant anti-proliferative activity in human colon cancer cells (Kim et al., 2007) and was able to induce apoptosis in human breast cancer cells (Cao et al., 2010). The same surfactin concentration is also capable of inhibiting the immunostimulatory function of macrophages (Park & Kim, 2009).

The LD_{50} (Lethal Dose, 50%; the dose required to kill half the members of a tested population) of surfactin is at > 100 mg/kg, *i.v.* in mice (Kikuchi & Hasumi, 2002). An oral intake of up to 500 mg/kg per day of the lipopeptide did not show apparent toxicities. Surfactin demonstrated no maternal toxicity, fetotoxicity, and teratogenicity in ICR mice (Hwang et al., 2008c). Surfactin did not show any toxicological effects at dose 2500 mg/kg after a single oral administration in rats. The no-observed-adverse-effect level (NOAEL) of surfactin was established to be 500 mg/kg following repeat (4 weeks) oral administration. No surfactin-related toxicities in survival, clinical signs, haematological parameters and histopathological observations of haematopoietic organs were found (Hwang et al., 2009).

Surfactin did not influence the viability of HUVEC (human umbilical vein endothelial cells) up to 30 μg/ml after 24 h. Surfactin was also regarded as being less toxic than other surfactants, as judged from the results of an acute toxicity study in mice (Takahashi et al., 2006) and also as a safer anti-endotoxin agent in comparison with polymyxin B (Hwang et al., 2007).

Another option for reducing surfactin toxicity is to design a tailor-made molecule. Minor alterations in the chemical structure of the molecule may lead to a dramatic adjustment in the toxicity profile of any compound. Genetic engineering of the surfactin synthetase resulted in the production of a novel antimicrobial agent. Reduced toxicity against erythrocytes concomitant with an increased inhibitory effect on bacterial growth was observed (Symmank et al., 2002). Similarly, linear forms of surfactin have lower surface and haemolytic activities and can even protect red blood cells against the action of other detergents. Linear surfactin analogues could be incorporated into cyclic surfactin in order to take advantage of its protective effect (Dufour et al., 2005). An alternative approach is to deliver cyclic surfactin in a liposome of a specific phospholipid constitution into different kinds of target cells (Bouffioux et al., 2007). Thus, similar surfactin derivatives may exhibit reduced toxicity against eukaryotic cells, which could improve their therapeutic applications. These synthetic analogues appear as an interesting research tool to investigate the subtle structure-function variations on the membrane activity of surfactin. In the future, it is expected that potential applications will be found in the biomedical and biotechnological fields, enabling the design of new surfactants with tuneable, well-defined properties (Francius et al., 2008).

Surfactin can be also regarded as a toxic agent that can insult the producing microorganism membrane. All antibiotic-producing bacteria ensure their self-resistance by coding for various means of self-defense mechanisms that are activated in parallel with antibiotic biosynthetic pathways; their expression subsequently increases in time in order to avoid suicide. The cytoplasmic membrane can be reasonably supposed to be the site of self-resistance against surfactin. The major advantage of drugs targeting the integrity of the membrane constitutes the multistep modification of this structure, necessary to bring about cell resistance. On the other hand, any use of antibiotics could lead to the selection of resistant variants of pathogens at some level. Nowadays, only limited information is available concerning the molecular background of surfactin tolerance in producing bacteria. However, as the ultimate source of resistance genes are almost certainly the producers (Hopwood, 2007), the elucidation of the self-protective resistance mechanism in the producer *B. subtilis* at the level of surfactin target site – the cytoplasmic membrane – is inevitably important.

The extracytoplasmic transcription σ^{W} factor, controlling genes that provide intrinsic resistance to antimicrobial compounds produced by *Bacilli*, was recently identified (Butcher & Helmann, 2006). Nevertheless, none of these resistance systems were proven to be engaged in surfactin resistance. The only gene plausibly involved in surfactin resistance is swrC (Tsuge et al., 2001; Kearns et al., 2004). It codes for the first published example of an RND family of the proton-dependent multidrug efflux pumps in Gram-positive bacteria and contributes to the secretion of surfactin. However, surfactin production was observed even in a swrC-deficient strains that persistently survived at concentrations higher than 10,000 µg/ml (Tsuge et al., 2001). This finding suggests the existence of other additional mechanisms that participate in the surfactin self-resistance of the producer.

In order to examine the self-protective mechanisms of the cytoplasmic membrane against the deleterious effect of surfactin, we have constructed a mutant derivative with an abolished ability to synthesize surfactin (Fig. 3) complementary to the wild type surfactin producer *B. subtilis* ATCC 21332 (Seydlova et al., 2009). In this mutant, the sfp gene essential to the synthesis of surfactin was replaced with its inactive counterpart from the non-producing strain *B. subtilis* 168, bearing a frame shift mutation (Nakano et al., 1992). This isogenic pair of strains, differing only in surfactin production, represents a key tool for the comparative study of surfactin-induced changes in the cytoplasmic membrane of *B.* subtilis producing surfactin. Our preliminary data show that the synthesis of surfactin coincides with the substantial reconstruction of phospholipid polar headgroups, leading to a more stable bilayer. On the other hand, GC/MS analysis revealed a minor alteration in membrane fatty acids, implying that surfactin operates mainly in the polar region, which is in agreement with recent findings observed *in vitro* (Shen et al., 2010b).

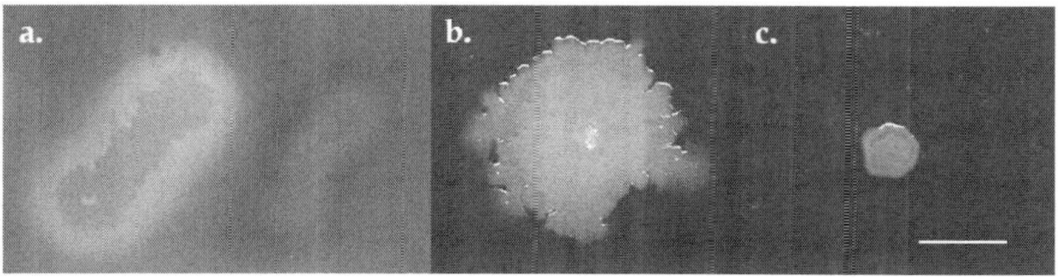

Fig. 3. The *B. subtilis* ATCC 21332 surfactin-producing strain and its mutant derivative minus surfactin production, accompanied by the absence of haemolysis (a - right) and swarming motility (b – wild type, c - mutant; bar 10 mm)

6.2 Economics of surfactin production

The high production cost of biosurfactants, which cannot compete with chemical surfactants, has been a major concern in commercial applications. Different strategies have been proposed to make the process more cost-effective, such as the optimization of fermentative conditions and downstream recovery processes, use of cheap and waste substrates and the development of overproducing strains (Banat et al., 2010).

Several advances in the optimization of culture conditions and downstream processing have been published recently. The amount and type of a raw material can contribute by 10-30% to total production costs in most biotechnological processes (Mukherjee et al., 2006). Interesting, cheap and renewable sources have been described from agroindustrial crops and residues. A promising perspective for large-scale industrial application was shown using the already commercialized, cottonseed-derived Pharmamedia medium (Al-Ajlani et al., 2007) or cashew apple juice for surfactin production (Ponte Rocha et al., 2009) reaching high yields of 2000 mg/l and 3500 mg/l, respectively.

A number of studies also deal with the improvement of culture and environmental parameters, the optimization of medium components and trace elements for the fermentation of surfactin. Carbon source (glucose), nitrogen source (ammonium nitrate), iron and manganese were found to be significant factors. It was reported that the addition of 4 mmol/l Fe^{2+} leads to a 10-fold increase in surfactin yield (Wei et al., 2004) and the addition of Mn^{2+} ions enhances lipopeptide production by a factor of 2.6 (Kim et al., 2010).

Apart from wild-type surfactin-producing strains, a few mutants have been selected and tested for surfactin production. Physical mutagenesis by ion beam implantation was used successfully to prepare a mutant that produced up to 12.2 g/l of crude surfactin (Gong et al., 2009). Another recombinant strain was obtained using random mutagenesis with N-methyl-N'-nitro-N-nitrosoguanidine, reaching a maximum production level of 50 g/l (Yoneda et al., 2006).

Downstream processing such as recovery, concentration and purification account for the greater part of the total cost of a biotechnological product (Mukherjee et al., 2006). The most common isolation techniques for biosurfactants use precipitation, solvent extraction and chromatographic purification. These techniques are already well established for lab-scale applications, but cost hinders their use in industrial production. Lately, many advances have been reported for the recovery and purification of surfactin, including different combinations of ultrafiltration and nanofiltration through polymeric membranes with molecular weight cut-off. High surfactin recovery and purification were achieved, showing potential for application (Isa et al., 2007; Chen et al., 2008; Juang et al., 2008; Shaligram & Singhal, 2010).

7. Conclusion

Surfactin, as a natural product with a multitude of auspicious features applicable in biomedicine, has attracted the intense attention of many research entities during the last decade. This systematic effort has resulted in substantial progress in understanding the different aspects of surfactin physicochemical properties, interactions with cell membranes and even its physiological role for the producer itself. A number of activities, such as antimicrobial, immunosuppressive, antitumor and antiparasitic activities, have been described and explored. This is of particular importance, especially at time when drug resistance among causal organisms for many life-threatening diseases is on the rise; other means of therapy are needed, or are entirely absent.

In spite of its immense potential, surfactin use remains restricted thus far. Further research needs to be carried out into the interaction of surfactin with target membranes and its global effect on the macroorganism and natural microbiota in order to validate the use of surfactin in biomedical and health-related areas. Last but not least, the mechanism of surfactin resistance also presents a crucial challenge. Nevertheless, it is only a matter of time before surfactin and its great biomedical potential are harnessed.

8. Acknowledgements

This work was supported by grant of the Grant Agency of Charles University in Prague 156/2006 and by grant SVV UK 261212/2010.

9. References

Abdel-Mawgoud, A. M.; Aboulwafa, M. M. & Hassouna, N. A. H. (2008). Characterization of surfactin produced by Bacillus subtilis isolate BS5. *Applied Biochemistry and Biotechnology*, Vol. 150, No. 3, (289-303), 0273-2289

Ahn, C. Y.; Joung, S. H., Jeon, J. W., Kim, H. S., Yoon, B. D. & Oh, H. M. (2003). Selective control of cyanobacteria by surfactin-containing culture broth of Bacillus subtilis C1. *Biotechnology Letters*, Vol. 25, No. 14, (1137-1142), 0141-5492

Al-Ajlani, M. M.; Sheikh, M. A., Ahmad, Z. & Hasnain, S. (2007). Production of surfactin from Bacillus subtilis MZ-7 grown on pharmamedia commercial medium. *Microbial Cell Factories*, Vol. 6, No. 17, 1475-2859

Angelini, T. E.; Roper, M., Kolter, R., Weitz, D. A. & Brenner, M. P. (2009). Bacillus subtilis spreads by surfing on waves of surfactant. *Proceedings of the National Academy of Sciences of U S A*, Vol. 106, No. 43, (18109-18113), 1091-6490

Arima, K.; Kakinuma, A. & Tamura, G. (1968). Surfactin, a crystalline peptidelipid surfactant produced by Bacillus subtilis: isolation, characterization and its inhibition of fibrin clot formation. *Biochemical and Biophysical Research Communications*, Vol. 31, No. 3, (488-494), 0006-291X

Banat, I. M.; Franzetti, A., Gandolfi, I., Bestetti, G., Martinotti, M. G., Fracchia, L., Smyth, T. J. & Marchant, R. (2010). Microbial biosurfactants production, applications and future potential. *Applied Microbiology and Biotechnology*, Vol. 87, No. 2, (427-444), 0175-7598

Barry, A. L.; Fuchs, P. C. & Brown, S. D. (2001). Relative potency of telithromycin, azithromycin and erythromycin against recent clinical isolates of gram-positive cocci. *European Journal of Clinical Microbiology and Infectious Diseases*, Vol. 20, No. 7, (494-497), 0934-9723

Bernheim, A. W. & Avigad, L. S. (1970). Nature and properties of a cytolytic agent produced by Bacillus subtilis. *Journal of General Microbiology*, Vol. 61, No., (361-366), 0022-1287

Boettcher, C.; Kell, H., Holzwarth, J. F. & Vater, J. (2010). Flexible loops of thread-like micelles are formed upon interaction of L-alpha-dimyristoyl-phosphatidylcholine with the biosurfactant surfactin as revealed by cryo-electron tomography. *Biophysical Chemistry*, Vol. 149, No. 1-2, (22-27), 1873-4200

Bonmatin, J. M.; Genest, M., Labbe, H. & Ptak, M. (1994). Solution three-dimensional structure of surfactin: a cyclic lipopeptide studied by 1H-NMR, distance geometry, and molecular dynamics. *Biopolymers*, Vol. 34, No. 7, (975-986), 0006-3525

Bonmatin, J. M.; Labbe, H., Grangemard, I., Peypoux, F., Magetdana, R., Ptak, M. & Michel, G. (1995). Production, isolation and characterization of [Leu(4)]surfactins and [Ile(4)]surfactins from Bacillus subtilis. *Letters in Peptide Science*, Vol. 2, No. 1, (41-47), 0929-5666

Bonmatin, J. M.; Laprevote, O. & Peypoux, F. (2003). Diversity among microbial cyclic lipopeptides: iturins and surfactins. Activity-structure relationships to design new bioactive agents. *Combinatorial Chemistry and High Throughput Screening*, Vol. 6, No. 6, (541-556), 1386-2073

Bouffioux, O.; Berquand, A., Eeman, M., Paquot, M., Dufrene, Y. F., Brasseur, R. & Deleu, M. (2007). Molecular organization of surfactin-phospholipid monolayers: effect of phospholipid chain length and polar head. *Biochimica et Biophysica Acta*, Vol. 1768, No. 7, (1758-1768), 0006-3002

Brasseur, R.; Braun, N., El Kirat, K., Deleu, M., Mingeot-Leclercq, M. P. & Dufrene, Y. F. (2007). The biologically important surfactin lipopeptide induces nanoripples in supported lipid bilayers. *Langmuir*, Vol. 23, No. 19, (9769-9772), 0743-7463

Brasseur, R.; Deleu, M., Mingeot-Leclercq, M. P., Francius, G. & Dufrene, Y. F. (2008). Probing peptide-membrane interactions using AFM *Surface and Interface Analysis*, Vol. 40, No. 3-4, (151-156), 0142-2421

Buchoux, S.; Lai-Kee-Him, J., Garnier, M., Tsan, P., Besson, F., Brisson, A. & Dufourc, E. J. (2008). Surfactin-triggered small vesicle formation of negatively charged membranes: A novel membrane-lysis mechanism. *Biophysical Journal*, Vol. 95, No. 8, (3840-3849), 0006-3495

Butcher, B. G. & Helmann, J. D. (2006). identification of Bacillus subtilis sigma(W)-dependent genes that provide intrinsic resistance to antimicrobial compounds produced by Bacilli. *Molecular Microbiology*, Vol. 60, No. 3, (765-782), 0950-382X

Byeon, S. E.; Lee, Y. G., Kim, B. H., Shen, T., Lee, S. Y., Park, H. J., Park, S. C., Rhee, M. H. & Cho, J. Y. (2008). Surfactin blocks NO production in lipopolysaccharide-activated macrophages by inhibiting NF-kappaB activation *Journal of Microbiology and Biotechnology*, Vol. 18, No. 12, (1984-1989), 1017-7825

Cao, X. H.; Wang, A. H., Wang, C. L., Mao, D. Z., Lu, M. F., Cui, Y. Q. & Jiao, R. Z. (2010). Surfactin induces apoptosis in human breast cancer MCF-7 cells through a

ROS/JNK-mediated mitochondrial/caspase pathway. *Chemico-Biological Interactions*, Vol. 183, No. 3, (357-362), 0009-2797

Carrillo, C.; Teruel, J. A., Aranda, F. J. & Ortiz, A. (2003). Molecular mechanism of membrane permeabilization by the peptide antibiotic surfactin. *Biochimica et Biophysica Acta*, Vol. 1611, No. 1-2, (91-97), 0006-3002

das Neves, L. C. M.; Kobayashi, M. J., Rodrigues, T. M., Converti, A. & Penna, T. C. V. (2009). Biomonitoring of biosurfactant production by green fluorescent protein-marked Bacillus subtilis W1012. *Journal of Chemical Technology and Biotechnology*, Vol. 84, No. 1, (112-118), 0268-2575

Das, P.; Mukherjee, S. & Sen, R. (2008). Antimicrobial potential of a lipopeptide biosurfactant derived from a marine Bacillus circulans. *Journal of Applied Microbiology*, Vol. 104, No. 6, (1675-1684), 1364-5072

Debois, D.; Hamze, K., Guerineau, V., Le Caer, J. P., Holland, I. B., Lopes, P., Ouazzani, J., Seror, S. J., Brunelle, A. & Laprevote, O. (2008). In situ localisation and quantification of surfactins in a Bacillus subtilis swarming community by imaging mass spectrometry. *Proteomics*, Vol. 8, No. 18, (3682-3691), 1615-9861

Deleu, M.; Nott, K., Brasseur, R., Jacques, P., Thonart, P. & Dufrene, Y. F. (2001). Imaging mixed lipid monolayers by dynamic atomic force microscopy. *Biochimica et Biophysica Acta*, Vol. 1513, No. 1, (55-62), 0006-3002

Dufour, S.; Deleu, M., Nott, K., Wathelet, B., Thonart, P. & Paquot, M. (2005). Hemolytic activity of new linear surfactin analogs in relation to their physico-chemical properties. *Biochimica et Biophysica Acta*, Vol. 1726, No. 1, (87-95), 0006-3002

Eeman, M.; Berquand, A., Dufrene, Y. F., Paquot, M., Dufour, S. & Deleu, M. (2006). Penetration of surfactin into phospholipid monolayers: nanoscale interfacial organization. *Langmuir*, Vol. 22, No. 26, (11337-11345), 0743-7463

Etchegaray, A.; Bueno, C. D., de Melo, I. S., Tsai, S., Fiore, M. D., Silva-Stenico, M. E., de Moraes, L. A. B. & Teschke, O. (2008). Effect of a highly concentrated lipopeptide extract of Bacillus subtilis on fungal and bacterial cells. *Archives of Microbiology*, Vol. 190, No. 6, (611-622), 0302-8933

Fassi Fehri, L.; Wroblewski, H. & Blanchard, A. (2007). Activities of antimicrobial peptides and synergy with enrofloxacin against Mycoplasma pulmonis. *Antimicrobial Agents and Chemotherapy*, Vol. 51, No. 2, (468-474), 0066-4804

Fernandes, P. A. V.; de Arruda, I. R., dos Santos, A. F. A. B., de Araujo, A. A., Maior, A. M. S. & Ximenes, E. A. (2007). Antimicrobial activity of surfactants produced by Bacillus subtilis R14 against multidrug-resistant bacteria. *Brazilian Journal of Microbiology*, Vol. 38, No. 4, (704-709), 1517-8382

Francius, G.; Dufour, S., Deleu, M., Papot, M., Mingeot-Leclercq, M. P. & Dufrene, Y. F. (2008). Nanoscale membrane activity of surfactins: Influence of geometry, charge and hydrophobicity. *Biochimica et Biophysica Acta-Biomembranes*, Vol. 1778, No. 10, (2058-2068), 0005-2736

Fujita, M.; Gonzalez-Pastor, J. E. & Losick, R. (2005). High- and low-threshold genes in the Spo0A regulon of Bacillus subtilis. *Journal of Bacteriology*, Vol. 187, No. 4, (1357-1368), 0021-9193

Geetha, I.; Manonmani, A. M. & Paily, K. P. (2010). Identification and characterization of a mosquito pupicidal metabolite of a Bacillus subtilis subsp. subtilis strain. *Applied Microbiology and Biotechnology*, Vol. 86, No. 6, (1737-1744), 1432-0614

Goldberg, J. (2001). Cyclic peptide antibiotics; self-assembly required. *Trends in Biotechnology*, Vol. 19, No. 10, (379-379), 0167-7799

Gong, G. H.; Zheng, Z. M., Chen, H., Yuan, C. L., Wang, P., Yao, L. M. & Yu, Z. L. (2009). Enhanced Production of Surfactin by Bacillus subtilis E8 Mutant Obtained by Ion Beam Implantation. *Food technology and biotechnology*, Vol. 47, No. 1, (27-31), 1330-9862

Grau, A.; Gomez Fernandez, J. C., Peypoux, F. & Ortiz, A. (1999). A study on the interactions of surfactin with phospholipid vesicles. *Biochimica et Biophysica Acta*, Vol. 1418, No. 2, (307-319), 0006-3002

Hadley, C. (2004). Overcoming resistance. *Embo Reports*, Vol. 5, No. 6, (550-552), 1469-221X

Han, Y. C.; Huang, X., Cao, M. W. & Wang, Y. L. (2008). Micellization of Surfactin and Its Effect on the Aggregate Conformation of Amyloid beta(1-40). *Journal of Physical Chemistry B*, Vol. 112, No. 47, (15195-15201), 1520-6106

Heerklotz, H. & Seelig, J. (2001). Detergent-like action of the antibiotic peptide surfactin on lipid membranes. *Biophysical Journal*, Vol. 81, No. 3, (1547-1554), 0006-3495

Hong, H. A.; Duc, L. H. & Cutting, S. M. (2005). The use of bacterial spore formers as probiotics. *Fems Microbiology Reviews*, Vol. 29, No. 4, (813-835), 0168-6445

Hopwood, D. A. (2007). How do antibiotic-producing bacteria ensure their self-resistance before antibiotic biosynthesis incapacitates them? *Molecular Microbiology*, Vol. 63, No. 4, (937-940), 0950-382X

Hosono, K. & Suzuki, H. (1983). Acylpeptides, the inhibitors of cyclic adenosine-3',5'-monophosphate phosphodiesterase. 3. Inhibition of cyclic-AMP phosphodiesterase. *Journal of Antibiotics*, Vol. 36, No. 6, (679-683), 0021-8820

Huang, X.; Wei, Z., Zhao, G., Gao, X., Yang, S. & Cui, Y. (2008). Optimization of sterilization of Escherichia coli in milk by surfactin and fengycin using a response surface method. *Current Microbiology*, Vol. 56, No. 4, (376-381), 0343-8651

Huang, X. Q.; Gao, X. P., Zheng, L. Y. & Hao, G. Z. (2009). Optimization of Sterilization of Salmonella enteritidis in Meat by Surfactin and Iturin Using a Response Surface Method. *International Journal of Peptide Research and Therapeutics*, Vol. 15, No. 1, (61-67), 1573-3149

Huang, X. Q.; Lu, Z. X., Bie, X. M., Lu, F. X., Zhao, H. Z. & Yang, S. J. (2007). Optimization of inactivation of endospores of Bacillus cereus by antimicrobial lipopeptides from Bacillus subtilis fmbj strains using a response surface method. *Applied Microbiology and Biotechnology*, Vol. 74, No. 2, (454-461), 0175-7598

Huang, X. Q.; Lu, Z. X., Zhao, H. Z., Bie, X. M., Lu, F. X. & Yang, S. J. (2006). Antiviral activity of antimicrobial lipopeptide from Bacillus subtilis fmbj against Pseudorabies Virus, Porcine Parvovirus, Newcastle Disease Virus and Infectious Bursal Disease Virus in vitro. *International Journal of Peptide Research and Therapeutics*, Vol. 12, No. 4, (373-377), 1573-3149

Huang, X. Q.; Wang, Y. F., Cui, Y. H. & Hua, X. (2010). Optimization of Antifungal Effect of Surfactin and Iturin to Penicillium notatum in Syrup of Peach by RSM. *International Journal of Peptide Research and Therapeutics*, Vol. 16, No. 2, (63-69), 1573-3149

Hue, N.; Serani, L. & Laprevote, O. (2001). Structural investigation of cyclic peptidolipids from Bacillus subtilis by high-energy tandem mass spectrometry. *Rapid Communications in Mass Spectrometry*, Vol. 15, No. 3, (203-209), 0951-4198

Hwang, M. H.; Chang, Z. Q., Kang, E. H., Lim, J. H., Yun, H. I., Rhee, M. H., Jeong, K. S. & Park, S. C. (2008a). Surfactin C inhibits Mycoplasma hyopneumoniae-induced transcription of proinflammatory cytokines and nitric oxide production in murine RAW 264.7 cells. *Biotechnology Letters*, Vol. 30, No. 2, (229-233), 0141-5492

Hwang, M. H.; Kim, M. H., Gebru, E., Jung, B. Y., Lee, S. P. & Park, S. C. (2008b). Killing rate curve and combination effects of surfactin C produced from Bacillus subtilis complex BC1212 against pathogenic Mycoplasma hyopneumoniae. *World Journal of Microbiology and Biotechnology*, Vol. 24, No. 10, (2277-2282), 0959-3993

Hwang, M. H.; Lim, J. H., Yun, H. I., Rhee, M. H., Cho, J. Y., Hsu, W. H. & Park, S. C. (2005). Surfactin C inhibits the lipopolysaccharide-induced transcription of interleukin-1beta and inducible nitric oxide synthase and nitric oxide production in murine RAW 264.7 cells. *Biotechnology Letters*, Vol. 27, No. 20, (1605-1608), 0141-5492

Hwang, Y. H.; Kim, M. S., Song, I. B., Park, B. K., Lim, J. H., Park, S. C. & Yun, H. I. (2009). Subacute (28 day) Toxicity of Surfactin C, a Lipopeptide Produced by Bacillus subtilis, in Rats. *Journal of Health Science*, Vol. 55, No. 3, (351-355), 1344-9702

Hwang, Y. H.; Park, B. K., Lim, J. H., Kim, M. S., Park, S. C., Hwang, M. H. & Yun, H. I. (2007). Lipopolysaccharide-binding and neutralizing activities of surfactin C in experimental models of septic shock. *European Journal of Pharmacology*, Vol. 556, No. 1-3, (166-171), 0014-2999

Hwang, Y. H.; Park, B. K., Lim, J. H., Kim, M. S., Song, I. B., Park, S. C. & Yun, H. I. (2008c). Evaluation of genetic and developmental toxicity of surfactin C from Bacillus subtilis BC1212. *Journal of Health Science*, Vol. 54, No. 1, (101-106), 1344-9702

Chakrabarty, S. P.; Saikumari, Y. K., Bopanna, M. P. & Balaram, H. (2008). Biochemical characterization of Plasmodium falciparum Sir2, a NAD(+)-dependent deacetylase. *Molecular and Biochemical Parasitology*, Vol. 158, No. 2, (139-151), 0166-6851

Chen, H.; Wang, L., Su, C. X., Gong, G. H., Wang, P. & Yu, Z. L. (2008). Isolation and characterization of lipopeptide antibiotics produced by Bacillus subtilis. *Letters in Applied Microbiology*, Vol. 47, No. 3, (180-186), 0266-8254

Isa, M. H. M.; Coraglia, D. E., Frazier, R. A. & Jauregi, P. (2007). Recovery and purification of surfactin from fermentation broth by a two-step ultrafiltration process. *Journal of Membrane Science*, Vol. 296, No. 1-2, (51-57), 0376-7388

Ishigami, Y.; Osman, M., Nakahara, H., Sano, Y., Ishiguro, R. & Matsumoto, M. (1995). Significance of beta-sheet formation for micellization and surface-adsorption of surfactin. *Colloids and Surfaces B-Biointerfaces*, Vol. 4, No. 6, (341-348), 0927-7765

Juang, R. S.; Chen, H. L. & Chen, Y. S. (2008). Resistance-in-series analysis in cross-flow ultrafiltration of fermentation broths of Bacillus subtilis culture. *Journal of Membrane Science*, Vol. 323, No. 1, (193-200), 0376-7388

Julkowska, D.; Obuchowski, M., Holland, I. B. & Seror, S. J. (2005). Comparative analysis of the development of swarming communities of Bacillus subtilis 168 and a natural wild type: critical effects of surfactin and the composition of the medium. *Journal of Bacteriology*, Vol. 187, No. 1, (65-76), 0021-9193

Kakinuma, A.; Hori, M., Isono, M., Tamura, G. & Arima, K. (1969). Determination of amino acid sequence in surfactin, a crystalline peptidelipid surfactant produced by Bacillus subtilis. *Agricultural and Biological Chemistry*, Vol. 33, No. 6, (971-979), 0002-1369

Kameda, Y.; Ouhira, S., Matsui, K., Kanatomo, S., Hase, T. & Atsusaka, T. (1974). Antitumor activity of Bacillus natto. 5. Isolation and characterization of surfactin in culture medium of Bacillus natto KMD 2311. *Chemical and Pharmaceutical Bulletin*, Vol. 22, No. 4, (938-944), 0009-2363

Kearns, D. B.; Chu, F., Rudner, R. & Losick, R. (2004). Genes governing swarming in Bacillus subtilis and evidence for a phase variation mechanism controlling surface motility. *Molecular Microbiology*, Vol. 52, No. 2, (357-369), 0950-382X

Kell, H.; Holzwarth, J. F., Boettcher, C., Heenan, R. K. & Vater, J. (2007). Physicochemical studies of the interaction of the lipoheptapeptide surfactin with lipid bilayers of L-alpha-dimyristoyl phosphatidylcholine. *Biophysical Chemistry*, Vol. 128, No. 2-3, (114-124), 0301-4622

Kikuchi, T. & Hasumi, K. (2002). Enhancement of plasminogen activation by surfactin C: augmentation of fibrinolysis in vitro and in vivo. *Biochimica et Biophysica Acta*, Vol. 1596, No. 2, (234-245), 0006-3002

Kikuchi, T. & Hasumi, K. (2003). Enhancement of reciprocal activation of prourokinase and plasminogen by the bacterial lipopeptide surfactins and iturin Cs. *Journal of Antibiotics*, Vol. 56, No. 1, (34-37), 0021-8820

Kim, K.; Jung, S. Y., Lee, D. K., Jung, J. K., Park, J. K., Kim, D. K. & Lee, C. H. (1998). Suppression of inflammatory responses by surfactin a selective inhibitor of platelet cytosolic phospholipase A2. *Biochemical Pharmacology*, Vol. 55, No. 7, (975-985), 0006-2952

Kim, P. I.; Ryu, J., Kim, Y. H. & Chi, Y. T. (2010). Production of biosurfactant lipopeptides Iturin A, fengycin and surfactin A from Bacillus subtilis CMB32 for control of Colletotrichum gloeosporioides. *Journal of Microbiology and Biotechnology*, Vol. 20, No. 1, (138-145), 1017-7825

Kim, S. D.; Park, S. K., Cho, J. Y., Park, H. J., Lim, J. H., Yun, H. I., Park, S C., Lee, K. Y., Kim, S. K. & Rhee, M. H. (2006). Surfactin C inhibits platelet aggregation. *Journal of Pharmacy and Pharmacology*, Vol. 58, No. 6, (867-870), 0022-3573

Kim, S. Y.; Kim, J. Y., Kim, S. H., Bae, H. J., Yi, H., Yoon, S. H., Koo, B. S., Kwon, M., Cho, J. Y., Lee, C. E. & Hong, S. (2007). Surfactin from Bacillus subtilis displays anti-proliferative effect via apoptosis induction, cell cycle arrest and survival signaling suppression. *FEBS Letters*, Vol. 581, No. 5, (865-871), 0014-5793

Kinsinger, R. F.; Kearns, D. B., Hale, M. & Fall, R. (2005). Genetic requirements for potassium ion-dependent colony spreading in Bacillus subtilis. *Journal of Bacteriology*, Vol. 187, No. 24, (8462-8469), 0021-9193

Kinsinger, R. F.; Shirk, M. C. & Fall, R. (2003). Rapid surface motility in Bacillus subtilis is dependent on extracellular surfactin and potassium ion. *Journal of Bacteriology*, Vol. 185, No. 18, (5627-5631), 0021-9193

Kolter, R. (2010). Biofilms in lab and nature: a molecular geneticist's voyage to microbial ecology. *International Microbiology*, Vol. 13, No. 1, (1-7), 1139-6709

Kracht, M.; Rokos, H., Ozel, M., Kowall, M., Pauli, G. & Vater, J. (1999). Antiviral and hemolytic activities of surfactin isoforms and their methyl ester derivatives. *Journal of Antibiotics*, Vol. 52, No. 7, (613-619), 0021-8820

Kumarasamy, K. K.; Toleman, M. A., Walsh, T. R., Bagaria, J., Butt, F., Balakrishnan, R., Chaudhary, U., Doumith, M., Giske, C. G., Irfan, S., Krishnan, P., Kumar, A. V., Maharjan, S., Mushtaq, S., Noorie, T., Paterson, D. L., Pearson, A., Perry, C., Pike, R., Rao, B., Ray, U., Sarma, J. B., Sharma, M., Sheridan, E., Thirunarayan, M. A., Turton, J., Upadhyay, S., Warner, M., Welfare, W., Livermore, D. M. & Woodford, N. (2010). Emergence of a new antibiotic resistance mechanism in India, Pakistan, and the UK: a molecular, biological, and epidemiological study. *The Lancet Infectious Diseases*, Vol. 10, No. 9, (597-602), 1473-3099

Li, Y.; Ye, R. Q. & Mu, B. Z. (2009a). Influence of Sodium Ions on Micelles of Surfactin-C-16 in Solution. *Journal of Surfactants and Detergents*, Vol. 12, No. 1, (31-36), 1097-3958

Li, Y.; Zou, A. H., Ye, R. Q. & Mu, B. Z. (2009b). Counterion-Induced Changes to the Micellization of Surfactin-C-16 Aqueous Solution. *Journal of Physical Chemistry B*, Vol. 113, No. 46, (15272-15277), 1520-6106

Lim, J. H.; Park, B. K., Kim, M. S., Hwang, M. H., Rhee, M. H., Park, S. C. & Yun, H. I. (2005). The anti-thrombotic activity of surfactins. *Journal of Veterinary Science*, Vol. 6, No. 4, (353-355), 1229-845X

Liu, J.; Zou, A. H. & Mu, B. Z. (2010). Surfactin effect on the physicochemical property of PC liposome. *Colloids and Surfaces a-Physicochemical and Engineering Aspects*, Vol. 361, No. 1-3, (90-95), 0927-7757

Lopez, D.; Fischbach, M. A., Chu, F., Losick, R. & Kolter, R. (2009a). Structurally diverse natural products that cause potassium leakage trigger multicellularity in Bacillus subtilis. *Proceedings of the National Academy of Sciences of U S A*, Vol. 106, No. 1, (280-285), 1091-6490

Lopez, D. & Kolter, R. (2010). Extracellular signals that define distinct and coexisting cell fates in Bacillus subtilis. *Fems Microbiology Reviews*, Vol. 34, No. 2, (134-149), 0168-6445

Lopez, D.; Vlamakis, H. & Kolter, R. (2009b). Generation of multiple cell types in Bacillus subtilis. *Fems Microbiology Reviews*, Vol. 33, No. 1, (152-163), 0168-6445

Lopez, D.; Vlamakis, H., Losick, R. & Kolter, R. (2009c). Cannibalism enhances biofilm development in Bacillus subtilis. *Molecular Microbiology*, Vol. 74, No. 3, (609-618), 1365-2958

Lopez, D.; Vlamakis, H., Losick, R. & Kolter, R. (2009d). Paracrine signaling in a bacterium. *Genes and Development*, Vol. 23, No. 14, (1631-1638), 1549-5477

Maget-Dana, R. & Ptak, M. (1992). Interfacial properties of surfactin. *Journal of Colloid and Interface Science*, Vol. 153, No. 1, (285-291), 0021-9797

Maget-Dana, R. & Ptak, M. (1995). Interactions of surfactin with membrane models. *Biophysical Journal*, Vol. 68, No. 5, (1937-1943), 0006-3495

Mireles, J. R., 2nd; Toguchi, A. & Harshey, R. M. (2001). Salmonella enterica serovar typhimurium swarming mutants with altered biofilm-forming abilities: surfactin inhibits biofilm formation. *Journal of Bacteriology*, Vol. 183, No. 20, (5848-5854), 0021-9193

Morikawa, M. (2006). Beneficial biofilm formation by industrial bacteria Bacillus subtilis and related species. *Journal of Bioscience and Bioengineering*, Vol. 101, No. 1, (1-8), 1389-1723

Morikawa, M.; Hirata, Y. & Imanaka, T. (2000). A study on the structure-function relationship of lipopeptide biosurfactants. *Biochimica et Biophysica Acta*, Vol. 1488, No. 3, (211-218), 0006-3002

Mukherjee, S.; Das, P. & Sen, R. (2006). Towards commercial production of microbial surfactants. *Trends in Biotechnology*, Vol. 24, No. 11, (509-515), 0167-7799

Mulligan, C. N. (2009). Recent advances in the environmental applications of biosurfactants. *Current Opinion in Colloid and Interface Science*, Vol. 14, No. 5, (372-378), 1359-0294

Nakano, M. M.; Corbell, N., Besson, J. & Zuber, P. (1992). Isolation and characterization of sfp: a gene that functions in the production of the lipopeptide biosurfactant, surfactin, in Bacillus subtilis. *Molecular and General Genetics*, Vol. 232, No. 2, (313-321), 0026-8925

Nitschke, M.; Araujo, L. V., Costa, S. G., Pires, R. C., Zeraik, A. E., Fernandes, A. C., Freire, D. M. & Contiero, J. (2009). Surfactin reduces the adhesion of food-borne pathogenic bacteria to solid surfaces. *Letters in Applied Microbiology*, Vol. 49, No. 2, (241-247), 0266-8254

Nitschke, M. & Costa, S. (2007). Biosurfactants in food industry. *Trends in Food Science & Technology*, Vol. 18, No. 5, (252-259), 0924-2244

Park, S. Y. & Kim, Y. (2009). Surfactin inhibits immunostimulatory function of macrophages through blocking NK-kappaB, MAPK and Akt pathway. *International Immunopharmacology*, Vol. 9, No. 7-8, (886-893), 1878-1705

Patrick, J. E. & Kearns, D. B. (2009). Laboratory Strains of Bacillus subtilis Do Not Exhibit Swarming Motility. *Journal of Bacteriology*, Vol. 191, No. 22, (7129-7133), 0021-9193

Peypoux, F.; Bonmatin, J. M. & Wallach, J. (1999). Recent trends in the biochemistry of surfactin. *Applied Microbiology and Biotechnology*, Vol. 51, No. 5, (553-563), 0175-7598

Ponte Rocha, M. V.; Gomes Barreto, R. V., Melo, V. M. & Barros Gonçalves, L. R. (2009). Evaluation of cashew apple juice for surfactin production by Bacillus subtilis LAMI008. *Applied Biochemistry and Biotechnology*, Vol. 155, No. 1-3, (366-378), 1559-0291

Porrini, M. P.; Audisio, M. C., Sabate, D. C., Ibarguren, C., Medici, S. K., Sarlo, E. G., Garrido, P. M. & Eguaras, M. J. (2010). Effect of bacterial metabolites on microsporidian Nosema ceranae and on its host Apis mellifera. *Parasitology Research*, Vol. 107, No. 2, (381-388), 0932-0113

Razafindralambo, H.; Dufour, S., Paquot, M. & Deleu, M. (2009). Thermodynamic studies of the binding interactions of surfactin analogues to lipid vesicles. Application of isothermal titration calorimetry. *Journal of Thermal Analysis and Calorimetry*, Vol. 95, No. 3, (817-821), 1388-6150

Rivardo, F.; Martinotti, M. G., Turner, R. J. & Ceri, H. (2010). The activity of silver against Escherichia coli biofilm is increased by a lipopeptide biosurfactant. *Canadian Journal of Microbiology*, Vol. 56, No. 3, (272-278), 0008-4166

Rivardo, F.; Turner, R. J., Allegrone, G., Ceri, H. & Martinotti, M. G. (2009). Anti-adhesion activity of two biosurfactants produced by Bacillus spp. prevents biofilm formation of human bacterial pathogens. *Applied Microbiology and Biotechnology*, Vol. 83, No. 3, (541-553), 0175-7598

Rodrigues, L.; Banat, I. M., Teixeira, J. & Oliveira, R. (2006). Biosurfactants: potential applications in medicine. *Journal of Antimicrobial Chemotherapy*, Vol. 57, No. 4, (609-618), 0305-7453

Rosenberg, E. & Ron, E. Z. (1999). High- and low-molecular-mass microbial surfactants. *Applied Microbiology and Biotechnology*, Vol. 52, No. 2, (154-162), 0175-7598

Sabate, D. C.; Carrillo, L. & Audisio, M. C. (2009). Inhibition of Paenibacillus larvae and Ascosphaera apis by Bacillus subtilis isolated from honeybee gut and honey samples. *Research in Microbiology*, Vol. 160, No. 3, (193-199), 0923-2508

Selvam, R.; Maheswari, P., Kavitha, P., Ravichandran, M., Sas, B. & Ramchand, C. N. (2009). Effect of Bacillus subtilis PB6, a natural probiotic on colon mucosal inflammation and plasma cytokines levels in inflammatory bowel disease. *Indian Journal of Biochemistry and Biophysics*, Vol. 46, No. 1, (79-85), 0301-1208

Seydlova, G.; Patek, M. & Svobodova, J. (2009). Construction of a surfactin non-producing mutant of Bacillus subtilis as a tool for membrane resistance study. *Febs Journal*, Vol. 276, No., (222-222), 1742-464X

Seydlova, G. & Svobodova, J. (2008a). Development of membrane lipids in the surfactin producer Bacillus subtilis. *Folia Microbiologica*, Vol. 53, No. 4, (303-307), 0015-5632

Seydlova, G. & Svobodova, J. (2008b). Review of surfactin chemical properties and the potential biomedical applications. *Central European Journal of Medicine*, Vol. 3, No. 2, (123-133), 1895-1058

Shaligram, N. S. & Singhal, R. S. (2010). Surfactin - A review on biosynthesis, fermentation, purification and applications. *Food technology and biotechnology*, Vol. 48, No. 2, (119-134), 1330-9862

Shen, H. H.; Thomas, R. K., Chen, C. Y., Darton, R. C., Baker, S. C. & Penfold, J. (2009). Aggregation of the Naturally Occurring Lipopeptide, Surfactin, at Interfaces and in Solution: An Unusual Type of Surfactant? *Langmuir*, Vol. 25, No. 7, (4211-4218), 0743-7463

Shen, H. H.; Thomas, R. K., Penfold, J. & Fragneto, G. (2010a). Destruction and Solubilization of Supported Phospholipid Bilayers on Silica by the Biosurfactant Surfactin. *Langmuir*, Vol. 26, No. 10, (7334-7342), 0743-7463

Shen, H. H.; Thomas, R. K. & Taylor, P. (2010b). The Location of the Biosurfactant Surfactin in Phospholipid Bilayers Supported on Silica Using Neutron Reflectometry. *Langmuir*, Vol. 26, No. 1, (320-327), 0743-7463

Singh, P. & Cameotra, S. S. (2004). Potential applications of microbial surfactants in biomedical sciences. *Trends in Biotechnology*, Vol. 22, No. 3, (142-146), 0167-7799

Souto, G. I.; Correa, O. S., Montecchia, M. S., Kerber, N. L., Pucheu, N. L., Bachur, M. & Garcia, A. F. (2004). Genetic and functional characterization of a Bacillus sp. strain excreting surfactin and antifungal metabolites partially identified as iturin-like compounds. *Journal of Applied Microbiology*, Vol. 97, No. 6, (1247-1256), 1364-5072

Stanley, N. R. & Lazazzera, B. A. (2004). Environmental signals and reglatory pathways that influence biofilm formation. *Molecular Microbiology*, Vol. 52, No. 4, (917-924)

Stein, T. (2005). Bacillus subtilis antibiotics: structures, syntheses and specific functions. *Molecular Microbiology*, Vol. 56, No. 4, (845-857), 0950-382X

Straight, P. D.; Willey, J. M. & Kolter, R. (2006). Interactions between Streptomyces coelicolor and Bacillus subtilis: Role of surfactants in raising aerial structures. *Journal of Bacteriology*, Vol. 188, No. 13, (4918-4925), 0021-9193

Symmank, H.; Franke, P., Saenger, W. & Bernhard, F. (2002). Modification of biologically active peptides: production of a novel lipohexapeptide after engineering of Bacillus subtilis surfactin synthetase. *Protein Engineering*, Vol. 15, No. 11, (913-921), 0269-2139

Takahashi, T.; Ohno, O., Ikeda, Y., Sawa, R., Homma, Y., Igarashi, M. & Umezawa, K. (2006). Inhibition of lipopolysaccharide activity by a bacterial cyclic lipopeptide surfactin. *Journal of Antibiotics*, Vol. 59, No. 1, (35-43), 0021-8820

Tang, J. S.; Gao, H., Hong, K., Yu, Y., Jiang, M. M., Lin, H. P., Ye, W. C. & Yao, X. S. (2007). Complete assignments of H-1 and C-13 NMR spectral data of nine surfactin isomers. *Magnetic Resonance in Chemistry*, Vol. 45, No. 9, (792-796), 0749-1581

Thimon, L.; Peypoux, F., Maget-Dana, R., Roux, B. & Michel, G. (1992). Interactions of bioactive lipopeptides, iturin A and surfactin from Bacillus subtilis. *Biotechnology and Applied Biochemistry*, Vol. 16, No. 2, (144-151), 0885-4513

Tsan, P.; Volpon, L., Besson, F. & Lancelin, J. M. (2007). Structure and dynamics of surfactin studied by NMR in micellar media. *Journal of the American Chemical Society*, Vol. 129, No. 7, (1968-1977), 0002-7863

Tsuge, K.; Ohata, Y. & Shoda, M. (2001). Gene yerP, involved in surfactin self-resistance in Bacillus subtilis. *Antimicrobial Agents and Chemotherapy*, Vol. 45, No. 12, (3566-3573), 0066-4804

Vollenbroich, D.; Ozel, M., Vater, J., Kamp, R. M. & Pauli, G. (1997a). Mechanism of inactivation of enveloped viruses by the biosurfactant surfactin from Bacillus subtilis. *Biologicals*, Vol. 25, No. 3, (289-297), 1045-1056

Vollenbroich, D.; Pauli, G., Ozel, M. & Vater, J. (1997b). Antimycoplasma properties and application in cell culture of surfactin, a lipopeptide antibiotic from Bacillus subtilis. *Applied and Environmental Microbiology*, Vol. 63, No. 1, (44-49), 0099-2240

Wei, Y. H.; Wang, L. F. & Chang, J. S. (2004). Optimizing iron supplement strategies for enhanced surfactin production with Bacillus subtilis. *Biotechnology Progress*, Vol. 20, No. 3, (979-983), 8756-7938

Yoneda, T.; Miyota, Y., Furuya, K. & Tsuzuki, T. (2006). Production process of surfactin. US patent 7011969.

Yoneyama, H. & Katsumata, R. (2006). Antibiotic resistance in bacteria and its future for novel antibiotic development. *Bioscience Biotechnology and Biochemistry*, Vol. 70, No. 5, (1060-1075), 0916-8451

Yong, D.; Toleman, M. A., Giske, C. G., Cho, H. S., Sundman, K., Lee, K. & Walsh, T. R. (2009). Characterization of a New Metallo-beta-Lactamase Gene, bla(NDM-1), and a Novel Erythromycin Esterase Gene Carried on a Unique Genetic Structure in Klebsiella pneumoniae Sequence Type 14 from India. *Antimicrobial Agents and Chemotherapy*, Vol. 53, No. 12, (5046-5054), 0066-4804

Zeraik, A. E. & Nitschke, M. (2010). Biosurfactants as Agents to Reduce Adhesion of Pathogenic Bacteria to Polystyrene Surfaces: Effect of Temperature and Hydrophobicity. *Current Microbiology*, Vol., No., 1432-0991

Zou, A.; Liu, J., Garamus, V. M., Yang, Y., Willumeit, R. & Mu, B. (2010). Micellization activity of the natural lipopeptide [Glu1, Asp5] surfactin-C15 in aqueous solution. *The Journal of Physical Chemistry B*, Vol. 114, No. 8, (2712-2718), 1520-5207

14

Molecular and Cellular Mechanism Studies on Anticancer Effects of Chinese Medicine

Yigang Feng[1], Ning Wang[2], Fan Cheung[2], Meifen Zhu[2], Hongyun Li[1] and Yibin Feng[2*]

[1]*Guanhau School of Stomatology, Hospital of Stomatology, Sun Yat-sen University, Guangzhou,*

[2]*School of Chinese Medicine, The University of Hong Kong, 10 Sassoon Road, Pokfulam, Hong Kong, PR China*

1. Introduction

Chinese medicine is an unique medical system, among which Chinese medicines (including Chinese medicinal plants, Chinese animal drugs, Chinese mineral drugs and composite formulae) have been used in main stream medical health care in China for years of thousands and have been accepted by many countries as complemental and alternative medicine. As one of the major traditional medicines and Ethnomedicines in the world, Chinese medicines as a resource and materials for unmet medical needs have been attracted by scientists in medical, pharmaceutical, biomedical engineering and life sciences. The challenges in safety (such as Aristolochic acid nephropathy, Chinese medicines adverse reaction and herb-drug interaction), quality control (like batch-to-batch reliable, contamination pesticide and heavy metals) and green enviroments (protection of endangerous species from animal and plants) have also become emerging issues. In the past decades, chemical and pharmacological profiles of many Chinese medicines have been extensively studied. In this chapter, we focus on advanced progress in molecular and celluar mechanism studies on anticancer action of Chinese medicines by trend prediction from top journals of Chinese medicine, ethnomedicine, alternative and complemental medicine. 12 representative Chinese medicines were selected in this chapter (Rhizoma coptidis, arsenic, Rhizoma Curcuma longae, Radis stephaniae tetrandrae, Radix tripterygii wilfordii, Radix scutellariae, Herba artemisiae annuae, Radix ginseng, Radix notoginseng, Radix astragali, Radix angelicae senensis and Radix salviae miltiorrhizae) and we reviewed the recent progress in order to understand their pharmacological action, active chemical ingredients and application of new approaches (genomics, proteomics and metabolics). We concentrated on the cellular and molecular mechanisms of the therapeutic actions of these Chinese medicines and introduced the major active chemical ingredients in relation to therapeutic values. These Chinese medicines can be used in treatment of cancer. After reviewing hot Chinese medicines in treatment of cancer in this chapter, we hope it will lead to further exploration of Chinese medicines by advanced scientific technology in drug discovery for treating cancer.

* Corresponding author: E-mail: yfeng@hku.hk

2. Important

This chapter reviewed the recent progress on Chinese medicines in the cellular and molecular mechanism studies and the major active chemical ingredients of Chinese medicines in relation to therapeutic values in order to understand their pharmacological action, active chemical ingredients and application of new approaches. We noted that the cellular and molecular mechanisms and the major active chemical ingredients of Chinese medicines have been deeply and widely studied which provide a useful information for new drug development and Chinese medicine clinical practice, but the challenges in safety (such as Aristolochic acid nephropathy, Chinese medicines adverse reaction and herb-drug interaction), quality control (like batch-to-batch reliable, contamination pesticide and heavy metals) and green enviroments (protection of endangerous species from animal and plants) have also become emerging issues. On the other hand, research mainly focused on sigle Chinese medicines in the past decades, we should do more studies on composite fomulae (consist of over two single Chinese medicines) by using new technologies, such as "Omics" technologics and system biology to get more evidences for Chinese medicine practice and new drug development in the future.

3. The structure of this chapter

The selected twelve Chinese medicines cover the following contents:

i. Name of the herb: Common names, botanical name, family, origin, distribution, commercially cultivated or wild, traditional use in Chinese medicine clinical practice
ii. General chemical and pharmacological profiles
iii. Mechanism studies on anticancer effect of Chinese medicines in in vitro and in vivo study
iv. Adverse reactions
v. References

4. The contents of this chapter

4.1 Rhizoma coptidis (Huanglian in Chinese)

Coptis Rhizome (CR) is the dried rhizome of Coptis chinensis Franch (Ranunculaceae). Its Chinese name is huanglian, which was first recorded in Shen Nong Ben Cao Jing (Shen Nong's Materia Medica, 220 A.D.) Other two species of Coptis Rhizome (Coptis deltoidea C. Y. Cheng et Hsiao. and Coptis teetoides C. Y. Cheng (or Coptis teeta Wall.) were also specified in the Chinese Pharmacopoeia (The State Pharmacopoeia Commission of the P.R. China, 2005). It is native to Sichuan, Hubei, Xizang, Shanxi, and Jiangxi Province of China. The source of Huanglian can be obtained from wild species of or cultivated plants. The GAP base of Huanglian in China is located in Chongqing, Hubei. Traditionally, CR can be used in treatment of diseases like diarrhea, inflammation of the eye, and women's abdomen ailments caused by damp-heat.

Raw material of CR mainly includes a series of alkaloids, such as berberine, coptisine, epiberberine, berberrubine, palmatine, columbamine, jarorrhizine, worenine, magnoflorine, groelandicine, berberastine, oxyberberine and thalifendine ect. Other chemicals in CR include ferulic acid, obakunone and obakulactone etc. Berberine is the main component and is credited as criteria for quality control of CR in China Pharmacopeia (Edition 2005). CR and berberine have been used for treatment of intestinal infections (acute gastroenteritis, cholera and bacterial diarrhea) by their antibacterial and antiviral effects, treatment of hypercholesterolemic patients and type 2 diabetes by hypolipidemic effects, and various experimental heart diseases, such as heart failure,cardiac dysfunction, pressure-overload induced cardiac hypertrophy (Feng et al., 2010). Berberine may help in neuropsychiatric diseases by inhibiting Prolylligopeptidase, a peptidase associated to schizophrenia, bipolar affective disorder and related conditions (Tarrago et al., 2007).

Recently, the most attractive pharmacological effect of CR and berberine is its anticancer activities (Tang et al., 2009). CR and berberine were used for prevention and treatment of human cancers, such as nasopharyngeal carcinoma (NPC), cholangecarsinoma with complication of liver cancer, and phase I study of CR (Chinese Herb) in patients with advanced solid tumors (Tian et al., 2000; Feng et al., 2008; http://cancer.gov/clinicaltrials/MSKCC-00061). Berberine is the principal active compound of anticancer effect in CR (Hara et al., 2005). There are many reports showing that berberine could inhibit proliferation of cancer cells in gastric cancer, leukemia, melanoma, liver cancer, colorectal cancer, pancreas cancer, oral cancer, breast cancer, cervical cancer, lung cancer, NPC and prostate cancer cell line models and may have potential chemotherapeutic properties against human cancers (Lin et al., 2006; Jantova et al., 2003; Serafim et al., 2008; Piyanuch et al., 2007; Katiyar et al., 2009; Lin et al., 2004; Lee et al., 2006; Liu et al., 2005; Kim et al., 2004). Current studies broadly indicate the involvement of cell cytotoxicity, cell cycle regulatory machinery, inflammation and cell death signalling pathways as targets of anticancer by berberine and Huanglian. It was demonstrated that CR extract can inhibit cancer cell growth by suppressing the expression of cyclin B1 and inhibiting CDC2 kinase activity in human cancer cells and induce apoptosis by up-regulation of interferon-beta and TNF-alpha (Low et al., 2002; Li et al., 2000; Kang et al., 2005). Multiple mechanisms underlying the anti-cancer action of CR and berberine have been reported and may involved inhibition of NFkappa-b pathways, induction of cell cycle arrest and apoptosis (Pandey et al., 2008; Hsu et al., 2007; Mantena et al., 2006). Anti-metastatic effects of berberine have been reported and inhibition of urokinase-plasminogen activator and matrix metalloproteinase-2 was implicated (Peng et al., 2006). It was also reported that berberine inhibits HIF-1alpha expression via enhanced proteolysis (Lin et al., 2004). Anti-inflammation may be another profile of CR and berberine in treatment of Cancers. The anti-inflammatory efficacy of berberine is due to its inhibition of prostaglandin E2 (PGE2) followed by the reduction of COX-2 protein in vivo and in vitro of malignant tumor (Kuo et al., 2004). Berberine could suppress inflammatory agents-induced interleukin-1β (IL-1β) and Tumor necrosis factor-α (TNF-α) productions via inhibiting the phosphorylation and degradation of inhibitor of kappa B-α (IκB-α) (Lee et al., 2007). We provide a new mechanism for anti-invasion of berberine which is to inhibit RhoA signaling pathway, an upstream of NF-kappa B (Tsang et al., 2009). In this study, we found that berberine distribution in cell nuclear and cytoplasm in dose dependent manner, so anti-invasion of berberine may inhibit RhoA signaling pathway at low dose while apoptosis are induced by berberine via G2 arrest at high dose in NPC cell lines. Furthermore, at low dose we use liver cancer cell lines (MHCC97-L) to demonstrate that CR extract has better anti-invasion than berberine and clarify that anti-invasive effect of CR extract on MHCC97-L cell line specific acts on F-actin via Rho/ROCK signaling pathway, but not other metastasis-related molecules such as integrin beta4, E-cadherine, u-PA and MMPs (Wang et al., 2010). At high dose, we use liver cancer cell lines (MHCC97-L and HepG2) to demonstrate that berberine can induce both apoptotic and autophagic cell death, in which apoptosis is major cell death type (Wang et al., 2010). Our results suggests that CR and berberine are promise alternative therapy in treatment of cancers. Computer–aided molecular design and prediction of cell response to CR, berberine and analogs, and genomics and proteomics, microRNA approaches to study antineoplastic effects of berberine and Huanglian are expected in the future. The relatively low toxicities at therapeutic level for both Huanglian and berberine also show additional benefit for their further development.

Adverse responses of berberine include constipation, laxative, anaphylaxis and other skin allergies such as dermatitis and rashes, and overdose may cause respiratory and circulatory system problems (Bao, 1983). Furthermore, berberine could displace bilirubin from serum-binding proteins, causing jaundice, kernicterus, and brain damage in infants (Bateman et al., 1998; Chan, 1993, 1994).

4.2 Arsenic (Pishuang in Chinese)

In Chinese medicine, arsenic was first recorded in Chinese book "KAI BAO BAN CAO" (Kai Bao of Materia Nedica, 973 A.D.). Arsenic has various forms. The most important compounds of arsenic are arsenic trioxide, As2O3, ("white arsenic"), the yellow sulfide orpiment (As2S3) and red realgar (As2S2). In 2006 and 2007, China was the top producer of arsenic trioxide with almost 50% world share, followed by Chile, Morocco and Peru, reports the United States Geological Survey [U.S. Geological Survey, 2008]. In modern society, arsenic and its compounds are used as pesticides, herbicides, insecticides and in various alloys, while arsenic compounds used as anti-cancer agents are a fascinating story. Arsenic has a long history of use in Chinese and Western medicine for cancer treatment. Contemporary clinical use of arsenic trioxide is largely due to purification of this compound from traditional mixtures, and the definition of effective, low-dose regimens for the treatment of acute promyelocytic leukemia (APL) [Chen et al., 2002].

In the 90's years of last century, two arsenic components including arsenic trioxide (As203) [Sun et al., 1992] and arsenic disulfide [Huang et al., 1995] used in some traditional Chinese formulae have been shown very effective in patients with acute promyelocytic leukemia (APL) treatment. Using NB4 cells model, cellular and molecular mechanisms of arsenic trioxide treatment have been clarified by modulation of bcl-2, as well as PML-RAR alpha and/ or PML proteins and induction of apoptosis, which is independent from the retinoid pathway [Chen et al., 1996]. Further studies indicated that As2O3 had dose-dependent dual effects on APL cells: inducing preferentially apoptosis at relatively high concentrations (0.5 to 2 micromol/L) and inducing partial differentiation at low concentrations (0.1 to 0.5 micromol/L) [Chen, et al., 1997], and As2O3 treatment is also an effective and relatively safe drug in APL patients refractory to all-trans retinoic acid (ATRA) and conventional chemotherapy [Shen et al., 1997]. Differentiation and apoptosis induction therapy in APL was established by combination therapy of ATRA and As2O3 [Giannì et al., 1998; Wang et al., 2000]. Synergic effects of arsenic trioxide and other drugs on APL, chronic myeloid leukemia and other solid cancers, such as in patients with primary hepatocellular and gallbladder tumors were also recommended [Chen et al., 2002; Du et al., 2006; Wang et al., 2008; Hu et al., 2009]. PML and PML-RARalpha (a fusion protein containing sequences from the PML zinc finger protein and retinoic acid receptor alpha) degradation is triggered by their SUMOylation, but the mechanism by which arsenic trioxide induces this posttranslational modification is unclear. Recently, Chen's group reported in Science demonstrated that PML is a direct target of arsenic trioxide providing new insights into the drug's mechanism of action and its specificity for APL. They showed that arsenic binds directly to cysteine residues in zinc fingers located within the RBCC domain of PML-RAR and PML. Arsenic binding induces PML oligomerization, which increases its interaction with the small ubiquitin-like protein modifier (SUMO)-conjugating enzyme UBC9, resulting in enhanced SUMOylation and degradation [Zhang et al., 2010].

Arsenic and many of its compounds are potent poisons. The International Agency for Research on Cancer (IARC) recognizes arsenic and arsenic compounds as group 1 carcinogens, as their toxic mechanisms, arsenic disrupts ATP production through several pathways [Klaassen C, Watkins J. 2003].

Arsenic is known to cause arsenicosis owing to its manifestation in drinking water. The study of chemolithoautotrophic As(III) oxidizers and the heterotrophic As(V) reducers can help the understanding of the oxidation and/or reduction of arsenic [Croal et al., 2004]. Treatment of chronic arsenic poisoning has been accomplished [The Psychiatric, Psychogenic and Somatopsychic Disorders Handbook. 1978].

4.3 Rhizoma Curcumae longae (Jiang Huang in Chinese)

Rhizoma Curcumae longae is the dried rhizome of Curcuma longa L. (Zingiberaceae), mainly produced in Sichuan, Fujian, Jiangxi and Yunnan. It was first recorded in Xin Xiu Ben cao (659 A.D.). The rhizome is collected in autumn and winter when the aerial part wither, washed clean, boiled or steamed thoroughly, dried in the sun, removed from fibrous root, and cut into slices. Traditionally, Rhizoma Curcumae longae can be used in treatment of pains and tumour induced by Qi and blood stasis.

Major chemical components in Rhizoma Curcumae longae are volatile oil (6%) composed of a number of monoterpenes and sesquiterpenes, including zingiberene, curcumene, α- and β-turmerone and others. The colouring principles (5%) are curcuminoids, 50–60% of which are a mixture of curcumin, monodesmethoxycurcumin and bisdesmethoxycurcumin (WHO Monographs on Selected Medicinal Plants). Recent pharmacological studies show that Rhizoma Curcumae longae has various kinds of action, including anti-inflammation, anti-microbial, anti-oxidation, cholagogue, antihyperlipidemics and cardiovasucular action.

There has been a long history for studies focusing on anti-tumor effect of Rhizoma Curcumae longae since Kuttan and his collegues firstly reported its anti-cancer potential in 1985 (Kuttan et al., 1985). Recent study reveals the anti-tumor activity of radix curcumae extract on human cervical cancer cells in vitro and in vivo by inducing, G1 cycle arrest, apoptosis and inhibiting proliferation. Molecular events invovled include retinoblastoma protein dephosphorylation, reduced amounts of cyclins D1 and D3, and cyclin-dependent kinase 4 and 6 proteins, caspase activation and PARP cleavage, mitochondrial membrane potential loss by Mcl-1 and Bcl-xL reduction and reduced PTEN, AKT, and STAT3 phosphorylation and downregulation of NFkappaB signaling (Lim et al., 2010). The anti-carcinogenic effect of Curcuma longa was further demonstrated in MNNG-induced tumorogenesis model, where the herbal extract reduces the expressions of VEGF, COX-2 and PCNA and inhibits gastric cancer growth (Lu, et al., 2010). Moreover, recent study exhibits the immunostimulatory activities of polysaccharide extract of Curcuma longa, indicating its potential as an adjuvant supplement for cancer patients, whose immune activities were suppressed during chemotherapies (Yue et al., 2010) As the major active compound discovered in Curcuma longa, curcumin is also under extensive study on its anti-tumor activity and underlying mechanism. Sahu et al reported that curcumin is able to induce G2/M cell cycle arrest in human pancreatic cancer cells. Phosphorylation of Chk1 at

Ser-345, Cdc25C at Ser-216 and a subtle increase in ATM phosphorylation at Ser-1981 are observed and silencing the Chk1/ATM pathway attenuated curcumin's effect on cancer cell cycle (Sahu et al., 2009). Another study also exhibits curcumin's action on G1/S phase of cell cycle in human prostate cancer cells, whcih is correlated with curcumin-induced expression of cyclin-dependent kinase (CDK) inhibitors p16(/INK4a), p21(/WAF1/CIP1) and p27(/KIP1), and the suppression of cyclin E and cyclin D1, and hyperphosphorylation of retinoblastoma (Rb) protein (Srivastava, et al., 2007). Curcumin could also depolymerizes mitotic microtubules, perturbes microtubule-kinetochore attachment and disturbes the mitotic spindle structure. Pertubed localization of the kinesin protein Eg5 and subsequent monopolar spindle formation is induced by curcumin. Further, curcumin increases the accumulation of Mad2 and BubR1 at the kinetochores and activate the mitotic checkpoint to induce apoptosis (Banerjee et al., 2010). Curcumin is able to induce apoptosis by some other pathways. Chen et al shows that curcumin could activate Bax expression and suppress Bcl-2 to change the Bax/Bcl-2 ratio, and decrease the motochondrial membrane potential to led to Cytochrome C release, caspase-9 and -3 activation and PARP cleavage. Blockade of caspase pathway attenuates curcumin's effect on apoptosis induction in human A549 lung adenocarcinoma cells (Chen et al., 2010). Curcumin also induces apoptosis through activate FAS and FADD, and triggers caspase-3 independent apoptotic cell death (Lu et al., 2009). Moreover, Curcumin was reported to inhibit tumor growth through some other different pathways. Choi et al states that curcumin interrupts the interaction between the androgen receptor and Wnt/beta-catenin signaling pathway in LNCaP prostate cancer cells by suppressing the beta-catenin expression, and therefore inhibits the prostate tumor grwoth (Choi et al., 2010). Another study reveals that curcumin's inhibitory effect of tumor growth is correlated with Sp transcrption factor-regulated decreased expression of NF-kappaB and its downstream genes such as cyclin D1, survivin, and vascular endothelial growth factor that contribute to the cancer phenotype (Jutorru et al., 2010). Ning et al reports that curcumin is able to down-regulate the Notch1 Intracellular Domain and inhibits the Notch1 signaling, which is correlated with the induction of cleaved poly ADP-ribose polymerase (PARP), the degradation of cyclin D1 and increase in cyclin-dependent kinase p21. This notch1 inhibtion contributes to curcumin's inhibitory effect on hepatocellular carcinoma growth (Ning et al., 2010).

Oxdiative stress is also involve as an important mechanism of curcumin's anti-tumor effect. Curcumin could potentiate paraptosis in human breast cancer cells by promoting vacuolation from swelling and fusion of mitochondria and/or the endoplasmic reticulum (ER). The paratosis inhibitor AIP-1/Alix protein was downregulated by curcumin, and AIP-1/Alix overexpression attenuated curcumin-induced death in these cells (Yoon et al., 2010). Reactive oxygen species induced by curcumin in human non-small cell lung cancer cell triggers Bcl-2 protein's degrdation, and sensitizes cells to detachment-induced anoikis (Pongrakhananon et al., 2010). However, curcumin was also reported to be an anti-tumor agent in oxidation-resistant cells, and gamma- glutamyltranspeptidase inhibition play the major role in curcumin's effect (Quiroga et al., 2010). In addition, curcumin is also reported to induce an apoptosis-independent cell death in human cancer cells (O'Sullivan-Coyne et al., 2009). Moreover, curcumin exhibits its anti-migration action on nasopharyngeal carcinoma cells through up-regulation of E-cadherin, indicating its potential as an anti-metastasis agent (Wong et al., 2010).

As a novel molecular event in cancer progress, microRNA has been demonstrated for its important role in regulating human tumoriogenesis. Curcumin was also reported to target to miRNA to exert its anti-tumor activity. Zhang et al reports that curcumin down-regulates the expression of miR-186* in and overexpression of miR-186* significantly inhibited curcumin-induced apoptosis in A549/DDP cells (Zhang et al., 2010). Curcumin could also alter miRNA expression in human pancreatic cells, up-regulating miRNA-22 and down-regulating miRNA-199a*, and up-regulation of miRNA-22 expression by curcumin in pancreatic cancer cells suppresses expression of its target genes SP1 transcription factor (SP1) and estrogen receptor 1 (ESR1), which may be correlated with curcumin's anti-cancer activity (Sun et al., 2008).

Similar to the crude extract, curcumin exhibits immunomodulatory property in suppressing the induction of indoleamine 2,3-dioxygenase by blocking the Janus-activated kinase-protein kinase Cdelta-STAT1 signaling pathway, and showed its potential as an adjuvant agent in cancer chemotherapy (Jeong et al., 2009)

4.4 Radix stephaniae tetrandrae (Han Fangji in Chinese)

Radix stephaniae tetrandrae is the dried root of Stephania tetrandra S. Moore (Menispermaceae). With its Chinese name as Han Fangji, it was firstly recorded in Shennong Bencao Jing. Commonly called as Stephania root or Tetrandra root, the Radix stephaniae tetrandrae is considered to be bitter, cold and pungent, and belongs to the meridians of Urinary bladder, kidney and spleen. Han Fangji is distributed in Shanxi, Yunnan and Guangxi Province of China. It is used to dispel wind and dampness, and to relieve edema and pain in Chinese Medicine clinical practice.

The phytochemical study on Radix stephaniae tetrandrae exhibits that it contains several kinds of alkaloids, including Tetrandrine, Fangchinoline, Cyclanoline and Trilobine. Recent pharmacological studies show that Radix stephaniae tetrandrae and its compounds has anti-inflammatory (Shen et al., 2001), antihypertensive, anti-arrhythmic (Yu et al., 2004), and cardiovascular action (Wong et al., 2000).

The whole extract or chemical fraction of Radix stephaniae tetrandrae was rarely reported for its anti-tumor activity either in vitro or in vivo. The reason behind may be that one of other plants, Aristolochia fangchi, was used as an substitution of Stephania tetrandra due to their similar name in Chinese (Guang Fangji for Aristolochia fangchi and Han Fangji for Stephania tetrandra). Several years ago, several studies reported that urothelial carcinoma is associated with the use of Aristolochia fangchi, which contains nephrotoxic and carcinogenic aristolochic acids, to replace Stephania tetrandra (Nortier et al., 2000). However, a recent report that a Stephania tetrandra-containing Chinese Herb Formula, SENL, could reduce the expression of mutildrug resistance- associated protein and increase the intracellular accumulation of chemotherapeutic agent, Adriamycin, in human lung cancer cell line SW1573/2R120 (Xu et al., 2010), indicating Stephania tetrandra could be used as a complementary agent in chemotherapy to enhancing cancer cell sensitivity to chemotherapeutic agents. In contrast, as the major compound isolated from Stephania tetrandra, tetrandrine is extensively reported for its anti-tumor activity in various human cancers. Tetrandrine induces human cancer cell cycle arrest at G1 by first, inhibiting cyclin-dependent kinase 2 (CDK2)/cyclin E and CDK4 and second, inducing the proteolysis of CDK4, CDK6, cyclin D1, and E2F1 in HT-29 cells (Meng et al., 2004). Consistent observation of G1 arrest action of tetrandrine could be also found in another study and may be attributable to tetrandrine's inhibitory effect on AKT pathway. Inhibition of Akt could subsequently activate GSK3β and upregulate p27 (Chen et al., 2008). Tetrandrine was also reported to be capable of inducing cell apoptosis in various kinds of human cancers, including lung carcinoma (Lee, et al., 2002), leukemia (Jang et al., 2004), hepatoma (Ng et al.,

2006), nasopharyngeal carcinoma (Sun et al., 2006) and colon cancer (Chen et al., 2008). Jang et al. stated that tetradrine could induce early oxidative stress and produce ROS in human U937 cells and this result in activation of JNK pathway. However, the activation of JNK is not responsible for tetrandrine-induced apoptosis but caspase-dependent generation of a catalytically active fragment of PKC-delta may play a role (Jang et al., 2004). Sun et al. reported that tetradrine is able to induced apoptosis in human nasopharyngeal carcinoma cells CNE and this effect results from the increased expression of pro-apoptotic Bax mRNA transcript and decreased expression of anti-apoptotic factor Bcl-2 mRNA transcript (Sun et al., 2006). Wu et al. showed that apoptosis could be induced by tetrandrine in colon cancers and the increased expression of Erk1/2 and p38 MAPK are observed. However, only p38 MAPK is responsible for tetrandrine-induced apoptosis in CT-26 cells (Wu et al., 2010). However, Cho et al. stated that tetrandrine selectively inhibits the proliferation of lung cancer cells by blocking Akt activation and increases apoptosis by inhibiting ERK in human lung carcinoma cellA549 (Cho et al., 2009). These studies indicate the multiple targets of tetrandrine in treating human cancers. In addition, tetrandrine was reported to inhibit gliomas angiogenesis by suppressing the VEGF expression in gliomas cells (Chen et al., 2004) and suppress pulmonary metastases of colorectal adenocarcinoma (Chang et al., 2004), where F-actin and microtubule remodeling may be involved (Lee et al., 2002). Moreover, tetrandrine was extensively reported for its capacity in reducing multidrug resistance (MDR) by inhibiting MDR-related protein P-gp at either expression or enzymatic level and increasing the efficacy of chemotherapeutic agent (Shen et al., 2010). However, it is contradictory to observe no significant difference between the doxorubicin pharmacokinetic parameters obtained in mice received doxorubicin only and doxorubicin combined with tetrandrine (Dai et al., 2007). Further study may be required to assure the exact action and mechanism of tetrandrine in helping chemotherapeutic agents to overcome the MDR in human cancer. Another major compound in Radix stephaniae tetrandrae, fangchinoline, also exhibits reversal effect on the MDR of cancer cells in response to chemotherapeutic agents paclitaxel and vinblastin via modulation of P-gp (Chio et al., 1998; Wang et al., 2005), however, very few studies were focusing on its anti-tumor mechanism. A recent investigation reports that fangchinoline could induce G1/S phase cycle arrest via inhibiting Cyclin D1 and overexpressing p27 in human prostate cancer cell PC3. In addition, fangchinline is able to potentiate cancer cell apoptosis by inducing pro-apoptotic Bax and down-regulating anti-apoptotic Bcl-2. Inhibition of prostate cancer in xenograft model by fangchinline was also observed (Wang et al., 2010). Our on-going study shows that fangchinoline could not induce apoptosis in human hepatocellular carcinoma cells though the potent cell death could be observed when exposed to low dose of fangchinoline, indicating an althernative cell death model may be involved in fangchinoline's effect. We found that autophagic cell death may be the substitute and activation of AMPK signaling may play a role.

There is no report on the adverse reaction of Radix stephaniae tetrandrae, but overdose of Radix stephaniae tetrandrae (4.5-9 grams in decoction is appropriate) may induce vomiting, tremor, ataxia, convulsions, quadriplegia, hypertonicity, and respiratory failure.

4.5 Radix tripterygii wilfordii (Lei Gongteng in Chinese)

Radix Tripteryii Wilfordii is the dried root of Triptrygium Wifordii Hook F. It is a native plant that grows widely in China, distributed in Zhejiang, Anhui, Jiangxi, Hu'nan, Guangdong, Guangxi, Fujian, Taiwan and Yunnan province. It is used to dispel wind and dampness, and to relieve arthritis and pain in Chinese Medicine clinical practice. Anticancer application is a new use for Radix tripterygii wilfordii.

The phytochemical study on Radix tripterygii wilfordii indicates that it contains various kinds of alkaloids, including wilfordine, wilforine, wilforidine, wilforgine, wilfortrine, wilforzine, wilformine, wilfornine, euonine, celacinnine, celafurine, celabenzine, neowilforine, regilidine and terpenoids, including triptolide T13, tripdiolide, tripterolide, triptonide, triptolidenol T9, hypolide, triptonoterpenol, triptophenolide methylether, neotriptophenolide, isotriptophenolide, isoneotriptophenolide, triptonoterpene, triptonoterpene methylether, tripdioltonide, tripdiolide T8, triptriolide T11, triptolide T10, wilforlide AT1, triptotriterpenoidal lactone A, wilforlide B, triptotriterpenic acid AT3, triptotriterpenic acid BT2, triptoterpenic acid CT28, selaspermic acid, wilfornide, triptofordin A,B,C-1,C-2, D (Xian et al., 1997).

Tripteryii Wilfordii was traditionally used as an important medicine for thousand of years in Chinese Medicine to treat the syndrome associated with immune- inflammatory diseases (Jia, 1985). However, it has been shown to have multiple uses in Chinese medicine of not only immune-inflammatory diseases, but also cancers, neurodegenerative diseases and fertility regulation (Brinker et al., 2007).

Triptolide is the predominant bioacitive compound which is isolated from Radix Tripterygii wilfordii (Zhou et al., 2010). A lot of studies show that triptolide has the anti-cancer effect by inducing cell apoptosis in several kinds of cancers, including leukemia (Lou et al., 2004), colorectal cancer (Min, 2010; Xu et al., 2010), Cholangiocarcinoma (Clawon et al., 2010; Lou et al., 2004), pancreatic cancer (Chen et al., 2010; Chang et al., 2010) and breast cancer (Liu et al., 2009). The latest research showed that triptolide has the anti-cancer effect via inducing cell death in pancreatic cancer cells via autophagy and apoptosis (Mujumdar et al., 2010). Mujumdar et al. reported that triptolide could induce autophagy by some specific genes, atg5 or beclin 1. Some studies indicate that triptolide inactivated the Protein kinase B (Akt)/ mammalian target of Rapamycin/ p70S6K pathway and up-regulated the expression of Extracelluar Signal-Related kinase (ERK) 1/2 pathway to promote apoptosis in pancreatic cancer cell lines (Mujumdar et al., 2010). Wang et al. showed that triptolide has the anti-cancer effect on acute myeloid leukemia by causing down-regulation of C-KIT and inhibiting the JAK-STAT signaling, which is the same as the situation in colon cancer (Wang et al., 2009). Moreover, the expression of p65 was decreased by triptolide, which inhibits the DNA-binding activity of NF-kappaB. Triptolide also has been shown to have the ability of decreasing cell viability in all cell lines at 48h via activating caspase-3 (Clawon et al., 2010). In endometrial and ovarian cancer cells, triptolide has been reported to have the anti-growth activity via targeting some specific genes, such as LRAP, CDH4, SFRP1 and so on (Li et al., 2010). Besides, some studies indicate that triptolide could act as the inhibitor of RNA polymerase I and II-dependent transcription promoting some short-lived mRNA, for example cell cycle regulator CDC25A (Vispé et al., 2009).

Celastrol is another main component isolated from radix tripterygii wilfordii, which has been reported to have the anti-cancer effect in cancer cell lines including leukemia (Lu et al., 2010), glioma (Zhou et al., 2009) and so on. Lu et al. reported that celastrol could decrease the protein levels of Bcr-Abi and inhibit the growth in chronic myelogenous leukemia (Lu et al., 2010). Zhou et al. showed that celastrol has the anti-angiogenic effect in human glioma via in vitro and in vivo study (Zhou et al., 2009). The other studies denoted that celastrol could suppress the tumor growth mediated by angiogenesis by inhibiting AKT pathway (Pang et al., 2010).

The side effects of tripterygii wilfordii include gastrointestinal upset, infertility and suppression of lymphocyte proliferation (Chou et al., 1995).

4.6 Radix scutellariae (Huangqin in Chinese)

Radix scutellariae with the Chinese name of Huangqin, is the root of Scutellaria baicalensis Georgi (Labiatae). It is native to Jilin, Liaoning, Shanxi, Henan, Inner Mongolia and Hebei Province of China. Radix scutellariae can be obtained from wild or cultivated species. Roots of the herbs are dried for medical use. Fruits are also collected and used as herbal drugs. It can be used in treatment of symptomes induced by damp-heat or heat-toxicity which can be convinced to be diseases related to infection or inflammation in Chinese medicine clinical practice.

Radix scutellariae includes a series of flavones and their derivatives, such as baicalein, baicalin, chrysin, 5,6-dihydroxy-7-O-glucoside-flavone, 5,7,2'-trihydroxy-flavone, 5,7,2', 3'-tetraflavone, 5,7,2',6'- tetraflavone, 5,7,2'-trihydroxy-8-methoxyflavone, oroxylin-A-glucoronide, oroxylin-A, 5,7,2'-trihydroxy- 6-methoxyflavone, nor-wogonin, Wogonin, Wogonoside, 5,8,2'-trihydroxy-7-methoxyflavone, Wogonoside, Scutevulin, etc. Other chemicals in Huangqin include proline, acetophenone, palmitic acid, etc. According to China Pharmacopeia (Edition 2005), baicalin is used as quality criteria for raw Radix scutellariae, and the content of bacalin should not be lower than 9.0% for the raw material.

It was reported that the stem and leaves of Radix scutellariae reveals potent anti-bacterial effect in vitro study (Zhao et al., 2007). Some studies indicated that the ethyl acetate extracting fraction showed the best anti-bacterial effect among fractions isolated from Radix scutellaria (Ren et al., 2005). Total flavones from stem and leaf of Radix scutellaria showed preventive effect against experimental hyperlipidemia (Yi et al., 2005).

Modern studies denoted that Radix scutellaria has anti-cancer effect in various kinds of cancer cell lines including breast cancer cell (Zhou et al., 2009; Wang et al., 2010), lung cancer (Gao et al., 2010), leukemia (Kumagai et al., 2007), prostate cancer (Miocinovic et al., 2005) and so on.

It was reported that anti-proliferative and apoptotic activity against acute lymphocytic leukemia, lymphoma and myeloma cell lines (Kumagai et al., 2007). The predominant of the anti-cancer effect of baicalin has been shown to induce apoptosis (Lian et al., 2003). The investigation of baicalin showed that it could induce prostate cancer cell line DU 145 apoptosis in vitro via inhibiting Bcl-2 and Bax while up-regulating Fas (Gu et al., 2005). Wang et al. reported that baicalin induced breast cancer cells apoptosis by increasing the expression of p53 and Bax (Wang et al., 2008). Besides, some studies indicated that the cancer cell death and proliferation retardation may be induced by the inhibition of CDC2 kinase and survivin associated with opposite role of p38 mitogen-activated protein kinase and AKT (Chao et al., 2007). Moerover, Sun et al. showed that baicalin played the role of suppressing MDA-MB-435 human breast cancer cells invasion by decreasing matrix metalloproteinase-2/9 (Sun et al., 2009).

Another active compound, wogonin, has also been reported to induce apoptosis in cancer cell lines (Li, 2010). Lee et al. showed that wogonin could involve in the regulation of apoptosis in human cancer cells which may associate with p53, PUMA, and Bax (Lee et al., 2008). Zhao et al. also reported that wogonin exert anti-cancer effect via decreasing the expression of NF-KappaB which induced apoptosis (Zhao et al., 2010). Besides, wogonin has been shown to delay cancer cell growth through inhibiting Akt, GSK-3 and NF-KappaB signaling (Parajuli et al., 2010).

Clinical adverse reactions include: gastric discomfort and diarrhea; fever reaction after i.v. injection of baicalin at dose of 150 mg (Bi, 1998; Nemoto et al., 2002)

4.7 Herba artemisiae annuae (Qinghao in Chinese)

Qinghao is the aerial part of Artemisia annua L. (Compositae). It is native to Hebei, Shandong, Jiangsu, Hubei and Fujian Province of China. Qinghao can be obtained from wild or cultivated species. It is used for fever and antimalaria in Chinese medicine clinical practice.

Artemisinin, artemisinin I, artemisinin II, artemisinin III, artemisinin IV, artemisinin V arteannuic acid, aremisilactone and artenimol and their derivations are the main composition of raw material of Qinghao. The major pharmacological action of Qinghao includes antimalaria, antiviral, treatment of schistosomiasis and anticancer activity (Feng et al., 2010).

A systematic screening on the active components in Herba artemisiae annuae with cytotoxicity on serveral human tumor cell lines was investigated in 1994, which then started the cellular and molecular mechanism study of the anti-tumor activity of compounds from Herba artemisiae annuae. Artemisinin and quercetagetin 6,7,3',4'-tetramethyl ether showed significant cy-totoxicity against P-388, A-549, HT-29, MCF-7, and KB tumor cells in this study (Zheng, 1994). As the major component in Herba artemisiae annuae, artemisinin and its derivatives were extensively reported for their anti-tumor action and underlying mechanism. The general mechanism of the anti-tumor activity of artemisinin and its derivatives may be that artemisinin-like chemical could carry iron, which is required for the proliferation of cancer cells, and form free radicals to kill the cancer cell (Lai et al., 2005). However, there are some other particular mechanisms invovled. Artemisinin is able to induce G1 arrest of the cell cycle in human hepatoma cells via regulating cyclin D1, CDK2, CDK4 and serveral other CDK inhibitos (Hou, et al., 2008). Mechanism study shows that artemisinin could disrupt the interaction of transcription factor Sp1 and CDK4 promoter and therefore suppress the expression of CDK4 (Willoughby, et al., 2009). Artemisinin is able to induce apoptosis with a caspase-3 dependent manner in cancer cells (Nam et al., 2007), and could selectively decrease functional levels of estrogen receptor-alpha to suppress the proliferation of human breast cancer cells (Sundar et al., 2008). In addition, Artemisinin could reduce cell migration in human melonoma by suppressing alpha V beta 3 integrin and reducing metalloproteinase 2 production (Bucmmino, et al., 2009).

Another major compound is dihydroartemisnin. A study reported that dihydroartemisinin is able to induce G1 cell cycle arrest in human pancrate carcinoma cells though regulating cyclin E, cdk2, cdk4 and p27(Kip1) (Chen et al., 2010). Dihydroartemisinin induces apoptosis through potentiating the mitochondrial transmembrane permeability, releasing cytochrome c and activating of caspases (Lu, et al., 2009). The induction of apoptosis by dihydroartemisinin is Bak- or NOXA-dependent (Handrick et al., 2010). Another study reports that the anti-cancer activity of dihydroartemisinin is associated with induction of iron-dependent endoplasmic reticulum stress in colorectal carcinoma HCT116 cells (Lu, et al., 2010). In human prostate carcinoma cells, dihydroartemisinin was observed to induce tumor cell death via extrinsic and intrinsic pathway. Transcriptional activation of the death receptor 5 (DR5) and suppression of PI3-K/Akt and ERK cell survival pathways may play a role (He et al., 2010). Studies also reveal that dihydroartemisnin exhibits anti-migration effect on human fibrosarcoma cell HT-1080 through inhibition of PKCalpha/Raf/MAPKs and NF-kappaB/AP-1-dependent mechanisms (Hwang, et al., 2010). In addition, dihydroartemisinin improves the efficiency of chemotherapeutics in lung carcinomas in vivo, where dihydroartemisinin could help inhibit tumor growth through inducing apoptosis and suppress metastasis via down-regulating the expression of VEGF receptor KDR/flk-1 (Zhou, et al., 2010). To further expolre the active compounds in Herba artemisiae annuae, a study was carried out to compare the anti-tumor effect of compounds in Herba artemisiae annuae on chemoresistant cancer cells, and found artesunate being the most active (Michaelis et al., 2010). Artesunate was reported to induce DNA damage (Li, et al., 2008) and apoptosis (Michaelis et al., 2010) in cancer cells. Recently, an interesting investigation reported a caspase-independent mechanism of cell death induced by artesunate, an oncosis-like cell death in pancrate cancer cells. This kind of cell death is dependent on the loss of mitochondrial membrane potential and the presence of reactive oxygen species (ROS) (Du et al., 2010). Moreover, artesunate exhibits anti-angiogenic effect in human ovarian cancer through inhibiting the VEGF receptor KDR/flk-1 expression (Chen et al., 2004). Finally, recent study shows that the old member of the artemisinin derivates artemisone also exhibits significant anti-tumor effect (Gravett et al., 2010). These extensive studies reveal the potential of compounds from Herba artemisiae annuae for anti-cancer therapy in clinical practice.

4.8 Radix Ginseng (Renshen in Chinese)

Radix Ginseng, the dried root of Panax ginseng C.A. Meyer (Araliaceae), has been widely used as a tonic agent in traditional Chinese medicine for improvement in physical and mental capacities. The earliest written account of Radix Ginseng is from "Shen Nong Ben Cao Jing" (Shen Nong's Materia Medica, circa A.D. 100). Its species include Radix ginseng cruda, Radix ginseng rubra and Radix ginseng silvestris, and is mainly produced in Jilin, Liaoning, Heilongjiang Provinces of China and Korea. Wild ginseng is called "Shanshen", whereas the cultivated ones are known as "Yuanshen" (Garden Ginseng), of which, the sun-dried or bake-dried are called "Shengshaishen" (Sun-dried Ginseng). The fresh ginseng, which is made by steaming and then drying under the sun or heat, is called "Red Ginseng" (Radix ginseng rubra). The sun-dried and freezing-dried wild ginseng is named "Sun-dried Wild Ginseng" [Pharmacopoeia of the People's Republic of China, 2000].

Numerous constituents of radix ginseng such as ginsenosides (ginseng saponins), polysaccharides, peptides, polyacetylenic alcohols, aminoglycosides, and ginseng oils have been found and characterized. Among these, ginsenosides are believed to be the main active constituents in the pharmacological actions of ginseng. Ginsenosides are triterpenoid glycosides of dammarane and oleanane structures and so far more than 30 ginsenosides have been isolated from radix ginseng. According to the chemical structure characteristics, ginsenosides can be divided into three groups: panaxadiol, panaxatriol and oleanolic acid [Chang et al., 1992].

There is an increasing interest in radix ginseng regarding the human cancers. It is believed that the life-prolonging effect of radix ginseng may be because of the protective effect against various cancers such as prostate cancer, ovarian cancer and lung adenocarcinoma [Kim et al., 2004; Liu et al., 2000; Nakata et al., 1989]. Ginsenosides are the major antitumor constituents in radix ginseng. In a recent study in Korea, ginsenoside Rp1 was examined the anti-metastatic activities using in vitro assays and in vivo metastasis models [Tae et al., 2008]. This study suggested that ginsenoside Rp1 might act as an anti-cancer agent by strongly inhibiting cell viability and metastatic processes, presumably by inhibiting the adhesion of tumor cells and vessel formation. Another study in Hong Kong indicated that ginsenosides might act in a similar way as steroid hormones attributes to the effect in anti-cancer. The study found that ginsenosides can act as functional ligands to activate different steroid hormone receptors [Yue et al., 2007]. The results of the study showed that the anti-tumour effects of ginsenosides included its ability to induce cell death (such as apoptosis and necrosis), and having effects of anti-proliferation, anti-invasion and metastasis, and anti-angiogenesis. Moreover, ginseng has been found to be a therapeutic agent for renal cell carcinoma (RCC) [Jeongwon et al., 1998], a disease which many patients having been diagnosed to be in metastatic status at initial diagnosis [Lam et al., 2005]. It was suggested that lipid soluble components of ginseng inhibit the growth of RCC cell lines by blocking cell cycle progression at G1 to S phase transition. Furthermore, ginseng has been established as non-organ specific cancer prevention [Yun, 2001]. There was a dose-response relationship that was showed between the decreased risk of cancer with increased ginseng intake.

A "ginseng-abuse syndrome" was reported in 14 of 133 long-term ginseng users [Siegel, 1979]. These patients experienced hypertension, nervousness, sleep-lessness, skin eruptions and diarrhoea; some subjects also became euphoric and agitated. Doses of 15 g were associated with depersonalization and confusion, while depression was reported after more than 15 g per day. Moreover, estrogenic-like side effect of ginseng had been published [Punnone et al., 1978]. Furthermore, it was reported that ginseng might inhibit the effects of warfarin [Janetzky, 1997] and interact with the monoamine oxidize inhibitor phenelzine [Jones et al., 1987].

4.9 Radix notoginseng (Sanqi/Tienchi in Chinese)

Radix notoginseng is the dried root of Panax notogiseng (Burk.) F. H Chen (Araliaceae). It was first recorded in "Compendium of Materia Medica" ("Bencao Gangmu" in Chinese) by Li Shizhen (1518–1593 A.D.). Radix notoginseng has a long history of use as a traditional herbal medicine due to its blood circulation promotion, blood stasis removal and pain alleviation effects, and has been widely utilized for the prevention and treatment of microcirculatory disturbance in Oriental countries [Lee et al., 2009]. The herb is slightly bitter in favor, non-toxic and is mainly cultivated in Wenshan region, Yunnan province in China.

Similar to P. ginseng C. A. Meyer and P. quinquefolius L., P. notoginseng contains saponins as its main bioactive constituents, commonly referred to as ginsenosides, notoginsenosides and gypenosides. Other types of constituents extracted from Radix Notoginseng such as essential oils, amino acids, polysaccharides, dencichine and flavonoids are also pharmacologically active and have a function on some diseases [Modern Chinese Materia Medica, 2007].

Recently, several studies have demonstrated the inhibitory effects of Radix Notoginseng extract against a variety of human cancers, such as skin tumours, cervical cancer, prostate cancer, gastric cancer, colorectal cancer, sarcoma and breast cancer [Ng, 2006]. Laboratory studies on colorectal cancer suggested that Radix Notoginseng could be used alone or as adjuncts to existing chemotherapy to improve the outcomes of the chemotherapeutic treatment and reduce the adverse effects of chemotherapy [Wang et al., 2007; Wang et al., 2009; Sadeghi and Yazdanparast, 2005; Zhang et al., 2007]. These Studies found that the anti-proliferative activity of Radix Notoginseng extract was most probably because of cell cycle arrest, which the cancer cells were arrested in S phase and G2/M phase, and the induction of cancer cell apoptosis. Wang's group also suggested that the anti-proliferative effects of Radix Notoginseng were in a concentration-dependent manner. Nowadays, the induction of cancer cell apoptosis, which is a programmed cell death, is an important therapeutic mechanism in anti-cancer drug. The mechanism of the induction of apoptosis in human cancer cells, such as lung carcinoma cells, cervical cancer cells and gastric cancer cells, by Panax Notoginseng extracts (PNE) was investigated in the recent studies. The studies showed that PNE treatment significantly inhibited the cell viability and induced cancer cell death in a dose-dependent manner. Furthermore, the results of these studies indicated that the major regulators of PNE-induced apoptosis in human carcinoma cells are the Bcl-2 family and caspase-3, which are associated with mitochondrial dysfunction and dephosphorylation of the Akt signaling pathway [Park et al., 2009; Yang et al., 2006; Li et al., 2008]. Except the inhibition of cancer cell proliferation and the induction of apoptosis, the regulation of gap junctional intercellular communication (GJIC) was believed to play an important role in cancer prevention [Ruch, 1994]. Recently, a study on human hepatocarcinoma cells suggested that Radix Notoginseng saponins could up-regulate or recover GJIC function which was in a concentration-dependent manner [Shang et al., 2006]. Minor allergic effects of Radix Notoginseng were reported in some studies [Yang et al., 2002]. The allergic reactions were likely due to the low quality of Radix Notoginseng use.

4.10 Radix Astragali (Huangqi in Chinese)

Radix Astragali (RA) is derived from the dried roots of Astragalus membranaceus (Fisch.) (Leguminosae). Bunge and Astragalus membranaceus (Fisch.) Bunge var. mongholicus (Bunge) Hsiao are two commonly used species. RA is mostly prepared from cultivated ones, as wild ones are increasingly scarce, mainly produced in the northern part (Shanxi, Neimenggu, and Hebei) and the northeastern part (Heilongjiang) of China. Recent studies indicated that Shanxi of China produced the best quality of Radix Astragali [Ma et al., 2000].The earliest scientific description of RA was in Shen Nong Ben Cao Jing, a materia medica book edited in the 1st century. It has been traditionally used as a qi-tonifying drug or an adaptogenic herb in Chinese medicine for thousands of years. RA is prescribed as an immunostimulant, hepatoprotective, anti-perspirant, a diuretic or a tonic, and is used for treatment of many diseases in Chinese medicine clinical practice [Sinclair, 1998].

Regarding the chemical constituents of RA, more than 100 compounds have been isolated and identified up to now, and the most often associated with the biological activity of RA are isoflavonoids, triterpene saponins, polysaccharides, amino acids, and various trace elements [Chen et al., 2008; Gui et al., 2006; Lin et al., 2000]. Among these, astragaloside IV (one of the two main saponins), calycosin and formononetin (two of the three major active isoflavonoids) are normally being used as makers for RA's quality control [Song et al., 2004]. Sinclair's study found that RA has a wide range of immunopotentiating effects, and has been used extensively as an adjuvant in cancer therapy and as a phytochemical immune modulator. A study on the effects of RA extract reported that RA lowered the incidence of urinary bladder carcinoma in N-butyl-N'-butanolinitrosoamine treated mice by activating the cytotoxicity of lymphocytes and increasing the production of IL-2 and IFN-γ [Kurashige et al., 1999]. Another study indicated that RA extract significantly increased the activity of IL-2, of B cell growth factor and IL-6 in vitro and of phytoemagglutinin-induced proliferation of T lymphocytes from patients with IgG subclass deficiency [Tu et al., 1995]. Renal cell carcinoma has been shown to produce factors which may impair the normal functions of the immune system, such as macrophage function suppression. A laboratory study found evidence that RA restored the chemiluminescent oxidative burst activity of murine splenic macrophages which were shown to be suppressed by renal cell carcinoma. It

was also suggested that RA might have exerted its anti-tumor effect via augmentation of phagocyte and lymphokine-activated NK cell activities in vivo [Lau et al., 1994; Yang et al., 1998]. Guanine nucleotide exchange factors (GEFs) (oncogenes), such as Vav proteins (Vav1, Vav2 and Vav3) are hyperactive in various cancers. A recent study demonstrated that Vav3.1 expression was down-regulated by astragaloside IV in a dose- and time-dependent manner which might be highly correlated with the inhibition of the cellular malignant transformation. Thus, the study suggested that astragaloside IV might elicit anti-cancer activity via down-regulating the expression of oncogenes such as Vav3.1 [Qi et al., 2010]. It was revealed that RA could induce erythroleukemia cell lines to undergo cell differentiation and cell death which the up-regulation of Apaf-1, caspase-3 and AChE activation might play a crucial role during the process of apoptosis in cancer cells [Cheng et al., 2004]. Apart from the above actions, it was also showed that Astragalus polysaccharides could counteract the side effects of chemotherapeutic drugs, such as a significant reduction in the degree of myelosuppression in cancer patients [Tin et al., 2007].
In general, RA was safe without any distinct adverse effects [Sinclair 1998; Yu et al., 2007].

4.11 Radix angelicae sinensis (Danggui in Chinese)

Radix angelica sinensis (AS) is the dried root of Angelica sinensis (Oliv.) Diels (Umbelliferae) and is indigenous to China. AS is rarely available in the wild and is currently cultivated and harvested in late autumn after three years. It is mainly cultivated in Gansu province and partly in Yunnan, Sichuan, Shanxi, Hubei and Guizhou provinces of China. AS was first documented in Shen Nong Ben Cao Jing around 100 A.D.. According to the medicinal theory of traditional Chinese medicine, AS is used to tonify blood, improve blood circulation, regulate menstruation, and lubricate the bowels to alleviate constipation. Clinically, it has been commonly applied to the treatment of gynecological disorders (such as menstrual disorders, anemia, premenstrual syndrome and menopause), cardiovascular diseases, cerebrovascular diseases, cancer and high blood pressure for a long time. It was first introduced into western countries in 1899 by Merck in the form of a liquid extract named "Eumenol" and is presently marketed the United States as a dietary supplement, with numerous related commercial products for women's care worldwide [Deng et al., 2006].
Currently, over 70 compounds have been isolated from AS and identified [Dong et al., 2007]. The main chemical constituents of AS are ferulic acid, ligustilide, angelicide, brefeldin A, butylidenephthalide, butyphthalide, succinic acid, nicotinic acid, uracil, and adenine. The constituents most often associated with the pharmacological activities of AS are ferulic acid and ligustilide (predominantly the Z-isomer), both of which are usually used as chemical markers for the quality control of AS [Liu et al., 2000; Song, 1996].
Clinical studies showed that AS had anti-cancer capabilities in various human cancers. One study showed the inhibitory effect of AS on growth and proliferation of glioblastoma multiforme (GBM). The lipid-soluble ingredients of AS were extracted with acetone (AS-AC) or chlorophenol (AS-CH) and their antiproliferative and proapoptotic effects were studied in cultured GBM 8401 cells and in tumors in nude mice. Both extracts significantly inhibited the proliferative activity of GBM 8401 cultured cells by decreasing the expression of VEGF and the proapoptotic protein, cathepsin B, as this compound induced cancer cell cycle arrest at the G0-G1 phase which led to apoptosis. Both fractions significantly inhibited microvessel formation in the tumors of nude mice [Lee et al., 2006]. Growth suppression of malignant brain tumor cells by AS-CH resulted from cell cycle arrest and apoptosis. AS-CH up-

regulated expression of cdk inhibitors, including p21, to decrease phosphorylation of Rb proteins which resulted in cell cycle arrest at the G0-G1 phase in human DBTRG-05MG and rat RG2 cells. The apoptosis-associated proteins were dramatically increased and activated in DBTRG-05MG cells and RG2 cells by AS-AC but without p53 protein expression in RG2 cells. In vitro results showed that AS-AC triggered both p53-dependent and p53-independent pathways of apoptosis [Tsai et al., 2005, 2006]. AS-AC and AS-CH also significantly inhibited microvessel formation in vivo. All these findings suggested that AS possessed anti-tumor effects and might be useful in the treatment of high-grade astrocytomas. It has been found that neodiligustilide, Z-ligustilide, 11(S), 16(R)-dihydroxy-octadeca-9Z, 17-dien-12, 14-diyn-1-yl acetate and 3(R),8(S)-falcarindiol possess cytotoxic properties (Chen et al., 2007) .

N-Butylidenephthalide (BP), isolated from the chloroform extract of AS, was examined for its antitumor effects on hepatocellular carcinoma cells and might be a potential clinical use for improving the prognosis of hepatocellular carcinoma cells by inducing apoptosis in carcinoma cells in vitro and in vivo [Chen et al., 2008]. Invasion and metastasis are essential characteristics of malignant tumors. An experimental study suggested that total polysaccharide of AS (ASP) possessed anti-tumor effects on experimental tumor models in vivo and inhibitory effects on invasion and metastasis of hepatocellular carcinoma cells in vitro [Shang et al., 2003]. AP promoted the release of NO, TNF-α, and ROS and improved the activity of iNOS and lysozyme in macrophages. However, ASP had no direct cytotoxicity to tumor cells, but the culture medium of macrophages, pretreated with ASP, killed L929 tumor cells [Yang et al., 2004]. These results indicate that the extract may directly inhibit the invasion and metastasis of cancer cells, and indirectly stimulate immunological activity against cancer cell growth. Cell- mediated immune defense plays a key role in anti-tumor activity and is mediated specifically by T cells and non-specifically by macrophages and natural killer (NK) cells [Shan et al., 2002; Wang et al., 2004]. A study found that ASP had immunomodulatory activity by regulating expression of Th1 and Th2 related cytokines. The time–effect relation of cytokines response also suggested that macrophages and natural killer cells involved in nonspecific immunity were primarily activated, and helper T cell were secondarily affected by ASP [Yang et al., 2006].

AS contains several coumarin derivatives and should be used with caution in women on anticoagulants because of the increased risk of bleeding. AS also contains a carcinogenic essential oil, and some recommend that "all unnecessary exposure to dong quai should be avoided" [Israel et al., 1997]. The irritant agents in AS are believed to be the essential oils and Ligustilide is the most irritant within the essential oils of AS. An excess amount of ligustilide results in nausea, xeransis, and anesthesia of the oral cavity and tongue [Xie, 1997].

4.12 Radix Salvia miltiorrhizae (Red Sage Root, Danshen in Chinese)

Danshen is the root and rhizome of Salvia miltiorrhiza Bge. (Labiatae), mainly produced in Hebei, Shanxi, Inner Mongolia, Liaoning, and Jilin of China. The herb is collected in spring or autumn and dried in the sun. Traditinally, Danshen can be used in menstrual disorders, subcutaneous infection and insomnia by removing blood stasis, relieveing pain and easing the mind.

In photochemistry, at least 80 compounds have been separated and identified from Danshen, including lipophilic compounds and hydrophilic compounds. Tanshinone IIA and Salvianolic Acid B are the main component and are credited as criteria for quality control of

Danshen in China Pharmacopeia (Edition 2005).Danshen is one of the most popular herbs in China. It has been widely applied for many years to treat various diseases by its neuroprotective, antimicrobial, cardiovascular, hepatoprotective, antiinflammatory and immunomodulatory effects, especially in cardiovascular and cerebrovascular disease (Feng et al., 2010). In recent years, danshen and its active compounds also showed anticancer effects as mentioned follows.

The aqueous extract of Danshen can inhibit the proliferation of HepG2 cells (Jiang et al., 2005). Salvinal, a compound identified from aqueous extract, inhibiting tubulin polymerization, arresting the cell cycle at mitosis, and inducing apoptosis in multidrug-sensitive and -resistant human tumor cells (Chang et al., 2004). Another hydrophilic component Salvianolic acid B inhibits growth of head and neck squamous cell carcinoma in vitro and in vivo via inhibiting cyclooxygenase-2 expression (Hao et al., 2009). The chi-shen extract (CSE) from the water-soluble compounds of Salvia miltiorrhiza and Paeoniae radix shows anticancer effects which are related to the Bcl-2 family pathway and the activation of caspases-3 and -9 in HepG2 cells (Hu et al., 2007). Tanshinone IIA can induce apoptosis in HL60, CNE1, SPC-A-1, NB4, K562 and HepG2 cell lines, and the cytotoxicity partly through mitotic arrest or activation of capspase 3 (Yoon et al., 1999; Yuan et al., 2003; Lee et al., 2008; Zhou et al., 2008). Tanshinone IIA can inhibite the proliferation of non-small cell lung cancer A549 cells which is possibly by decreasing the MMP and inducing apoptosis due to the induction of a higher ratio of Bax/Bcl-2 (Chiu and Su 2010). Tanshinone I induces apoptosis, suppresses growth and invasion in MCF-7 and MDA-MB-231 breast cancer cell line, and its effect may be partly through activation of caspase 3 and regulation of some adhesion molecules, including intercellular adhesion molecule-1 (ICAM-1) and vascular cell adhesion molecule-1 (VCAM-1). Tanshinone I also exerts anticancer effect via mediation of interleukin-8, Ras-mitogen-activated protein kinase, and Rac1 signaling pathways in highly invasive human lung adenocarcinoma cell line, CL1-5 and CL1-5-bearing severe combined immunodeficient mice (Lee et al., 2008). Furthermore, other tanshinones, such as sibiriquinone A, sibiriquinone B, cryptotanshinone, and dihydrotanshinone I possess the anticancer activity partly through inhibition of HIF-1 accumulation (Dat et al., 2007). Recentlly, a novel compound, acetyltanshinone IIA (ATA) was obtained from chemical modifications of tanshinone TIIA (TIIA) which shows a higher growth inhibition ability on breast cancer especially HER2 positive cells than normal cells and it inhibites xenografted tumor growth in mice due to significant reactive oxygen species (ROS) generation, Bax translocation to mitochondria, resulting in mitochondria damage, cytochrome c release, caspase-3 activation and apoptotic cell death (Tian et al., 2010).

Denshen has low toxicity and less side effects in clinical practice. LD50 of Danshen water extract for mice: 25.807 g/kg by oral administration. This LD50 value is equivalent to 3934 times the intended clinical human oral dosage (6.56 mg of Danshen extract/kg). Treating rats with an oral dose of 2500 mg/kg Danshen extract (400 times human oral dosage) for 90 days have been found to be nontoxic (Tianjin Talisco Pharmaceutical Group Co. Ltd., 1998).

5. Conclusion

Chinese medicine is an unique medical system, among which Chinese medicines have been used in main stream medical health care in China for years of thousands and have been accepted by many countries as an complemental and alternative medicine. On the other hand, Chinese medicines are also as a resource in new drug develupment for unmet medical needs in some hard-to-cure diseases. In this chapter, we reviewed the recent progress of twelve representative Chinese medicines (Rhizoma coptidis, arsenic, Rhizoma Curcuma longae, Radis stephaniae tetrandrae, Radix tripterygii wilfordii, Radix scutellariae, Herba artemisiae annuae, Radix ginseng, Radix notoginseng, Radix astragali, Radix angelicae senensis and Radix salviae miltiorrhizae) on the anticancer cellular and molecular mechanisms, major active chemical ingredients and adverse effects. We noted that safety, quality control and sustainable develupment should be stressed in Chinese medicines research. On the other hand, research mainly focused on sigle Chinese medicines in the past decades, we should do more studies on composite fomulae in the future. After reviewing hot Chinese medicines in treatment of cancer in this chapter, we hope it will lead to further exploration of Chinese medicines by advanced scientific technology in drug discovery for treating cancer in the worldwide.

6. Reference

Banerjee, M.; Singh, P.& Panda, D. (2010). Curcumin suppresses the dynamic instability of microtubules, activates the mitotic checkpoint and induces apoptosis in MCF-7 cells, *FEBS J*, 277(16):3437-48.

Bao,YQ. (1983). Adverse reaction of berberine and Huanglian. *Shandong Medical Journal*, 7:53.

Bateman, J. (1998). Chapman RD, Simpson D. Possible toxicity of herbal remedies. *Scottish Medical Journal*, 43; 7-15.

Bi, YH. (1998). Pharmacology and clinical utilization of Huangqin. *Chinese Journal of Medicine*,38(3): 53-54.

Brinker, AM.; Ma, J.; Lipsky, PE.& Raskin, I. (2007). Medicinal chemistry and pharmacology of genus Tripterygium (Celastraceae), *Phytochemistry*, 68: 732–766.

Buommino, E.; Baroni, A.; Canozo, N.; Petrazzuolo, M.; Nicoletti R.; Vozza, A.&Tufano,MA. (2009). Artemisinin reduces human melanoma cell migration by down-regulating alpha V beta 3 integrin and reducing metalloproteinase 2 production. *Invest New Drugs*, 27(5):412-8.

Chan, E. (1993). Displacement of bilirubin from albumin by berberine. *Biology of the Neonate*, 63:201-8.

Chan, TKY. (1994). The prevalence, use, and harmful potential of some Chinese herbal medicines in babies and children. *Veterinary & Human Toxicology*, 36:238-40.

Chang, JY.; Chang, CY.; Kuo, CC.; Chen, LT.; Wein, YS. & Kuo, YH. (2004). Salvinal, a novel microtubule inhibitor isolated from Salviae miltiorrhiza Bunge (Danshen), with antimitotic activity in multidrug-sensitive and -resistant human tumor cells. *Mol. Pharmacol*, 65 (1): 77–84.

Chang, KH.; Liao, HF.; Chang, HH.; Chen, YY.; Yu, MC.; Chou, CJ.& Chen, YJ. (2004). Inhibitory effect of tetrandrine on pulmonary metastases in CT26 colorectal adenocarcinoma-bearing BALB/c mice. *Am J Chin Med*, 32(6):863-72.

Chang, WT.; Kang, JJ.; Lee, KY.; Wei, K.; Anderson, E.; Gotmare, S.; Ross, JA.& Rosen, GD. (2001). Triptolide and chemotherapy cooperate in tumor cell apoptosis. A role for the p53 pathway. *J of Biological Chemistry*, 276: 2221–2227.

Chang, XL..& Pei, GX. (1992). Recent advances on ginseng research in China. *J Ethnopharmacol*, 36(1):27-38.

Chao, JI.; Su, WC.& Liu, HF. (2007). Baicalein induces cancer cell death and proliferation retardation by the inhibition of CDC2 kinase and survivin associated with opposite role of p38 mitogen-activated protein kinase and AKT. *Mol Cancer Ther,* 6(11): 3039-3048.

Chen, GH. & Huang, WF. (2008). Progress in pharmacological effects of compositions of Astragalus membranaceus. *Chin J of New Drugs*, 17(17):1482-5.

Chen, GQ.;Shi, XG.; Tang, W.; Xiong, SM.; Zhu, J.; Cai, X.; Han, ZG., Ni, JH.; Shi, GY.;Jia, PM.; Liu, MM.; He, KL.; Niu, C.; Ma, J.; Zhang, P.; Zhang, TD.; Paul, P.; Naoe, T.; Kitamura, K.; Miller, W.; Waxman, S.; Wang, ZY.; de Th, H.; Chen, SJ.&Chen, Z. (1997) Use of arsenic trioxide (As2O3) in the treatment of acute promyelocytic leukemia (APL): I. As2O3 exerts dose-dependent dual effects on APL cells. *Blood,* 89(9):3345-53.

Chen, GQ.; Zhu, J.; Shi, XG.; Ni, JH.; Zhong, HJ.; Si, GY.; Jin, XL.; Tang, W.; Li, XS.; Xong, SM.; Shen, ZX.; Sun, GL.; Ma, J.; Zhang, P.; Zhang, TD.; Gazin, C.; Naoe, T.; Chen, SJ.; Wang, ZY.&Chen Z. (1996). In vitro studies on cellular and molecular mechanisms of arsenic trioxide (As2O3) in the treatment of acute promyelocytic leukemia: As2O3 induces NB4 cell apoptosis with downregulation of Bcl-2 expression and modulation of PML-RAR alpha/PML proteins *Blood,* 88(3):1052-61.

Chen, H.; Sun, B.; Wang, S.; Pan, S.; Gao, Y.; Bai, X.&Xue, D. (2010). Growth inhibitory effects of dihydroartemisinin on pancreatic cancer cells: involvement of cell cycle arrest and inactivation of nuclear factor-kappaB. *J Cancer Res Clin Oncol.* 136(6): 897-903.

Chen, HH.; Zhou, HJ.; Wu, GD.& Lou, XE. (2004). Inhibitory effects of artesunate on angiogenesis and on expressions of vascular endothelial growth factor and VEGF receptor KDR/flk-1. *Pharmacology.* 71(1):1-9.

Chen, Q.; Lu, ZZ.; Jin, YL.; Wu, YB.& Pan, JX. (2010). Triptolide inhibits Jak2 transcription and induces apoptosis in human myeloproliferative disorder cells bearing Jak2V617F through caspase-3-mediated cleavage of Mcl-1, *Cancer Lett,* 291(2): 246-55.

Chen, QC.; Lee, J.; Jin, W.; Youn, U.; Kim, H.; Lee, I.S.; Zhang, X.; Song, K.; Seong, Y. & Bae, K. (2007). Cytotoxic constituents from angelicae sinensis radix. *Arch Pharm Res,* 30 (5): 565-569.

Chen, QY.; Lu, GH.; Wu, YQ.; Zheng, Y.; Xu, K.; Wu, LJ.; Jiang, ZY.; Feng, R.& Zhou, JY. (2010). Curcumin induces mitochondria pathway mediated cell apoptosis in A549 lung adenocarcinoma cells. *Oncol Rep,* 23(5):1285-92

Chen, XL.; Ren, KH.; He, HW.& Shao, RG. (2008). Involvement of PI3K/AKT/GSK3beta pathway in tetrandrine-induced G1 arrest and apoptosis. *Cancer Biol Ther,* 7(7):1073-8. Epub 2008

Chen, Y.; Chen, JC.& Tseng,SH. (2009). Tetrandrine suppresses tumor growth and angiogenesis of gliomas in rats. *In t J Cancer,* 124(10):2260-9.

Chen, YL.; Jian, MH.; Lin, CC.; Kang, JC.; Chen, SP.; Lin, PC.; Hung, FJ.; Chen, JR.; Chang, WL.; Lin, SZ. & Harn, HJ. (2008). The induction of orphan nuclear receptor Nur77 expression by n-butylenephthalide as pharmaceuticals on hepatocellular carcinoma cell therapy. *Mol Pharmacol,* 74:1046-1058.

Chen, Z.; Chen, GQ.; Shen, ZX.; Sun, GL.; Tong, JH.; Wang, ZY.&Chen, SJ.(2002). Expanding the use of arsenic trioxide: leukemias and beyond. *Semin Hematol,* 39(2 Suppl 1):22-6.

Cheng, XD.; Hou, CH.; Zhang, XJ.; Xie, HY.; Zhou, WY.; Yang, L.; Zhang, SB. & Qian, RL. (2004). Effects of Huangqi (Hex) on Inducing Cell Differentiation and Cell Death in K562 and HEL Cells. *Acta Biochimica et Biophysica Sinica*, 36(3): 211–7.

Chiu, TL.& Su, CC.; (2010). Tanshinone IIA induces apoptosis in human lung cancer A549 cells through the induction of reactive oxygen species and decreasing the mitochondrial membrane potential, *Int J Mol Med.*;25(2):231-6.

Cho, HS.;Chang, SH.;Chung, YS.; Shin, JY.; Park, SJ.; Lee, ES.; Hwang, SK.; Kwon, JT.; Tehrani, AM.; Woo, M.; Noh, MS.; Hanifah, H.; Jin, H.; Xu, CX.& Cho, MH. (2009). Synergistic effect of ERK inhibition on tetrandrine-induced apoptosis in A549 human lung carcinoma cells. *J Vet Sci,* 10(1):23-8.

Choi, HY.; Lim, JE.& Hong, JH. (2010). Curcumin interrupts the interaction between the androgen receptor and Wnt/beta-catenin signaling pathway in LNCaP prostate cancer cells. *Prostate Cancer Prostatic Dis,* Aug 3

Choi, SU.; Park, SH.; Kim, KH.; Choi, EJ.; Kim, S.; Park, WK.; Zhang, YH.; Kim, HS.; Jung, NP.& Lee, CO. (1998). The bisbenzylisoquinoline alkaloids, tetrandine and fangchinoline, enhance the cytotoxicity of multidrug resistance-related drugs via modulation of P-glycoprotein. *Anticancer Drugs,* 9(3):255-61.

Chou, WC.; Wu, CC.; Yang, PC.& Lee, YT. (2010). Hypovolemic shock and mortality after ingestion of Tripterygium wilfordii hook F.: a case report. *Int J Cardiol,* 1995 49(2): 173-7.

Clawson KA, Borja-Cacho D, Antonoff MB, Saluja AK, Vickers SM. Triptolide and TRAIL Combination Enhances Apoptosis in Cholangiocarcinoma. *J Surg Res,* Apr 25. [Epub ahead of print].

Croal, LR.; Gralnick , JA.; Malasarn, D.& Newman, DK. (2004). The Genetics of Geochemisty. *Annual Review of Genetics*, 38:175–206.

Dai, CL.; Xiong, HY.; Tang, LF.; Zhang, X.; Liang, YJ.; Zeng, MS.; Chen, LM.; Wang, XH.& Fu,LW. (2007). Tetrandrine achieved plasma concentrations capable of reversing MDR in vitro and had no apparent effect on doxorubicin pharmacokinetics in mice. *Cancer Chemother Pharmacol,* 60(5):741-50.

Deng, SX,.; Chen, SN.; Yao, P.; Nikolic, D.; van Breemen, RB.; Bolton, JL.; Fong, HHS.; Farnsworth, NR. & Pauli, GF. (2006). Serotonergic Activity-Guided Phytochemical Investigation of the Roots of Angelica sinensis. *J Nat Prod*, 69:536-541.

Dong, L.; Deng, CH,.; Wang, B. & Shen, XZ. (2007). Fast determination of Z-ligustilide in plasma by gas chromatography/mass spectrometry following headspace single-drop microextraction. *J Sep Sci*, 30:1318-1325.

Du, JH.; Zhang, HD,; Ma, ZJ.& Ji, KM.(2010). Artesunate induces oncosis-like cell death in vitro and has antitumor activity against pancreatic cancer xenografts in vivo. *Cancer Chemother Pharmacol,* 65(5): 895-902.

Du, Y.; Wang, K.; Fang, H.; Li, J.; Xiao, D.; Zheng, P.; Chen, Y.; Fan, H.; Pan, X.; Zhao, C.; Zhang, Q.; Imbeaud, S.; Graudens, E.; Eveno, E.; Auffray, C.; Chen, S.; Chen, Z.& Zhang, J.(2006). Coordination of intrinsic, extrinsic, and endoplasmic reticulum-mediated apoptosis by imatinib mesylate combined with arsenic trioxide in chronic myeloid leukemia. *Blood*, 107(4):1582-90.

Feng, Y.,;Chen, XM..;Wang ,N. &Shen, JG.(2010). Current progress on medicinal plants and their biological properties in vontemporary China. Chapter in recent progress in medicinal plants Vol. 28: *Drug plants II*. Studium Press LLC, USA., pp513-7, pp526-9 and pp494-9.

Feng,,Y.; Luo,WQ&Zhu,SQ. (2008). Explore new clinical application of Huanglian and corresponding compound prescriptions from their traditional use. *China Journal of Chinese Materia Medica*, 33:1221-1225.

Gao J, Zhao H, Hylands PJ, Corcoran O. Secondary metabolite mapping identifies Scutellaria inhibitors of human lung cancer cells. *J Pharm Biomed Anal*, 2010 53(3): 723-8.

Gianni, M.; Koken, MH.; Chelbi-Alix, MK.; Benoit, G.; Lanotte, M.; Chen, Z.& de Thé, H. (1998). Combined arsenic and retinoic acid treatment enhances differentiation and apoptosis in arsenic- resistant NB4 cells. *Blood*, 91(11):4300-10.

Gravett, AM.; Liu, WM.; Krishna, S.; Chan, WC.; Haynes, RK.; Wilson, NL.& Dalgleish,,AG.(2010). In vitro study of the anti-cancer effects of artemisone alone or in combination with other chemotherapeutic agents. *Cancer Chemother Pharmacol*, May 19. [Epub ahead of print]

Gu, ZQ.; Sun, YH.; Xu, CL.& Liu, Y. (2005). Study of baicalin in inducing prostate cancer cell line DU145 apoptosis in vitro. *Zhongguo Zhong Yao Za Zhi*, 30(1): 63-6.

Gui, SY.; Wei, W.; Wang, H.; Sun, WY.; Chen, WB. & Wu, CY. (2006). Effects and mechanisms of crude astragalosides fraction on liver fibrosis in rats. *J Ethnopharmacol*, 103(2):154–9.

Handrick, R.; Ontikatze, T.; Bauer, KD.; Freier, F.; Rübel, A.; Dürig, J.; Belka, C.; Jendrossek, V. (2010). hydroartemisinin induces apoptosis by a bak-dependent intrinsic pathway. *Mol Cancer Ther*, 9(9):2497-510.

Hao, Y.; Xie, T.; Korotcov, A.; Zhou, Y.; Pang, X.; Shan, L.; Ji, H.; Sridhar, R.; Wang, P.; Califano, J. & Gu, X. (2009). Salvianolic acid B inhibits growth of head and neck squamous cell carcinoma in vitro and in vivo via cyclooxygenase-2 and apoptotic pathways. *Int J Cancer*, 124(9):2200-9.

Hara, A.; Iizuka, N.; Hamamoto, Y,.; Uchimura , S.; Miyamoto, T.; Tsunedomi, R..; Miyamoto, K,.; Hazama, S.; Okita, K.&Oka M.(2005). Molecular dissection of a medicinal herb with anti-tumor activity by oligonucleotide microarray. *Life Sci*, 77: 991-1002.

He, Q.; Shi, J.; Shen, XL.; An, J.; Sun, H.; Wang, L.; Hu, YJ ; Sun, Q.; Fu, LC.; Sheikh, MS.& Huang, Y. (2010). Dihydroartemisinin upregulates death receptor 5 expression and cooperates with TRAIL to induce apoptosis in human prostate cancer cells. *Cancer Biol Ther*, 9(10):819-24.

Hou, J.; Wang, D.; Zhang, R.& Wang, H. (2008). Experimental therapy of hepatoma with artemisinin and its derivatives: in vitro and in vivo activity, chemosensitization, and mechanisms of action. *Clin Cancer Res*, 14(17):5519-30.

Hsu, WH.; Hsieh, YS.; Kuo, HC.; Teng , CY,; Huang, HI.; Wang , CJ.; Yang , SF.; Liou, YS.&Kuo WH. (2007). Berberine induces apoptosis in SW620 human colonic carcinoma cells through generation of reactive oxygen species and activation of JNK/p38 MAPK and FasL. *Arch Toxicol*, 81(10):719-728.

Hu, J.; Liu, YF.; Wu, CF.; Xu, F.; Shen, ZX.; Zhu, YM.; Li, JM.; Tang, W.; Zhao, WL.; Wu, W.; Sun, HP.; Chen, QS.; Chen, B.; Zhou, GB.; Zelent, A.; Waxman, S.; Wang, ZY.; Chen, SJ.&(2009). Chen, Z. Long- term efficacy and safety of all-trans retinoic acid/arsenic trioxide-based therapy in newly diagnosed acute promyelocytic leukemia. *Proc Natl Acad Sci USA*, 106(9):3342- 7.

Hu, S.; Chen, SM.; Li, XK.; Qin, R.& Mei, ZN. (2007). Antitumor effects of chi-shen extract from Salvia miltiorrhiza and Paeoniae radix on human hepatocellular carcinoma cells. *Acta Pharmacol Sin,* 28(8):1215-23.

Huang, SL.; Guo, AX.; Xiang, Y.; Wang, XB.; HJ, Ling.& L, Fu. (1995). Clinical study on the treatment of APL mainly with composite Indigo Naturalis tablets. *Chin J Hematol*, 16:26.

Hwang, YP.; Yun, HJ.; Kim, HG.; Han, EH.; Lee, GW.& Jeong, HG. (2010). Suppression of PMA-induced tumor cell invasion by dihydroartemisinin via inhibition of PKCalpha/Raf/MAPKs and NF-kappaB/AP-1-dependent mechanisms. *Biochem Pharmacol*. 79(12):1714-26.

Israel, D. & Youngkin EQ. (1997). Herbal therapies for perimenopausal and menopausal complaints. *Pharmacotherapy*, 17:970-984.

Janetzky, K.& Morreale, AP. (1997). Probable interaction between warfarin and ginseng. *Am J Health Syst Pharm*, 54:692-3.

Jang, BC.; Lim, KJ.; Paik, JH.; Cho, JW.; Baek, WK.; Suh, MH.; Park, JB.; Kwon, TK.; Park, JW.; Kim, SP.; Shin, DH.; Song, DK.; Bae, JH.; Mun, KC.& Suh, SI. (2004). Tetrandrine-induced apoptosis is mediated by activation of caspases and PKC-delta in U937 cells. *Biochem Pharmacol,* 67(10):1819-29.

Jantova, S.; Cipak, L.; Cernakova, M.&Kost'alova, D.(2003). Effect of berberine on proliferation, cell cycle and apoptosis in HeLa and L1210 cells. *J Pharm Pharmacol*, 55:1143-1149.

Jeong, YI.; Kim, SW.; Jung, ID.; Lee, JS.; Chang, JH.; Lee, CM.; Chun, SH.; Yoon. MS.; Kim, GT.; Ryu, SW.; Kim, JS.; Shin, YK.; Lee, WS.; Shin, HK.; Lee, JD.& Park, YM. (2009). Curcumin suppresses the induction of indoleamine 2,3-dioxygenase by blocking the Janus-activated kinase-protein kinase Cdelta-STAT1 signaling pathway in interferon-gamma-stimulated murine dendritic cells. *J Biol Chem,* 284(6):3700-8.

Jeongwon, S.; Lee, CH.; Chung, DJ.; Park, SH.; Kim, I.& Hwang WI. (1998) Effect of petroleum ether extract of Panax ginseng roots on proliferation and cell cycle progression of human renal cell carcinoma cells. *Exp Mol Med*, 30(1): 47-51.

Jia, L. (1985). Chemistry and pharmacology and clinical application of the plants of Tripterygium family. *Yao Xue Tong Bao,* 20: 1001–1005.

Jones, BD.;& Runkis, AM.;(1987). Interaction of ginseng with phenelzine. *J Clin Psychopharmacol*, 7:201-202.

Jutooru, I.; Chadalapaka, G.; Lei, P.& Safe S. (2010).Inhibition of NFkappaB and pancreatic cancer cell and tumor growth by curcumin is dependent on specificity protein down-regulation. *J Biol Chem,* 285(33):25332-44.

Kang, JX.; Liu, J.; Wang, J.; He, C.&Li FP. (2005). The extract of huanglian, a medicinal herb, induces cell growth arrest and apoptosis by upregulation of interferon-beta and TNF-alpha in human breast cancer cells. *Carcinogenesis*, 26(11):1934-1939.

Katiyar, SK.; Meeran, SM.; Katiyar, N.&Akhtar S. (2009). p53 cooperates berberine-induced growth inhibition and apoptosis of non-small cell human lung cancer cells in vitro and tumor xenograft growth in vivo. *Mol Carcinog,* 48(1):24-37.

Kim, HS.; Lee, EH.; Ko, SR.; Choi, KJ.; Park, JH.; & Im, DS. (2004). Effects of ginsenosides Rg3 and Rh2 on the proliferation of prostate cancer cells. *Arch Pharm Res*, 27:429-435.

Kim, YJ.; Kang, SA.; Hong, MS.; Park, HJ.; Kim, MJ.; Park, HJ.&Kim HK. (2004). Coptidis rhizoma induces apoptosis in human colorectal cancer cells SNU-C4. *Am J Chin Med*, 32(6):873-882.

Klaassen, C.& Watkins, J. (2003). Casarett and Doull's Essentials of Toxicology. *McGraw-Hill.*. pp512.

Kumagai T, Müller CI, Desmond JC, Imai Y, Heber D, Koeffler HP. Scutellaria baicalensis, a herbal medicine: anti-proliferative and apoptotic activity against acute lymphocytic leukemia, lymphoma and myeloma cell lines. *Leuk Res*, 2007 31(4): 523-30.

Kuo, CL.; Chi, CW.&Liu, TY.(2004). The anti-inflammatory potential of berberine in vitro and in vivo. *Cancer Lett*, 203(2):127-137.

Kurashige, S.; Akuzawa, Y. & Endo, F. (1999). Effects of Astragali Radix Extract on Carcinogenesis, Cytokine Production, and Cytotoxicity in Mice Treated with a Carcinogen, N-Butyl-N'- butanolnitrosoamine. *Cancer Investigation*, 17(1):30-5.

Kuttan, R.; Bhanumathy, P.; Nirmala, K.& George, MC. (1985).Potential anticancer activity of turmeric (Curcuma longa). *Cancer Lett*, 29(2):197-202.

Lai, H.; Sasaki, T.; Singh. NP. (2005). Targeted treatment of cancer with artemisinin and artemisinin-tagged iron-carrying compounds. *Expert Opin Ther Targets*, 9(5):995-1007.

Lam, JS.; Shvarts,O.; Leppert, JT.; Figlin, RA.; &Belldegrun, AS.; (2005). Renal cell carcinoma 2005: new frontiers in staging, prognostication and targeted molecular therapy. *J Urol*, 173:1853-1862.

Lau, BH.; Ruckle, HC.; Botolazzo, T. & Lui, PD. (1994). Chinese Medicinal Herbs Inhibit Growth of Murine Renal Cell Carcinoma. *Cancer Biother*, 9(2):153-161.

Lee, CH.; Chen, JC.; Hsiang, CY.; Wu, SL.; Wu, HC.&Ho TY. (2007). Berberine suppresses inflammatory agents-induced interleukin-1beta and tumor necrosis factor-alpha productions via the inhibition of IkappaB degradation in human lung cells. *Pharmacol Res*, 56(3):193-201.

Lee, CY.,; Sher, H.F.; Chen, HW.; Liu, CC.; Chen, CH.; Lin, CS.; Yang, PC..; Tsay, H.S. &Chen, J.J. (2008). Anticancer effects of tanshinone I in human non-small cell lung cancer, *Mol Cancer Ther*, 7 (11): 3527-38.

Lee, DH.; Kim, C.; Zhang, L. & Lee YJ. (2008). Role of p53, PUMA, and Bax in wogonin-induced apoptosis in human cancer cells. *Biochem Pharmaco*, *l*75(10): 2020-2033.

Lee, HJ.; Son, DH.; Lee, SK.; Lee, J.; Jun, CD.; Jeon, BH.; Lee, SK.&Kim EC. (2006). Extract of Coptidis rhizoma induces cytochrome-c dependent apoptosis in immortalized and malignant human oral keratinocytes. *Phytother Res*, 20(9):773-779.

Lee, J.; Zhao, YQ.; &Liang, XJ.;(2009). Current Evaluation of the Millennium Phytomedicine-Ginseng (II): Collected Chemical Entities, Modern Pharmacology, and Clinical Applications Emanated from Traditional Chinese Medicine. *Curr Med Chem*, 16(22):2924–42.

Lee, JH.; Kang, GH.; Kim, KC.; Kim, KM.; Park, DI.; Choi, BT.; Kang, HS.; Lee, YT.& Choi , YH. (2002). Tetrandrine-induced cell cycle arrest and apoptosis in A549 human lung carcinoma cells. *Int J Oncol*, 21(6):1239-44.

Lee, WH.; Jin, JS.; Tsai, WC.; Chen, YT.; Chang, WL.; Yao. CW.; Sheu, LF. & Chen, A. (2006). Biological inhibitory effects of the Chinese herb Danggui on Brain Astrocytoma. *Pathobiology*, 73:141-148.

Lee, WY.; Chiu, LC.& Yeung, JH. (2008). Cytotoxicity of major tanshinones isolated from Danshen (Salvia miltiorrhiza) on HepG2 cells in relation to glutathione perturbation.*Food Chem. Toxico*, 46 (1): 328-38.

Li, H.; Takai, N.; Yuge, A.; Furukawa, Y.; Tsuno, A.; Tsukamoto, Y.; Kong, S.; Moriyama, M.& Narahara, H. (2010). Novel target genes responsive to the anti-growth activity of triptolide in endometrial and ovarian cancer cells. *Cancer Lett*, 297(2):198-206.

Li, JX.; Wang, ZB.; Zhu, LQ.; Niu, FL.; & Cui, W.; (2008). Effects of Radix Notoginseng extracts drug- containing serum on expressions of bcl-2, Bax and p21WAF1 proteins in MNNG transformed GES-1 cells. *J Chin Integ Med*, 6(8):817-20.

Li, PC.; Lam, E.; Roos, WP.; Zdzienicka, MZ.; Kaina, B.& Efferth T. (2008). Artesunate derived from traditional Chinese medicine induces DNA damage and repair. *Cancer Res*, 68(11):4347-51.

Li-Weber, M. (2010). Targeting apoptosis pathways in cancer by Chinese medicine. *Cancer Lett.* [Epub ahead of print].

Li, XK.; Motwani, M.; Tong, W.; Bornmann, W.; Schwartz, GK.& Huanglian.(2000). A chinese herbal extract, inhibits cell growth by suppressing the expression of cyclin B1 and inhibiting CDC2 kinase activity in human cancer cells. *Mol Pharmacol*, 58: 1287-1293.

Lian, Z.; Niwa , K.; Gao, J.; Tagami, K.; Mori, H.& Tamaya, T. (2003). Association of cellular apoptosis with anti-tumor effects of the Chinese herbal complex in endocrine-resistant cancer cell line. *Cancer Detect Prev*, 27(2): 147-54.

Lim, CB.; Ky, N.; Ng, HM.; Hamza, MS.& Zhao, Y. (2010). Curcuma wenyujin extract induces apoptosis and inhibits proliferation of human cervical cancer cells in vitro and in vivo. *Integr Cancer Ther*, 9(1):36-49.

Lin, CC.; Lin, SY.; Chung, JG.; Lin, JP.; Chen, GW.&Kao ST.(2006). Down-regulation of cyclin B1 and up-regulation of Wee1 by berberine promotes entry of leukemia cells into the G2/M-phase of the cell cycle. *Anticancer Res*, 26: 1097-1104.

Lin, JP.; Yang, JS.; Lee, JH.; Hsieh, WT,.&Chung JG. (2006). Berberine induces cell cycle arrest and apoptosis in human gastric carcinoma SNU-5 cell line. *World J Gastroenterol*, 12: 21-28.

Lin, LZ.; He, XG.; Lindenmaier, M.; Nolan, G.; Yang, J.; Cleary, M.; Qiu, SX. & Cordell, GA. (2000). Liquid chromatography- electrospray ionization mass spectrometry study of the flavonoids of the roots of Astragalus mongholicus and A. membranaceus. *J Chromatogr A*, 876:87–95

Lin, S.; Tsai, SC.; Lee, CC.; Wang, BW.; Liou, JY.&Shyu KG. (2004) Berberine inhibits HIF-1alpha expression via enhanced proteolysis. *Mol Pharmacol*, 66: 612-619.

Liu, CX.; Xiao, PG. & Li, DP. (2000). Modern Research and Application of Chinese Medicinal Plants. Hong Kong Medical Publisher: *Hong Kong China*, pp166-169.

Liu, J.; Jiang, Z.; Xiao, J.; Zhang, Y.; Lin, S.; Duan, W.; Yao, J.; Liu, C.; Huang, X.; Wang, T.; Liang, Z.; Wang, R.; Zhang, S.& Zhang, L. (2009). Effects of triptolide from Tripterygium wilfordii on ERalpha and p53 expression in two human breast cancer cell lines. *Phytomedicine*. 16(11): 1006-13.

Liu, K.; Xu,SX.; & Che, CT.; (2000). Anti-proliferative effect of ginseng saponins on human prostate cancer cell line. *Life Sci*, 67:1297-1306.

Lou, YJ.& Jin, J. (2004). Triptolide down-regulates bcr-abl expression and induces apoptosis in chronic myelogenous leukemia cells. *Leukemia & Lymphoma*, 45:373–376.

Lu, B.; Yu, L.; Xu, L.; Chen, H.; Zhang, L.& Zeng,Y. (2010) The effects of radix curcumae extract on expressions of VEGF, COX-2 and PCNA in gastric mucosa of rats fed with MNNG. *Curr Pharm Biotechnol*, 11(3):313-7.

Lu, HF.; Lai, KC.; Hsu, SC.; Lin, HJ.; Yang, MD.; Chen, YL.; Fan, MJ. Yang, JS.; Cheng, PY.; Kuo, CL.& Chung, JG. (2009). Curcumin induces apoptosis through FAS and FADD, in caspase-3- dependent and -independent pathways in the N18 mouse-rat hybrid retina ganglion cells. *Oncol Rep*, 22(1):97-104.

Lu, JJ.; Chen, SM.; Zhang, XW.; Ding, J.& Meng, LH. (2010). The anti-cancer activity of dihydroartemisinin is associated with induction of iron-dependent endoplasmic reticulum stress in colorectal carcinoma HCT116 cells. *Invest New Drugs*. [Epub ahead of print]

Lu, YY.; Chen, TS.; Qu, JL.; Pan, WL.; Sun, L.& Wei, XB. (2009). Dihydroartemisinin (DHA) induces caspase-3-dependent apoptosis in human lung adenocarcinoma ASTC-a-1 cells. *J Biomed Sci*, 16:16.

Lu, Z.; Jin, Y.; Qiu, L.; Lai, Y.& Pan, J. (2010). Celastrol, a novel HSP90 inhibitor, depletes Bcr-Abl and induces apoptosis in imatinib-resistant chronic myelogenous leukemia cells harboring T315I mutation. *Cancer Lett*, 290(2): 182-91.

Luo, WQ.; Hui, SC.; Chan, TY.&Feng, Y. (2002). Inhibitory effect of water extract from golden thread (Huanglian) on Leukemia L-1210 cells cultured in vitro. *Pharmacologist*, 44: A126.

Ma, XQ.; Duan, JA.; Zhu, DY.; Dong, TTX. & Tsim, KWK. (2000). Chemical comparison of Astragali Radix (Huangqi) from different regions of China. *Nat Med*, 54: 213-8.

Mantena, SK.; Sharma, SD.& Katiyar SK. (2006). Berberine inhibits growth, induces G1 arrest and apoptosis in human epidermoid carcinoma A431 cells by regulating Cdki-Cdk-cyclin cascade, disruption of mitochondrial membrane potential and cleavage of caspase 3 and PARP. *Carcinogenesis*, 27(10):2018-27.

Meng, LH.; Zhang, H.; Hayward, L.; Takemura, H.; Shao, RG.& Pommier, Y. (2004). Tetrandrine induces early G1 arrest in human colon carcinoma cells by down-regulating the activity and inducing the degradation of G1-S-specific cyclin-dependent kinases and by inducing p53 and p21Cip1. *Cancer Res*, 64(24):9086-92.

Michaelis M, Kleinschmidt MC, Barth S, Rothweiler F, Geiler J, Breitling R, Mayer B, Deubzer H, Witt O.; Kreuter, J.; Doerr, HW.; Cinatl, J.; Cinatl. J,Jr. (2010). Anti-cancer effects of artesunate in a panel of chemoresistant neuroblastoma cell lines. *Biochem Pharmacol*, 79(2):130-6.

Min, LW. (2010). Targeting apoptosis pathways in cancer by Chinese medicine, *Cancer Lett*, 297(2): 198-206.

Miocinovic, R.; McCabe, NP.; Keck, RW.; Jankun, J.; Hampton, JA.& Selman, SH.(2002). In vivo and in vitro effect of baicalein on human prostate cancer cells. *Int J Oncol*, 2005 26(1): 241-6.

Mujumdar, N.; Mackenzie, TN.; Dudeja, V.; Chugh, R.; Antonoff, MB.; Borja-Cacho, D.; Sangwan, V.; Dawra, R.; Vickers, SM.& Saluja, AK. (2010). Triptolide Induces Cell

Death in Pancreatic Cancer Cells by Apoptotic and Autophagic Pathways. *Gastroenterology*, 139(2): 598-608.

Nakata, H.; Kikuchi, Y.; Tode, T.; Hirata, J.; Kita, T.; Ishii, K.; Kudoh, K.; Nagata, I,.;;;& Shinomiya, N.; (1989). Inhibitory effects of ginsenoside Rh2 on tumor growth in nude mice bearing human ovarian cancer cells. *Jpn J Cancer Res*, 89:733-740.

Nam, W.; Tak, J.; Ryu, JK.; Jung, M, Yook.; JI, Kim.HJ, Cha, IH. (2007). Effects of artemisinin and its derivatives on growth inhibition and apoptosis of oral cancer cells. *Head Neck*, 29(4):335-40.

Nemoto, Y.; Satoh, K.; Toriizuka, K.; Hirai, Y.; Tobe, T.; Sakagami, H.; Nakashimam, H.& Ida, Y. Cytotoxic and radical scavenging activity of blended herbal extracts. *In Vivo*, 16(5): 327-332.

Ng, LT.; Chiang, LC.; Lin, YT.& Lin, CC. (2006). Antiproliferative and apoptotic effects of tetrandrine on different human hepatoma cell lines. *Am J Chin Med*, 34(1):125-35.

Ng, TB.; (2006). Pharmacological activity of sanchi ginseng (Panax notoginseng). *J Pharm Pharmacol*, 58: 1007–1019.

Ning, L.; Wentworth, L.; Chen, H.& Weber, SM. (2009). Down-regulation of Notch1 signaling inhibits tumor growth in human hepatocellular carcinoma. *Am J Transl Res*, 1(4):358-66.

Nortier, JL.; Martinez, MC.; Schmeiser, HH.; Arlt, VM.; Bieler, CA.; Petein, M.; Depierreux , MF.; De Pauw, L.; Abramowicz, D.; Vereerstraeten, P.& Vanherweghem, JL. (2000). Urothelial carcinoma associated with the use of a Chinese herb (Aristolochia fangchi). *N Engl J Med*, Jun 8;342(23):1686-92.

O'Sullivan-Coyne, G.; O'Sullivan, GC.; O'Donovan, TR.; Piwocka, K.& McKenna, SL. (2009). Curcumin induces apoptosis-independent death in oesophageal cancer cells. *Br J Cancer*, 101(9):1585-95.

Pandey, MK.; Sung, B.; Kunnumakkara, AB.; Sethi, G.; Chaturvedi, MM.&Aggarwal BB. (2008). Berberine modifies cysteine 179 of IkappaBalpha kinase, suppresses nuclear factor-kappaB-regulated antiapoptotic gene products, and potentiates apoptosis. *Cancer Res*, 68: 5370-5379.

Pang, X.; Yi,; Z.; Zhang, J.; Lu, B.; Sung, B.; Qu, W.; Aggarwal, BB.& Liu, M. Celastrol suppresses angiogenesis-mediated tumor growth through inhibition of AKT/mammalian target of rapamycin pathway. *Cancer Res*, 70(5): 1951-9.

Parajuli, P.; Joshee, N.; Chinni, SR.; Rimando, AM.; Mittal, S.; Sethi, S.& Yadav, AK. (2010). Delayed growth of glioma by Scutellaria flavonoids involve inhibition of Akt, GSK-3 and NF-kappaB signaling. *J Neurooncol*, May 14. [Epub ahead of print]

Park, CS.; Yoo, HS.; Park, C.; Cho, CK.; Kim, GY.; Kim, WJ.; Lee, YW.;& Choi, YH.; (2009). Induction of apoptosis in human lung carcinoma cells by the water extract of Panax notoginseng is associated with the activation of caspase-3 through downregulation of Akt. *Int J Oncol*, 35:121-7.

Peng, PL.; Hsieh, YS.; Wang, CJ.; Hsu, JL.&Chou FP. (2006). Inhibitory effect of berberine on the invasion of human lung cancer cells via decreased productions of urokinase-plasminogen activator and matrix metalloproteinase-2. *Toxicol Appl Pharmacol*, 214: 8-15.

Piyanuch, R.; Sukhthankar, M.; Wandee, G.&Baek, S.J.(2007). Berberine, a natural isoquinoline alkaloid, induces NAG-1 and ATF3 expression in human colorectal cancer cells. *Cancer Lett*, 258: 230-240.

Pongrakhananon, V.; Nimmannit, U.; Luanpitpong, S.; Rojanasakul, Y.& Chanvorachote, P. (2010). Curcumin sensitizes non-small cell lung cancer cell anoikis through reactive oxygen species-mediated Bcl-2 downregulation. *Apoptosis*, 15(5):574-85.

Punnone, R.;&Lukola, A.; (1978). Oestrogen like effect of ginseng. *BMJ*, 1:1284.

Qi, HY.; Wei, L.; Han, YF.; Zhang, QL.; Lau, SY. & Rong, JH. (2010). Proteomic characterization of the cellular response to chemopreventive triterpenoid astragaloside IV in human hepatocellular carcinoma cell line HepG2. *Int J Oncol*, 36:725-35.

Quiroga, A.; Quiroga, PL.; Martínez, E,.; Soria, EA.& Valentich, MA. (2010). Anti-breast cancer activity of curcumin on the human oxidation-resistant cells ZR-75-1 with gamma- glutamyltranspeptidase inhibition. *J Exp Ther Oncol*, 3(3):261-6.

Ren, LL.; Zhang, CZ.; Chen, JP.& Liang, XM. (2005). Anti-m icrobia lActivity of Scutellaria Baicalensis Georgi and HPLC Analysis. *Fine Chemcials*, 22(8): 589-591.

Ruch, RJ.; (1994). The role of gap junctional intercellular communication in neoplasia. *Annals of Clinical & Laboratory Science*, 24(3) 216-231.

Sadeghi, H.; & Yazdanparast, R.; (2005). Isolation and structure elucidation of a new potent anti- neoplastic diterpene from Dendrostellera lessertii. *Am J Chin Med*, 33(5):831-7.

Sahu, RP.; Batra, S,.& Srivastava, SK. (2009) Activation of ATM/Chk1 by curcumin causes cell cycle arrest and apoptosis in human pancreatic cancer cells. *Br J Cancer*, 100(9):1425-33.

Shan, JJ.; Wang, Y.; Wang, SC.; Liu, D. & Hu, ZB. (2002). Effect of Angelica sinensis polysaccharides on lymphocyte proliferation and induction of IFN-gamma. *Acta Pharmaceutica Sinica*, 37(7):497-500.

Shang, P. Qian, AR.; Yang, TH.; Jia, M.; Mei, QB.; Cho, CH.; Zhao, WM.; Chen, ZN.(2003 Experimental study of anti-tumor effects of polysaccharides from Angelica sinensis. *World J Gastroenterol*, 9(9):1963-7.

Shang, XL.; Fu, HQ.; Liu, L.;& Li, XD.; (2006). Inhibitory effects on human hepatocarcinoma cells with panax notoginseng saponins. *Chinese Journal of Clinical Rehabilitation*, 10(23):121-3.

Shen, H.; Xu, W.; Chen, Q.; Wu, Z.; Tang, H.& Wang, F. (2010). Tetrandrine prevents acquired drug resistance of K562 cells through inhibition of mdr1 gene transcription. *J Cancer Res Clin Oncol*. 136(5):659-65.

Shen, YC.; Chou, CJ.; Chiou, WF.& Chen, CF. (2001). Anti-inflammatory effects of the partially purified extract of radix Stephaniae tetrandrae: comparative studies of its active principles tetrandrine and fangchinoline on human polymorphonuclear leukocyte functions. *Mol Pharmacol*, 60(5):1083-90.

Shen, ZX.; Chen, GQ.; Ni, JH.; Li, XS.; Xiong, SM.; Qiu, QY.; Zhu, J., Tang, W.; Sun, GL.; Yang, KQ.; Chen, Y.; Zhou, L.; Fang, ZW.; Wang, YT.; Ma, J.; Zhang, P.; Zhang, TD.; Chen, SJ.; Chen, Z.& Wang, ZY. (1997). Use of arsenic trioxide (As2O3) in the treatment of acute promyelocytic leukemia (APL): II. Clinical efficacy and pharmacokinetics in relapsed patients. *Blood*, May 1;89(9):3354-60.

Siegel, RK.;(1979). Ginseng abuse syndrome. Problems with the panacea. *JAMA*, 241(15):1614-5.

Sinclair, S. (1998). Chinese herbs: a clinical review of Astragalus, Lingusticum, and Schizandrae. *Altern Med Rev*, 3(5):338-44.

Song, ZH.; Ji, ZN.; Lo, CK.; Dong, TT.; Zhao, KJ.; Li, OT.; Haines, CJ.; Kung, SD. & Tsim, KW. (2004). Chemical and biological assessment of a traditional chinese herbal decoction prepared from Radix Astragali and Radix Angelicae Sinensis: orthogonal array design to optimize the extraction of chemical constituents. *Planta Med,* 70(12):1222-7.

Song, ZY. (1996). The Modern Studies on the Chinese Meteria Medica; Peking Union Medical College and Beijing Medical University Press: Beijing China, Vol. 2, pp 1-25.

Srivastava, RK.; Chen, Q.; Siddiqui, I.; Sarva, K. & Shankar, S. (2007). Linkage of curcumin-induced cell cycle arrest and apoptosis by cyclin-dependent kinase inhibitor p21(/WAF1/CIP1). *Cell Cycle,* 6(23):2953-61.

Sun, HD.; Ma, L,.; Hu, XC.& Zhang, TD. (1992). Ai-Lin I treated 32 cases of acute promyelocytic leukemia. *Chin J Integrat of Chinese and Western Medicine,* 12:170.

Sun, M.; Estrov, Z,; Ji, Y.; Coombes, KR,.; Harris, DH.& Kurzrock, R. (2008). Curcumin (diferuloylmethane) alters the expression profiles of microRNAs in human pancreatic cancer cells. *Mol Cancer Ther,* 7(3):464-73.

Sun, X.; Xu, R.; Deng, Y.; Cheng, H.; Ma, J.; Ji, J. & Zhou, Y. (2007). Effects of tetrandrine on apoptosis and radiosensitivity of nasopharyngeal carcinoma cell line CNE. *Acta Biochim Biophys Sin (Shanghai),* 39(11):869-78.

Sun, Y.; Lu, N.; Ling, Y.; Gao, Y.; Chen, Y.; Wang, L.; Hu, R,.; Qi, Q.; Liu, W.; Yang, Y.; You, Q.& Guo, Q. (2009). Oroxylin A suppresses invasion through down-regulating the expression of matrix metalloproteinase-2/9 in MDA-MB-435 human breast cancer cells. *Eur J Pharmacol,* 603(1-3): 22-8.

Sundar, SN.; Marconett, CN.; Doan, VB.; Willoughby, JA Sr.& Firestone, GL. (2008). Artemisinin selectively decreases functional levels of estrogen receptor-alpha and ablates estrogen-induced proliferation in human breast cancer cells. *Carcinogenesis,* 29(12):2252-8.

Tae, YP.; Myung, HP.; Won, CS.; Man, HR.; Dong, WS.; Jae, YC.; & Hwan, MK.; (2008). Anti-metastatic Potential of Ginsenoside Rp1, a Novel Ginsenoside Derivative. *Biol. Pharm. Bull,* 31(9):1802-5.

Tang, J.; Feng, Y.; Tsao, S.; Wang, N.; Curtain, R.&Wang Y. (2009). Berberine and Coptidis Rhizoma as novel antineoplastic agents: a review of traditional use and biomedical investigations. *J Ethnopharmacol.,* 126:5-17.

Tarrago, T.; Kichik, N.; Segui, J.&Giralt E.(2007). The Natural Product Berberine is a Human Prolyl Oligopeptidase Inhibitor. *Chem Med Chem,* 2(3):354-359.

The Psychiatric, Psychogenic and Somatopsychic Disorders Handbook. New Hyde Park, NY: *Medical Examination Publishing Co.* 1978. pp81–82.

Tian, DF.; Tang, FQ.; Chen, XY.&Jian, YZ. (2000) A clinical observation on the inhibitory effect of Yiqijiedu Granules to the infection activity of EBV in population highly susceptible to NPC. *Journal of Hunan University of TCM,* 20:47-49.

Tian, HL.; Yu, T.; Xu, NN.; Feng, C.; Zhou, LY.; Luo, HW.; Chang,, DC.; Le. XF.; Luo. KQ. (2010). A novel compound modified from tanshinone inhibits tumor growth in vivo via activation of the intrinsic apoptotic pathway. *Cancer Lett,* 297(1):18-30.

Tianjin Talisco Pharmaceutical Group Co. Ltd. (1998). Approval of Compound DanshenDripping Pill (DSP) by FDA through pre-IND for clinical trials, *Proceedings of Forum of Internationalized Chinese Materia Medica,* 18-30.

Tin, MM.; Cho, CH.; Chan, K.; James, AE. & Ko, JK. (2007). Astragalus saponins induce growth inhibition and apoptosis in human colon cancer cells and tumor xenograft. *Carcinogenesis*, 28(6):1347-55.

Tsai, NM.; Chen, YL.; Lee, CC.; Lin, PC.; Chen, SP, Cheng, YL.; Chang, WL.; Lin, SZ. & Harn, HJ. (2006). The natural compound n-butylidenephthalide derived from Angelica sinensis inhibits malignant brain tumor growth in vitro and in vivo. *J Neurochem*, 99:1251-262.

Tsai, NM.; Lin, SZ.; Lee, CC.; Chen, SP.; Su, HC.; Chang, WL. & Harn, HJ. (2005). The Antitumor Effects of Angelica sinensis on Malignant Brain Tumors In vitro and In vivo. *Clin Cancer Res*, 11(9):3475-3484.

Tsang, CM.; Lau, EP.; Di, K.; Cheung, PY.; Hau, PM.; Ching, YP.; Wong, YC.; Cheung, AL.; Wan, TS.; Tong, Y.; Tsao, SW.& Feng, Y. (2009). Berberine inhibits Rho GTPases and cell migration at low doses but induces G2 arrest and apoptosis at high doses in human cancer cells. *Int J Mol Med.*, 24:131-138.

Tu, WW.; Yang, YQ.; Wang, LJ.; Zhang, YW. & Shen, J. (1995). In vivo effects of Astragalus membranaceus on immunoglobulin G subclass deficiency. *Chin J Immunol*, 11:34-7.

U.S. Geological Survey, Mineral Commodity Summaries, January 2008. *Arsenic*, pp26-27

Vispé, S.; DeVries, L.; Créancier, L.; Besse, J.; Bréand, S.; Hobson, DJ.; Svejstrup, JQ.; Annereau, JP.; Cussac, D.; Dumontet, C.; Guilbaud, N.; Barret, JM.& Bailly, C. (2009). Triptolide is an inhibitor of RNA polymerase I and II-dependent transcription leading predominantly to down-regulation of short-lived mRNA. *Mol Cancer Ther*, 8(10): 2780-90.

Wang, CD.; Huang, JG .; Gao, X.; Li, Y.; Zhou, SY.; Yan X., Zou, A.; Chang, JL.; Wang, YS.; Yang, GX.& He , GY. (2010). Fangchinoline induced G1/S arrest by modulating expression of p27, PCNA, and cyclin D in human prostate carcinoma cancer PC3 cells and tumor xenograft. *Biosci Biotechnol Biochem* 74(3):488-93.

Wang, CZ.; Li, XL.; Wang, QF.; Mehendale, SR.& Yuan,CS. (2010). Selective fraction of Scutellaria baicalensis and its chemopreventive effects on MCF-7 human breast cancer cells. *Phytomedicine*, 17(1): 63-8.

Wang, CZ.; Xie, JT.; Zhang, B.; Ni, M.; Fishbein, A.; Aung, HH.; Mehendale, SR.; Du, W.; He, TC.;& Yuan, CS.; (2007). Chemopreventive effects of Panax notoginseng and its major constituents on SW480 human colorectal cancer cells. *Int J Oncol*, 31(5):1149-56.

Wang, CZ.; Xie, JT.; Fishbein, A.; Aung, HH.; He, H.; Mehendale, SR.; He, TC.;;; Du, W.;& Yuan, CS.; (2009). Antiproliferative Effects of Different Plant Parts of Panax notoginseng on SW480 Human Colorectal Cancer Cells. *Phytother Res*, 23:6-13.

Wang, FP.; Wang, L.; Yang, JS.; Nomura M.& Miyamoto, K. (2005). Reversal of P-glycoprotein- dependent resistance to vinblastine by newly synthesized bisbenzylisoquinoline alkaloids in mouse leukemia P388 cells. *Biol Pharm Bull*, 28(10):1979-82.

Wang, J.; Xia, XY.; Peng, RX. & Chen X. (2004). Activation of the immunologic function of rat Kupffer cells by the polysaccharides of Angelica sinensis. *Acta Pharmaceutica Sinica*, 39(3):168-171.

Wang, L.; Zhou, GB.; Liu, P.; Song, JH.; Liang Y.; Yan, XJ.; Xu, F.; Wang, BS.; Mao, JH.; Shen, ZX.; Chen, SJ.& Chen, Z. (2008). Dissection of mechanisms of Chinese medicinal formula Realgar-Indigo naturalis as an effective treatment for promyelocytic leukemia. *Proc Natl Acad Sci U S A*, 105(12):4826-31.

Wang, N.; Feng, Y.; Lau, PW.; Tsang, CM,.; Ching, YP.; Man, K.; Tong, Y.; Nagamatsu, T.; Su, W.&Tsao, SW. (2010). F-actin reorganization and inactivation of Rho signaling pathway involved in the inhibitory effect of Coptidis Rhizoma on hepatoma cell migration. *Integr Cancer Ther*, In press.

Wang, N.; Feng, Y.; Zhu, M.; Tsang, CM.; Man, K.; Tong, Y.&Tsao SW. (2010). Berberine induces autophagic cell death and mitochondrial apoptosis in liver cancer cells: the cellular mechanism. *J Cell Biochem*, In press.

Wang, N.; Tang, LJ.; Zhu, GQ.; Peng, DY.; Wang, L.; Sun, FN.& Li, QL. (2008). Apoptosis induced by baicalin involving up-regulation of P53 and bax in MCF-7 cells. *J Asian Nat Prod Res*, 10(11-12): 1129-35.

Wang, ZP.; Jin, HF.; Xu, R.; Mei, QB.& Fan, DM. (2009). Triptolide downregulates Rac1 and the JAK/STAT3 pathway and inhibits colitis-related colon cancer progression. *Exp Mol Med*, 41(10): 717–727.

Willoughby, JA Sr,.; Sundar, SN.; Cheung, M.; Tin, AS.; Modiano, J..& Firestone, GL. (2009). Artemisinin blocks prostate cancer growth and cell cycle progression by disrupting Sp1 interactions with the cyclin-dependent kinase-4 (CDK4) promoter and inhibiting CDK4 gene expression. *J Biol Chem*, 284(4):2203-13.

Wong, TM.; Wu, S.; Yu, XC.& Li,HY. (2000). Cardiovascular actions of Radix Stephaniae Tetrandrae: a comparison with its main component, tetrandrine. Acta Pharmacol Sin, 21(12):1083-8.

Wong, TS.; Chan, WS.; Li, CH.; Liu, RW.; Tang, WW.; Tsao, SW.; Tsang, RK.; Ho, WK.; Wei, WI.;& Chan, JY. (2010). Curcumin alters the migratory phenotype of nasopharyngeal carcinoma cells through up-regulation of E-cadherin. *Anticancer Res*, 30(7):2851-6.

Wu, JM.; Chen, Y.; Chen, JC.; Lin, TY.& Tseng, SH. (2010). Tetrandrine induces apoptosis and growth suppression of colon cancer cells in mice. *Cancer Lett*, 287(2):187-95.

Xian, D.; Zhong, YY. & Li, X. (1997). Contemporary Pharmacology of Chinese *Herbs*, 413.

Xie, M. (1997). Modern study of the medical formulae in traditional Chinese medicine. *Xueyuan Press*, Beijing China, pp 603-4.

Xu, B.; Xiao, XG.; Sumi, M.;Angel, LA.; James, C.; John, LD.& Wang, W. (2010). Triptolide simultaneously induces reactive oxygen species, inhibits NF-κB activity and sensitizes 5-fluorouracil in colorectal cancer cell lines, *Cancer Lett*, 291(2): 200-8.

Xu, M.; Sheng, LH.; Zhu, XH.; Zeng, SB.& Zhang, GJ. (2010). Reversal effect of Stephania tetrandra- containing Chinese herb formula SENL on multidrug resistance in lung cancer cell line SW1573/2R120. *Am J Chin Med*, 38(2):401-13.

Yan, D.; Jin, C.; Xiao, XH.&Dong XP. (2008). Antimicrobial properties of berberines alkaloids in Coptis chinensis Franch by microcalorimetry. *J Biochem Biophys Methods*, 70 (6):845-849.

Yang, HX. & Zhao G. (1998). Death and apoptosis of LAK cell during immunologic assault and the rescuing effects of APS. *Chin J Clin Oncol*, 25:669-72.

Yang, TH.; Jia, M.; Meng, Jia.; Wu, H. & Mei, QB. (2006). Immunomodulatory activity of polysaccharide isolated from Angelica sinensis. *Int J Bio Macromol*, 39:179-184.

Yang, XB.; Mei, QB.; Zhou, SY.; Teng, ZH. & Wang, HF. (2004). The role of Angelica polysaccharides in inducing effector molecule release by peritoneal macrophages. *Chin J Cell Mol Immunol*, 20(6):747-9.

Yang, XG.; Lu, BQ.;& Guo, YP.; (2002). A literature review on the side effect of Radix Notoginseng, *Zhong Yao Cai*, 25(3):216-8.

Yang, ZG.; Sun, HX.;& Ye, YP.; (2006). Ginsenoside Rd from Panax notoginseng Is Cytotoxic towards HeLa Cancer Cells and Induces Apoptosis. *Chem Biodivers*, 3(2):187-197.

Yi, WJ.; Tong, JM.; Su, BF.& Lu, YL. (2005). Preventive effect of total flavones from stem and leaf of scutellaria baicalensis on experimental hyperlipidemia in rats. *Chinese J of Clinical Rehabilitation,* 9(27): 228-229.

Yoon, MJ.; Kim, EH.; Lim, JH.; Kwon, TK.& Choi, KS. (2010). Superoxide anion and proteasomal dysfunction contribute to curcumin-induced paraptosis of malignant breast cancer cells. *Free Radic Biol Med,* 48(5):713-26.

Yoon, Y.; Kim, YO.; Jeon, WK.; Park, HJ. & Sung, HJ. (1999). Tanshinone IIA isolated from Salvia miltiorrhiza Bunge induced apoptosis in HL60 human premyelocytic leukemia cell line. *J Ethnopharmaco*, 68 (1-3): 121–127.

Yu, SY.; Ou Yang, HT.; Yang, JY.; Huang, XL.; Yang, T.; Duan, JP.; Cheng, JP.; Chen, YX.; Yang, YJ. & Qiong P. (2007). Subchronic toxicity studies of Radix Astragali extract in rats and dogs. *J Ethnopharmacol*, 110:352–5.

Yu, XC.; Wu, S.; Chen, CF.; Pang, KT.& Wong, TM. (2004). Antihypertensive and anti-arrhythmic effects of an extract of Radix Stephaniae Tetrandrae in the rat. *J Pharm Pharmacol,* 56(1):115-22.

Yuan, SL.; Wang, XJ. & Wei, YQ. (2003). Anticancer effect of tanshinone and its mechanisms.*Ai Zheng,* 22(12):1363-6.

Yuan, SL.; Wei, YQ.; Wang, XJ.; Xiao, F.; Li, SF.& Zhang, J. (2004). Growth inhibition and apoptosis induction of tanshinone II-A on human hepatocellular carcinoma cells. *World J Gastroenterol,* 10(14): 2024-8.

Yue, GG.; Chan, BC.; Hon, PM.; Kennelly, EJ.; Yeung, SK.; Cassileth, BR.; Fung, KP.; Leung , PC.& Lau, CB. (2010). Immunostimulatory activities of polysaccharide extract isolated from Curcuma longa. *Int J Biol Macromol,* 47(3):342-7.

Yue, YK.; Mak, NK.; Cheng, YK.; Leung, KW.; Ng, TB.; Fan, TP.; Yeung, HW.; & Wong, NS..; (2007). Pharmacogenomics and the Yin/Yang actions of ginseng:anti-tumor, angiomodulating and steroid-like activities of ginsenosides. *Chin Med*, 2:6.

Yun, TK.; (2001). Panax ginseng - a non-organ-specific cancer preventive? *Lancet Oncol*. 2:49-55.

Yun, TK.; (2003). Experimental and epidemiological evidence on non-organ specific cancer preventive effect of Korean ginseng and identification of active compounds. *Mutat Res*, 523-524, 63-74

Zhang, J.; Zhang, T.; Ti, X.; Shi, J.; Wu, C.; Ren, X.& Yin, H. (2010). Curcumin promotes apoptosis in A549/DDP multidrug-resistant human lung adenocarcinoma cells through an miRNA signaling pathway. *Biochem Biophys Res Commun,* 399(1):1-6

Zhang, M.; Liu, X.; Li, J.; He, L.;& Tripathy, D.; (2007). Chinese medicinal herbs to treat the side-effect of chemotherapy in breast cancer patients. *Cochrane Database Syst Rev,* 2:CD004921.

Zhang, XW.; Yan, XJ.; Zhou, ZR.; Yang, FF.; Wu, ZY.; Sun, HB.; Liang, WX.; Song, AX.; Lallemand- Breitenbach, V.; Jeanne, M.; Zhang, QY.; Yang, HY.; Huang, QH.; Zhou,

GB.; Tong JH.; Zhang, Y.; Wu, JH. Hu, HY.; de Thé, H.; Chen, SJ.& Chen, Z. (2010). Arsenic trioxide controls the fate of the PML-RARalpha oncoprotein by directly binding PML. *Science*, 328(5975): 240-3.

Zhao, Q.; Wang, J.; Zou, MJ.; Hu, R.; Zhao, L.; Qiang, L.; Rong, JJ.; You, QD.& Guo,QL. (2010).Wogonin potentiates the antitumor effects of low dose 5-fluorouracil against gastric cancer through induction of apoptosis by down-regulation of NF-kappaB and regulation of its metabolism. *Toxicol Lett,* 197(3): 201-10.

Zhao, TH.; Deng, SH.; Yang, HS.& Chen SP. (2007). Study of antibacterial activity of active fraction from stems and leaves of Scutellaria baicalensis Georg. *Chinese Pharmacology Bulletin,* 23(7):882-886.

Zheng, GQ. (1994) Cytotoxic terpenoids and flavonoids from Artemisia annua. *Planta Med.* 60(1):54-7.

Zhou, GS.; Hu, Z.; Fang, HT.; Zhang, FX.; Pan, XF.; Chen, XQ.; Hu, AM.; Ling, Xu.& Zhou GB. (2010). Biologic activity of triptolide in t(8;21) acute myeloid leukemia cells, *Leuk Res,* Aug 4. [Epub ahead of print]

Zhou, HJ.; Zhang, JL,.; Li, A.; Wang, Z.& Lou. XE. 2010Dihydroartemisinin improves the efficiency of chemotherapeutics in lung carcinomas in vivo and inhibits murine Lewis lung carcinoma cell line growth in vitro. *Cancer Chemother Pharmacol,* 66(1):21-9.

Zhou, L.; Chan, WK.; Xu, N.; Xiao, K.; Luo, H.; Luo, K.Q. & Chang, D.C. (2008). Tanshinone IIA, an isolated compound from Salvia miltiorrhiza Bunge, induces apoptosis in HeLa cells through mitotic arrest .*Life Sci,* 183 (11-12): 394-403.

Zhou, YX.& Huang, YL. (2009). Antiangiogenic effect of celastrol on the growth of human glioma: an in vitro and in vivo study. *Chin Med J,* 122(14): 1666-73.

Zhou , M.; Wang, S.; Zhang, H.; Lu, YY.; Wang, XF.; Motoo, Y.& Su SB. (2009). The combination of baicalin and baicalein enhances apoptosis via the ERK/p38 MAPK pathway in human breast cancer cells. *Acta Pharmacol Sin,* 30(12): 1648-58.

15

Analytical Methods for Characterizing Bioactive Terpene Lactones in *Ginkgo Biloba* Extracts and Performing Pharmacokinetic Studies in Animal and Human

Rossana Rossi, Fabrizio Basilico,
Antonella De Palma and Pierluigi Mauri
*Institute for Biomedical Technologies,
Proteomics and Metabolomics Unit - CNR Segrate (Milan),
Italy*

1. Introduction

Ginkgo biloba is an ancient Chinese tree, appeared more than 250 million years ago, and the only surviving member of Ginkgoacea family [Schmid, 1997]. *Ginkgo biloba* was used as herbal remedy for many centuries in China, and now its extracts are one of the most widely used herbal products in the world, especially in the United States and in Europe [Blumenthal, 2000; Mahadevan & Park, 2008]. *Ginkgo biloba* extract is considered an alternative medicine for the treatment and/or the prevention of different pathologies and in some cases it could be suggested to be used as complementary of the mainstream medicine [Ernst, 2000]. In fact, over the past decades, there was a steady growth trend in the use of these alternative treatments. In particular, concentrated and partially purified products, containing *Ginkgo biloba* active constituents, have been marketed widely in the world for the treatment of cognitive deficits and other age-associated impairments [Kanowski et al., 1996; Le Bars et al., 1997]. Furthermore, it has been used as therapeutic compound for many other chronic and acute forms of diseases such as cardiovascular and bronchial pathologies [Diamond et al., 2000].

In view of the large market as well as the keen interest in the use and rediscovery of these herbal products throughout the world, the quality control of *Ginkgo biloba* extracts becomes necessary, in order to guarantee their clinical efficacy and safety. Therefore, it is important to monitor simultaneously the bioactive constituents present in *Ginkgo biloba* extracts, optimizing the analysis time and reducing costs. In fact, in the recent years, numerous groups reported in literature different analytical methods, using various chromatographic conditions and spectophotometric technologies, to create quick, accurate and applicable analytical approaches for the identification and the chemical structure characterization of *Ginkgo biloba* constituents.

Ginkgo biloba extracts contain a large number of representative constituents such as terpenoids, polyphenols, allyl phenol, organic acids, carbohydrates, fatty acids and lipids, inorganic salts and amino acids. However, the pharmacological activity of *Ginkgo biloba* extracts was attributed to the synergistic action of two distinct classes of chemical compounds, the flavonoids and the terpene trilactones [Sticher, 1993; Stiker et al., 2000; Li & Fitzloff, 2002a; Van Beek, 2002; Smith & Luo, 2004]. The flavonoids comprise a large group of polyphenols and include flavone and flavonol glycosides, acylated flavonol glycosides, biflavonoids, flavan-3-ols and proanthocyanidins. Of these, flavonol glycosides are more abundant than the other ones. Moreover, numerous flavonol glycosides were identified in *Ginkgo biloba* extracts as derivatives of the aglycones such as quercetin, kaempferol and isorhamnetin that are usually present in the leaves in relatively small amounts [Haslet et al., 1992; Van Beek, 2002]. The flavonoids are known to act mainly as antioxidants [Goh et al., 2003], free radical scavengers [Ellnain-Wojtaszek et al., 2003] and cation chelators [Gohil & Packer, 2002]. Finally, they could play a protective role in the prevention of certain kind of cancer as suggested in different studies on animal models [Kuo, 1997; Kandaswami et al., 2005].

The second group is represented by the terpene trilactones, which include diterpenoid (ginkgolides) and a sesquiterpenoid (bilobalide) compounds. Ginkgolides A, B, C, J, K, L and M are potent and selective antagonist of platelet activating factor (PAF) [Braquet, 1987; Van Beek et al., 1991; Smith et al., 1996; Hu et al., 1999]. PAF is an endogenous and highly active mediator of inflammation in the human body; it is produced by a variety of inflammatory cells and for this reason it is implicated in various disease states. So, the ginkgolides, used as the PAF antagonist, are able to prevent and treat thrombosis, illness of blood vessel of heart and brain, arhythmia, asthma, bronchitis and allergic reactions [Chavez & Chavez, 1998; Sticher, 1999; Diamond et al., 2000; Koch, 2005].

On the other hand, the sesquiterpene bilobalide exhibits neuroprotective properties [Chandrasekaran et al., 2001; Defeudis, 2002]. It is widely employed to treat symptoms associated with mild-to-moderate dementia, impairment of other cognitive functions associated with ageing and senility and related neurosensory problems [Blumental et al., 2000]. In fact, numerous studies, based on in vivo models, indicated that the administration of bilobalide can reduce cerebral edema due to triethyltin, decrease cortical infarct volume as verified in certain stroke models and reduce damage caused by cerebral ischemia [Chandrasekaran et al., 2001; Defeudis, 2002].

All the mentioned pharmacological actions of the compounds isolated from *Ginkgo biloba* were clarified over the years and helped to highlight the diversity of their potential activities on human health. In particular, in the present chapter we focused our attention to review the neuroprotective role of *Ginkgo biloba* extracts. In fact some publications, reporting the pharmacokinetic behaviours and in vitro and in vivo clinical results of *Ginkgo biloba* extracts, shown that they are an important ingredient to treat cognitive disturbance, although the molecular mechanism of their action is still ambiguous. In particular we examined bilobalide, the bioactive compound of *Ginkgo biloba* that is probable the principal responsible for this effect.

Finally, this chapter aims to provide an overview on the main techniques and methods used for the assay of *Ginkgo biloba* components.

2. Neuroprotective properties of *Ginkgo biloba* extracts and Bilobalide

Gingko biloba extract (GBE) presents a wide range of biological/therapeutical effects. Concerning its pharmacological activity on the central nervous system it seems due to synergic action of its main constituents: flavonoid-glycosides and terpene-lactones.

The investigations of neuroprotective effects of *Ginkgo biloba* have used its standardized extract. The extract standardized contains about 24% flavonoid glycosides and 6% terpene lactone.

Specifically *Ginkgo biloba* extract (GBE) is described to have different biological effects. For example, several authors reported that GBE may be a molecular target of amyloid precursor protein (APP) [Luo et al., 2002; Agustin et al., 2009; Jin et al., 2009] and it determined beneficial effects on brain function.

Other authors investigated the action of GBE on oxidative damage [Bridi et al., 2001; Naik et al., 2006; Sener et al., 2007], specifically in relation to ischemia/reperfusion [Urikova et al., 2006; Domorakova et al., 2009]. In addition, it is reported that GBE protects against mitochondrial dysfunction in platelets and hippocampi [Shi et al., 2010a; Shi et al., 2010b].

Ginkgo biloba extract it was also reported to have a positive effect on memory in healthy animals [Gong et al., 2006; Yamamoto et al., 2007; Blecharz-Klin et al., 2009] and humans [Kennedy et al., 2007].

Of course a number of authors concern the effect of GBE on typical neuro-degeneration diseases, such as Alzheimer [Agustin et al., 2009; Luo, 2006 Ahlemeyer & Krieglstein, 2003; Luo, 2001] and Parkinson [Beal, 2003; Kim et al., 2004; Ahmad et al., 2005; Chen et al., 2007; Rojas et al., 2008].

Regarding the flavonoid fraction of GBE only few studies have been performed and they concern prevention of membrane damage caused by free radicals. In particular, flavonoid fraction protects cultures of neurons against oxidative stress due to hydrogen peroxide and iron sulfate [Sloley et al., 2000], as well as neural tissue against cerebral ischemia lesion [Dajas et al., 2003]. Moreover, it was described that flavonoid fraction inhibited sodium nitroprusside-induced death in primary hippocampal cultures of rat [Saija et al., 1995], and the authors suggested that flavone glycosides, as radical scavengers, block the formation of peroxynitrite as a product of NO and superoxide anion reaction.

Concerning the terpene-lactones, studies mainly regard bilobalide. In vitro and ex vivo investigations indicate that bilobalide has multiple actions, such as preservation of mitochondrial ATP synthesis [Janssens et al., 1995], inhibition of apoptotic damage [Ahlemeyer et al., 1999], suppression of hypoxia-induced membrane deterioration [Klein et al., 1997] and increasing the expression of the mitochondrial DNA-encoded COX III [Chandrasekaran et al., 2001].

Specifically, the sesquiterpene reduces the edema formation in hippocampal slices exposed to N-methyl-D-aspartate (NMDA) [Kiewert et al., 2007], or obtained by oxygen-glucose deprivation (OGD) [Mdzinarishvii et al., 2007]. The neuroprotective effect of bilobalide is partially correlated to its GABAergic antagonism, but it doesn't fully explain the bilobalide's action [Kiewert et al., 2007]. More recently, it has been reported that glycine, at 10-100 mM level, contrasts the effect of bilobalide. In particular, bilobalide reduces the release of glycine during ischemia but it does not interact with glycine receptors [Kiewert et al., 2008].

Because bilobalide is instable, it has been prepared a stable derivative called NV-31. This modified compound resulted to reduce by 50% the cellular ROS content in chick neurons submitted to serum deprivation and staurosporine-induced apoptosis [Ahlemeyer et al., 2001]. Moreover NV-31 has been reported to potentiate hippocampal neuron recombinant glycine receptor Cl channels [Lynch & Chen, 2008].

The protective effect of bilobalide against convulsion was observed by Sasaki et al. (2000) using 4-O-methylpyroxidine (MPN) for changing the levels of gamma-aminobutyric acid (GABA) and glutamic acid decarboxylase (GAD) activity in hippocampus cerebral cortex.

Finally, gingkolide B (GB) was used in neuroprotective studies. In particular, this terpen-lactone reduced up-regolation of constitutive and inducible nitric oxide synthase in hyperthermic brain injury [Sharma et al., 2000].

3. Structural characterization of *Ginkgo biloba's* main compounds

Ginkgo biloba is characterized by the presence of numerous constituents belonging to different chemical classes, which are well investigated over the years. In fact, there are many studies that report the various groups of components present in its extracts [Van Beek, 2002; Singh et al., 2008; Van Beek & Montoro, 2009]. However, depending on their chemical structures, the major bioactive compounds can be classified into two groups: flavonoids and terpene lactones [Li & Fitzloff, 2002a; Li & Fitzloff, 2002b].
The flavonoids, also called phenylbenzopyrines or phenylchromones, comprise a large group of structurally related compounds, characterized by the presence of two aromatic rings and a heterocyclic ring with one oxygen atom; this group include flavonol glycosides, biflavonoids, biflavones, proanthocyanidins and isoflavonoids. Specifically, the flavonoids most commonly present in *Ginkgo biloba* extracts are the flavonol glycosides, in which one or more hydroxyl group of the aglycones are bound to a carbohydrate moiety, usually via the 3 or 7 position (Fig.1). Numerous flavonol glycosides were identified as derivatives of the phenolic aglycones (quercetin, kaempferol or isorhamnetin) that, when alone, are present in relatively low concentration [Hasler et al., 1992; Sticher, 1999]. However, the *Ginkgo biloba* contains also a large number of biflavonoids, which are flavonoid–flavonoid dimers connected by a C–O–C or C–C bond.

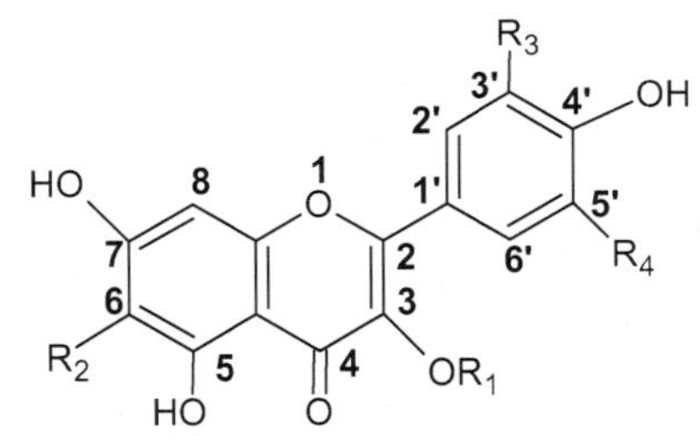

Fig. 1. Structural skeleton of flavonoids.

Terpene lactones include 20-carbon diterpene lactone derivatives (ginkgolides) and a 15-carbon sesquiterpene (bilobalide). These compounds are the unique natural products to possess a tert-butil group in their structure [Van Beek, 2005) (Fig.2). In particular, ginkgolides contain a rigid carbon skeleton consisting of six fused 5-membered carbocyclic rings, that is, a spiro [4.4] nonane carbocyclin ring, three lactones and a tetraydrofuran. On the contrary bilobalide has a more flexible structure containing only 5-membered rings [Nakanish et al., 1971].

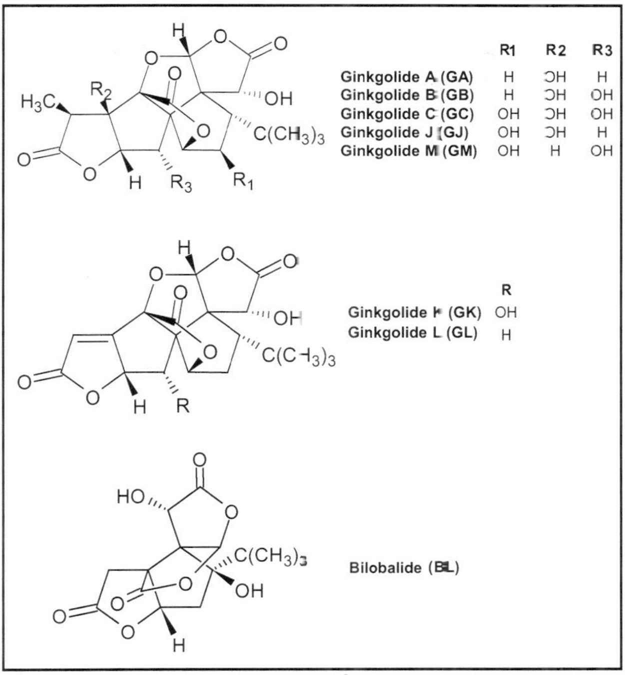

Fig. 2. Chemical structures of the terpene trilactones of *Ginkgo biloba* extract.

By far the terpene lactones received a great attention for the chemical uniqueness, due to their cage like structure. Ginkgolide A, B, C and M were isolated for the fist time from *Ginkgo biloba* root bark and described by Furukawa in 1932 (1932), and only later, ginkgolides A, B and C were reported to be present in the leaves too. Ginkgolide J was identified, by Weings et al. in 1987 (1987), as a minor constituent present in the leaves of *Ginkgo biloba*. In addition, Wang et al. (2001) reported the identification of other two ginkgolides (K and L) containing a further double bond. In fact, Yuan et al. (2008) recently described ginkgolide K as the dehydrated form of ginkgolide B. Similarly, ginkgolide L should derived from the dehydratation of ginkgolide A, although this hypothesis is not confirmed in literature.

A thorough mass spectrometric investigation of this class of compounds is very important for their identification and characterization.

The fragmentation pathway of bilobalide observed in our laboratory is shown in Fig.3. It was based on data obtained by means of LC-MS/MS analysis with an APCI source and an ion trap analyzer (ITMS), in negative ion mode. These results are in good agreement with those observed by Sun et al. (2005) using an electrospray interface. Instead, the fragmentation of bilobalide obtained by LC-ESI-MS/MS using a triple quadrupole (QqQ) analyzer, shows differences related to the relative abundances of the fragmented ions. Specifically, the most abundant fragments are *m/z* 163 and 251 from QqQ and ITMS, respectively.

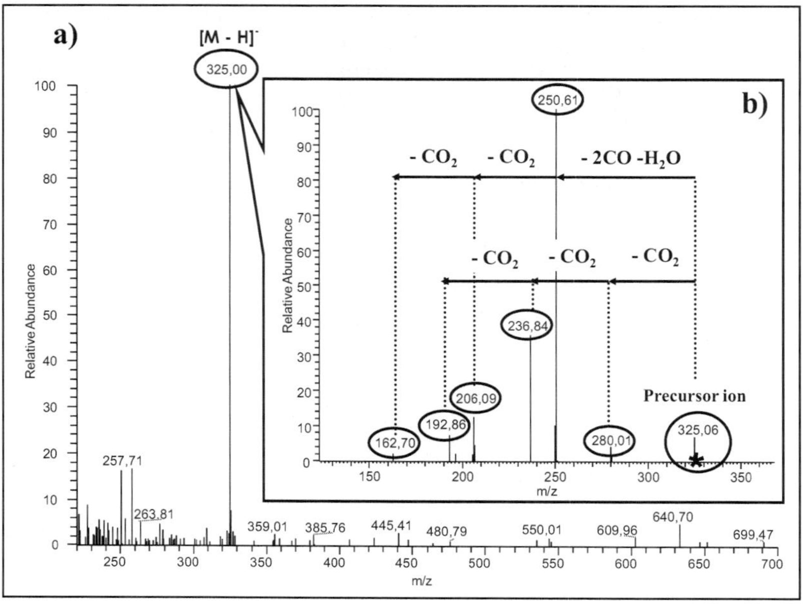

Fig. 3. **a)** APCI-MS and **b)** APCI-MS/MS spectra of $[M-H]^-$ at 325 m/z.

Table 1 reports the fragmentated bilobalide ions obtained by ion trap and triple quadrupole. In particular, ion product at *m/z* 325 is due to the loss of a ter-butyl and a hydroxyl group, while fragmentation at *m/z* 163 is related to the loss of two carbon dioxide molecules.

Ion	Bilobalide *m/z*	% relative abundance	
		HPLC/ESI-MS/MS [Sun et al.; 2005]	HPLC/APCI-MS/MS
$[M-H]^-$	325	30	6
$[M-H-CO_2]^-$	281	0	4
$[M-H-2CO_2]^-$	237	25	36
$[M-H-3CO_2]^-$	193	30	8
$[M-H-2CO-H_2O]^-$	251	30	100
$[M-H-CO-H_2O-2CO_2]^-$	206	10	14
$[M-H-2CO-H_2O-2CO_2]^-$	163	100	2

Table 1. Comparison of the major product ions of the bilobalide obtained by using ESI-MS/MS and APCI-MS/MS methods.

On the other hand, the ginkgolides show fragmentation pathways similar among them. Generally, the most favourable fragmentation way of the deprotonated ginkgolides is the loss of single and multiple carbon monoxide molecules. In each cases, the most abundant fragment ion derived from the loss of two carbon monoxide molecule, $[M-H-2CO]^-$. For example the MS/MS spectrum obtained from the ginkgolide A molecule ion $[M-H]^-$ 407 *m/z* gives a prominent ion product at *m/z* 351, resulting from the loss of two carbon dioxide molecules and a three less intense product ions at *m/z* 379, 363 and 319 due to the loss of one carbon monoxide molecule, one and two molecules of carbon dioxide, respectively [Van Beek, 2005; Sun et al., 2005].

4. Analytical methods for quality control of *Ginkgo biloba* extracts

Chemical fingerprint analysis represents a comprehensive approach for the quality assessment purpose of traditional Chinese herbs. In fact, most herbal medicines are complex mixtures whose therapeutic effect is often attributed to the cumulative effects of many components. For this reason, it is important to achieve an overall view of all the components present in the extracts to evaluate the quality of the plant products. Moreover, it is necessary and important to develop a reliable and applicable quality control method for the constituents present in most herbal extracts. To this end, different analytical methods are proposed for the quality and the stability evaluation of herbal medicines.

As described above, for the analysis of the flavonoids and terpene lactones, the main bioactive compounds present in *Ginkgo biloba* extracts, the scientific literature report a lot of methods. The great number of these methods is based on high-performance liquid chromatography (HPLC) coupled to UV [Pietta et al., 1990; Pietta et al., 1992; Hasler, et al., 1992], refractive index (RI) [Van Beek et al.. 1991; Chen et al., 1998; Wang & Ju, 2000], or ELSD [Li & Fitzloff, 2002] detection and gas chromatography (GC) combined to flame ionisation (FID) [Huch & Staba, 1993; Van Beek, 2002; Yang et al., 2002] or mass spectrometry (MS) [Chauret et al., 1991; Deng & Zito, 2003] detection.

High-performance liquid chromatography coupled to the ultra-violet detection (HPLC-UV) is the technique of choice for the fingerprinting analysis of the total flavonoids of *Ginkgo biloba* L. extracts [Hasler et al., 1992], while it presents several limitations for the qualitative and quantitative determination of terpenes, due to their low UV absorption and the impurities present in the complex matrix of *Ginkgo biloba* L. extracts. However, Pietta et al. (1990; 1992) described a new procedure for the preparation of samples that, using HPLC combined to UV detector, permits the identification of terpene compounds of *Ginkgo biloba* L. extracts. In particular, in the study proposed by Pietta et al. in 1990 was developed an efficient method for the purification of terpene compounds in *Ginkgo biloba* L. extracts based on the separation of the ginkgolides fractions by means of prepacked alumina columns. The resulting cleaned samples were separated by isocratic elution on Microsorb C18 columns (analytical: 100 x 4.6 mm i.d., 3μm; Rainin Instrument Co., Woburn, MA, USA - semi-preparative: 250 x 10 mm i.d., 5 μm; Biolab Instrument) using 10% isopropanol and analyzed with an UV photodiode detector. These results show that combining a new sample purification process together with the optimization of the chromatographic conditions, it is possible to obtain a simple method suitable for the determination of bilobalide, ginkgolide A, B and C in *Ginkgo biloba* L. extracts.

Several investigators instead applied refractive index (RI) as an alternative detection method [Van Beek et al., 1991; Chen et al., 1998; Wang & Ju, 2000]. As an example, Wang and Ju (2000) developed a rapid analytical method that, using HPLC on a C18 column with methanol-water-orthophosphoric acid as eluents combined to refractive index (RI) detector, permits the quantification of terpene lactones (bilobalide and ginkgolide A, B, C, J) in *Ginkgo biloba* L. extracts in only 20 min of analysis time. This method resulted to be more suitable and was employed with considerable success, although the sensitivity and the baseline stability still remain a problem.

On the contrary, evaporative light scattering detection (ELSD) seems to solve the problems related to the baseline stability and permits to reach higher sensitivity, requiring small solvent consumption. So, even if it is a non-selective detector, this technique has gained in popularity over the last decades, due to its capacity to detect the number and size of non-volatile compounds. In fact, several papers reported the application of HPLC with ELSD detector for the routine determination of ginkgolides and bilobalide [Li & Fitzloff, 2002b; Tang et al., 2003; Dubber & Kanfer, 2006]. As an example, Tang et al. (2003), applied RP-HPLC-ELSD method for the quantitation analysis of terpene lactones in *Ginkgo biloba* extracts. These authors by means of a Dinamic C18 column, using methanol and water under isocratic conditions as mobile phase (33:67, v/v), obtained the separation of five terpene lactones in 40 min of analysis time (bilobalide and ginkgolide A, B, C, J). This method represented a big advantage in terms of selectivity and precision; however the narrow linearity intervals (from 100 to 800μg/ml) produced through ELSD response represent the major inconvenience of such kind of detectors.

Another excellent separation technique for terpene lactones is represented by gas-chromatography coupled to flame ionization detection (GC-FID) [Huch & Staba, 1993; Lang & Wai, 1999; Van Beek, 2002; Yang et al., 2002] which is very reliable for the sensitivity and reproducibility. However, the sensitivity and selectivity of this separative technique could be further increased by the coupling with mass spectrometer detectors (MS) [Chauret et al., 1991; Biber & Koch, 1999; Deng & Zito, 2003]. Nevertheless GC-based methods require complicated and time-consuming sample preparation steps and compound derivatization.

In the recent years, these problems are solved with the development of several mass spectrometry instruments and taking advantage of the combination of these ones with HPLC separation systems. In fact, in literature are reported many works in which different MS techniques were coupled to HPLC for analysing *Ginkgo biloba* extracts.

In particular, different investigators developed HPLC methods combined to MS detection, using a thermospray interface (TSP) (Pietta et al., 1994; Caponovo et al., 1995). Briefly, Pietta et al. (1994), applied high-performance liquid chromatography interfaced with a thermospray ion source mass spectrometer (LC-TSP/MS) for the identification of various flavonol glycosides from *Ginkgo biloba*. While, Caponovo et al. in 1995, employed LC-TSP/MS analytical techniques for the rapid detection of ginkgo terpene lactones. LC-TPS/MS method is not very precise due to variability and poor stability of the TSP interface.

On the contrary, the discovery of the API (atmospheric pressure ionization) interfaces and in particular of electrospray ionisation sources (ESI) allowed a soft ionization and a stable combination between HPLC separation and MS detection. As reported by Mauri et al. (1999), the method based on liquid chromatography coupled with electrospray mass spectrometry (LC-ESI-MS) is specific, reproducible, rapid and permits quantitative analyses of terpenoids in *Ginkgo biloba* extracts. In particular LC-ESI-MS method permitted the monitory of terpene lactones in *Ginkgo biloba* extracts by means of quadrupole instrument (positive mode) coupled to a C18 columns and 20 min of analysis time in isocratic separation [Mauri et al., 1999].

Similar results were obtained by Jensen et al. (2002) using a triple quadrupole equipped with an atmospheric pressure chemical ionization (APCI) interface in the negative ion mode and a methanol gradient. For increasing the sensitivity quadrupole needs selectively detection of single ion monitoring (SIM).

However, in this way, increasing the number of selected ions monitored, the sensitivity decreases and it is not possible to monitor unexpected ions. These problems were solved with the introduction of ion trap mass spectrometer (ITMS). In fact ITMS present the same sensitivity in full scan and SIM modes. Ding et al. (2008a) characterized the flavonoid and terpene compounds of *Ginkgo biloba* products by using a C18 capillary column coupled to ion trap MS. The use of the negative ion mode combined to the data depending scan for MS/MS acquisition lead to the characterization of more than 70 components from the *Ginkgo biloba* in 140 min of analysis time. As another example Chen et al. (2005) used a 28 min HPLC separation, based on a C18 analytical column, coupled to sonic spray ionization source (SSI) and a mass spectrometer equipped with a ion trap analyzer for characterizing terpene lactones constituents from *Ginkgo biloba* extracts in positive ion mode. On the other hand, Mauri et al. (2001) used liquid chromatography/atmospheric pressure chemical ionization for coupling HPLC with ion trap mass spectrometry (LC/APCI-IT-MS) to study the pharmacokinetics of terpene lactones in human. In particular, in this study chromatographic separation was achieved in less than 8 min and calibration curve was linear over a concentration range of 5-2000 ng/ml.

In addition to the ion trap analyzer, Ding et al. (2008b) employed a quadrupole time-of-flight (QTOF) mass spectrometer for characterizing terpene lactones (bilobalide and ginkgolide A, B, C,) in *Ginkgo biloba* L. extracts [Ding et al., 2008b]. Specifically, the authors used both analyzers to obtain two specific goals: ion trap MS for the characterization of the terpene fragmentation pathways and QTOF for the estimation of fragment ion mass accuracy (3-5 ppm) and the confirmation of the structural identification.

More recently, in our laboratory, the accurate mass measurement of the *Ginkgo biloba* terpene lactones was performed by means of the Exactive (Thermo Electron Corporation, San Josè, CA, USA) a non -hybrid mass spectrometer based on the Orbitrap technology. This instrument, equipped with a nanoelectrospray ion source, allows the acquisition of accurate mass data together with the improvement of sensitivity.

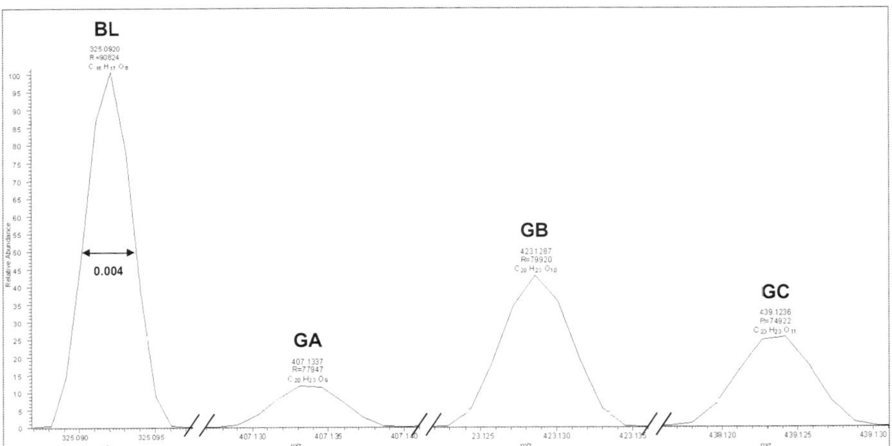

Fig. 4. MS spectra zoom of [M-H]- ions of bilobalide and ginkgolides A,B,C.

Fig. 4 reports the MS spectrum of [M-H]- ions of bilobalide and ginkgolides A,B,C. The full scan spectra were acquired at a resolution setting of 100,000 in an infusion experiment calibration (i.e. no lock masses were used) and a high dynamic range. In particular, for all the terpene lactone ions showed in Fig. 4 it was possible to achieve narrow peak widths with a mass accuracy and a resolving power of around 0,2 ppm and 8 x 10^5, respectively.
High resolution, accurate mass measurement together with high dynamic range are required for unequivocal characterization of mixtures even in the absence of precursor ion mass selection. However, if it is needed, additional informations can be provided by high resolution/ high mass accuracy MS/MS experiments in an "all ion fragmentation" mode.
In fact, the Exactive mass spectrometer allows high efficiency "all ion fragmentation" experiments by means of Higher energy Collision induced Dissociation (HCD) [Olsen et al., 2007].
All these performance characteristics make this mass spectrometer well suited for discovery analyses, screening applications, quantitative estimation and elemental composition determination, solving the limitation of the ion trap technology and representing a good alternative to the ion trap based hybrid instruments.

5. Pharmacokinetic analysis

Pharmacokinetic and metabolic studies of *Ginkgo biloba* extracts concern the investigations of the main bioactive compounds, flavonoids and terpene-lactones.
Concerning flavonoids, few metabolic studies are available. In particular, Hackett (1986) described correlation between flavonoids and their metabolites using selected standard analyzed by means of Thin-layer chromatography (TLC). Of course, TLC technique didn't permit the investigation of complex extracts. Wang et al. (2003) developed a method based on liquid chromatography coupled to UV detector (λ=380 nm) for determining kaempferol and quercetin in human urine samples after orally administrated *Ginkgo biloba* extract.
Other authors used LC-UV and mass spectrometry for characterizing the metabolites of flavonoids in rat [Pietta et al, 1995] and human [Pietta et al., 1997] urine samples due to administration of standardized *Ginkgo biloba* extract. The main metabolite resulted to be conjugates of 4-hydroxybenzoic, vanillic and 4-hydroxyhippuric acids.
Recently, Ding et al. (2006) prepared an analytical method, based on ion trap mass spectrometry in negative ion mode, for assaying flavonoids in urine from volunteers after up-take with *Ginkgo biloba* extract. In addition, the authors monitored terpene-lactones simultaneously elution at a flowrate of 4 μL/min (LOD around 2 and 10 ng/mL for flavonoids and terpenes, respectively). This method is interesting, but requires a long gradient (> 2 hours) and standard deviation resulted higher than 10%.
Concerning pharmacokinetics studies of terpene-lactones, many works are available. For example Biber [Biber & Koch; 1999] and co-workers [Furtillan et al.; 1995] used gas chromatography mass spectrometry for determining, after oral administration, the main ginkgolides in plasma from both humans [Furtillan et al., 1995] and rats [Biber & Koch, 1999]. In particular, in rats the half life of ginkgolides resulted to be around 2 h; at the contrary, in human differences were noted for ginkgolide A, ginkgolide B and bilobalide (4.5, 10.5, and 3.2 hours, respectively).
In 2001 Mauri et al. (2001) proposed a fast (within 8 min) method based on atmospheric pressure chemical ionization (APCI) interface coupled to an ion trap mass spectrometer to

monitor (LOD about 2 ng/mL) terpenes in plasma of volunteers after administration of two different *Ginkgo biloba* formulations (free and phospholipids complex formulations). When supplied in the phospholipid complex form, both Cmax and AUC (Area Under the Curve) of terpene lactones increased, suggesting that this formulation may increase their bioavailability.

The same approach was extended to investigate pharmacokinetics of terpene-lactones in rats and guinea pigs after acute and chronic oral administrations [Mauri et al., 2003]. Other authors used APCI interface combined with a triple quadrupole analyzer for investigating the bioavailability of ginkgolides after intravenous administration to rats [Xie et al., 2008] Specifically, multiple reaction monitoring (MRM) was used and the limit of quantification resulted around 2 ng/mL.

In alternative to APCI, Hua et al. (2006) proposed electrospray interface coupled to Q-array-Octapole-Quadrupole mass analyzer (QoQ) for investigating the intragastric administration of pure ginkgolide B (0.1 ng/kg) in Beagle dogs. The authors reported a LOD around 0.1 ng/mL while Tmax and t1/2 resulted to be 0.5 h and 2.8 h, respectively.

Other authors have studied the bioavailability of pure ginkgolide B after oral administration and Tmax resulted around 2 and 4 h for phytosomic and free forms, respectively [Mauri et al., 2003].

Concerning ginkgolide C, different authors observed a very low recovery from plasma of this terpene-lactone. This is accompanied by the increase of methylated metabolite observed in plasma of both animals and humans [Mauri et al, 2006].

All in-vivo studies of terpene-lactones from *Ginkgo biloba* concern plasma or urine samples. However, very recently it has been published a study about the identification of bilobalide in rat brain after single oral dose [Rossi et al., 2009]. In particular, it has been observed that bilobalide presents different profiles in brain and plasma samples. In fact, in plasma the bilobalide levels increase with the administered dose; while the brain levels increase for dose up to 10 mg/kg; and decrease for higher doses. These results support the studies that described the positive cognitive efforts on brain due to *Ginkgo biloba* extracts (Lee et al., 2002; Kennedy et al., 2007). Moreover the absorption of bilobalide could be explained by a specific mechanism of transport and by an inhibition effect due to an overloading of transporter after its administration at high doses.

6. Conclusion

Ginkgo biloba contains mainly two types of constituents, the flavonoids and terpene lactones, which together have been proven to be responsible of the polyvalent activities of *Ginkgo biloba* herbal and *Ginkgo biloba*-containing preparations. In fact, for many centuries *Ginkgo biloba* was used for the treatment of several pathologies, but in recent years its interest increased in relation to the neuroprotective activities ascribed to terpene lactones. To this end, the development of many analytical technologies improved fingerprinting authentication and quantitative determination of target analytes, as well as the pharmacokinetic and pharmacodynamic studies on the active components of *Ginkgo biloba* and its finished products. This is because of selectivity and specificity achieved by both the chromatographic and mass spectrometry detection systems. In particular, LC-MS approach appeared to be the method of choice for the measurement of target analytes in biological samples. In fact, the separation efficiency and fastness of the new HPLC systems combined to the high resolution and accurate measurements of the recent mass spectrometry detectors permit an unequivocal characterization of bioactive compounds from *Ginkgo biloba* extracts. These analytical tools will be very important for elucidating the transport and pharmacological *in vivo* mechanisms of terpene lactones and flavonoids.

7. References

Ahlemeyer, B.; Mowes, A. & Krieglstein, J. (1999). Inhibition of serum deprivation- and staurosporosine-induced neuronal apoptosis by Ginkgo biloba extract and some of its constituents. *Eur. J. Pharmacol.*, Vol. 367, N. 2-3, (Feb 1999), 423-430.

Ahlemeyer, B. & Krieglstein, J. (2003). Pharmacological studies supporting the therapeutic use of Ginkgo biloba extract for Alzheimer's disease. *Pharmacopsychiatry*, Vol. 36, N. Suppl. 1, (Jun 2003), S8-S14.

Ahlemeyer, B., Junker, V., Huhne, R. & Krieglstein, J. (2001). Neuroprotective effects of NV-31, a bilobalide-derived compound: evidence for an antioxidative mechanism. *Brain Res.*, Vol. 890, N. 2, (Feb 2001), 338-342.

Ahmad, M., Saleem, S., Ahmad, A.S., Yousuf, S., Ansari, M.A., Kan, M.B., Ishrat, T., Chaturvedi, R.K., Agrawal, A.K. & Islam F. (2005). Ginkgo biloba affords dose-dependent protection against 6-hydroxydopamine-induced parkinsonism in rats: neurobehavioural, neurochemical and immunohistochemical evidences. *J. Neurochem.*, Vol. 93, N. 1, (Apr 2005), 94-104.

Augustin, S., Rimbach, G., Augustin, K., Schliebs, R., Wolffram, S. & cermak, R. (2009). Effect of a short- and long-term treatment with Ginkgo biloba extract on amyloid precursor protein levels in a transgenic mouse model relevant to Alzheimer's disease. *Arch. Biochem. Biophys.*, Vol. 481, N. 2, (Jan 2009), 177-182.

Beal, M.F. (2003). Bioenergic approaches for neuroprotection in Parkinson's disease. *Ann. Neurol.*, Vol. 53, N. Suppl 3, (2003), S39-S47.

Biber, A. & Koch, E. (1999). Bioavailability of ginkgolides and bilobalide from extracts of ginkgo biloba using GC/MS. *Planta Med.*, Vol. 65, N. 2, (Mar 1999), 192-193.

Blecharz-Klin, K., Piechal, A., Joniec, I., Pyrzanowska, J. & Widy-Tyszkiewicz, E. (2009). Pharmacological and biochemical effects of Ginkgo biloba extract on learning memory consolidationand motor activity in old rats. *Acta Neurobiol. Exp. (Wars)*, Vol. 69, N. 2, (2009), 217-231.

Blumental, M., Goldberg, A. & Brinckman, J. (2000). Herbal medicine expanded commission E monographs. Integrative medicine Communications, Boston, Massachusetts. American Botany Council, Austin, TX, USA, 160-169.

Blumenthal, M. (2000). Herb Sales Down 15 percent in Mainstream Market. *HerbalGram.*, Vol. 51, (Winter 2000), 69.

Braquet, P (1987). The ginkgolides: potent platelet-activating factor antagonists isolated from Ginkgo biloba L.: chemistry, pharmacology and clinical applications. *Drug of the Future*, Vol, 12, N. 7, (1987), 643-699.

Bridi, R., Crossetti, F.P., Steffen, V.M. & Henriques, A.T. (2001). The antioxidant activity of standardized exctract of Ginkgo biloba (EGb 761) in rats. *Phytother. Res.*, Vol. 15, N. 5, (Aug 2001), 449-451.

Bruno, C., Cuppini, R., Sartini, S., Cecchini, T., Ambrogini, P. & Bombardelli, E. (1993). Regeneration of motor nerves in bilobalide-treated rats. *Planta Med.*, Vol. 59, N. 4, (Aug 1993), 302-307.

Caponovo, F.F., Wolfender, J.L., Maillard, M.P.M, Potterat, O. & Hostettmann, K. (1995). Evaporative light scattering and thermospray mass spectrometry: Two alternative methods for detection and quantitative liquid chromatographic determination of ginkgolides and bilobalide in Ginkgo biloba leaf extracts and phytopharmaceuticals. *Phytochemical Analysis*, Vol. 6, N. 3, (May-Jun 1995), 141–148.

Chandrasekaran, K., Mehrabian, Z., Spinnewyn, B., Drieu, K. & Fiskum, G. (2001). Neuroprotective effects of bilobalide, a component of the Ginkgo biloba extract (EGb 761), in gerbil global brain ischemia. Brain Res., Vol. 922, N. 2, (Dec 2001), 282-292.

Chauret, N., Carrier, J., Mancini, M., Neufeld, R., Weber, M. & Archambault, J. (1991). Gas chromatographic-mass spectrometric analysis of ginkgolides produced by Ginkgo biloba cell culture. *J. Chromatogr.*, Vol. 588, N. 1-2, (Dec 1991), 281-287.

Chavez, M.L & Chavez,.P.I. (1998). Ginkgo (part 1): history, use, and pharmacologic properties. *Hosp. Pharm.*, Vol 33, (1998), 658-672.

Chen, E., Ding, C. & Lindsay, R.C. (2005). Qualitative and quantitative analyses of ginkgo terpene trilactones by liquid chromatography/sonic spray ionization ion trap mass spectrometry. *Anal Chem.*, Vol. 77, N. 9, (May 2005), 2966-2970.

Chen, L.W., Wang, Y.Q., Wie, L.C., Shi, M. & Chan, Y.S. (2007). Chinese herbs and herbal extracts for neuroprotection of dopaminergic neurons and potential therapeutic treatment of Parkinson's disease. *CNS Neurol. Disord. Drug Targets*, Vol. 6, N. 4, (Aug 2007), 273-281.

Chen, P., Su, X. L., Nie, L. H., Yao, S. Z. & Zeng J. G. (1998). Analysis of Ginkgolides and Bilobalides in Ginkgo biloba L. Extract for Its Production Process Control by High-Performance Liquid Chromatography. *J. Chrom. Sci.*. Vol. 36, N.4, (1998), 197-200.

Dajas, F., Rivera, F., Blasina, F., Arredondo, F., Echeverry, C., Lafon, L., Morquio, A. & Heizen, H. (2003). Cell colture protection and in vivo neuroprotective capacity of flavonoids. *Neurotox. Res.*, Vol. 5, N. 6, (2003) 425-432.

Defeudis, F.V. (2002). Bilobalide and neuroprotection. *Pharmacol. Res.*, Vol. 46, N. 6, (Dec 2002), 565-568.

Deng, F. & Zito, S.W. (2003). Development and validation of a gas chromatographic-mass spectrometric method for simultaneous identification and quantification of marker compounds including bilobalide, ginkgolides and flavonoids in Ginkgo biloba L. extract and pharmaceutical preparations. *J. Chromatogr A*, Vol. 986, N. 1, (Jan 2003), 121-127.

Diamond, B.J., Schiflett, S.C., Fiewel, N., Matheis, R.J., Noskin, O., Richards, J.A. & Schoenberger, N.E. (2000). Ginkgo biloba extract: mechanisms and clinical indications. *Arch. Phys. Med. Rehabil.*, Vol. 81, N. 5, (May 2000), 668-678.

Ding, S., Dudley, E., Chen, L., Plummer, S., Tang, J., Newton, R.P. & Brenton, A.G. (2006). Determination of active components of Ginkgo biloba in human urine by capillary high-performance liquid chromatography/mass spectrometry with on-line column-switching purification. *Rapid Commun Mass Spectrom.*, Vol. 20, N. 24, (Dec 2006), 3619-3624.

Ding, S., Dudley, E., Plummer, S., Tang, J., Newton, R.P. & Brenton, A.G. (2008a). Fingerprint profile of Ginkgo biloba nutritional supplements by LC/ESI-MS/MS. *Phytochemistry*, Vol. 69, Vol. 7, (Mar 2008), 1555-1564.

Ding, S., Dudley, E., Song, Q., Plummer, S., Tang, J., Newton, R.P. & Brenton A.G. (2008b). Mass spectrometry analysis of terpene lactones in Ginkgo biloba. Rapid *Commun. Mass Spectrom.*, Vol. 22, N. 6, (Mar 2008), 766-772.

Domorakova, I., Mechirova, E., Dankova, M., Danielisova, V. & Burda, J. (2009). Effect of antioxidant treatment in global ischemia and ischemic postcondictioning in the rat hippocampus. *Cell. Mol. Neurobiol.*, Vol. 29, N. 6-7, (Sep 2009), 837-844.

Dubber, M.J. & Kanfer, I. (2006). Determination of terpene trilactones in Ginkgo biloba solid oral dosage forms using HPLC with evaporative light scattering detection. *J. Pharm. Biomed. Anal.*, Vol. 41, N. 1, (Apr 2006), 135-140.

Ellnain-Wojtaszek, M., Kruczynski, Z. & Kasprzak, J. (2003) Investigation of the free radical scavenging activity of Ginkgo biloba L. leaves. *Fitoterapia*, Vol. 74, N.1-2, (Feb 2003), 1-6.

Ernest, E. (2000). The role of complementary and alternative medicine. *Br. Med. J*, Vol. 321, N. 7269, (Nov 2000), 1133-1135.

Furtillan, G.J., Brisson, A.M., Girault, J., Ingrand, I., Decourt, J.P., Drieu, K,. Jouenne, P. & Biber, A. (1995). Pharmacokinetic properties of Bilobalide and Ginkgolides A and B in healthy subjects after intravenous and oral administration of Ginkgo biloba extract (EGb 761). *Therapie*, Vol. 50, N. 2, (Mar-Apr 1995), 137-144.

Furukawa, S. (1932). Constituents of Ginkgo biloba leaves. *Scientific Papers of the Institute of Physical and Chemical Research*, Vol. 19, (1932), 27.

Goh, L.M., Barlow, P.J. & Yong, C.S. (2003). Examination of antioxidant activity of Ginkgo biloba leaf infusions. *Food chem.*, Vol. 82, N. 2, (2003), 275-282.

Gohil, K. & Packer L. (2002). Global.gene expression analysis identifies cell and tissue specific actions of Ginkgo biloba extract, EGb 761. *Cell. Mol. Biol.*, Vol. 48, N. 6, (Sep 2002), 625-631.

Gong, Q.H., Wu, Q., Huang, X.N., Sun, A.S., Nie, J. & Shi, J.S. (2006). Protective effect of Ginkgo biloba leaf extract on learning and memory deficit induced by aluminium in model rats. *Chin. J. Integ. Med.*, Vol. 12, N. 1, (Mar 2006), 37-41.

Ha, S.W., Yi, C.J., Cho, C.K., Cho, M.J., Shin, K.H. & Park, C.I. (1996). Enhancement of radiation effect by Ginkgo biloba extract in C3H mouse fibrosarcoma. *Radiother Oncol.* Vol. 41, N. 2, (Nov 1996), 163-167.

Hackett, A.M. (1986). The metabolism of flavonoid compounds in mammals. In Plant Flavonoids in Biology and Medicine: Biochemical, Pharmacological and Structure-Activity Relationship, Alan R. Liss, New York , 177-194.

Hasler, A., Sticher, O. & Meier, B. (1992). Identification and determination of the flavonoids from Ginkgo biloba by high-performance liquid chromatography. *J Chromatogr A*, Vol. 605, N. 1, (Jul 1992), 41-48.

Hu, L., Chen, Z., Cheng, X. & Xie, Y.(1999). Chemistry of ginkgolides: structure-activity relationship as PAF antagonists. *Pure Appl. Chem.*, Vol. 71, N. 6, (1999), 1153-1156.

Hua, L., Guangji, W., Hao, L., Minwen, H., Haitang, X., Chenrong, H., Jianguo, S. & Tian, L. (2006). Sensitive and selective liquid chromatography-electrospray ionization mass spectrometry analysis of ginkgolide B in dog plasma. *J. Pharm. Biomed. Anal.*, Vol. 40, N. 1, (Jan 2006), 88-94.

Huch, H. & Staba E. (1993). Ontogenic Aspects of Ginkgolide Production in Ginkgo biloba. *Planta med.*, Vol. 59, N. 3, (Jun 1993), 232-239.

Itokawa, H., Totsuka, N., Nakahara, K., Maezuru, M., Takeya, K., Kondo, M., Inamatsu, M. & Morita, H. (1989). A quantitative structure-activity relationship for antitumor activity of long-chain phenols from Ginkgo biloba L. *Chem Pharm Bull (Tokyo)*, Vol. 37, N. 6, (Jun 1989), 1619-1621.

Janssens, D., Micheils, C., Delaive, E., Eliaers, F., Drieu, K. & Ramacle, J. (1995). Protection of hypoxia-induced ATP decrease in endothelial cell by Ginkgo biloba extract and bilobalide. *Biochem. Pharmacol.*, Vol. 50, N. 7, (Sep 1995), 991-999.

Jensen, A.G., Ndjoko, K., Wolfender, J.L., Hostettmann, K., Camponovo, F. & Soldati, F. (2002). Liquid chromatography-atmospheric pressure chemical ionisation/mass spectrometry: a rapid and selective method for the quantitative determination of ginkgolides and bilobalide in ginkgo leaf extracts and phytopharmaceuticals. *Phytochem Anal.*, Vol. 13, N.1, (Jan-Feb 2002), 31-38

Jin, C.H., Shin, E.J., Park, J.B., Jang, C.G., Li, Z., Kim, M.S., Koo, K.H., Yoon, H.J., Park, S.J., Choi, W.C., Yamada, K. Nabeshima, T. & Kim, H.C. (2009). Fustin flavonoid attenuates beta-amyloid (1-42)-induced learning impairment *J. Neurosci. Res.*, Vol. 87, N. 16, (Dec 2009), 3658-3670.

Kandaswami, C., Lee, L.T., Lee, P.P., Hwang, J.J., Ke, F.C., Huang, Y.T. & Lee, M.T. (2005). The antitumor activities of flavonoids. *In Vivo*, Vol. 19, N. 5, (Sep-Oct 2005), 895-909.

Kanowski, S., Herrmann, W.M., Stephan, K., Wierich, W. & Hörr, R. (1996). Proof of efficacy of the Ginkgo biloba special extract EGb 761 in outpatients suffering from mild to moderate primary degenerative dementia of the Alzheimer type or multi-infarct dementia. *Pharmacopsychiatry*, Vol. 29, N. 2, (Mar 1996), 47-56.

Kennedy, D.O., Haskell, C.F., Mauri, P.L. & Sholey, A.B. (2007). Acute cognitive effects of standardised Ginkgo biloba extract complexed with phosphatidylserine. *Hum. Psychopharmacol.*, Vol. 22, N. 4, (Jun 2007), 199-210.

Kiewert, C., Kumar, V., Hidmann, O., Hartmann, J., Hillert, M. & Klein, J. (2008). Role of glycine receptors and glycine release for the neuroprotective activity of bilobalide. *Brain Res.*, Vol. 1201, (Mar 2008), 143-150.

Kiewert, C., Kumar, V., Hildmann, O., Rueda, M., Hartmann, J., Naik, R.S. & Klein, J. (2007). Role of GABAergic antagonism in the neuroprotective effects of bilobalide. *Brain Res.*, Vol. 1128, N. 1, (Jan 2007), 70-78.

Kim, M.S., Lee, J.I., Lee, W.Y. & Kim S.E. (2004). Neuroprotective effect of Ginkgo biloba L. extract in a rat model of Parkinson's disease. *Phytother. Res.*, Vol. 18, N. 8, (Aug 2004) 663-666.

Klein, J., Chatterjee, S.S. & Loffelholz, K. (1997). Phospholipid breakdown and choline release under hypoxic conditions: inhibition by bilobalide, a constituent of ginkgo biloba. *Brain Res.*, Vol. 755, N. 2, (May 1997), 347-350.

Koch, E. (2005). Inhibition of platelet activating factor (PAF)-induced aggregation of human thrombocytes by ginkgolides: considerations on possible bleeding complications after oral intake of Ginkgo biloba extracts. *Phytomed.*, Vol.12, N. 1-2, (Jan 2005), 10-16.

Kuo, S.M. (1997). Dietary flavonoid and cancer prevention: evidence and potential mechanism. *Crit. Rev. Oncog.*, Vol. 8, N. 1 (Sep 1997), 47-69.

Lang, Q. & Wai, M. (1999). An extraction method for determination of ginkgolides and bilobalide in Ginkgo leaf extracts. *Anal. Chem.*, Vol. 71, N. 14, (Jul. 1999), 2929-2933.

Le Bars P.L., Kats, M.M, Berman, N., Itil, T.M., Freedman, A.F. & Schatzberg J. (1997). A placebo-controlled, double-blind, randomized trial of an extract of Ginkgo biloba for dementia. North American EGb Study Group. *J. Am Assoc.*, Vol. 278, N. 16, (Oct 1997), 1327-1332.

Lee, E.J., Chen, H.Y., Wu, T.Y. & Maynard, K.L. (2002). Acute administration of Ginkgo biloba extract (EGb 761) affords neuroprotection against permanent and transient focal cerebral ischemia in Sprague-Dawley rats. *J. Neurosci. Res.*, Vol. 68, N. 5, (Jun 2002), 636-645.

Li, W. & Fitzloff, J.F. (2002a). HPLC determination of flavonoids and terpene lactones in commercial Ginkgo biloba products. *J. Liq. Chrom. Rel. Technol.*, Vol. 25, N. 16, (2002), 2501-2514.

Li, W. & Fitzloff, J.F. (2002b). Simultaneous determination of terpene lactones and flavonoid aglycones in Ginkgo biloba by high-performance liquid chromatography with evaporative light scattering detection. *J. Pharm Biomed. Anal.*, Vol. 30, N. 1, (Aug 2002), 67–75.

Liang, X., Zhang, L., Zhang, X., Dai, W., Li, H., Hu, L., Liu, H., Su, J. & Zhang, W. (2010). Qualitative and quantitative analysis of traditional Chinese medicine Niu Huang Jie Du Pill using ultra performance liquid chromatography coupled with tunable UV detector and rapid resolution liquid chromatography coupled with time-of-flight tandem mass spectrometry. *J. Pharm. Biomed. Anal.*, Vol. 51, N. 3, (Feb 2010), 565-571.

Luo, Y. (2001). Ginkgo biloba neuroprotection: Therapeutic implication in Alzheimer's disease. *J. Alzheimers Dis.*, Vol. 3, N. 4, (Aug 2001), 401-407.

Luo, Y. (2006) Alzheimer's disease, the nematode Caenorhabditis elegans, and Ginkgo biloba leaf extract. *Life Sci.*, Vol. 78, N. 18, (Mar 2006), 2066-2072.

Luo, Y., Smith, J.V., Paramasivam, V., Burdick, A., Curry, K.J., Buford, J.P., Khan, I., Netzer, W.J., Xu, H. & Butko, P. (2002). Inhibition of amyloid-beta aggregation and caspase-3 activation by the Gingo biloba extract EGb761. *Proc Natl. Acad. Sci. USA.*, Vol. 99, N. 19, (Sep 2002), 12197-12202.

Lynch, J.W. & Chen, X. (2008). Subunit-specific potentation of recombinant glycine receptors by NV-31, a bilobalide-derived compound. *Neurosci. Lett.*, Vol. 435, N. 2, (Apr 2008), 147-151.

Mahadevan, S. & Park., Y.(2008). Multifaceted Therapeutic Benefits of Ginkgo biloba L.: Chemistry, Efficacy, Safety, and Uses. *J. Food Sci,* Vol. 73, N. 1, (Jan 2008), R14-19.

Makarov, A., Denisov, E. & Lange O. (2009). Performance evaluation of a high-field Orbitrap mass analyzer. *J. Am. Soc. Mass Spectrom.*, Vol. 20, N. 8, (Aug 2009), 1391-1396.

Mauri, P., Migliazza, B. & Pietta, P. (1999). Liquid chromatography/electrospray mass spectrometry of bioactive terpenoids in Ginkgo biloba *L. J. Mass Spectrom.*, Vol. 34, N. 12, (Dec 1999), 1361-1367.

Mauri, P., Simonetti, P., Gardana, C., Minoggio, M., Morazzoni, P., Bombardelli, E. & Pietta, P. (2001). Liquid chromatography/atmospheric pressure chemical ionization mass spectrometry of terpene lactones in plasma of volunteers dosed with Ginkgo biloba L. extracts. *Rapid Commun. Mass Spectrom.*, Vol. 15, N. 12, (May 2001), 929-934.

Mauri, P.L, Minoggio, M., Iemoli, L., Rossoni, G., Morazzoni, P., Bombardelli, E. & Pietta P.G. (2003). Liquid chromatography/atmospheric pressure chemical ionization ion trap mass spectrometry of terpene lactones in plasma of animals. *J. Pharm. Biomed. Anal.*, Vol. 32, N. 4-5, (Aug 2003), 633-639.

Mauri, P.L., De Palma, A., Pozzi, F., Basilico, F , Riva, A., Morazzoni, P., Bombardelli, E. & Rossoni, G. (2006). LC–MS characterization of terpene lactones in plasma of experimental animals treated with Ginkgo biloba extracts: Correlation with pharmacological activity. *J. Pharm. Biomed. Anal.*, Vol. 40, N. 3, (Feb 2006), 763-768.

Mdzinarishvili, A., Kiewert, C., Kumar, V., Hillert, M. & Klein, J. (2007). Bilobalide prevents ischemia-induced edema formation in vitro and in vivo. *Neuroscience*, Vol. 144, N. 1, (Jan 2007), 217-222.

Naik, S.R., Pilgaonkar, V.W. & Panda, V.S. (2006). Evaluation of antioxidant activity of Ginkgo biloba phytosomes in rat brain. *Phytoter. Res.*, Vol. 20, N. 11, (Nov 2006), 1013-1016.

Nakanishi, K., Habaguchi, K., Nakadaira, Y., Woods, M.C., Maruyama, M., Major, R.T., Alauddin, M., Patel, A.R., Weinges, K & Bahr, W. (1971) Structure of bilobalide, a rare tert-butyl containing sesquiterpenoid related to the C20-ginkgolides. *J Am Chem Soc*, Vol. 93, (1971), 3544–3546.

Olsen, J.V., Macek, B., Lange, O., Makarov, A., Horning, S. & Mann, M. (2007). Higher-energy C-trap dissociation for peptide modification analysis. *Nat. Methods.*, Vol. 4, N. 9, (Sep 2007), 709-712.

Pietta, P., Facino R, Carini, M. & Mauri P. (1994). Thermospray liquid chromatography-mass spectrometry of flavonol glycosides from medicinal plants. *J. Chromatogr. A*, V. 661, N.1-2, (Feb 1994), 121-126.

Pietta, P., Mauri, P. & Rava, A. (1992). Rapid liquid chromatography of terpenes in Ginkgo biloba L. extracts and products. *J. Pharm. Biomed. Anal.*, Vol. 10, N. 10-12, (Oct-Dec 1992), 1077-1079.

Pietta, P.G, Gardana, C., Mauri, P.L., Maffei-Facino, R. & Carini, M. (1995). Identification of flavonoid metabolites after oral administration to rats of a Ginkgo biloba extract. *J. Chromatogr. B Biomed. Appl.*, Vol. 673, N. 1, (Nov 1995), 75-80.

Pietta, P.G., Gardana, C. & Mauri, P.L. (1997). Identification of Gingko biloba flavonol metabolites after oral administration to humans. *J. Chromatogr B Biomed. Sci. Appl.*, Vol. 693, N. 1, (May 1997), 249-255.

Pietta, P.G., Mauri, P.L. & Rava, A. (1990). Analysis of terpenes from Ginkgo biloba L. extracts by reversed phase high-performance liquid chromatography. *Chromatographia*, Vo.29, N. 5-6, (Mar 1990), 251-253.

Rojas, P., Serrano-Garcia, N., Mares-Samano, J.J., Medina-Campos, O.S., Pedraza-Chaverri, J. & Ogren S.O. (2008). EGb761 protect against nigrostrial dopaminergic neurotoxicy in 1-methyl-4-phenyl-1,2,3,6-tetrahydropyridine-induced Parkinsonism in mice: role of oxidative stress. *Eur. J. Neurosci.*, Vol. 28, N. 1, (Jul 2008), 41-50.

Rossi, R., Basilico, F., Rossoni, G., Riva, A., Morazzoni, P. & Mauri, P.L. (2009). Liquid chromatography/atmospheric pressure chemical ionization ion trap mass spectrometry of bilobalide in plasma and brain of rats after oral administration of its phospholipidic complex. *J. Pharm. Biomed. Anal.*, Vol. 50, N.2, (Sep 2009), 224-227.

Ryu, K.H., Han, H.Y., Lee, S.Y., Jeon, S.D., Im, G.J., Lee, B.Y., Kim, K., Lim, K.M. & Chung, J.H. (2009). Ginkgo biloba extract enhances antiplatelet and antithrombotic effects of cilostazol without prolongation of bleeding time. *Thromb Res. Jul,* Vol. 124, N. 3, (Apr 2009), 328-334.

Saija, A., Scalese, M., Lanza, M., Marzullo, D., Bonina, F. & Castelli, F. (1995). Flavonoid as antioxidant agents: importance of their interaction with biomembrane. *Free Radic. Biol. Med.*, Vol. 19, N. 4, (Oct 1995), 481-486.

Sasaki, K., Hatta, S., Wada, K., Ohshika, H. & Haga, M. (2000). Bilobalide prevents reduction of gamma-aminobutyric acid levels and glutamic acid decarboxylase activity induced by 4-O-methylpyridoxine in mouse hippocampus. *Life Sci.*, Vol. 67, N. 6, (Jun 2000), 705-715.

Schmid, W. (1997). Ginkgo thrives. *Nature,* Vol. 386, N. 6627, (Apr 1997), 755.

Sener, G., Sehirili, O., Tozan, A., Velioğlu-Ovunç, A., Gedik, N. & Omurtag, G.Z. (2007). Ginkgo biloba extract protects against mercury(II)-induced oxidative tissue damnage in rats. *Food Chem. Toxicol.*, Vol. 45, N. 4, (Apr 2007) 543-550.

Sharma, H.S. Drieu, K., alm, P. & Westman, J. (2000). Role of nitric oxide in blood –brain barrier permeability, brain edema and cell damage followinghyperthermic brain injury. An experimental study using EGB-761 and Gingkolide B pretreatment in the rat. *Acta neurochir. Suppl.*, Vol. 76, (2000), 81-86.

Shi, C., Fang, L., Yew, D.T., Yao, Z., & Xu, J. (2010a). Ginkgo biloba extract EGb761 protects against mitochondrial dysfunction in platelets and hippocampi in ovariectomized rats. *Platelets,* Vol. 21, N. 1, (Feb 2010), 53-59.

Shi, C., Xiao, S., Liu, J., Guo, K., Wu, F., Yew, D.T. & Xu, J. (2010b). Ginkgo biloba extract EGb761 protects against aging-associated mitochondrial dysfunction in platelets and hippocampi of SAMP8 mice. *Platelets,* Vol. 21, N. 5, (2010b), 379-379.

Singh, B., Kaur, P., Gopichand, R.D. & Ahuja, P,S. (2008). Biology and chemistry of Ginkgo biloba. *Fitoterapia,* Vol. 79, N. 6, (Sep 2008),401-418.

Sloley, B.D., Urichuk, L.J., Morley, P., Durkin, J., Shan, j.J., Pang, P.K. & Coutts, R.T. (2000). Identification of kaempferol as a monoamine oxidase inhibitor and potential Neuroprotectant in extracts of Ginkgo biloba. *J. Pharm. Pharmacol.*, Vol. 52, N. 4, (Apr 2000), 451-459.

Smith, J.V. & Luo Y. (2004). Studies on molecular mechanisms of Ginkgo biloba extract. *Appl Microbiol Biotechnol.*, Vol. 64, N. 4, (May 2004), 465-472.

Smith, P.F., Maclennan, K. & Darlington, C. L. (1996). The neuroprotective properties of the Ginkgo biloba leaf: a review of the possible relationship to platelet-activating factor (PAF). *J. Ethnopharmacol.*, Vol. 50, N. 3, (Mar 1996), 131-139.

Sticher, O. (1993). Quality of Ginkgo preparations. *Planta Med.*, Vol. 59. N. 1, (Feb 1993), 2-11.

Sticher, O. (1999). Herbal Medicines for Neuropsychiatric Diseases, Ginkgo Preparations: Biochemical, Pharmaceutical, and Medical Perspectives, *in: S. Kanba, E. Richelson (Eds.) Seiwa Shoten Publishers*, Tokyo, 83.

Stiker, O., Meier, B. & Hasler, A. (2000). The analysis of ginkgo flavonoids, *in van Beek TA (ed), Ginkgo biloba*. Harwood, Amsterdam, 179–202.

Sun, Y., Li, W., Fitzloff, J.F. & Van Breemen, R,B. (2005). Liquid chromatography/electrospray tandem mass spectrometry of terpenoid lactones in Ginkgo biloba. *J. Mass Spectrom.*, Vol. 40, N. 3, (Mar 2005), 373-379.

Tang, C., Wei, X. & Yin C. (2003). Analysis of ginkgolides and bilobalide in Ginkgo biloba L. extract injections by high-performance liquid chromatography with evaporative light scattering detection. *J. Pharm. Biomed. Anal.*, Vol. 33, N. 4, (Nov2003), 811-817.

Urikova, A., Babusikova, E., Dobrota, A, Drgova, A., Kaplan, P., Tatarkova, Z. & Lehotsky, J. (2006). Impact of Ginkgo Biloba Extract EGb 761 on ischemia/reperfusion - induced oxidative stress products formation in rat forebrain. *Cell. Mol. Neurobiol.*, Vol. 26, N. 7-8, (Oct-Nov 2006), 1343-1353.

Van Beek, T.A. & Montoro, P. (2009). Chemical analysis and quality control of Ginkgo biloba leaves, extracts, and phytopharmaceuticals. *J. Chromatogr. A.*, Vol.1216, N. 11, (Mar 2009), 2002-2032

Van Beek, T.A. (2002), Chemical analysis of Ginkgo biloba leaves and extracts. *J Chromatogr. A.*, Vo. 967, N. 1, (Aug 2002), 21-55.

Van Beek, T.A. (2005). Ginkgolides and bilobalide: their physical, chromatographic and spectroscopic properties. *Bioorg. Med. Chem.*, Vol. 13. N. 17, (Sep 2005), 5001-5012.

Van Beek, T.A., Scheeren, H.A., Rantio, T., Melger, W.C. & Lelyveld, G.P. (1991). Determination of Ginkgolides and Bilobalide in Ginkgo biloba Leaves and Phytopharmaceuticals. *J. Chromatography*, Vol. 543, (1991), 375-387.

Wang, F.M., Yao, T.W. & Zeng, S. (2003). Determination of quercetin and kaempferol in human urine after orally administrated tablet of ginkgo biloba extract by HPLC. *J. Pharm. Biomed. Anal.*, Vol. 13; N. 2, (Sep. 2003), 317-321.

Wang, G.X., Cao, F.L & Chen, J. (2006). Progress in researches on the pharmaceutical mechanism and clinical application on Ginkgo biloba extract on various kinds of diseases. *Chin. J. Integr. Med.*, Vol. 12, N. 3, (Sep 2006), 234-239.

Wang, H.F. & Ju, X.R. (2000). Rapid analysis of terpene lactones in extract of Ginkgo biloba L by high performance liquid chromatography. *Se Pu*. Vol. 15, N. 5, (Sep 2000), 394-397.

Wang, Y., Sheng, L.S. & Lou, F.C. (2001). Analysis and structure identification of trace constituent in the total ginkgolide by using LC/DAD/ESI/MS. *Acta Pharmcol. Sin.*,Vol. 36 N. 8,(Aug 2001) 606-608

Weinges, K., Hepp, M. & Jaggy, H. (1987). Chemistry of ginkgolides. II. Isolation and structural elucidation of a new ginkgolide. *Liebigs Ann. Chem.*,Vol. 6, (1987), 521-526

Xie, J., Ding, C., Ge, Q., Zhou, Z. & Zhi X. (2008). Simultaneous determination of ginkgolides A, B, C and bilobalide in plasma by LC-MS/MS and its application to the pharmacokinetic study of Ginkgo biloba extract in rats. *J. Chromatogr. B Analyt.* Technol. Biomed. *Life Sci.*, Vol. 864, N. 1-2, (Mar 2008), 87-94.

Yamamoto, Y., Adachi, Y., Fujii, Y. & Kamei C. (2007). Ginkgo biloba extract improves spatial memory in rats mainly but not exclusively via a histaminergic mechanism. *Brain Res.*, Vol. 1129, N. 9, (Jan 2007), 161-165.

Yang, C., Xu, Y.R. & Yao, W.X. (2002). Extraction of Pharmaceutical Components from Ginkgo biloba Leaves Using Supercritical Carbon Dioxide. J. Agric. Foods Chem., Vol 50, N. 4, (Feb 2002), 846-849.

Yuan, C., Pan, J. & Hu, X. (2008). Determination of the derivative from ginkgolide B. *Nat. Prod. Res.*, Vol. 22, N. 15, (Oct 2008), 1333-1338.

Zhou, W., Chai, H., Lin, P.H., Lumsden, A.B., Yao, Q. & Chen, C. (2004). Clinical use and molecular mechanism of action of extract of Ginkgo biloba leaves in cardiovascular diseases. *Cardiovascular. Drug Rev.*, Vol. 22, N. 4, (Winter 2004), 309-319.

16

Fish Lipids as a Source of Healthy Components: Fatty Acids from Mediterranean Fish

Lara Batičić[1], Neven Varljen[2] and Jadranka Varljen[1*]

[1]*Department of Chemistry and Biochemistry,*

[2]*Department of Physical Medicine and Rehabilitation, Thalassotherapy Hospital;*

School of Medicine. University of Rijeka,

Croatia

1. Introduction

From the time when the epidemiological work on Greenland Eskimos suggested a possible correlation between low incidence of heart disease and the consumption of seafood (Bang et al., 1971), a considerable number of studies have been done on the role of n-3 polyunsaturated fatty acids (n-3 PUFA) in human health and diseases. A substantial number of experiments have indicated that consumption of fish oils rich in n-3 PUFA has different health benefits including cardiovarscular health improving, proper fetal development, anti-inflammatory effects and chronic disease alleviation (Harris, 2010; Itua & Naderali, 2010; Lloret, 2010; Massaro et al., 2010; Roberts et al., 2010). The natural sources of n-3 PUFA are foremost fish lipids, especially those of marine origin. The two most important n-3 PUFA are eicosapentaenoic acid (20:5 n-3, EPA) and docosahexaenoic acid (22:6 n-3, DHA). EPA and DHA have been largely investigated and their positive biological effects have been demonstrated from feeding studies with fish or fish oil supplements (Smutna et al., 2009). Therefore, the nutritional importance of fish consumption is associated with their n-3 PUFA contents. These findings have created a new market for fish oil as a source of healthy components. Many products based on fish oil fatty acids such as dietary supplements and pharmaceuticals as well as other products with technical and cosmetic applications based on fish oil fatty acids have been developed and produced commercially (Driscoll et al., 2009; Martin et al., 2008; Raatz et al., 2009; Smutna et al., 2009). Knowledge about the presence of important constituents and the fatty acid composition of different lipid fractions is essential in the assessment of diet evaluation. Likewise, fatty acid compositional data are needed by food scientists and nutritionists for dietary formulation, processing and product development. In the last decade a significant number of fatty acid compositional data for a number of fish from different parts of the world have been published. However, the fatty acid composition of Adriatic Sea fish species lipids has not been investigated thoroughly. Therefore, the aim of our study was to determine the edible muscle tissue and/or liver fatty

* Corresponding author; Address: Braće Branchetta 20, 51000 Rijeka, Croatia
E-mail: vjadran@medri.hr

acid composition of the white sea bream, *Diplodus sargus*, L., the common two-banded sea bream, *Diplodus vulgaris*, L. and the sea eel, *Conger conger*, L. These are all appreciated fish species in the Mediterranean diet, which occupy an important place in the fishing activity of Croatia and other Mediterranean countries. This review summarizes some published data from our previous research (Baticic et al., 2009; Varljen et al., 2004; Varljen et al., 2003), and some new, unpublished data regarding the fatty acid characterization of fish liver and/or edible muscle tissue lipid fractions. The fatty acid compositions of neutral (triacylglycerols, TAG) and polar (phosphatidylinositol, PI; phosphatidylserine, PS; phosphatidylcholine, PC; and phosphatidylethanolamine, PE) lipid classes were described and their potential relevance as source of healthy components is proposed.

2. Materials and methods

The entire procedure of fish sample collection and preparation likewise the analytical procedures described below were previously published in details in the Journal of the American Oil Chemists' Society (Varljen et al., 2004).

2.1 Collection of fish species

Samples of two-banded sea bream (*Diplodus vulgaris*, L.), white sea bream (*Diplodus sargus*, L.) and sea eel (*Conger conger*, L.) were collected from the Kvarner Bay and the Šibenik basin, in the Adriatic Sea, Croatia by long-line at a depth of 10–15 m, overnight. Specimens of similar body weight and length were selected from all the captured specimens. Biological characteristics, namely body weight (g) and length (cm), were noted, and the fish were dissected immediately after catch. The head, tails, fins, viscera and skin were removed. Intact fish livers were set aside for the determination of moisture, lipid content and fatty acid composition. Samples of about 5 g of white fish muscle (edible muscle tissue) were taken from the left lateral region of the body prior to analysis, while about 1 g of muscle tissue samples were taken for moisture content analysis. Each sample was put into a plastic tube, sealed, and marked, then transported on ice to the laboratory of the Department of Chemistry and Biochemistry at the Faculty of Medicine, Rijeka. Samples for lipid extraction and determination of fatty acid composition in different fractions were preserved at –20°C for further analysis.

2.2 Water content analysis

The water content was determined in fish muscle tissue and liver samples having an average mass of 1 g. The samples, that were separated for water content analysis were preserved overnight at +4°C and analyzed immediately the following day, so as to obtain reliable results. The analyses were performed after drying the tissue at 105°C to a constant mass.

2.3 Extraction of total lipids

Total lipids were extracted from fish muscle tissue samples according to Folch et al. (1957). Briefly, a chloroform/methanol solvent mixture (2:1, vol/vol) was added to frozen samples in the ratio solvent/tissue of 20:1 (vol/wt). The samples were homogenized three times and each homogenization step was followed by cooling of the sample for 1 h at +4°C. The chloroform/methanol extracts were incubated overnight at +4°C to allow the organic (containing the extract of total lipids) and aqueous layers to separate completely. The upper (aqueous) layer was removed, and the lower (organic) layer was rinsed with chloroform/methanol (2:1 vol/vol), then placed into a glass tube. The total lipid fraction was obtained by evaporating the lower phase. The solvent was removed in a rotary evaporator under vacuum at +40°C. These extracts, representing the total lipids, were weighed, and results were noted for each fish. Total lipid contents were determined gravimetrically. After that, each extract was dissolved once again in 2 mL of chloroform/methanol (2:1 vol/vol). The resulting extract of total lipids was stored at +4°C until further analysis.

2.4 Analysis of lipid classes

Polar and neutral lipid fractions were separated from the total lipid extract by thin layer chromatography. Chromatograms were developed on silica gel plates [Allurole Silica gel F254; Merck, Darmstadt, Germany; 20 × 20 cm, 0.2 mm, using petroleum ether/diethyl ether (80:20, vol/vol)] up to 18 cm, so as to allow the separation of polar and neutral lipids. A small quantity of the sample was applied separately at the edge of the plate. That part of the chromatogram was cut off after development, and the bands were visualized by spraying with 50% sulfuric acid in ethanol followed by heating for 1 h at 180°C. Polar lipids remained at the start line, whereas neutral lipids moved along the plate. The position of the bands on the preparative part of the plate was determined by comparison with their position on the small, visualized part of the plate. Neutral lipids (TAG) were scraped off the plate together with the silica gel into tubes for methylation and further analysis. The same plate was put into the polar-lipid reagent (chloroform/methanol/ammonium hydroxide 65:35:5, by vol), up to the part where neutral lipids were scraped off. Polar lipid fractions (PE, PC, PI, PS) were visualized by iodine staining and scraped off the plate together with silica gel into tubes for methylation. Samples of polar and neutral lipid fractions, obtained as described, were used for fatty acid analysis.

2.5 Fatty acid analysis

Fatty acid compositions of polar and neutral lipid fractions of fish muscle tissue and liver samples were determined by gas cromatography of the corresponding methyl esters. Fatty acid methyl esters were obtained by acid methanolysis of lipid fractions extracts. A capillary gas chromatograph equipped with a flame ionization detector was used. A nonpolar capillary column, HP Innowax cross-linked polyethyleneglycol (HP-5, 30 m × 0.32mm; Agilent, Zagreb, Croatia) containing 5% diphenyl and 95% dimethylpolysiloxane, was used for analysis, which were performed in duplicates. Fatty acid methyl esters were identified by comparing their retention times with those of commercial fatty acid methyl esters standards (GLC 68B; Nu-Chek-Prep, Inc., Elysian, MN). The relative share of each identified fatty acid for each polar and neutral lipid fraction was calculated automatically. The degree of unsaturation, expressed as the unsaturation index, according to Kates and Baxter (1962), was calculated as follows: Δ/mol = [% monoene + 2 (% diene) + 3 (% triene) + 4 (% tetraene) + 5 (% pentaene) + 6 (% hexaene)]/100.

2.6 Statistical analysis

The results of fatty acid composition were expressed as mean ± SD for each fatty acid, representing a percentage of their total. Differences between selected parameters were tested by analysis of variance (ANOVA) followed by Scheffe post hoc test. The value of $P < 0.05$ was considered as statistically significant.

3. Results and discussion

Fish species described in this review were abundantly available throughout all seasons in the coastal region of the Kvarner Bay, North Adriatic Sea (*D. vulgaris* and *D. sargus*) and the Šibenik basin, middle Adriatic Sea, Croatia (*D. vulgaris* and *C. conger*). The two-banded sea bream, *D. vulgaris,* and the white sea bream, *D. sargus,* belonging to the same genus *Diplodus,* family *Sparidae,* are common marine teleosts in the Adriatic Sea, widely distributed along the Mediterranean and eastern Atlantic coasts. The sea eel, *C. conger* belongs to the family of *Congridae* and it is also relatively abundantly found in the Mediterranean, North and Irish Sea. The fatty acid compositions of the edible muscle tissue and/or liver were determined for different lipid fractions. Some analyses also included seasonal variations of fatty acid compositions.

3.1 Liver Fatty acid composition of fish originating from the North Adriatic Sea

3.1.1 *Diplodus sargus*, L.

Data regarding *D. sargus* length and mass, liver mass, total lipid content in liver, expressed as a fraction (%) on a wet mass basis, and moisture content in liver during four seasons are presented in Table 1.

	Winter	Spring	Summer	Autumn
Fish length (cm)	25.7 ± 2.0	29.4 ± 4.8	28.2 ± 1.3	20.4 ± 1.3
Fish body weight (g)	445.0 ± 97.1	435.0 ± 193.9	592.3 ± 32.2	354.1 ± 50.1
Liver weight (g)	3.79 ± 1.17	3.14 ± 0.33	3.38 ± 0.65	2.67 ± 0.36
Total lipids (%)	5.5 ± 1.5	6.5 ± 1.5	4.2 ± 1.0	4.6 ± 0.7
Moisture content (%)	71.5 ± 1.1	74.1 ± 0.6	76.9 ± 1.1	73.8 ± 2.4

Table 1. *Diplodus sargus,* L. biological characteristics in different seasons

Body mass and length of fish specimens analyzed in this study are within the limits reported in the literature (Jardas, 1996). The total lipid content in liver was the highest in spring ((6.5±1.5) %) and the lowest in summer ((4.2±1.0) %). The moisture content in the liver was the highest in summer ((76.9±1.1) %), while it was the lowest in winter ((71.5±1.1) %). The obtained results for *D. sargus* from the Adriatic Sea showed slightly lower values for total lipid content in the liver, while they are in agreement with the published results of moisture content for *D. sargus* from other parts of the Mediterranean Sea (Cejas et al., 2004; Perez et al., 2007).

The fatty acid compositions of neutral (TAG) and polar (PI/PS, PC, PE) lipid fractions of *D. sargus* liver, as well as other fatty acid parameters, have been determined during spring, summer, autumn and winter. Results are shown in Tables 2 to 5. The relative ratios of each fatty acid are expressed as mean values ± SD, representing the fraction (%) of total identified fatty acids. According to their characteristics and the nomenclature adopted in mariculture, the analyzed fatty acids were grouped as saturated (SFA), monounsaturated (MUFA), diunsaturated (DUFA), while tri-, tetra-, penta-, and hexaenoic fatty acids were grouped as polyunsaturated fatty acids (PUFA). The degree of unsaturation and the n-3/n-6 ratios were also determined.

Fatty acid component	Percentage of total fatty acids in TAG[1]			
	Winter	Spring	Summer	Autumn
14:0	3.4 ± 0.2	3.9 ± 0.9	5.7 ± 0.1	5.1 ± 1.1
14:1 n-5	0.8 ± 0.3	0.8 ± 0.5	0.7 ± 0.4	0.5 ± 0.2
16:0	16.8 ± 2.5	29.1 ± 2.1	25.4 ± 3.0	25.5 ± 2.0
16:1 n-7	10.0 ± 0.8	10.1 ± 1.2	8.4 ± 1.7	10.2 ± 1.3
18:0	4.4 ± 0.2	11.1 ± 4.2	9.1 ± 1.5	8.1 ± 0.8
18:1 n-9	19.3 ± 1.5	24.5 ± 7.2	11.4 ± 2.6	24.6 ± 3.5
18:2 n-6	3.6 ± 0.6	2.1 ± 1.5	0.8 ± 0.5	0.8 ± 0.3
20:0	0.1 ± 0.1	0.6 ± 0.5	0.6 ± 0.3	0.3 ± 0.2
18:3 n-3	1.0 ± 0.3	2.7 ± 2.5	0.1 ± 0.1	1.2 ± 1.5
20:1 n-9	2.3 ± 1.1	2.1 ± 1.7	2.7 ± 1.3	2.6 ± 1.7
22:0	0.3 ± 0.4	Trace	0.1 ± 0.1	1.7 ± 3.6
20:4 n-6	4.0 ± 1.3	2.7 ± 0.9	4.1 ± 2.7	4.4 ± 1.7
22:1 n-11	0.1 ± 0.2	0.8 ± 0.4	0.1 ± 0.1	0.1 ± 0.2
20:5 n-3	8.6± 0.8	3.0± 1.3	4.3± 2.6	4.8± 0.9
24:0	Trace[2]	0.3 ± 0.3	0.2 ± 0.0	0.1 ± 0.2
22:3 n-3	1.0 ± 1.0	1.7 ± 1.6	2.6 ± 1.5	1.9 ± 1.1
24:1 n-9	0.2 ± 0.2	0.4 ± 0.4	0.3 ± 0.2	1.7 ± 0.4
22:6 n-3	23.9 ± 5.2	4.3 ± 2.4	23.2 ± 5.9	6.6 ± 1.4
MUFA + DUFA	36.4 ± 4.1	40.7 ± 9.2	24.5 ± 2.8	40.4 ± 4.5
PUFA	38.6 ± 4.1	14.3 ± 4.9	34.4 ± 4.3	18.9 ± 2.8
Σ UFA	74.9 ± 3.1	55.0 ± 5.1	58.8 ± 4.7	59.3 ± 4.0
EPA + DHA	32.5 ± 5.6	7.3 ± 3.2	27.5 ± 5.7	11.4 ± 2.2
Σ SFA	25.1 ± 3.1	45.0 ± 5.1	41.2 ± 4.7	40.7 ± 4.0
Unsaturation index	2.49	1.07	2.11	1.32
n-3/n-6	4.53	2.43	6.07	2.79

Table 2. Fatty acid composition of triacylglycerols-TAG (neutral lipid fraction) of *Diplodus sargus,* L. liver with seasonal variation (expressed as percentage of total identified fatty acids). [1]Values are mean ± SD; [2]Trace, <0.1%.

	Percentage of total fatty acids in PI/PS[1]			
Fatty acid component	Winter	Spring	Summer	Autumn
14:0	1.6 ± 0.6	3.0 ± 0.8	0.9 ± 0.4	0.9 ± 0.2
14:1 n-5	0.8 ± 0.5	1.5 ± 0.8	0.4 ± 0.3	0.3 ± 0.1
16:0	26.0 ± 9.8	46.6 ± 5.3	23.2 ± 8.0	17.1 ± 3.0
16:1 n-7	3.9 ± 2.2	8.1 ± 2.1	1.8 ± 1.1	1.7 ± 0.9
18:0	30.0 ± 13.5	19.6 ± 8.6	40.7 ± 4.0	42.3 ± 6.7
18:1 n-9	10.0 ± 2.0	12.9 ± 1.5	9.4 ± 2.9	6.8 ± 0.7
18:2 n-6	0.6 ± 0.4	0.4 ± 0.2	1.1 ± 0.8	0.4 ± 0.2
20:0	0.2 ± 0.2	0.2 ± 0.3	0.5 ± 0.2	0.5 ± 0.2
18:3 n-3	Trace[2]	0.3 ± 0.0	Trace	Trace
20:1 n-9	0.7 ± 0.4	0.3 ± 0.2	0.8 ± 0.3	1.0 ± 0.5
22:0	0.2 ± 0.1	0.1 ± 0.1	0.2 ± 0.2	0.6 ± 1.3
20:4 n-6	12.0 ± 3.7	2.2 ± 1.9	10.2 ± 3.5	11.0 ± 4.0
22:1 n-11	Trace	0.1 ± 0.1	Trace	0.2 ± 0.3
20:5 n-3	4.5 ± 2.4	2.0 ± 2.3	1.6 ± 1.1	4.6 ± 2.3
24:0	Trace	Trace	0.3 ± 0.4	1.0 ± 1.2
22:3 n-3	1.2 ± 1.8	0.4 ± 0.4	4.0 ± 2.2	5.3 ± 2.2
24:1 n-9	0.1 ± 0.2	Trace	Trace	0.8 ± 0.6
22:6 n-3	8.1 ± 4.2	2.3 ± 2.6	4.8 ± 2.0	5.5 ± 2.7
MUFA + DUFA	16.1 ± 2.0	23.3 ± 2.7	13.6 ± 1.7	11.2 ± 1.9
PUFA	25.8 ± 3.8	7.2 ± 7.2	20.7 ± 4.4	26.4 ± 9.1
Σ UFA	41.9 ± 5.1	30.5 ± 7.9	34.3 ± 4.3	37.6 ± 9.5
EPA + DHA	12.1 ± 6.1	4.3 ± 4.8	6.5 ± 2.3	10.1 ± 4.9
Σ SFA	58.1 ± 5.1	69.5 ± 7.9	65.7 ± 4.3	62.4 ± 9.5
Unsaturation index	1.40	0.58	1.05	1.28
n-3/n-6	1.33	1.99	0.94	1.35

Table 3. Fatty acid composition of phosphatidylinositol-PI/phosphatidylserine-PS (polar lipid fractions) of *Diplodus sargus*, L. liver with seasonal variation (expressed as percentage of total identified fatty acids). [1]Values are mean ± SD; [2]Trace, <0.1%.

	Percentage of total fatty acids in PC[1]			
Fatty acid component	Winter	Spring	Summer	Autumn
14:0	2.3 ± 0.8	2.4 ± 0.9	2.0 ± 1.2	1.8 ± 0.6
14:1 n-5	1.2 ± 0.6	0.5 ± 0.2	1.1 ± 0.1	0.8 ± 0.7
16:0	34.7 ± 5.9	24.1 ± 1.4	40.4 ± 4.4	37.0 ± 9.1
16:1 n-7	8.0 ± 2.2	2.9 ± 1.8	4.7 ± 2.5	4.8 ± 2.1
18:0	5.6 ± 0.7	35.6 ± 2.5	8.0 ± 0.6	6.5 ± 1.2
18:1 n-9	9.8 ± 1.5	11.8 ± 4.5	6.1 ± 3.6	8.4 ± 2.4
18:2 n-6	2.4 ± 2.9	0.3 ± 0.4	0.3 ± 0.0	0.8 ± 1.1
20:0	0.1 ± 0.0	Trace	0.4 ± 0.2	0.1 ± 0.2
18:3 n-3	0.2 ± 0.0	0.7 ± 0.2	Trace	0.1 ± 0.2
20:1 n-9	0.3 ± 0.1	0.5 ± 0.5	0.4 ± 0.3	0.5 ± 0.4
22:0	0.1 ± 0.0	0.1 ± 0.1	Trace	0.2 ± 0.1
20:4 n-6	4.6 ± 1.3	2.3 ± 0.8	6.3 ± 2.1	8.7 ± 1.7
22:1 n-11	Trace[2]	0.1 ± 0.1	Trace	Trace
20:5 n-3	7.6 ± 2.6	2.2 ± 1.3	6.6 ± 0.7	8.5 ± 2.5
24:0	0.1 ± 0.1	Trace	Trace	Trace
22:3 n-3	0.4 ± 0.1	0.5 ± 0.2	0.4 ± 0.3	0.9 ± 0.4
24:1 n-9	0.3 ± 0.5	Trace	0.7 ± 0.5	1.3 ± 0.7
22:6 n-3	22.3 ± 4.8	15.5 ± 5.4	22.7 ± 5.7	19.5 ± 6.5
MUFA + DUFA	22.1 ± 2.1	16.7 ± 5.2	13.3 ± 3.7	16.6 ± 3.6
PUFA	35.1 ± 6.5	21.1 ± 5.9	36.0 ± 6.8	37.7 ± 9.9
Σ UFA	57.2 ± 6.7	37.8 ± 1.0	49.3 ± 4.6	54.3 ± 9.8
EPA + DHA	29.9 ± 6.3	17.7 ± 5.9	29.3 ± 5.8	28.0 ± 8.6
Σ SFA	42.2 ± 6.7	62.2 ± 1.0	50.7 ± 4.6	45.7 ± 9.8
Unsaturation index	2.16	2.16	2.09	2.15
n-3/n-6	1.82	6.22	4.52	3.04

Table 4. Fatty acid composition of phosphatidylcholine-PC (polar lipid fraction) of *Diplodus sargus,* L. liver with seasonal variation (expressed as percentage of total identified fatty acids). [1]Values are mean ± SD; [2]Trace, <0.1%.

	Percentage of total fatty acids in PE[1]			
Fatty acid component	Winter	Spring	Summer	Autumn
14:0	1.0 ± 0.5	2.8 ± 0.4	1.6 ± 0.4	1.3 ± 0.5
14:1 n-5	0.5 ± 0.2	1.6 ± 0.2	0.6 ± 0.3	0.4 ± 0.3
16:0	21.0 ± 3.7	38.0 ± 2.8	22.2 ± 3.5	23.4 ± 8.2
16:1 n-7	5.4 ± 1.9	8.2 ± 1.0	6.3 ± 1.2	4.9 ± 1.9
18:0	11.1 ± 1.0	13.9 ± 3.0	11.8 ± 0.4	13.4 ± 4.4
18:1 n-9	17.3 ± 3.9	12.5 ± 2.4	13.6 ± 2.7	12.3 ± 3.5
18:2 n-6	4.5 ± 4.7	0.4 ± 0.3	0.5 ± 0.3	0.9 ± 0.3
20:0	0.2 ± 0.2	0.1 ± 0.1	0.1 ± 0.1	0.2 ± 0.2
18:3 n-3	1.5 ± 1.0	0.3 ± 0.2	0.4 ± 0.7	0.7 ± 0.7
20:1 n-9	0.4 ± 0.3	0.3 ± 0.1	0.8 ± 0.8	0.7 ± 0.8
22:0	0.2 ± 0.2	0.1 ± 0.0	Trace	0.7 ± 0.9
20:4 n-6	9.4 ± 2.7	6.2 ± 0.8	10.8 ± 1.4	8.2 ± 2.5
22:1 n-11	0.2 ± 0.3	Trace	0.3 ± 0.6	0.1 ± 0.3
20:5 n-3	7.7 ± 2.8	5.6 ± 2.2	7.4 ± 0.7	5.5 ± 3.6
24:0	Trace[2]	0.1 ± 0.3	0.3 ± 0.6	0.3 ± 0.9
22:3 n-3	1.1 ± 0.6	0.9 ± 0.3	0.8 ± 0.7	2.7 ± 3.6
24:1 n-9	0.3 ± 0.2	0.1 ± 0.1	0.4 ± 0.5	1.8 ± 1.4
22:6 n-3	18.5 ± 1.1	9.0 ± 4.7	22.0 ± 1.6	22.4 ± 9.9
MUFA + DUFA	28.4 ± 6.7	23.0 ± 2.3	22.6 ± 2.6	21.2 ± 4.6
PUFA	38.2 ± 5.5	22.0 ± 7.3	41.4 ± 1.2	39.5 ± 12.6
Σ UFA	66.6 ± 4.8	45.1 ± 5.3	64.0 ± 3.4	60.7 ± 10.4
EPA + DHA	26.2 ± 3.1	14.7 ± 6.4	29.4 ± 1.3	27.9 ± 11.3
Σ SFA	33.4 ± 4.8	54.9 ± 5.3	36.0 ± 3.4	39.3 ± 10.4
Unsaturation index	2.30	1.34	2.39	2.27
n-3/n-6	2.08	2.40	2.72	3.45

Table 5. Fatty acid composition of phosphatidylethanolamine-PE (polar lipid fraction) of *Diplodus sargus,* L. liver with seasonal variation (expressed as percentage of total identified fatty acids). [1]Values are mean ± SD; [2]Trace, <0.1%.

3.1.2 *Diplodus vulgaris,* L.

The fatty acid compositions of neutral (TAG) and polar (PI/PS, PC, PE) lipid fractions of *D. vulgaris* liver, as well as other fatty acid parameters, have been determined during four different seasons. Results are shown in Tables 6 to 9. The relative ratios of each fatty acid are expressed as mean values ± SD, representing the fraction (%) of total identified fatty acids. The degree of unsaturation, expressed as unsaturation index and the n-3/n-6 ratio were also determined.

	Percentage of total fatty acids in TAG[1]			
Fatty acid component	Winter	Spring	Summer	Autumn
14:0	5.5 ± 1.1	3.3 ± 1.7	5.2 ± 1.4	4.9 ± 2.1
14:1 n-5	0.9 ± 0.6	0.6 ± 0.1	0.7 ± 0.4	0.9 ± 0.7
16:0	21.8 ± 3.2	25.0 ± 4.5	24.4 ± 3.8	27.4 ± 4.5
16:1 n-7	9.1 ± 1.9	8.1 ± 4.0	9.0 ± 3.8	6.7 ± 2.9
18:0	6.8 ± 2.6	9.3 ± 4.1	11.6 ± 5.0	12.1 ± 4.0
18:1 n-9	20.6 ± 4.8	23.7 ± 5.3	22.4 ± 5.0	16.0 ± 5.3
18:2 n-6	1.1 ± 0.7	0.9 ± 0.3	0.8 ± 0.5	1.5 ± 1.1
20:0	0.4 ± 0.2	0.3 ± 0.3	0.2 ± 0.1	0.9 ± 0.8
18:3 n-3	0.8 ± 1.1	1.4 ± 1.5	0.1 ± 0.2	2.2 ± 1.0
20:1 n-9	0.9 ± 0.7	0.6 ± 0.7	1.3 ± 1.6	0.3 ± 0.2
22:0	0.3 ± 0.2	0.4 ± 0.2	0.4 ± 0.4	1.0 ± 0.7
20:4 n-6	4.5 ± 1.3	5.5 ± 2.0	4.7 ± 1.5	4.7 ± 1.0
22:1 n-11	0.2 ± 0.7	0.2 ± 0.7	Trace	Trace
20:5 n-3	5.6 ± 1.5	5.7 ± 3.4	7.4 ± 3.3	6.4 ± 3.3
24:0	0.3 ± 0.7	Trace[2]	0.2 ± 0.4	0.4 ± 0.8
22:3 n-3	2.6 ± 1.9	2.7 ± 1.2	2.2 ± 1.8	4.2 ± 1.8
24:1 n-9	0.2 ± 0.3	0.1 ± 0.1	Trace	Trace
22:6 n-3	18.3 ± 4.3	12.4 ± 4.7	9.1 ± 2.6	10.4 ± 4.2
MUFA + DUFA	33.0 ± 7.0	34.2 ± 6.0	34.3 ± 7.8	25.5 ± 6.0
PUFA	31.9 ± 7.2	27.7 ± 9.1	23.6 ± 3.7	27.9 ± 6.3
Σ UFA	64.9 ± 6.2	61.9 ± 8.1	57.9 ± 8.5	51.7 ± 7.5
EPA + DHA	23.9 ± 4.7	18.1 ± 6.5	16.5 ± 4.0	16.7 ± 5.8
Σ SFA	35.0 ± 5.8	38.2 ± 8.0	42.1 ± 8.5	46.6 ± 5.1
Unsaturation index	2.01	1.72	1.53	1.59
n-3/n-6	4.92	3.50	3.49	3.77

Table 6. Fatty acid composition of triacylglycerols-TAG (neutral lipid fraction) of *Diplodus vulgaris,* L. liver with seasonal variation (expressed as percentage of total identified fatty acids). [1]Values are mean ± SD; [2]Trace, <0.1%.

	Percentage of total fatty acids in PI/PS[1]			
Fatty acid component	Winter	Spring	Summer	Autumn
14:0	1.4 ± 0.7	3.0 ± 1.5	2.0 ± 0.9	1.4 ± 0.6
14:1 n-5	0.1 ± 0.1	0.7 ± 0.3	0.8 ± 0.5	0.1 ± 0.1
16:0	14.4 ± 1.6	38.9 ± 7.0	43.0 ± 9.4	14.4 ± 1.4
16:1 n-7	1.3 ± 0.7	2.6 ± 1.2	2.7 ± 0.6	1.3 ± 0.6
18:0	38.6 ± 5.0	33.4 ± 4.7	30.8 ± 8.2	39.7 ± 5.2
18:1 n-9	13.9 ± 5.2	9.9 ± 4.9	8.2 ± 3.0	13.6 ± 4.6
18:2 n-6	0.7 ± 0.7	0.8 ± 0.5	0.6 ± 0.7	0.7 ± 0.6
20:0	0.6 ± 0.2	0.4 ± 0.1	0.5 ± 0.6	0.7 ± 0.3
18:3 n-3	0.2 ± 0.5	0.2 ± 0.2	0.1 ± 0.2	0.2 ± 0.4
20:1 n-9	0.8 ± 0.6	1.4 ± 0.8	0.4 ± 0.4	0.9 ± 0.6
22:0	0.7 ± 0.4	1.4 ± 1.4	0.6 ± 0.5	0.8 ± 0.4
20:4 n-6	8.8 ± 5.4	1.5 ± 1.9	3.9 ± 4.1	8.1 ± 5.0
22:1 n-11	0.1 ± 0.2	0.1 ± 0.1	Trace	0.4 ± 0.7
20:5 n-3	3.1 ± 1.7	1.1 ± 0.9	1.8 ± 1.7	2.6 ± 1.8
24:0	0.8 ± 1.1	0.2 ± 0.3	0.2 ± 0.6	0.7 ± 1.0
22:3 n-3	7.8 ± 3.5	2.6 ± 1.3	1.5 ± 1.4	8.5 ± 3.5
24:1 n-9	0.2	0.3 ± 0.3	Trace	0.1 ± 0.2
22:6 n-3	6.5 ± 2.7	1.5 ± 1.1	2.8 ± 2.5	5.7 ± 3.0
MUFA + DUFA	17.1 ± 5.1	15.8 ± 4.4	12.9 ± 2.8	17.2 ± 4.5
PUFA	26.4 ± 7.9	6.8 ± 3.1	10.1 ± 6.3	25.0 ± 7.6
Σ UFA	43.5 ± 5.6	22.7 ± 7.2	23.0 ± 8.4	42.2 ± 5.7
EPA + DHA	9.6 ± 3.5	2.6 ± 1.8	4.6 ± 3.1	8.3 ± 4.1
Σ SFA	56.5 ± 5.6	77.4 ± 7.2	77,0 ± 8.4	57.8 ± 5.7
Unsaturation index	1.32	0.45	0.60	1.23
n-3/n-6	2.54	1.70	2.19	2.54

Table 7. Fatty acid composition of phosphatidylinositol-PI/phosphatidylserine-PS (polar lipid fractions) of *Diplodus vulgaris,* L. liver with seasonal variation (expressed as percentage of total identified fatty acids). [1]Values are mean ± SD; [2]Trace, <0.1%.

	Percentage of total fatty acids in PC[1]			
Fatty acid component	Winter	Spring	Summer	Autumn
14:0	3.2 ± 1.1	2.4 ± 0.6	2.0 ± 0.5	0.8 ± 0.6
14:1 n-5	0.8 ± 0.5	0.7 ± 0.5	0.8 ± 0.3	0.2 ± 0.1
16:0	37.0 ± 5.3	35.5 ± 7.8	37.2 ± 6.4	12.7 ± 1.4
16:1 n-7	5.5 ± 1.8	5.5 ± 2.6	3.9 ± 2.9	1.8 ± 0.3
18:0	8.7 ± 4.8	12.8 ± 9.2	13.7 ± 4.1	33.8 ± 7.4
18:1 n-9	13.8 ± 5.4	15.1 ± 3.7	11.0 ± 1.3	8.2 ± 1.2
18:2 n-6	0.7 ± 0.4	0.4 ± 0.4	0.7 ± 0.5	0.4 ± 0.2
20:0	0.3 ± 0.3	0.1 ± 0.1	0.2 ± 0.2	0.1 ± 0.1
18:3 n-3	0.2 ± 0.4	0.1 ± 0.3	0.6 ± 0.5	0.7 ± 0.5
20:1 n-9	0.4 ± 0.5	0.5 ± 0.3	0.7 ± 0.5	0.3 ± 0.3
22:0	0.1 ± 0.1	0.4 ± 0.4	0.2 ± 0.2	0.8 ± 0.6
20:4 n-6	3.9 ± 1.4	7.1 ± 1.7	7.5 ± 3.3	12.3 ± 3.7
22:1 n-11	0.1 ± 0.2	0.3 ± 0.6	0.1 ± 0.1	0.8 ± 1.0
20:5 n-3	6.3 ± 1.6	6.2 ± 0.9	5.9 ± 1.7	4.5 ± 1.1
24:0	Trace[2]	0.1 ± 0.1	Trace	0.4 ± 0.5
22:3 n-3	1.1 ± 0.5	0.7 ± 0.5	1.2 ± 0.7	7.5 ± 4.9
24:1 n-9	0.2 ± 0.2	0.4 ± 0.3	0.4 ± 0.4	Trace
22:6 n-3	17.6 ± 6.9	11.5 ± 6.7	14.1 ± 5.1	14.7 ± 5.2
MUFA + DUFA	21.4 ± 6.4	23.0 ± 1.1	17.6 ± 2.7	11.7 ± 1.2
PUFA	29.2 ± 8.7	24.3 ± 8.8	29.2 ± 7.7	39.6 ± 7.2
Σ UFA	50.6 ± 5.1	47.3 ± 8.5	46.8 ± 5.5	51.4 ± 7.2
EPA + DHA	24.0 ± 8.0	16.2 ± 8.4	20.0 ± 5.7	19.1 ± 5.8
Σ SFA	49.4 ± 5.1	52.4 ± 8.1	53.2 ± 5.5	48.6 ± 7.2
Unsaturation index	1.79	1.54	1.67	1.96
n-3/n-6	5.67	2.68	2.37	2.43

Table 8. Fatty acid composition of phosphatidylcholine-PC (polar lipid fraction) of *Diplodus vulgaris,* L. liver with seasonal variation (expressed as percentage of total identified fatty acids). [1]Values are mean ± SD; [2]Trace, <0.1%.

	Percentage of total fatty acids in PE[1]			
Fatty acid component	Winter	Spring	Summer	Autumn
14:0	1.1 ± 0.3	2.2 ± 0.5	2.0 ± 0.5	2.0 ± 0.8
14:1 n-5	0.2 ± 0.1	0.6 ± 0.3	0.8 ± 0.3	0.5 ± 0.3
16:0	21.5 ± 2.8	37.0 ± 8.5	37.2 ± 6.4	26.0 ± 3.0
16:1 n-7	4.6 ± 0.9	7.2 ± 0.2	3.9 ± 2.9	6.9 ± 2.3
18:0	14.2 ± 4.1	11.8 ± 1.4	13.7 ± 4.1	14.9 ± 2.0
18:1 n-9	24.2 ± 4.5	17.8 ± 2.6	11.0 ± 1.3	11.4 ± 2.0
18:2 n-6	0.5 ± 0.3	0.6 ± 0.4	0.7 ± 0.5	0.7 ± 0.3
20:0	0.3 ± 0.1	0.1 ± 0.1	0.2 ± 0.2	0.2 ± 0.1
18:3 n-3	1.0 ± 1.3	0.3 ± 0.4	0.6 ± 0.5	0.2 ± 0.1
20:1 n-9	0.5 ± 0.8	0.7 ± 0.2	0.7 ± 0.5	0.2 ± 0.2
22:0	0.1 ± 0.1	0.3 ± 0.1	0.2 ± 0.2	0.3 ± 0.1
20:4 n-6	5.6 ± 3.7	4.9 ± 2.2	7.5 ± 3.3	6.7 ± 1.5
22:1 n-11	Trace[2]	Trace	0.1 ± 0.1	0.2 ± 0.2
20:5 n-3	5.2 ± 1.6	5.4 ± 1.9	3.8 ± 2.1	5.3 ± 1.1
24:0	Trace	0.1 ± 0.2	Trace	Trace
22:3 n-3	1.5 ± 0.8	1.1 ± 0.4	1.8 ± 1.4	1.7 ± 0.8
24:1 n-9	0.4 ± 0.5	0.3 ± 0.3	0.1 ± 0.2	Trace
22:6 n-3	19.0 ± 7.1	9.7 ± 4.7	8.5 ± 4.2	22.9 ± 2.7
MUFA + DUFA	30.4 ± 3.6	27.2 ± 2.5	26.4 ± 5.9	19.9 ± 3.9
PUFA	32.3 ± 9.2	21.3 ± 8.8	20.4 ± 6.5	36.8 ± 4.0
Σ UFA	62.7 ± 6.4	48.5 ± 9.4	46.8 ± 7.7	56.7 ± 2.6
EPA + DHA	24.1 ± 7.3	15.1 ± 6.4	12.3 ± 4.7	28.2 ± 3.1
Σ SFA	37.3 ± 6.4	51.5 ± 9.4	53.2 ± 5.5	43.3 ± 2.6
Unsaturation index	2.01	1.36	1.67	2.17
n-3/n-6	4.37	3.12	2.37	4.23

Table 9. Fatty acid composition of phosphatidylethanolamine-PE (polar lipid fraction) of *Diplodus vulgaris*, L. liver with seasonal variation (expressed as percentage of total identified fatty acids). [1]Values are mean ± SD; [2]Trace, <0.1%.

Eighteen different fatty acids were identified in analyzed *D. sargus* and *D. vulgaris* liver lipid fractions samples. The major constituents of total fatty acids were saturates: palmitic (16:0) and stearic acid (18:0); monounsaturated fatty acids: oleic (18:1 n-9) and palmitoleic acid (16:1 n-7), while arachidonic acid (20:4 n-6), EPA (20:5 n-3) and DHA (22:6 n-3) were the major constituents among polyunsaturated fatty acids. The fatty acid amounts and ratios differed significantly among seasons. Palmitic acid was the predominant saturated fatty acid. Oleic acid and DHA were the predominant unsaturated fatty acids. An accentuated seasonality pattern was found for these fatty acids. The same observation was made for *D. sargus* captured along the eastern Mediterranean coast of Turkey (Ozyurt et al., 2005; Imre & Saglik, 1998). The seasonal changes in the contents of these fatty acids were previously recorded for gilthead sea bream (*Sparus aurata*) (Grigorakis et al., 2002), for Baltic herring (*Clupea harengus membras*) (Aro et al., 2000), and some other fish species (Luzia et al., 2003; Tanakol et al., 1999). Furthermore, observations regarding the seasonality of fatty acid composition in *D. vulgaris* caught in other areas of the Mediterranean Sea that were previously published (Donato et al., 1984) are in agreement with the results of this study.

The results of our study revealed that total unsaturated fatty acids (UFAs) in all analyzed lipid fractions were the highest in the winter period in both *D. sargus* and *D. vulgaris*, except for PC in *D. vulgaris* where slightly higher total UFAs were found in the autumn perion. Likewise, the EPA+DHA values were the highest for all lipid fractions in both fish in the winter period, except for PE in *D. sargus*, where EPA+DHA values were slightly higher in the summer period while in *D. vulgaris* in the autumn period. In contrast, saturated fatty acids (SFA) were the highest in the spring and summer period in all analyzed lipid fractions. Neutral lipid fractions contained more UFAs in comparison with polar lipid fractions during the year, except for PE in summer and autumn (*D. sargus*) and autumn period (*D. vulgaris*). The decrease in the amount of UFAs in the analyzed fractions from winter to spring was noticed, followed by an increase in the UFA content in summer and autumn. In TAG, the UFAs were lower in all seasons in comparison with their highest values achieved in winter in both fish species. In PE, the content of UFAs was higher in all seasons compared to the lowest values in the spring also in both fish species. Similarly, PUFA content also showed seasonal variations, having an even more accentuated pattern of seasonality. Similar findings were reported by Donato et al. (1997) for *D. sargus* originating from the Mediterranean Sea. We noticed that PI/PS had the highest content of SFAs in all seasons with the highest values in the spring in both fish species. The lowest total SFA in *D. sargus* and *D. vulgaris* were found in winter in all lipid fractions, except for PC in *D. vulgaris*, where the lowest content of SFAs was determined in the autumn period. These results are in agreement with previously reported findings for this fish species from other catch areas among the Mediterranean coasts (Ozyurt et al., 2005). The observed decrease in total SFA in the winter period is most probably due to the catabolization of SFA in order to ensure the additional metabolic energy required in that period. Likewise, they could be necessary for the increase in PUFA required for spawning in spring and used in gonadal development.

The degree of fatty acid unsaturation, expressed as unsaturation index, differed among the analyzed lipid fractions in both fish species thorough the year. It was the highest for TAG in winter and the lowest for PI/PS in spring both in *D. sargus* and *D. vulgaris*, which reflects the fatty acid compositions in those seasons. It was observed that unsaturation indices in different lipid fractions achieved their highest values mostly in the winter period. This is in agreement with the previously published observation that a decrease in water temperature results in an increase in the degree of unsaturation (Henderson & Tocher, 1987). This could be explained by the fact that a higher degree of fatty acid unsaturation is essential to maintain the flexibility of membrane phospholipids at lower temperatures (Lovell, 1991).

The content of n-3 PUFA, EPA and DHA is especially important for their beneficial effects. The highest EPA+DHA values were noticed in TAG in the winter period in both fish species, except for PE in *D. vulgaris,* where the highest EPA+DHA values were determined in the autumn period. On the other hand, the lowest but still appreciable EPA+DHA values were always detected in PI/PS, and also showed seasonal variations. Considerable amounts of EPA+DHA in *D. sargus* and *D. vulgaris* liver make them potentially important for exploitation in pharmaceutical and other industries as a potential raw material for dietary omega-3 supplements and other fish-based oil products.

Growing scientific evidence shows that n-3 fatty acids are important in the prevention and amelioration of different chronic disorders (Lloret, 2010). Increasing knowledge suggests that the n-3/n-6 ratio could be used as a biomedical index. The n-3/n-6 ratios were calculated for all lipid fractions in both fish liver samples. Fatty acids of *D. sargus* and *D. vulgaris* liver lipids have an n-3/n-6 ratio between 1 and 6, which is mostly in agreement with previously reported findings for these fish genus (Donato et al. 1997). The n-3/n-6 ratio is also a good marker for comparing nutritional value of fish oils. It is considered to be the most important indicator of fish lipid quality, which best reflects the quality of fish as food (Hu et al., 2002).

3.2 Edible muscle tissue fatty acid composition of fish originating from north Adriatic Sea

3.2.1 *Diplodus vulgaris*, L.

D. vulgaris edible muscle tissue was analyzed and fatty acid compositions of neutral and polar lipid fractions in winter and summer were determined. Body weights of analyzed *D. vulgaris* specimens ranged from 200 to 400 g, with average lengths from 16 to 20 cm. Those values are within the limits reported in the literature (Jardas, 1996). The total lipid content, expressed on a wet weight basis (%, w/w), amounted to 1.0 ± 0.4% in the winter period and 0.9 ± 0.3% in the summer period. According to the lipid content classification, this fish species belongs to low-fat fish (Ackman, 1989). The water content in fish tissue samples amounted to 77.8 ± 2.7% in the winter period and 76.6 ± 1.7% in the summer period.

The fatty acid compositions of neutral (TAG) and polar (PI/PS, PC, PE) lipid fractions of *D. vulgaris* edible muscle tissue, as well as other fatty acid parameters, have been determined during summer and winter periods. Results are presented in Table 10 and 11. The relative ratios of each fatty acid are expressed as mean values ± SD, representing the fraction (%) of total identified fatty acids. The analyzed fatty acids were also grouped as saturated (SFA), monounsaturated (MUFA), diunsaturated (DUFA), while tri-, tetra-, penta-, and hexaenoic fatty acids were grouped as polyunsaturated fatty acids (PUFA). The degree of unsaturation, expressed as unsaturation index, and the n-3/n-6 ratio were also determined.

Fatty acid component	Percentage of total fatty acids in winter period[1]			
	TAG	PI/PS	PC	PE
14:0	5.9 ± 1.0	2.2 ± 1.9	1.4 ± 0.3	4.6 ± 4.3
16:0	21.9 ± 3.6	24.0 ± 8.5	44.7 ± 7.6	25.2 ± 7.0
16:1 n-7	10.7 ± 1.7	1.8 ± 2.0	5.3 ± 0.5	4.3 ± 1.9
18:0	6.6 ± 0.9	17.2 ± 6.1	9.5 ± 4.0	20.7 ± 10.5
18:1 n-9	32.8 ± 3.9	24.4 ± 15.0	19.9 ± 6.8	19.9 ± 5.8
18:2 n-6	1.9 ± 0.7	1.8 ± 1.8	1.6 ± 0.8	3.9 ± 4.0
20:0	0.6 ± 0.4	0.2 ± 0.5	0.2 ± 0.3	0.8 ± 0.9
18:3 n-3	2.6 ± 2.3	Trace[2]	0.8 ± 0.9	1.2 ± 1.5
20:1 n-9	2.5 ± 1.8	4.2 ± 3.9	0.9 ± 0.4	2.2 ± 1.4
22:0	0.3 ± 0.5	1.5 ± 2.0	1.5 ± 2.3	1.0 ± 2.5
20:4 n-6	4.3 ± 1.8	7.4 ± 6.3	4.2 ± 4.8	6.7 ± 2.0
22:1 n-11	1.0 ± 1.6	2.1 ± 2.6	1.3 ± 2.5	0.3 ± 0.7
20:5 n-3	4.1 ± 0.9	0.9 ± 1.6	3.7 ± 2.7	2.7 ± 1.3
24:0	0.1 ± 0.2	1.0 ± 1.6	0.4 ± 0.4	0.4 ± 0.8
22:3 n-3	2.2 ± 1.2	9.9 ± 9.1	1.1 ± 1.0	0.9 ± 0.8
22:6 n-3	2.6 ± 1.8	1.3 ± 2.3	3.6 ± 2.7	5.3 ± 2.4
MUFA + DUFA	48.8 ± 4.9	34.3 ± 14.8	29.0 ± 7.0	30.6 ± 7.9
PUFA	15.7 ± 4.0	19.5 ± 12.3	13.3 ± 10.0	16.8 ± 7.9
Σ UFA	64.5 ± 3.3	53.8 ± 6.3	42.3 ± 9.1	47.4 ± 15.8
EPA + DHA	6.7 ± 2.6	2.2 ± 3.8	7.3 ± 4.5	8.0 ± 3.7
Σ SFA	35.4 ± 3.3	42.6 ± 6.3	57.7 ± 9.1	52.7 ± 26.0
Unsaturation index	1.18	1.08	0.93	1.13
n-3/n-6	1.85	1.32	1.59	0.95

Table 10. Fatty acid composition of neutral (triacylglycerols, TAG) and polar (phosphatidylinositol, PI; phosphatidylserine, PS; phosphatidylcholine, PC; and phosphatidylethanolamine, PE) lipid fractions of *Diplodus vulgaris*, L. edible muscle tissue in the winter period (expressed as percentage of total identified fatty acids). [1]Values are mean ± SD; [2]Trace, <0.1%.

	Percentage of total fatty acids in summer period[1]			
Fatty acid component	TAG	PI/PS	PC	PE
14:0	4.9 ± 1.1	1.5 ± 0.9	2.2 ± 1.7	0.7 ± 0.1
16:0	23.1 ± 2.4	29.6 ± 5.0	22.5 ± 8.9	39.6 ± 10.3
16:1 n-7	7.3 ± 2.2	2.6 ± 2.9	3.6 ± 3.6	2.9 ± 0.9
18:0	11.4 ± 2.2	32.6 ± 16.3	36.5 ± 16.8	24.3 ± 20.4
18:1 n-9	21.7 ± 2.5	5.9 ± 6.4	11.7 ± 8.5	15.0 ± 1.1
18:2 n-6	2.8 ± 0.9	1.1 ± 1.0	1.5 ± 1.1	0.4 ± 0.3
20:0	0.3 ± 0.2	0.8 ± 0.1	0.5 ± 0.4	Trace
18:3 n-3	0.5 ± 0.6	0.8 ± 1.1	0.4 ± 0.5	0.1 ± 0.2
20:1 n-9	1.8 ± 1.7	0.8 ± 1.4	0.5 ± 0.4	0.2 ± 0.2
22:0	0.7 ± 0.3	1.8 ± 1.4	1.1 ± 0.5	0.5 ± 0.7
20:4 n-6	6.6 ± 2.7	7.7 ± 9.9	5.7 ± 4.2	4.9 ± 5.5
22:1 n-11	Trace[2]	1.0 ± 1.4	Trace	0.1 ± 0.1
20:5 n-3	6.0 ± 2.0	1.7 ± 2.2	1.4 ± 1.6	2.1 ± 2.8
24:0	0.1 ± 0.2	1.9 ± 4.0	0.3 ± 0.2	0.1 ± 0.1
22:3 n-3	5.1 ± 0.5	6.6 ± 3.3	7.5 ± 2.1	3.6 ± 2.3
22:6 n-3	7.9 ± 1.0	3.7 ± 5.3	4.7 ± 2.9	5.5 ± 5.7
MUFA + DUFA	33.6 ± 2.5	11.3 ± 6.9	17.4 ± 11.6	18.5 ± 1.3
PUFA	26.0 ± 4.8	20.5 ± 13.7	19.7 ± 5.9	15.9 ± 13.4
Σ UFA	59.6 ± 4.3	31.8 ± 14.1	37.1 ± 11.8	34.4 ± 14.3
EPA + DHA	13.8 ± 2.8	5.4 ± 6.4	6.1 ± 3.8	7.3 ± 8..6
Σ SFA	40.4 ± 4.3	68.2 ± 14.1	64.5 ± 10.8	65.3 ± 14.1
Unsaturation index	1.56	0.96	1.01	0.93
n-3/n-6	2.07	1.45	1.94	2.13

Table 11. Fatty acid composition of neutral (triacylglycerols, TAG) and polar (phosphatidylinositol, PI; phosphatidylserine, PS; phosphatidylcholine, PC; and phosphatidylethanolamine, PE) lipid fractions of *Diplodus vulgaris,* L. edible muscle tissue in the summer period (expressed as percentage of total identified fatty acids). [1]Values are mean ± SD; [2]Trace, <0.1%.

Sixteen different fatty acids were identified in *D. vulgaris* edible muscle tissue lipid fractions. The major constituents of total FA in winter and summer were saturates: palmitic (16:0) and stearic acids (18:0); monoenes: oleic (18:1n-9) and palmitoleic acids (16:1); and polyunsaturates: arachidonic acid (20:4n-6), EPA (20:5n-3), and DHA (22:6n-3). The amounts and ratios of major FA identified in our study (16:0, 18:0, and 18:1n-9) differed significantly between the two seasons and between lipid fractions. A similar observation for this fish species in other areas of catch in the Adriatic Sea is available in literature (Donato et al., 1984). A statistically significant difference (P < 0.0001) in oleic acid (18:1n-9) content was found between summer and winter. This FA showed the greatest seasonal variation in our study, followed by 18:0 and 16:0. Values for 18:0 in TAG and PC were found to be statistically different (P < 0.0001) during the two periods. The content of 18:0 was considerably higher in summer, when the relative ratio of 18:0 was almost two times higher for TAG and almost four times higher for PC than in the winter period. No statistically significant seasonal variation was detected in the relative ratio of 16:0 in TAG and PI/PS, but it was noticeable in PC and PE (P < 0.05). Values for 16:0 were twice as high in winter in PC. In contrast, for PE the relative ratio of 16:0 was much higher in the summer. The content of 18:1n-9 significantly decreased from winter to summer (P < 0.05). These results are also in agreement with the results of Donato et al. (1984) for *D. vulgaris* originating from the Adriatic Sea.

The concentrations of n-3 PUFA, EPA, and DHA are significant for their confirmed biomedical importance. Greater amounts in EPA and DHA were found in TAG in the summer period. No such enhanced difference was found in polar lipid fractions. EPA + DHA values were twice as high in the summer period in TAG and PI/PS. Appreciable quantities of 20:4n-6 and 22:3n-3 were also found in all the lipid fractions, with statistically significant seasonal differences (P < 0.0001) in TAG, PC, and PE for 22:3n-3. Seasonal variation in the content of 20:4n-6 was significant only in TAG (P < 0.05).

Generally, MUFA + DUFA values were significantly higher in winter. On the other hand, PUFA values were higher in summer, especially in TAG. SFA values were also higher in summer. The diminution of the MUFA content in the summer was clearly accompanied by an increase in PUFA content. This is in agreement with the observations of Donato et al. (1984).

The TAGs serve as a store for SFA for energy purposes, and they also may be a temporary PUFA reservoir (Napolitano et al., 1988). They could be forwarded to the synthesis of structural lipids or directed to specific metabolic pathways. Statistically significant seasonal differences (P < 0.05 and P < 0.0001) were most conspicuous in TAG for all detected FA except 16:0, 20:0, 18:3n-3, 20:1n-9, 22:1n-11 and 24:0. Pazos et al. (1996) reported a similar observation. On the other hand, statistically significant differences (P < 0.05 and P < 0.0001) in polar lipid fractions (PI/PS, PC, and PE) were found to be less noticeable, especially in PI/PS, where statistically significant seasonal variation was found only for 18:1n-9 (P < 0.0001).

The degree of unsaturation, expressed as the unsaturation index, also differed between neutral and polar lipid fractions. It was highest in TAG during the summer while the lowest index was determined in PC n the winter and PE in the summer period.

Emphases on n-3 PUFA over n-6 PUFA propose that the n-3/n-6 ratio could be applied as a biomedical index. Therefore, the n-3/n-6 ratio is a biomedical marker for fish lipids. N-3/n-6 ratios were calculated for all the lipid fractions in analyzed fish muscle tissue samples. FA in *D. vulgaris* muscle tissue lipids have an n-3/n-6 ratio between 1 and 2, which is relatively good. But it must be emphasized that all the ratios were higher in the summer period.

Results of our study indicate that *D. vulgaris* is a good source of natural n-3 PUFA and would therefore be suitable for inclusion in highly unsaturated low-fat diets. Our results are in agreement with other published results for teleost fish species originating from the Mediterranean and Adriatic Sea (Donato et al., 1984; Passi et al., 2002).

Seasonal variations of FA composition have previously been studied for different fish species (Mayzaud et al., 1999; Pazos et al., 1996, Donato et al. 1984). An inverse relationship between water temperature and the amount of PUFA in tissue lipids of fish and invertebrates has been shown (Hazel, 1979). Seasonal variation of n-3 PUFA seems to be linked to the diet as well as the reproductive cycle (Donato et al., 1984).

In this study, the FA composition in edible muscle tissue of *D. vulgaris* showed a significant variation from winter to summer. The seasonal variations in *D. vulgaris* lipids reflected fluctuations mainly in TAG. But it must also be emphasized that the reproductive cycle of *D. vulgaris* correlates with those seasons, since previtellogenesis occurs in winter and vitellogenesis occurs in summer (Donato et al., 1984). It can be concluded that, although the FA composition of fish is complex and depends on many factors, it clearly shows a seasonal pattern of distribution.

3.3 Edible muscle tissue fatty acid composition of fish originating from middle Adriatic Sea

Diplodus vulgaris, L. and *Conger conger*, L. edible muscle tissue fatty acid compositions were also determined. Fish were caught in the Šibenik basin, Middle Adriatic Sea as previously described. Data on moisture content, total lipids, polar and neutral lipid contents, expressed as a percentage (%) in analysed fish muscle tissue samples, are shown in Table 12. It was found that the total lipids (TL, percentage of wet weight of muscle tissues) in *C. conger* (3.7 ± 0.2 %) were almost three times higher than in *D. vulgaris* (1.3 ± 0.2 %). Moisture content was also higher in *C. conger* (77.5 ± 2.1 %) in comparison with *D. vulgaris* (76.7 ± 1.3 %). Polar lipids (PL, % of total lipids) were almost twice higher in *D. vulgaris* (28.1 ± 4.2) than in *C. conger* (15.5 ± 0.2 %). Neutral lipids (NL, % of total lipids) were present in higher proportions, (71.9 ± 4.2 %) in *D. vulgaris* and (84.5 ± 0.2 %) in *C. conger*.

Fish species	Moisture content (%)	Total lipids (%)	Polar lipids (%)	Neutral lipids (%)
Diplodus vulgaris. L.	76.7 ± 1.3	1.3 ± 0.2	28.1 ± 4.2	71.9 ± 4.2
Conger conger, L.	77.5 ± 2.1	3.7 ± 0.2	15.5 ± 0.2	84.5 ± 0.2

Table 12. Moisture content, total lipids, polar lipids and neutral lipids in *Diplodus vulgaris*, L. and *Conger conger*, L. edible muscle tissue.

Fatty acid component	Percentage of total fatty acids[1]			
	TAG	PI/PS	PC	PE
14:0	7.0 ± 1.5	0.8 ± 0.9	2.3 ± 0.2	4.4 ± 1.5
14:1	Trace[2]	Trace	Trace	Trace
15:0	0.7 ± 0.6	0.4 ± 0.8	1.9 ± 0.5	0.8 ± 1.1
16:0	25.4 ± 4.0	41.0 ± 22.2	63.9 ± 17.7	38.8 ± 13.1
16:1	12.5 ± 2.3	1.1 ± 1.5	3.7 ± 0.8	4.6 ± 3.3
17:0	1.4 ± 0.9	0.7 ± 1.0	2.3 ± 0.7	0.9 ± 1.3
17:1	0.3 ± 0.4	Trace	Trace	Trace
18:0	10.5 ± 3.1	43.4 ± 30.0	14.9 ± 17.4	19.6 ± 7.7
18:1 n-9t	0.2 ± 0.5	Trace	Trace	Trace
18:1 n-9c	20.4 ± 3.0	5.5 ± 1.8	8.8 ± 1.7	10.5 ± 1.4
18:2 n-6c	1.3 ± 0.8	Trace	Trace	0.2 ± 0.5
18:3 n-6	0.1 ± 0.1	Trace	Trace	Trace
20:0	0.5 ± 0.5	Trace	Trace	0.1 ± 0.3
18:3 n-3	0.1 ± 0.3	Trace	Trace	0.2 ± 0.4
20:1 n-9	1.3 ± 1.0	Trace	Trace	0.1 ± 0.3
21:0	Trace	Trace	Trace	Trace
20:2	0.4 ± 0.5	Trace	Trace	2.0 ± 4.1
20:3 n-3	0.1 ± 0.2	Trace	Trace	Trace
20:3 n-6	4.8 ± 1.6	1.2 ± 2.0	Trace	1.4 ± 1.8
22:1 n-9	0.1 ± 0.1	Trace	Trace	Trace
20:4 n-6	7.8 ± 3.5	0.7 ± 1.5	Trace	1.8 ± 2.6
22:2	Trace	Trace	1.0 ± 2.0	Trace
20:5 n-3	1.4 ± 1.6	Trace	Trace	3.8 ± 5.7
24:1 n-9	0.7 ± 1.1	3.2 ± 5.0	0.8 ± 1.5	4.0 ± 4.0
22:6 n-3	3.0 ± 4.1	2.2 ± 3.1	0.5 ± 1.0	6.9 ± 12.5
MUFA + DUFA	37.2 ± 1.4	9.7 ± 5.1	14.2 ± 3.4	21.5 ± 3.0
PUFA	17.2 ± 5.5	4.1 ± 5.8	0.5 ± 1.0	14.0 ± 22.9
Σ UFA	54.4 ± 5.9	13.3 ± 7.0	14.7 ± 3.8	35.5 ± 21.2
EPA + DHA	4.3 ± 3.0	2.2 ± 3.1	0.5 ± 1.0	10.7 ± 18.1
Σ SFA	45.6 ± 5.9	86.1 ± 7.0	85.3 ± 3.9	64.5 ± 21.4
Unsaturation index	1.10	0.29	0.18	0.96
n-3/n-6	0.34	1.21	-	3.25

Table 13. Fatty acid composition of neutral (triacylglycerols, TAG) and polar (phosphatidylinositol, PI; phosphatidylserine, PS; phosphatidylcholine, PC; and phosphatidylethanolamine, PE) lipid fractions of *Diplodus vulgaris*, L. edible muscle tissue (expressed as percentage of total identified fatty acids). [1]Values are mean ± SD; [2]Trace, <0.1%.

	Percentage of total fatty acids[1]			
Fatty acid component	TAG	PI/PS	PC	PE
14:0	5.6 ± 1.1	Trace	3.4 ± 0.4	5.8 ± 0.6
14:1	0.1 ± 0.2	Trace	Trace	Trace
15:0	0.9 ± 0.3	Trace	1.2 ± 1.2	5.3 ± 0.8
16:0	20.3 ± 1.3	18.9 ± 5.7	62.8 ± 6.3	44.8 ± 2.5
16:1	10.3 ± 2.0	Trace	4.3 ± 1.1	3.0 ± 4.2
17:0	0.8 ± 0.2	0.5 ± 1.2	0.5 ± 0.7	1.4 ± 2.0
17:1	0.6 ± 0.3	Trace	Trace	Trace
18:0	5.5 ± 0.7	58.7 ± 3.3	6.8 ± 1.4	22.1 ± 7.0
18:1 n-9c	23.1 ± 6.0	3.8 ± 3.8	13.6 ± 2.6	15.8 ± 3.2
18:2 n-6c	2.6 ± 0.9	Trace	Trace	Trace
20:0	0.4 ± 0.2	Trace	Trace	Trace
18:3 n-6	1.1 ± 0.6	Trace	Trace	Trace
20:1 n-9	0.7 ± 0.7	Trace	Trace	Trace
20:2	0.6 ± 0.4	Trace	Trace	Trace
20:3 n-3	0.2 ± 0.2	Trace	Trace	Trace
20:3 n-6	2.7 ± 0.7	Trace	1.5 ± 3.6	Trace
22:1 n-9	Trace[2]	Trace	Trace	Trace
20:4 n-6	6.8 ± 2.2	Trace	1.9 ± 3.6	Trace
20:5 n-3	1.6 ± 1.7	5.3 ± 6.3	1.2 ± 1.7	2.0 ± 2.8
24:1 n-9	0.9 ± 0.6	4.8 ± 7.4	Trace	Trace
22:6 n-3	15.4 ± 5.2	8.1 ± 10.7	2.9 ± 2.0	Trace
MUFA + DUFA	38.8 ± 7.9	8.6 ± 4.8	17.8 ± 2.2	18.8 ± 1.1
PUFA	27.7 ± 7.0	13.3 ± 9.3	7.6 ± 8.2	2.0 ± 2.8
Σ UFA	66.6 ± 1.3	22.0 ± 6.9	25.4 ± 6.1	20.8 ± 3.8
EPA + DHA	17.0 ± 5.0	13.3 ± 9.3	4.2 ± 2.7	2.0 ± 2.8
Σ SFA	33.7 ± 1.4	78.1 ± 7.0	74.6 ± 6.1	79.4 ± 3.9
Unsaturation index	1.81	0.83	0.54	0.29
n-3/n-6	1.53	-	1.20	-

Table 14. Fatty acid composition of neutral (triacylglycerols, TAG) and polar (phosphatidylinositol, PI; phosphatidylserine, PS; phosphatidylcholine, PC; and phosphatidylethanolamine, PE) lipid fractions of *Conger conger,* L. edible muscle tissue (expressed as percentage of total identified fatty acids). [1]Values are mean ± SD; [2]Trace, <0.1%.

D. vulgaris and *C. conger* belong to low-fat type fish, according to the lipid content classification (Ackman, 1989). Total lipid content as well as polar and neutral lipid contents in *D. vulgaris* and *C. conger* accord with the results for different Mediterranean marine fish species (Passi et al., 2002).

TAG formed the dominant lipid fraction in fish muscle lipids and contained an entire spectrum of detected fatty acids in both analysed fish species. On the contrary, the fatty acid composition of polar lipid classes was much less complex. Our results are in agreement with previously published results which showed that TAG are the main part of stored lipids (Corraze & Kaushik, 1999).

Major fatty acids detected in *D. vulgaris* and *C. conger* in this study were palmitic (16:0), palmitoleic (16:1), stearic (18:0) and oleic (18:1 n-9c) acid in all lipid classes, but their amounts and ratios differed significantly. Palmitic acid (16:0) and oleic acid (18:1n-9c) were the predominant saturate and monoene, respectively. PUFA values were higher in neutral lipid fractions, especially in *C. conger*. However, high concentrations of stearic acid (18:0) were found in polar lipid fractions for both fishes (*D. vulgaris*: 1.9–43.4 %, *C. conger*: 6.8–58.7 %), which are not usually found in marine vertebrates. Our results showed much higher content of SFAs in polar lipids fractions in comparison with other marine fish from the Adriatic and the Mediterranean Sea (Passi et al., 2002). This departs from the observation that phospholipids are characteristically rich in long chain PUFA, with EPA and DHA often being the major fatty acids. TAG showed more favourable fatty acid composition when compared to polar lipid fractions for both analysed fishes, containing more UFAs.

Fatty acid contents of *D. vulgaris* and *C. conger* from the Middle Adriatic Sea show a very heterogeneous distribution. When comparing the fatty acid composition data between these two fish species, statistically significant differences ($P < 0.05$) were found in neutral lipids, in the contents of 16:0, 18:0, 18:2n-6c, 18:3n-3, 20:3n-3, 22:6n-3 in TAG. When analysing polar lipid fractions, statistically significant differences were found only in PC, in the amounts of 14:0, 18:1n-9c and 22:6n-3. Generally, *C. conger* showed a greater content of UFA, especially EPA and DHA, which makes its fatty acid profile more favourable. This could be due to different nutritional habits of the two fish species, but also because of a natural variation in the accumulation of fatty acids and the differences in environmental conditions. The most accentuated changes in total lipid and fatty acid composition of fish were previously noticed by other researchers during the reproduction period, when the storage of lipids and other compounds are mobilized from muscle, liver and visceral organs to gonads (Guler et al., 2007; Perez et al., 2007).

N-3/n-6 ratios were calculated for fatty acids in analysed fish edible muscle tissue samples. These ratios amounted between 0.34 and 3.25, also showing different values between analysed lipid classes and between analysed fish species. All n-3/n-6 ratios for different lipid fractions were higher than 1, except for *D. vulgaris* TAG. This findings accord with the observation reported for different Mediterranean marine species of fish and shellfish (Passi et al., 2002), confirming the great importance of fish as a significant dietary source of n-3 PUFAs.

4. Conclusion

This review summarizes data about our research of fatty acid compositions in different lipid fractions of marine fish from the Adriatic Sea, Croatia. Due to the relatively high content of unsaturated fatty acids, Adriatic Sea fish edible muscle tissue could be recommended for inclusion in the Mediterranean type of diet, as low-fat food with elevated content of highly unsaturated fatty acids. Furthermore, livers from those fish, which are even more rich in polyunsaturated fatty acids in all lipid fractions, could be a good source of biomedically significant components if used as a raw material for products based on fish oil fatty acids such as dietary supplements and pharmaceuticals. Obtained results indicate that fatty acid composition in Adriatic Sea marine fish edible muscle tissue and liver lipid fractions show an accentuated pattern of seasonality. The fatty acid composition of marine fish lipids is multifarious and changes are complex, depending on fish biological and physiological conditions, diet, water temperature, fishing ground and season. Therefore, the influence of season and other factors should be taken into consideration in order to obtain the most appropriate fatty acid composition for industrial and pharmaceutical needs.

5. References

Ackman, R.G. (1989). *Fatty Acids. In: Marine Biogenic Lipids, Fats and Oils*, edited by R.G. Ackman, ISBN: 0849348897, CRC Press, Boca Raton, USA.

Aro, T., Tahvonen, R., Mattila, T., Nurmi, J., Sivonen, T., & Kallio, H. (2000). Effects of season and processing on oil content and fatty acids of Baltic herring (Clupea harengus membras). *Journal of Agricultural & Food Chemistry, 48*(12), 6085-6093. ISSN: 0021-8561.

Bang, H. O., Dyerberg, J., & Nielsen, A. B. (1971). Plasma lipid and lipoprotein pattern in Greenlandic West-coast Eskimos. *Lancet, 1*(7710), 1143-1145. ISSN: 0140-6736.

Baticic, L., Varljen, N., Butorac, M. Z., Kapovic, M., & Varljen, J. (2009). Potential Value of Hepatic Lipids from White Sea Bream (Diplodus sargus, L.) as a Good Source of Biomedical Components: Seasonal Variations. *Food Technology & Biotechnology 47(3 Special Issue, 47*(3 Special Issue SI), 260-268. ISSN: 1330-9862.

Cejas, J. R., Almansa, E., Jerez, S., Bolanos, A., Samper, M., & Lorenzo, A. (2004). Lipid and fatty acid composition of muscle and liver from wild and captive mature female broodstocks of white seabream, Diplodus sargus. *Comp Biochem Physiol B Biochem Mol Biol, 138*(1), 91-102. ISSN: 1096-4959.

Corraze, G., & Kaushik, S. (1999). Lipids from marine and freshwater fish [French]. *Ocl-Oleagineux Corps Gras Lipides, 6*(1), 111-115. ISSN: 1258-8210.

Donato, A., Dugo, G., Mauceri, A., & Verzera, A. (1984). Changes in Fatty Acids Composition in Diplodus vulgaris Liver in Relation to Sexual Maturation, *Riv. Ital. Sostanze Grasse 59*, 349–353. ISSN: 0035-6808.

Donato, A., Salpietro, L., Verzera, A., & Trozzi, A. (1997). Hepatic fatty acid composition of Diplodus sargus caught along the coast of Messina strait during spermatogenesis, *Riv. Ital. Sostanze Grasse, 74*, 79–83. ISSN: 0035-6808

Driscoll, D. F., Ling, P. R., & Bistrian, B. R. (2009). Pharmacopeial compliance of fish oil-containing parenteral lipid emulsion mixtures: Globule size distribution (GSD) and fatty acid analyses. *Int J Pharm, 379*(1), 125-130. ISSN: 1873-3476.

Folch, J., Lees, M., & Sloane Stanley, G. H. (1957). A simple method for the isolation and purification of total lipides from animal tissues. *J Biol Chem, 226*(1), 497-509. ISSN: 0021-9258.

Grigorakis, K., Alexis, M. N., Taylor, K. D. A., & Hole, M. (2002). Comparison of wild and cultured gilthead sea bream (Sparus aurata); composition, appearance and seasonal variations. *International Journal of Food Science & Technology, 37*(5), 477-484. ISSN: 0950-5423.

Guler, G. O., Aktumsek, A., Citil, O. B., Arslan, A., & Torlak, E. (2007). Seasonal variations on total fatty acid composition of fillets of zander (Sander lucioperca) in Beysehir Lake (Turkey). *Food Chemistry, 103*(4), 1241-1246. ISSN: 0308-8146.

Harris, W. S. (2010). Marine Omega-3 Fatty Acids and Plaque Stabilization. *Curr Atheroscler Rep. 12*(6), 357-358. ISSN: 1534-6242.

Hazel, J. R. (1979). Influence of thermal acclimation on membrane lipid composition of rainbow trout liver. *Am J Physiol, 236*(1), R91-101. ISSN: 0002-9513.

Henderson, R. J., & Tocher, D. R. (1987) The lipid composition and biochemistry of freshwater fish. *Prog Lipid Res, 26*(4), 281-347. ISSN: 0163-7827.

Hu, F. B., Bronner, L., Willett, W. C., Stampfer, M. J., Rexrode, K. M., Albert, C. M., Hunter, D., & Manson, J. E. (2002). Fish and omega-3 fatty acid intake and risk of coronary heart disease in women. *Jama, 287*(14), 1815-1821. ISSN: 0098-7484.

Imre, S., & Saglik, S. (1998). Fatty Acid Composition and Cholesterol Content of Some Turkish Fish Species. *Turkish Journal of Chemistry, 22*(4), 321-324. ISSN: 1010-7614.

Itua, I., & Naderali, E. K. (2010). Review: omega-3 and memory function: to eat or not to eat. *Am J Alzheimers Dis Other Demen, 25*(6), 479-482. ISSN: 1938-2731.

Jardas, I. (1996). *Adriatic Ichthyofauna*, edited by J.M. Dragarović, ISBN 953-0-61501-9, Školska knjiga, Zagreb, Croatia. (in Croatian).

Kates, M., & Baxter, R.M. (1962). Lipid composition of mesophilic and psychrophilic yeasts (Candida species) as influenced by environmental temperature, *Can. J. Biochem. Physiol.* 40, 1213–1227. ISSN: 0576-5544.

Lloret, J. (2010). Human health benefits supplied by Mediterranean marine biodiversity. *Mar Pollut Bull. 60*(10), 1640-1646. ISSN: 1879-3363.

Lovell, R. T. (1991). Nutrition of aquaculture species. *J Anim Sci, 69*(10), 4193-4200. ISSN: 0021-8812.

Luzia, L. A., Sampaio, G. R., Castellucci, C. M. N., & Torres, E. (2003). The influence of season on the lipid profiles of five commercially important species of Brazilian fish. *Food Chemistry, 83*(1), 93-97. ISSN: 0308-8146.

Martin, L., Zarn, D., Hansen, A. M., Wismer, W., & Mazurak, V. (2008). Food products as vehicles for n-3 fatty acid supplementation. *Can J Diet Pract Res, 69*(4), 203-207. ISSN: 1486-3847.

Massaro, M., Scoditti, E., Carluccio, M. A., & De Caterina, R. (2010). Nutraceuticals and prevention of atherosclerosis: focus on omega-3 polyunsaturated fatty acids and Mediterranean diet polyphenols. *Cardiovasc Ther, 28*(4), e13-19. ISSN: 1755-5922.

Mayzaud, P., Virtue, P., & Albessard, E. (1999). Seasonal variations in the lipid and fatty acid composition of the euphausiid Meganyctiphanes norvegica from the Ligurian Sea. *Marine Ecology-Progress Series, 186*, 199-210. ISSN: 0171-8630.

Napolitano, G. E., Ratnayake, W. M., & Ackman, R. G. (1988). Fatty acid components of larval Ostrea edulis (L.): importance of triacylglycerols as a fatty acid reserve. *Comp Biochem Physiol B, 90*(4), 875-883. ISSN: 0305-0491.

Ozyurt, G., Polat, A., & Ozkutuk, S. (2005). Seasonal changes in the fatty acids of gilthead sea bream (Sparus aurata) and white sea bream (Diplodus sargus) captured in Iskenderun Bay, eastern Mediterranean coast of Turkey. *European Food Research & Technology, 220*(2), 120-124. ISSN: 1438-2377.

Passi, S., Cataudella, S., Di Marco, P., De Simone, F., & Rastrelli, L. (2002). Fatty acid composition and antioxidant levels in muscle tissue of different Mediterranean marine species of fish and shellfish. *J Agric Food Chem, 50*(25), 7314-7322. ISSN: 0021-8561.

Pazos, A. J., Ruiz, C., Garciamartin, O., Abad, M., & Sanchez, J. L. (1996). Seasonal Variations of the Lipid Content and Fatty Acid Composition of Crassostrea Gigas Cultured in El Grove, Galicia, Nw Spain. *Comparative Biochemistry & Physiology -, 114*(2), Comparative Biochemistry. 114(112):171-179. ISSN: 0305-0491.

Perez, M. J., Rodriguez, C., Cejas, J. R., Martin, M. V., Jerez, S., & Lorenzo, A. (2007). Lipid and fatty acid content in wild white seabream (Diplodus sargus) broodstock at different stages of the reproductive cycle. *Comp Biochem Physiol B Biochem Mol Biol, 146*(2), 187-196. ISSN: 1096-4959.

Raatz, S. K., Redmon, J. B., Wimmergren, N., Donadio, J. V., & Bibus, D. M. (2009). Enhanced absorption of n-3 fatty acids from emulsified compared with encapsulated fish oil. *J Am Diet Assoc, 109*(6), 1076-1081. ISSN: 1878-3570.

Roberts, R. O., Cerhan, J. R., Geda, Y. E., Knopman, D. S., Cha, R. H., Christianson, T. J., Pankratz, V. S., Ivnik, R. J., O'Connor, H. M., & Petersen, R. C. (2010). Polyunsaturated Fatty Acids and Reduced Odds of MCI: The Mayo Clinic Study of Aging. *J Alzheimers Dis*. ISSN: 1875-8908.

Smutna, M., Kruzikova, K., Marsalek, P., Kopriva, V., & Svobodova, Z. (2009). Fish oil and cod liver as safe and healthy food supplements. *Neuro Endocrinol Lett, 30 Suppl 1*, 156-162. ISSN: 0172-780X.

Tanakol, R., Yazici, Z., Sener, E., & Sencer, E. (1999). Fatty acid composition of 19 species of fish from the Black Sea and the Marmara Sea. *Lipids, 34*(3), 291-297. ISSN: 0024-4201.

Varljen, J., Baticic, L., Sincic-Modric, G., Obersnel, V., & Kapovic, M. (2004). Composition and seasonal variation of fatty acids of Diplodus vulgaris L. from the Adriatic Sea. *Journal of the American Oil Chemists Society, 81*(8), 759-763. ISSN: 0003-021X.

Varljen, J., Sulic, S., Brmalj, J., Baticic, L., Obersnel, V., & Kapovic, M. (2003). Lipid classes and fatty acid composition of Diplodus vulgaris and Conger conger originating from the Adriatic Sea. *Food Technology & Biotechnology, 41*(2), 149-156. ISSN: 1330-9862.

17

Flax Engineering for Biomedical Application

Magdalena Czemplik[1], Aleksandra Boba[1], Kamil Kostyn[1],
Anna Kulma[1], Agnieszka Mituła[1], Monika Sztajnert[1],
Magdalena Wróbel- Kwiatkowska[2], Magdalena Żuk[1],
Jan Szopa[1] and Katarzyna Skórkowska- Telichowska[3]

[1]Faculty of Biotechnology, Wrocław University
[2] Department of Pharmaceutical Biology and Botany,
Medical University in Wrocław
[3]IVth Military Hospital in Wroclaw
[4]Linum Foundation, Wroclaw
Poland

1. Introduction

Flax (Linum usitatissimum) is an important crop plant that is widely distributed in the Mediterranean and temperate climate zones. It has great significance for industry as a valuable source of oil and fibres. A unique feature of flax is the possibility of whole plant exploitation with almost no waste products. For this reason, flax has quite significant potential for biotechnological application. To increase the valuable qualities of flax products, the flax genome has been genetically modified, with the specific aims to improve the plant's pathogen resistance, taste and nutritional properties, and to produce pharmaceuticals and other compounds. In this chapter, we describe the plant characteristics that show the biochemical and industrial importance of flax oil and fibres and their various possible applications and the relevant genetic modifications.

Since ancient times, flax has been known to be a source of oil and fibres, and it has been cultivated as a dual-purpose plant for a long time. Nowadays, it is a multi-purpose plant and its exploitation is not restricted to the production of linen fibre and oil. Actually, whole plant exploitation is possible, which justifies the name given to it by Linnaeus: *L. usitatissimum*, meaning "useful flax". There is a wide range of possible applications of flax (Fig.1). The long fibres are used in the textile industry, and the short fibres in paper production, isolation materials and biocomposite production. The wooden shives released during flax scutching can serve as an energy source. Flax seeds also have many important applications, and due to its high nutritional value, it is used in the food, pharmaceutical and health care industries. The seedcake, which is rich in antioxidants, is used in the pharmaceutical and cosmetic industries.

The development of molecular biology emerged as an important tool for the genetic modification of plants, and enabled the improvement of many different features of wild type plants. These modifications broadened the range of practical applications for flax, making the plant more valuable and more significant for the innovative biotechnological industry.

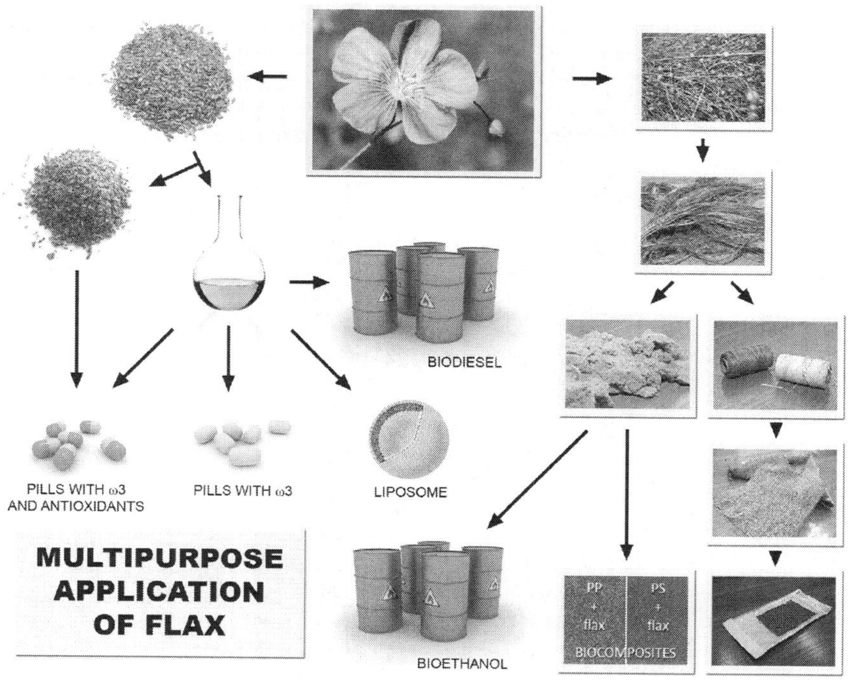

Fig. 1. The multipurpose application of flax

Flax is a good source of unsaturated fatty acids, dietary fibre and another nutrients. It is composed mainly of fat (41%), protein (20%) and dietary fibre (28%). The contents may vary depending on genetics, environment, seed processing and the analysis method. *Linum usitatissimum* is the best-known species with a high concentration of α-linolenic acid (ALA). Polyunsaturated fatty acids compose about 73% of the total fatty acid content. Flax proteins are rich in arginine, aspartic acid and glutamic acid. *Linum usitatissimum* is characterized with a high content of polysaccharidic mucilage. It confers from 6 to 8% of the dry weight. The acidic polysaccharide consists of L-rhamnose, L-galactose and D-galacturonic acid and the neutral polysaccharides L-arabinose, D-xylose and D-galactose. The amino acid composition of flax indicates that the most abundant are glutamic acid, aspartic acid and arginine. Moreover a series of cyclic polypeptides, which contains between eight and ten amino acids, have been identified in *Linum usitatissimum*. Some of them exhibit immunosuppressive activity. Phytochemicals that have been identified in flax mainly consist of lignans, isoprenoids, phenolic acids, flavonoids and cyanogenic glucosides. All these compounds, apart from cyanogenic glucosides are known to have antioxidant properties or inhibitory activity against carcinogen induced tumors.

2. Flax fibre quality improvement and its biomedical application

Flax fibres have many useful applications. They are flexible, lustrous and soft. Moreover, flax fibres are stronger than cotton but less elastic. They absorb humidity and are allergen-free. These properties make flax fibres useful in the textile industry but they are also used in the manufacture of car-door panels, plant pots and retaining mats. Recently, some research has been carried out to improve the quality of flax fibres and make them suitable for the biomedical industry. Innovative flax fibre-containing products have been developed with potential applications in the medical field. The main strategy was to make use of genetically modified flax fibres with unusual and unique properties.

2.1 Fibre quality improvement

Flax is a great source of fibre. Plant fibres are divided into three groups: the phloem stem fibres (phloem stem fibres or xylem stem fibres) of dicotyledonous plants; the leaf fibres of monocotyledonous plants; and the seed and fruit fibres (Ivessalo-Pfaffli, 1995). Flax fibres belong to the first group.

The flax stem is 70% composed of cellulose. These hollow tubes grow together as bundles and are held by complex carbohydrates such as pectins, gums and waxes. These function as a plant support. The fibre separation process from the non-fibre tissues is called retting (Antonov *et al.*, 2007). Retting is mainly the enzymatic action of polygalacturonase, which degradates the pectin polymers of the middle lamella into soluble galacturonic acid. This process is mainly carried out by plant pathogens like filamentous fungi. To obtain high-quality fibres, the proper degree of retting is necessary (Zhang *et al.*, 2000). The efficiency of retting depends on the method used, but traditional dew retting is still the most widely performed method. In this method, the flax stalks are left in the field after the harvesting of the flax seeds, and the soil microorganisms digest the cell matrix polysaccharides. The dew retting method is weather dependent, which makes it uncontrollable.

The chemical composition of the flax stems can affect the degree of retting. Fibres which have more lignins need a longer period of retting. However, a longer exposure to fungal and bacterial enzymes decomposes the cellulose and weakens the fibres. One solution to this problem is to harvest the flax before seed maturity when the level of stem lignification is still low. Another solution is to genetically manipulate the flax, yielding an improved retting process. It is known that the pectin and hemicellulose contents of the fibres influence the fibre processing. A new technology to modify the biosynthesis and degradation of pectins with beneficial consequences for the flax fibre properties has been recently developed. The flax plant was transformed with *Aspergillus aculeatus* genes coding for polygalacturonase (PGI) or rhamnogalacturonase (RHA), which are the enzymes required to break down pectin of the flax fibres. The transformants were characterized by an increased enzyme activity and a significant reduction of pectin content. The reduction in pectin content was in the range of 56–68% for both the PGI and RHA plants. These results correlated with the retting efficiency, which was more than 2-fold higher in the transgenic flax than in the control plants (Musialak *et al.*, 2007). Interestingly, the overexpression of the enzymes did not affect the fibre composition. No changes in the lignin or cellulose contents was observed in comparison to the control. Similarly, the levels of soluble sugars and starch were at the same levels as in the non-transformed flax. As the biochemical parameters of the cell wall components remained similar to those for the control plants and the fibre quality did not change, it is suggested that these modifications might be important for industrial and medical application.

Another strategy of improving flax fibre quality was reducing the level of lignin synthesis. Lignins are complex polymers of three aromatic alcohols: coniferyl, sinapyl and p-coumaryl (Amthor, 2003), and cinnamyl alcohol dehydrogenase (CAD) is an enzyme that catalyses the biosynthesis of lignin monomers (hydroxycinnamoylalcohols) from the corresponding aldehydes. CAD is the specific marker of lignification (Barakat *et al.*, 2009). Flax fibres comprise 3-5% lignins, and they are mainly responsible for mechanical resistance. They create a physical barrier against pathogen infection, and are highly accumulated and deposited in response to pathogen attack (Tobias *et al.*, 2005). The accumulation of lignins negatively influences the retting efficiency. To overcome this problem, transgenic flax with a silenced *cad* gene was created. In the generated plants, the CAD enzyme activity was 20-40% lower, and the lignin level decreased by up to 40 % (Wróbel- Kwiatkowska *et al.*, 2006). Moreover, this modification influenced the composition of the cell wall. The pectin content and the hemicellulose content was significantly lower. Decreasing the level of the above-mentioned compounds facilitated the retting process. Furthermore, the mechanical properties of the modified fibres were strongly improved, as the ratio of cellulose to lignin increased. Cellulose is the fibrous component of the cell wall, and the hemicellulose, pectins and lignins are the matrix components. An increased proportion of the fibrous to matrix components is the reason for the improvements in the mechanical properties of the stem. This data indicates that *via* genetic modification, it is possible to improve the mechanical properties of flax fibres and make them more useful for further application.

2.2 Biodegradable flax biocomposite material as a new medical polymer

Composites are materials made of matrix reinforced with natural fibres, and the term biocomposites is used for composites employed in bioengineering (Ramakrishna *et al.*, 2004). The development of biocomposites is attractive because the properties of two or more types of material can be combined, which influences the properties of the composites. Most medical devices used in medicine and made of a single material, such as a polymer, metal or ceramic, are too flexible or too weak or too stiff to host tissues, and some may also be sensitive to corrosion or cause allergic reactions (e.g. nickel and chromium). All these disadvantages led to the development of composite materials for medical use. Nowadays, composites are used in numerous biomedical applications: sutures, cardiovascular patches, wound dressings, regeneration devices and tissue engineering scaffolds (Misra *et al.*, 2006). Many composites have poor biomechanical properties and poor bioactivities. The composites containing biodegradable polymers can be divided into two groups: one based on natural polymers (e.g. starch, alginate, silk) containing as reinforcement natural fibres (lignocellulosic or cellulosic fibres); and the second based on synthetic polymers (polylactic acid PLA, polyglicolic acid PGA, poly-ε-caprolactone PCL) (Rezwan *et al.*, 2006). Natural fibres replace glass, ceramics or carbon fibres (Bax and Mussig, 2008). In the last decade biocomposites were used by the automotive industry for door panels, seat backs, headrests and package trays among other things (Fig. 2), (Suddel *et al.*, 2003; Bledzki *et al.*, 2006).

Biocomposites have favourable biomechanical properties and they can also have bioactive properties, for example antioxidative and bacteriostatic action. The main problem in preparing biocomposites is often the poor adhesion between the matrix and the fibres used as reinforcement. This influences the mechanical properties of the composites and remains a significant disadvantage. Better contact between the fibres and the matrix also enhances the hydrophobicity of the composite. The possible solution to this problem might be the production of a biocomposite containing transgenic flax fibres enriched with hydrophobic and thermoplastic poly-β-hydroxybutyrate (PHB). This non-toxic and water-insoluble compound displays chemical and physical properties similar to polypropylene. PHB is a biodegradable, ecologically friendly compound, and may be an alternative to conventional

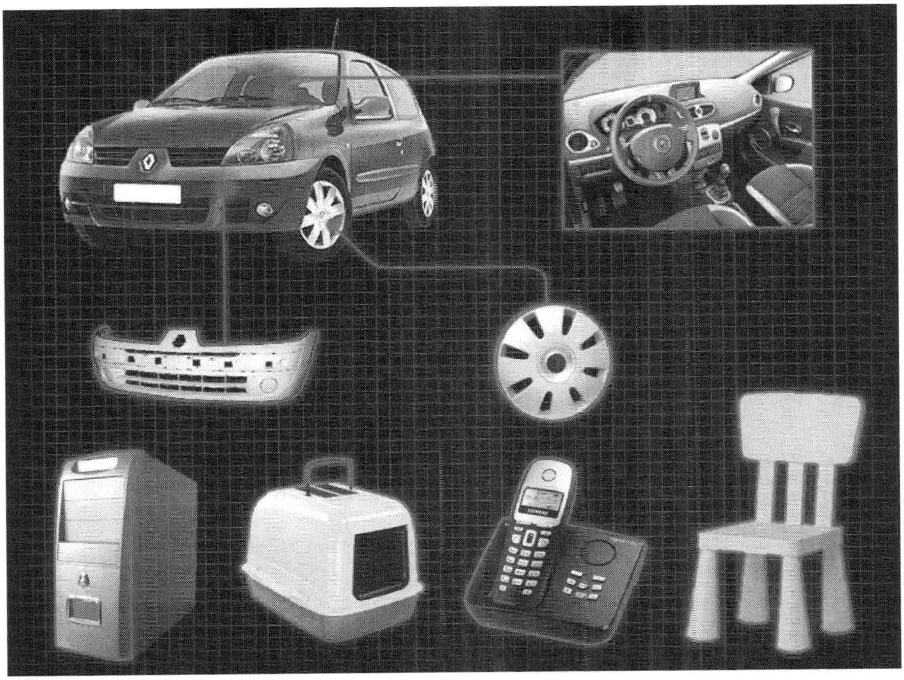

Fig. 2. Applications of biocomposites in industrial products

plastics used as the matrix component of composites, particularly those reinforced with fibres of natural origin (Peijs, 2002). PHB was discovered in the bacterium *Bacillus megaterium* and is found in other species of bacteria, including Alcaligenes, Azotobacter, Bacillus, Nocardia, Pseudomonas and Rhizobium. It is synthesized in a three-step reaction catalysed by β-ketothiolase (phbA), acetoacetyl-CoA reductase (phbB) and by PHB synthase (phbC) (Fig. 3), (Steinbuchel and Fuchtenbusch, 1998). In bacteria, PHB serves as a source of carbon and energy.

Isolating PHB from bacteria is expensive, so producing PHB in plants could be a promising method. Transgenic flax plants with overexpression of the three genes encoding PHB synthesis have been generated, and shown to be useful for biomedical applications. The stem-specific 14-3-3 promoter was used for the transformation. Three genes coding for β-ketothiolase, acetoacetyl-CoA reductase and PHB synthase were derived from *R. eutropha*. The generated plants (named M plants) exhibited a PHB content of up to 4.62 μg/gFW (Wróbel *et al.*, 2004). The electron-lucent granules of PHB were detected in the stroma of the plastids in the M plants. Moreover, the PHB synthesis affected the shape and size of the chloroplasts: the diameter of chloroplast increased, and they were characterized by a more oval shape. The accumulation of PHB resulted in changes in the stem's mechanical properties. These properties were measured using Young's modulus. This parameter was two-fold higher in the M plants, which indicates that transgenic fibres enriched with PHB have a higher average resistance to tensile loads and better elastic properties. The fibre composition of the M plants was examined using the infrared (IR) spectra method.

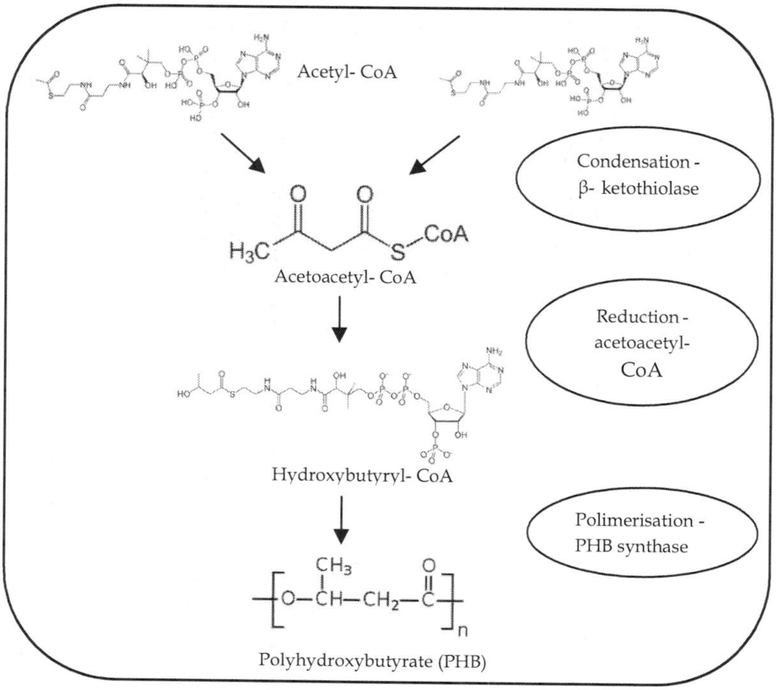

Fig. 3. Polyhydroxybutyrate (PHB) synthesis pathway

The greater structural disorder of the M fibres resulted from the formation of celluloses with an amorphous structure and from the shortening of the cellulose chain lengths. What is more, the M plants exhibited stronger coupling between the elementary fibres, which made them more stable (Wróbel- Kwiatkowska et al., 2009). Introducing PHB to flax fibres yielded the commercially utilized bast fibres. Fibres derived from those plants can be particularly used as the reinforcement in biocomposites (Fig.4).

First of all, the PHB in those fibres improves the adhesion between the fibres and the matrix, and secondly, such fibres remain a great source of phenolic acids, which possess antioxidative properties that are especially important when the fibres are used for medical purposes. Previous studies showed that composites of transgenic flax fibres enriched with PHB and polypropylene do not promote platelet aggregations in contrast to pure polypropylene (Szopa *et al.*, 2009). It was also noticed that those transgenic fibres have bacteriostatic properties (data not published).

A new generation of entirely biodegradable composites were made of polylactic acid (PLA) and alternatively of poly-ε-caprolactone (PCL) enriched with bioplastic flax fibres. Determining the level of platelet aggregations on the surface of the prepared composites and the level of colonization of bacteria (*E. coli*) to their surfaces showed the composites' anti-aggregational and bacteriostatic properties. The new composites also exhibited improved biomechanical properties in comparison to membranes made of pure PLA or PCL, and good *in vitro* biocompatibility, even though the cell viability of mouse fibroblast cells treated with

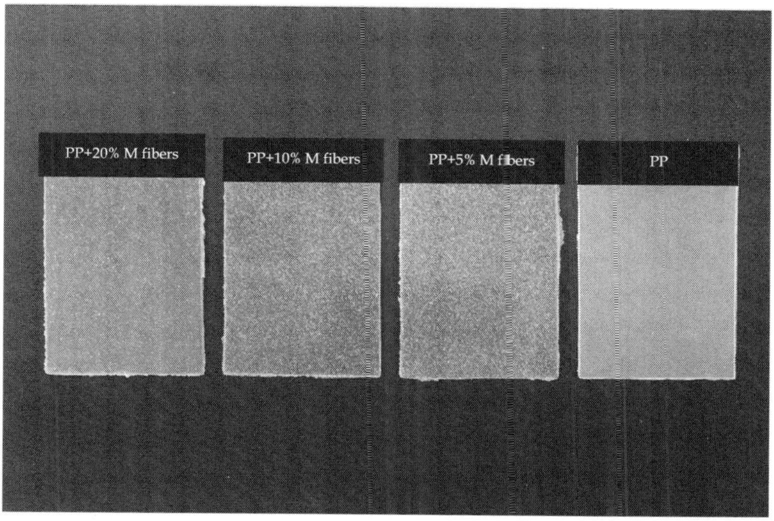

Fig. 4. Biodegradable flax composites made of polypropylene (PP) enriched with different content of bioplastic flax fibres (M plants). The control composite is made of polypropylene with no addition of flax fibres

these composites was slightly reduced and the amount of dead cells also slightly increased when compared to untreated cells (Gredes et al., 2010). It was also shown that implanting the tested biocomposites based on PLA and transgenic flax fibres into rat skeletal muscle had no influence on the gene expression of the most analysed genes, i.e. vascular endothelial growth factor (VEGF), insulin-like growth factor (IGF) and growth differentiation factor 8 (GDF8) (Gredes et al., 2010). The used implants composed of transgenic plastic fibres in a PLA matrix showed better biocompatibility than pure PLA or PHB implants, and they did not have any negative effect on muscle function and gene expression. Thus, the new biocomposites created with bioplastic flax fibres might be considered as a new material for tissue engineering and other branches of medicine.

2.3 The new bandage based on transgenic flax products

The number of patients with serious ulcer wounds is still increasing. This is a consequence of chronic diseases such as diabetes, obesity and atherosclerosis. An ulcer that is considered chronic, or non-healing, is one which takes more than eight weeks to heal despite optimal local and general treatment. Wound healing is a complex and dynamic process, divided into three overlapping stage: cleaning, proliferation, and wound constriction and cicatrisation. The complex treatment of ulcers mainly consists of wound diagnostics, casual treatment directed at the primary disease, the exclusion of other factors that inhibit healing processes, and general and local treatment (Abbade & Lastória, 2005). There are many factors that can influence wound healing, and using a proper wound dressing is among them. In recent years, many different specialized wound dressings were developed, such as hydroxycellulose, hydrocolloid, polyuretic-foam dressing, alginans, hydrogel dressing and dressing containing silver (Jones et al., 2006; Skórkowska-Telichowska et al., 2009). The purpose of a dressing is to isolate the wound, keep it at an optimal moisture level, remove excess exudates, help clean the wound of debris and necrotic tissue, help combat microbiological infection when necessary, and stimulate tissue regeneration.

One recently proposed wound dressing is made from genetically modified flax fabric (Fig.5). Flax has been used since ancient times for the production of linen cloth widely used for making clothes that are especially useful in humid climates due to certain flax fibre properties, the effects of which are called "wicking". This refers to their capillary action, which channels moisture away from the body (Muir & Westcott, 2003). This makes flax an attractive material for wound dressing, as it may be useful in keeping the wound at the optimal moisture level. Additionally, the loose weave of flax tissue enables wound purification from various contaminations.

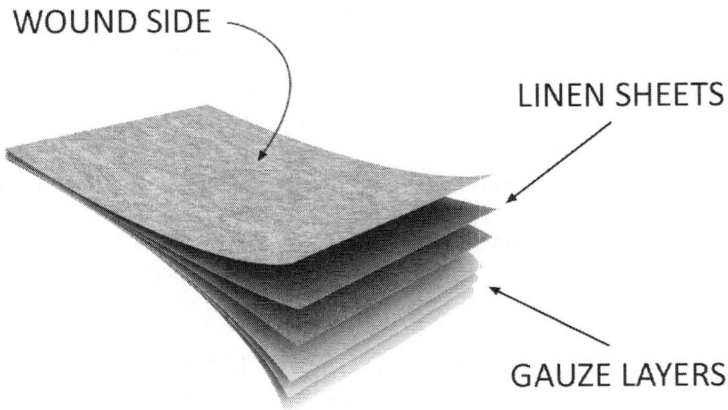

Fig. 5. Scheme of flax dressing

The biotechnological engineering was used to improve the flax fibres for medicinal use. After it was suggested that reactive oxygen species are responsible for chronic wound pathogenesis and anti-healing processes because they reduce the cell proliferation capacity (Chen et al., 2004; Wall et al., 2008), the use of flax fibres enriched in antioxidants in making of a wound dressing was proposed. Oxidative stress causes damage to cellular macromolecules; the deregulation of key proteins involved in DNA replication, the cell cycle, and cellular resistance to such stress; and the promotion of wound fibroblast apoptosis. Antioxidant-rich flax plants called W92 were created using three genes controlling the synthesis of plant secondary metabolites from the phenylopropanoid pathway: chalcone synthase, chalcone isomerase, and dihydroflavonol reductase. The introduction of those genes resulted in the accumulation of various antioxidative compounds like flavonoids, phenolic acids and lignans in the plant seeds and fibres (Lorenc-Kukuła et al., 2005). The antioxidant properties of these compounds might have a great significance for wound healing, because they inhibit enzymatic and non-enzymatic peroxidation. Flavonoids and phenolic acids also exhibit anti-inflammatory, antihistamine, antiviral and vasodilatory properties. It is suggested that the high level of phenylopropanoid compounds strengthens wound tissue defenses against biotic and abiotic stresses (Afaq et al., 2007; Chiang et al., 2005; Bae et al., 2009). The simultaneous use of fibres, oil emulsion and seedcake extract from genetically modified flax plants promoted the healing of chronic skin ulcerations (Skórkowska-Telichowska et al., 2010). In the pilot clinical trial, 30 patients with chronic skin ulceration (having lasted from 2 to 23 years) were treated with a linen dressing for 12 weeks. The treatment was divided into three phases: the dry phase with use of a highly hygroscopic linen dressing aimed at drying and cleaning the wounds; the second stage with linen dressing wetted with an oil emulsion derived from transgenic flax, with the aim to supply the wounds with polyunsaturated fatty acids (PUFA) and antioxidants; and the third stage with flax bandages wetted with seedcake extract rich in lignans, which are anti-inflammatory and cell proliferation promoting compounds. Such treatment effectively reduced the wound exudates in almost 67% of the subjects. Moreover, 93% of the patients exhibited a decrease in the fibrin level, which is one of the steps in wound healing. An important and objective parameter that was assessed was the wound size, and it emerged that in 80% of the patients, the ulcer size was reduced, of which 23% were totally cured (Fig.6). Interestingly and importantly, the bandage diminished the pain accompanying chronic venous ulceration as reported by patients.

It is believed that the effectiveness of a flax wound dressing is thanks to:

- the hygroscopic properties of the flax fibres providing an optimal moisture level and absorbing the excess of exudates;
- the phenolic acid and flavonoid content in the flax fibres reducing the inflammation in the wound;
- the unsaturated fatty acids which reinforce the integrity of the plasma membranes of the fibroblasts
- the presence of lignans stimulating fibroblast proliferation;
- the protection of the wound from mechanical irritation;
- the wound being kept clean and insulated from necrotic elements and contamination that move beyond the dressing surface.

Recently this new bandage, which is called Flax Aid, has become certified and is now offered by the Linum Foundation (www.leczenielnem.pl).

There is a proposal to replace the linen dressings from W92 plants with dressings from M plants (bioplastic fibres) because the induction of cell proliferation is very important for wound healing. For this reason, polyhydroxybutyrate (PHB) has received particular interest. Upon contact with body fluids, the polymer degrades to release D,L-β-hydroxybutyrate, promoting the proliferation of cells in high-density cultures by preventing apoptotic cell death (Cheng et al., 2006) making it an attractive candidate for tissue engineering applications, especially those requiring the regeneration of large numbers of cells as described in the previous section. The fabric, made from plants enriched in polyhydroxybutyrate (M plants), was tested for suitability as a wound dressing. In this case, only the first stage (flax fabric wetted with isotonic solution) was investigated and only the wound size was considered, and the results were compared to those obtained with the W92 type dressing. During the four weeks of flax dressing treatment (twenty cases with chronic ulcerations of venous origin), the majority of the subjects treated with M flax bandages showed a statistically significant reduction in wound size. The average reduction in the ulcer size within this group was 28% (6 cm2), which is a far better result than that (7.78%) obtained for dressings prepared from the fibres of W92 plants. Thus, it is suggested that the fabric from the fibres of M plants is more effective in wound healing than that from W92 plants. It should be pointed out that both transgenic fabrics inhibit the growth of pathogenic bacteria and fungi in *in vitro* studies and are more effective than control and cotton fibres.

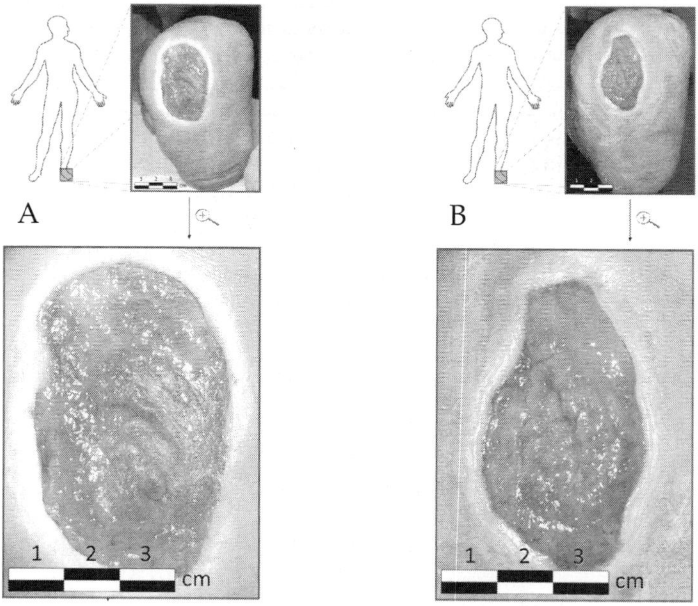

Fig. 6. Foot ulcer before (A) and after (B) twelve- week treatment with flax dressing

The antimicrobial activity of a flax fabric dressing is of great interest, as from clinical practice it is known that quite often long-term wounds can become infected. Very often this is caused by a antibiotic-resistant bacterial and fungal strains, so new ways to combat microbiological infections are needed. These results show that linen dressings obtained from GM flax have beneficial effects on wound healing and can be used as an innovative flax biotechnological product.

3. Transgenic flax as a source of bioactive compounds designated for therapy and health-promoting actions

Linseed oil has commercial value as a component of adhesives, paints and varnishes, plasticizers, inks and linoleum. It is also a precursor of nylon and composite materials. That said, the most important aspect for humans is the dietary properties of flax seeds. Linseed oil is one of the richest sources of α-linolenic acid (ALA), with a content of 44–57%; it also contains 15–29% linoleic acid and 13–29% oleic acid (Muir and Westcott, 2003). As the human body cannot produce ALA, which belongs to the ω-3 family, it is an essential fatty acid in our diet. Therefore, linseed oil plays an important role in the food, health care and pharmaceutical industries. The unsaturated fatty acids of linseed oil have a positive influence on the metabolism and peristalsis. They can lower the total and LDL cholesterol and glucose levels in the blood (Pellizzon et al., 2007).

The market value of linseed oil is limited by the lability of polyunsaturated fatty acids (PUFA), which are susceptible to peroxidation. Only a few cultivars of the flax with low

PUFA contents are suitable for commercial use as an edible oil. The rancidity and the development of an undesirable odor in linseed oil is mainly caused by the interaction of reactive oxygen species (ROS) with PUFA. Lipid peroxidation degrades unsaturated fatty acids and leads to the accumulation of dangerous products ROS are known to be associated with aging, inflammation, carcinogenesis and atherosclerosis (Choi et al., 2002). For this reason, the inactivation and elimination of ROS might be very beneficial not only in industrial but also in nutritional applications. To avoid oxidation, linseed oil is supplemented with vitamin E and stored in low temperature in dark bottles. However, these methods are not satisfactory. A promising strategy might be the genetic manipulation of flax to improve the oil quality and the stability of the PUFA, and thus the natural supplementation of protective antioxidant compounds in flax seeds. There are a few interesting approaches in which various antioxidant compounds were synthesized in transgenic plants. The goal of this research was to improve flax seed quality by increasing the level and stability of unsaturated fatty acids and antioxidant compounds *via* genetic engineering. The modifications were directed toward improving the beneficial effects of flax seeds.

3.1 Manipulation of the flax genes of the phenylopropanoid pathway

Breeding plants which are able to produce pharmaceuticals and other valuable compounds is one major reason for the genetic modification of plants. The phenylopropanoid pathway seems to be one of the most important metabolic pathways due to its involvement in the synthesis of a large range of natural products in plants, including lignans, lignin, flavonoids and anthocyanins. All of these compounds act as antioxidants, chelators of divalent cations, photoreceptors, and visual attractors. The pathway of flavonoid synthesis begins with chalcone synthesis catalysed by chalcone synthase (CHS) and flavonon and flavonol synthesis catalysed by chalcone isomerase (CHI), leading to flavan production in a reaction catalysed by dihydroflavonol reductase (DFR) (Fig.7). Flavan is direct precursor of anthocyanidins and proantocyanidins. The last step in flavonoid biosynthesis is their glycosylation by glycosyl transferase. The phenylopropanoid synthesis pathway is the source of different compounds of great biomedical application like phenolic acids, lignans catecholamines and lignins.

Many phenolic compounds (lignans, phenolic acids) have been identified in both the green parts and the seeds of flax plants, which is the irrefutable proof of the presence of an active phenylopropanoid pathway in this plant. The enzymes of the phenylpropanoid pathway are appropriate targets for genetic manipulation, and the modulation of their levels alters the content of secondary metabolites. There are two alternative ways to increase the phenolic compound contents in plants: increase the expression of the key enzymes of synthesis; and overexpress the enzymes regulating stability of these compounds.

The first strategy was used to create flax plants overexpressing three genes of the phenylopropanoid synthesis pathway: chalcone synthase (CHS), chalcone isomerase (CHI), and dihydroflavonol reductase (DFR). Such plants were characterized by a significant increase in the levels of flavonoids in the seeds, fibres and in the green parts of the plant (Lorenc-Kukuła et al., 2005). The major differences in the antioxidant levels were observed in the phenolic acid content, and more importantly for human consummates, flax seeds obtained from transgenic plants are rich in the strong antioxidants secoisolariciresinol diglucoside (SDG), kaempferol and quercetin. The results obtained for these plants are presented in Figure 8.

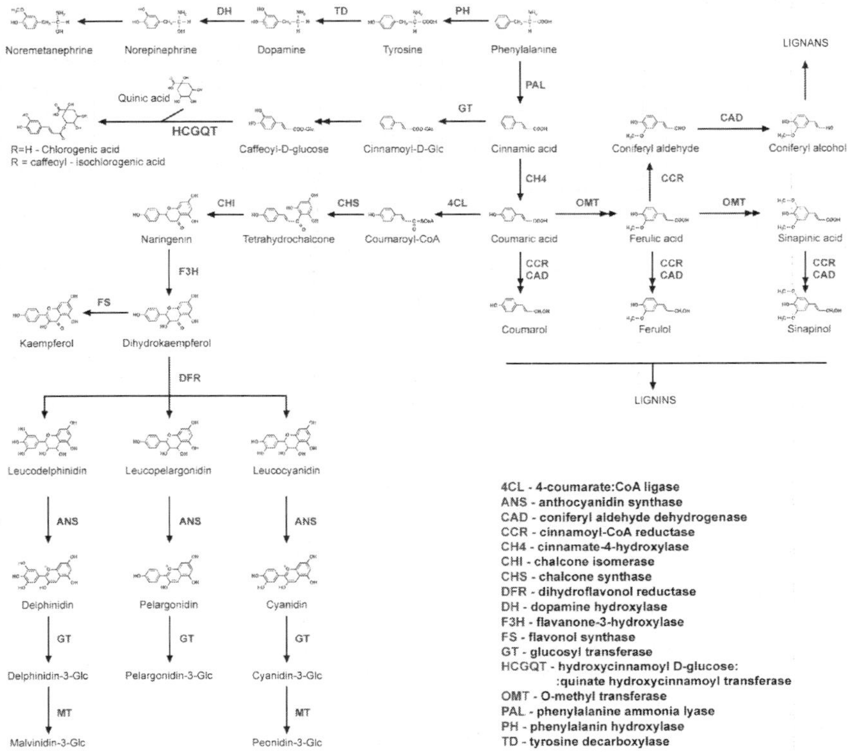

Fig. 7. The phenylopropanoid pathway

A similar effect was obtained for flax plants with overproduction of glycosyltransferase (the second strategy), which resulted in higher accumulation of proanthocyanin, lignans and phenolic acids compared to the control (Lorenc-Kukuła et al., 2009) (Fig 8). Linseed oil is one of the richest sources of unsaturated fatty acids, especially α-linolenic acid (ALA). Unfortunately, this product is unstable during long storage, because of the tendency to oxidation of fatty acids. Both modifications resulted in unsaturated fatty acid accumulation in the seeds. This observation suggests the involvement of polyphenol glycosides in the protection of unsaturated fatty acids against oxidation, which improves the oil.

The genetic engineering approach could involve the overproduction of various natural antioxidants within the flax grains. In addition to preventing fat rancidity, antioxidants such as flavonoids might also have a beneficial effect on human health and such plants are a very good source of compounds for biomedical applications. Recently, there has been a growing interest in the probiotic properties of flax and in its beneficial effects on coronary heart disease, some types of cancer, and neurological and hormonal disorders (Saffron, 2008; Huang & Ziboch, 2001; Simopoulos, 2002). Flax seeds are the richest source of the plant lignan secoisolariciresinol diglucoside (SDG), which can be metabolized by the colonic microflora to yield the mammalian lignans, enterodiol (ED) and enterolactone (EL)

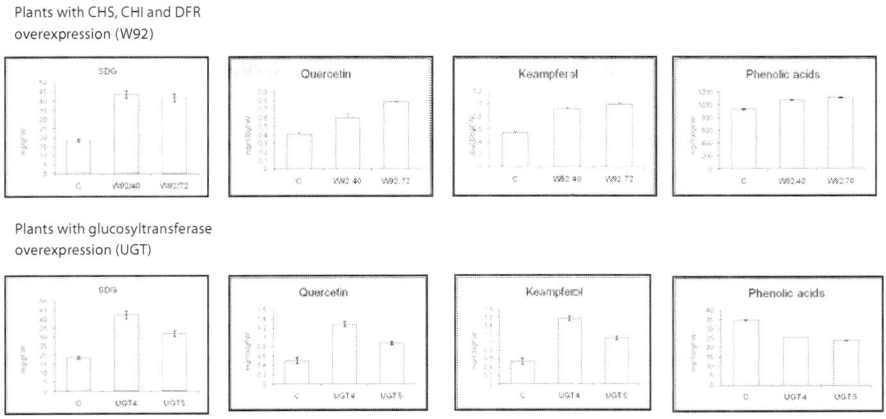

Fig. 8. The contents of compounds with potential biomedical applications in transgenic plants overexpressing genes from the phenylopropanoid pathway

Phytoestrogens such as lignans, which exhibit weak estrogenic and antiestrogenic properties in a tissue-specific manner, have potential in the prevention and treatment of breast cancer (Adlercreutz, H. & Herman, 2002). Flax seeds and their lignans have been reported to inhibit chemically induced mammary tumorigenesis at the preinitiation, early, and late promotion stages of carcinogenesis in rats (Thompson et al., 1996), and the growth and metastasis of human breast cancer in nude mice (Chen et al., 2002). The last published evidence also suggests that a dose of at least 500 mg SDG/day for approximately 8 weeks is enough to observe positive effects on cardiovascular risk factors in human patients. Flax seeds and their lignan extracts appear to be safe for most adult populations (Adolphe et al., 2010).
It is indicated that a diet rich in flavonoid compounds is strongly correlated with a lower risk of cancer (Ross and Kasum 2010). The compound with an especially higher anti-cancer action is quercetin, particularly in synergic action with keampferol (Brusselmans et al., 2005). In both prostate and breast cancer cells, a remarkable dose-response parallelism was observed between the flavonoid-induced inhibition of fatty acid synthesis, the inhibition of cell growth, and the induction of apoptosis. The dose which caused a reduction of the cancer cell proliferation to 19% is 100 µM quercetin; 100 µM kaempferol caused a reduction to 32% (Brusselmans *et al.*, 2005).

3.2 Flax with elevated levels of terpenoids

Terpenoids, also called isoprenoids, are group of about 40000 compounds. The group contains both primary and secondary metabolites of great significance for the growth and development of plants. Gibberellic acid, abscisic acid (phytohormons), carotenoids, chlorophyll, and ubiquinone can be distinguished among the primary metabolites (Aharoni *et al.*, 2008). The classification of terpenoids is based on the number of 5-carbon isoprene units, which compose the backbone of the molecule. Hemi-, mono-, sesqui-, di-, tri- and tetraterpenes correspond to 5-, 10-, 15-, 20-, 30- and 40-carbon terpenoids (Saremi and Arora, 2009). In plants, the isoprene units are produced from isopentenyl pyrophosphate (IPP) and dimethylallyl pyrophosphate (DMAPP), which may originate from different pathways (Fig. 9).

The mevalonate pathway occurs in the cytosol, and was discovered first. IPP synthesis begins with transformation of 2 molecules of acetyl-CoA to 3-Hydroxy-3-Methyl-Glutaryl-CoA (HMG-CoA), which is subsequently converted by HMG-CoA reductase to mevalonate. The mevalonate undergoes phosphorylation to mevalonyl phosphate (catalysed by mevalonyl kinase), and then to mevalonyl diphosphate (catalysed by mevalonyl phosphate kinase). Isopentenyl pyrophosphate (IPP) is formed *via* the action of mevalonyl phosphate decarboxylase. This is next transformed by isopentyl isomerase to dimethylallyl pyrophosphate (DMAPP) (Siemieniuk & Skrzydlewska, 2005). It is suggested that this pathway is the source for 15- and 30-carbon terpenoids (squalene, sterols, brassinosteroids).
The second, non-mevalonate pathway was discovered 10 years ago, and some of its steps are not fully known. It takes place in the plastids and is responsible for the synthesis of 10-, 20- and 40-carbon terpenoids (gibberellins, carotenoids, chlorophyll, tocopherol). The substrates are pyruvate and glyceraldehyde 3-phosphate, which are converted by DXS synthase to 1-deoxy-D-xylulose 5-phosphate (DXP). DXP is then transformed by DXR reductase into methylerytritol phosphate (MEP). The final step is the reduction of MEP to isopentenyl phosphate (IPP) (Cheng et al., 2007).

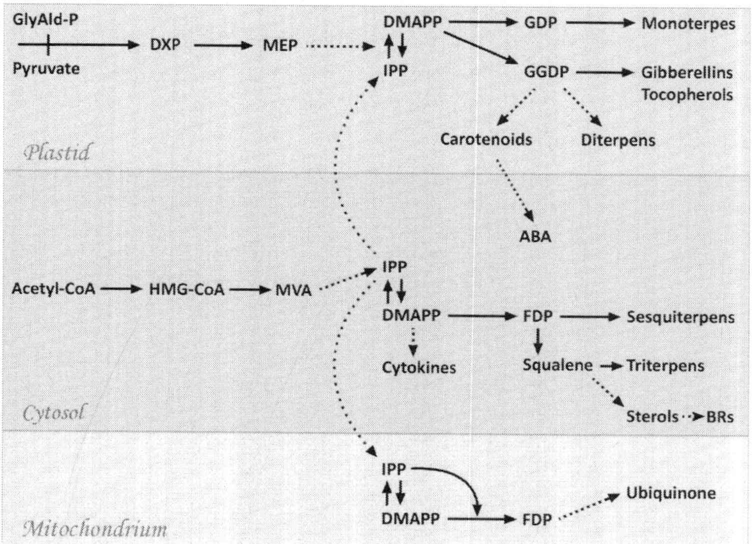

Fig. 9. The pathway of terpenoid biosynthesis

In the second step of terpenoid synthesis, 5-carbon molecule IPP and DMAPP undergo condensation due to the activity of prenyltransferases. The combination of one IPP and one DMAPP molecule yields geranyl diphosphate (in a reaction catalysed by GDP synthase), which is a precursor for monoterpenes. Two IPP molecules associated with DMAPP are transformed to farnesyl diphosphate (catalysed by FDP synthase), which gives a 15-carbon precursor of sesquiterpenes and triterpenes. Three molecules of IPP connected to DMAPP give geranylgeranyl diphosphate (catalysed by GGDP synthase), which is a precursor of the 20- and 40-carbon compounds. The last step of terpenoid synthesis comprises the transformation of prenyl diphosphates (GDP, FDP and GGDP) by the appropriate terpenoid synthases (e.g. squalene synthase) (Cheng et al., 2007).

In plants, terpenoids play mainly protective roles against various environmental stresses. Many of them possess antioxidative properties (carotenoids, tocopherols), bacterio- and mycostatic properties (menthol, camphor), and recently, anti-neoplastic and anti-inflammatory properties are frequently reported (squalene, tocopherols, carotenoids, taxol) (Peltier et al., 2006). The ability to quench free radicals produced both during normal cell functioning, as well as under stress conditions, also contributes to the inhibition of many free radical-based diseases, including neoplasms (Grassmann, 2005; Gershenzon and Dudareva, 2007). The above-mentioned properties of terpenoids make them attractive dietary supplements.

Stress, pollution, lack of movement and bad nutritional habits cause many diseases, including neoplasms. Pharmacies offer a plethora of vitamin preparations, but they are mainly composed of substances obtained *via* chemical synthesis. The newest results indicate that the assimilability of compounds obtained from natural sources is much higher. Therefore, instead of "swallowing" more pills, nutritionists advise the consumption of products rich in natural bioactive compounds. Without a doubt, linseed oil is such a product. It constitutes the main source of omega-3 and omega-6 fatty acids. A drawback of this oil is its lability, caused by the presence of highly unsaturated fatty acids. Enriching it in natural substances increases its stability (tocopherol, carotenoids) and improves its health-oriented properties (squalene), expanding its potential for use in prophylaxis against many diseases, including diseases of the circulatory system and eyesight. This may make flax more competitive in relation to imported oils. An innovative product with a broad spectrum of action will result from such modifications.

Carotenoids are a group of over 700 compounds of yellow or orange colour. The majority are tetraterpenes consisting of 8 isoprene units. The molecule consists of 40 carbon atoms. The human organism is unable to synthesize carotenoids, and thus must intake them with nutrients. Studies prove that a diet rich in these compounds, provided they are of natural origin, lowers the risk of several diseases, particularly neoplasms and eyesight diseases. The anti-cancer character of carotenoids is based on different mechanisms, such as their antioxidative activity, strengthening of the immunological system, stimulation of gap junction formation in intracellular communication, induction of detoxification enzymes, and inhibition of cell proliferation. The anti-cancer activity of carotenoids was mainly observed and studied in the case of lung cancer (β-carotene), prostate cancer (lycopene), gullet and larynx cancer (lycopene), stomach cancer (lycopene), and leukemia (β-carotene). Carotenoids are mainly accumulated in the testicles, epididymides and liver (mostly β-carotene and lycopene). Without a doubt, the best-known benefit of carotenoid intake is the fact that about 50% of them can be converted into vitamin A, and the most prominent pro-vitamin activity is shown by β-carotene. Vitamin A is transformed to retinen, which is an indispensable component of the retinal pigments, and which conditions normal sight. Intake of nourishment containing those carotenoids protects the retina from degradation and diseases connected with age (Johnson, 2002).

Carotenoids are insoluble in water, but they dissolve very well in fats. The production of flax plants with an elevated carotenoid content was recently described (Fujisawa *et al.*, 2008). Flax was successfully transformed with the phytoene synthase gene (*crtB*) derived from the soil bacterium *Pantoea ananatis* under the control of the constitutive cauliflower mosaic virus (CaMV) 35S promoter. The genetically modified flax produced orange seeds with a high accumulation of phytoene, α- and β-carotene. The carotenoid amounts in the seeds reached 63.4 to 156.3 μg/g of fresh weight, which was a 7.8 to 18.6-fold increase in comparison to non-transformed plants (Fujisawa *et al.*, 2008). It is suggested that the flux of phytoene synthesis from geranylgeranyl diphosphate was first promoted by the expressed crtB gene product, and then the phytoene was decomposed to the downstream metabolites as α- and β-carotene and lutein. It is expected that oil obtained from the seeds of those plants will contain an elevated pool of carotenoids. This will improve the stability and quality of the oil, rich in highly unsaturated fatty acids. *In vitro* studies showed that the addition of β-carotene to oils protects unsaturated fatty acids from oxidation. The oil is characterized with an elevated amount of vitamin A and lutein, and is a potential innovative product.

Squalene is a triterpene obtained via the mevalonate pathway. It is also a precursor for cholesterol biosynthesis (Reddy and Couvreur, 2009). For commercial purposes, it is acquired mainly from shark liver oil, though there are also plants rich in this compound, e.g. amaranth seeds, rice bran, wheat germs and olives. Its direct anti-tumour activity is based on inhibiting the catalytic activity of β-HMGCoA. Although it is a weak inhibitor of tumour-cell proliferation, it contributes directly or indirectly to cancer treatment by strengthening the influence of antigens, which bind to it. Thus, it is widely used in vaccines and medicines (Kelly, 1999). Squalene diminishes the side effects of chemotherapy (Reddy and Couvreur, 2009). In addition, it normalizes the level of cholesterol in blood.

Introducing a gene of lycopene β-cyclase from *Arabidopsis thaliana* to flax caused homological repression and lowered carotenoid content. At the same time, it redirected the substrates to produce the remaining terpenoids. The plants generated in this way turned out to be more resistant to *Fusarium* infection (unpublished data), which is an additional argument for the cultivation of this transgenic type.

Through the repression of carotenoid synthesis, flax with an elevated squalene content was obtained (Table 1). The seeds of the transformed flax (L plants) are richer in squalene (data not published). An important aspect of this modification is not only that plants rich in a health-oriented compound are obtained, but also that a new strategy can be proposed for the modification of the metabolism in a preferred direction *via* repression of a pathway or pathways which are not desired. This strategy is justified by the fact that repression of a gene in plants is much easier than its activation, as only a short DNA fragment (100-200 bp) homologous to the endogenous gene is required.

Terpenoid	Linola	L9	L18
Squalene	100%	80%	192%
Tocopherol alpha	100%	136%	217%
Tocopherol beta	100%	170%	818%
Gibberellic acid GA3	100%	85%	182%
Menthol	100%	156%	141%
β-carotene	100%	62,5%	50%
lutein	100%	98%	80%

Table 1. Percentage level of different terpenoids in flax plants with repression of lycopene beta cyclase gene (named L)

3.3 Modified flax oil as a precious source of unsaturated fatty acids

An increasing coefficient of morbidity of civilization diseases such as obesity, atherosclerosis, heart disease and hypertension was observed with the development of industry and the economy. The Western diet is characterized by high intakes of animal fat, saturated acids, omega-6 acids, and *trans*-fatty acids, and this contributes to civilization diseases. The consumption of flax seeds is suggested to be beneficial for human health. Flax seeds have about 40% fat in dry weight (Łukaszewicz et al., 2004). Linseed oil consists of about 16% linoleic acid and 54% linolenic acid, and is the richest source of these polyunsaturated fatty acids (PUFA), (Table 2).

Fatty acids	Olive oil	Rapeseed oil	Soybean oil	Sunflower oil	Corn oil	Grapeseed oil	Linseed oil
14:0	0	0	0.11	0.08	0	0	0
16:0	11.46	4.68	10.62	6.66	10.1	6.79	5.06
16:0	0.96	0	0.09	0.08	0	0.10	0
18:0	2.20	2.36	3.76	4.27	1.6	3.63	3.73
18 : 1 n-9	68.76	57.14	21.67	24.2	31.4	17.8	19.68
18 : 1 n-7	0	3.40	1.61	0.58	0	0	0.68
18 : 2 n-6	10.51	21.16	55.07	63.65	56.3	65.9	16.21
18 : 3 n-3	0.67	11.25	6.89	0.19	0.4	0.38	54.52

Table 2. The fatty acid composition of seed oils (%) in different plant oils
(http://www.biuletynfarmacji.wum.edu.pl/0501Jelinska/0Jelinska.html)

PUFA are divided into two main groups: omega-6 and omega-3. Their precursors are linoleic (LA) and α- linolenic acids (ALA), respectively. LA and ALA are numbered among essential fatty acids because they cannot be synthesized in mammals. LA and ALA delivered in food play an important role in the correct development and functioning of the human body. They are structural components of the cell membranes and substrates in the biosynthesis pathway of arachidonic acid (AA), eicosapentaenoic acid (EPA), docosahexaenoic acid (DHA), and their eicosanoids (Fig. 10). Biosynthesis of omega-6 and omega-3 fatty acids is catalyzed by the same enzymes. Through the conversion by desaturase and elongase enzymes, LA is transformed to arachidonic acid (AA), and ALA to eicosapentaenoic acid (EPA), and then to docosahexaenoic acid (DHA). Supplementing the diet with ALA promotes the omega-3 pathway, leading to the inhibition of synthesis of arachidonic acid and eicosanoids derived from AA, which stimulate inflammation (Muir and Westcott, 2003).

Numerous epidemiological and experimental studies have shown the positive effects of omega-3 fatty acids on the reduction in risk of cardiovascular disease, stroke and atherosclerosis. They revealed anti-cancer and anti-inflammatory activities (Saravanan et al., 2010).

PUFAs, especially α- linolenic acid, are susceptible to oxidation, which causes a change in taste and odour, and causes problems with long-term storage. A mutation in the *FAD3* genes, responsible for the conversion of linoleic acid to linolenic acid in flax, was achieved in order to minimize the oxidation processes. This led to a new type of flax seeds, described as the solin type (low α- linolenic acid content), which are suitable for the production of edible oil (Rowland, 1991). The mutation induced with methane sulphonate (EMS) resulted in a stable low linolenic acid mutant. The low linolenic character is controlled by recessive alleles at two independent loci, which are the result of a double mutation.

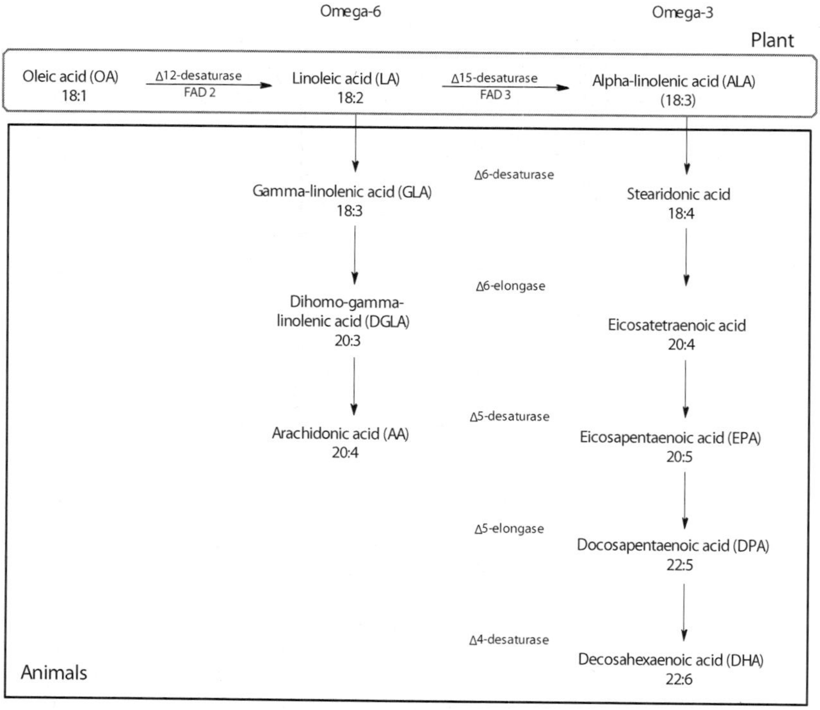

Fig. 10. The metabolic pathway of polyunsatured fatty acids. Linoleic acid and alpha-linolenic acid are the respective parents for the omega-6 and omega-3 fatty acids. They are synthesized in flax seeds by desaturation catalysed by a set of enzymes coded by the *FAD2* and *FAD3* genes

During the cold extraction of oil most of the natural antioxidants are lost. It is desirable to find a technology of oil production with improved oxidative protection. One possibility is oil supplementation with natural antioxidants. This supplementation was performed on flax seeds *via* various transgenic modifications. One of these modification was transformation with the *Solanum sogarandinum*-derived gene (designated SsGT1) coding for glycosyltransferase (UGT) under a seed-specific napin promoter. UGTs are large group of enzymes found in all living organisms which catalyse the transfer of a nucleotide diphosphate-activated monosaccharide unit (glucose, rhamnose, galactose, xylose, rutinose, and neohesperidose) to an acceptor molecule. Plant UGTs play a role in developmental and metabolic homeostasis, and also take part in detoxification processes. It is known that the glycosylation of low molecular weight compounds such as flavonoids makes the molecules more stable, increases their solubility in the vacuole, and can enhance the pathogen resistance of plants. Flax plants overexpressing SsGT1 accumulated higher levels of glucosylated flavonoids in the seeds, mainly the kaempferol and quercetin glycoside (Lorenc-Kukuła et al., 2009). Overproduction of SsGT1 in transgenic flax (named UGT plants) also resulted in proanthocyanin, phenolic acid and unsaturated fatty acid accumulation in the seeds. The linseed oil of UGT plants was examined *via* gas chromatography, which revealed an increase in unsaturated 18:1 (11-14%), 18:2 (9.5-24.7%), and 18:3 (23.7-54.5%) fatty acids. The antioxidant compounds are hydrophilic in nature. They accumulated in seeds, partially cross to the oil phase. Moreover, their level changes during the oil purification processes and remains the highest if cold-oil pressing is used. Various hydrophilic and hydrophobic compounds can stabilize linseed oil depending on their concentration, structure and proportions. The antioxidant compounds found in UGT plants were able to improve oil storage. It was observed that the rate of conjugated diene and aldehyde formation in the heated oils from transgenic seeds was lower than in the oil of the control plants (data not published). A similar positive effect on oil storage was achieved in flax oil derived from plants overexpressing three genes of the flavonoid route: *chs*, *chi* and *dfr*. As described in section 2.1 (Manipulation of flax genes of phenylopropanoid pathway), W92 transgenic flax was characterised by an elevated level of flavonoids and by an increased antioxidant capacity of the seeds (Lorenc-Kukuła et al., 2007). The accumulation of antioxidants in W92 plants had a positive effect on oil storage (Prescha et al., 2008).

Among the fatty acids that belong to the omega-3 group, EPA and DHA have beneficial effects on health. These PUFAs mostly occur in fish oil, but a drop in the quantity, and the contamination of this source has been continuously observed. A diet rich in ALA elevates erythrocyte EPA and DPA concentration in humans (Barceló-Coblijn et al., 2008). Another alternative was the expression of enzymes, such as Δ6-desaturase, Δ6-elongase, and Δ5-desaturase, which participate in biosynthesis of very-long-chain polyunsaturated fatty acids in flax. In spite of the high level of accumulation of C18 desaturated fatty acids, these products were channeled to triacyloglycerols, which led to a lack of substrates for Δ6-elongase. Only 5% C20 polyunsaturated fatty acids were obtained (Abbadi et al., 2004).

The oxidative stability of linseed oil is still the main goal to achieve. The high production and accumulation of very long-chain polyunsaturated fatty acids in linseed oil, especially EPA and DHA, is the next challenge.

Variation in oil lipid composition of the different flax cultivars is presented in Table 3.

It is worth mentioning the geometric and positional isomers of linoleic acid, the conjugated linoleic acids (CLA). The main sources of CLA are dairy products and the fat tissue of ruminant animals. Studies indicate that CLA has anti-cancer, anti-atherosclerotic, anti-diabetic, anti-inflammatory, and anti-obesity activities (Wahle et al., 2004). Linseed oil is still underestimated as a valuable source of compounds that are beneficial for human health. The wide range of action of polyunsaturated fatty acids make linseed oil a desirable and helpful product in medical treatment.

3.4 New anti-inflammatory and analgesic compounds derived from flax

The most recent studies on flax products' properties have revealed many health-beneficial actions in aspects of different diseases. One of the latest investigated activities is the anti-inflammatory nature of flax plant and product extracts. This aspect of the flax plant studies was based on promising results of flax bandage use in the healing of chronic wounds of different etiologies. The direct reasons for chronic ulcerations are always connected to the inflammation state of the organism, so inflammation-related processes are very important in wound healing.

Cultivar/fatty acid	16:0	18:0	18:1	18:2	18:3	20:0
Voroezski	6.11	4.6	22.0	14.9	52.2	0.24
Jenny	6.91	5.7	19.7	14.2	52.1	0.36
La Estanzuela AR	6.28	4.1	17.7	14.1	57.5	0.46
Opal	5.43	3.73	18.2	15.3	56.1	1.22
Szafir	5.19	3.28	14.1	11.9	65.4	0.11
Abby	5.99	3.4	13.3	18.2	58.9	0.11
Linola	6.28	1.91	13.5	74.5	3.27	0.28
W92.40	6.03	3.37	15.94	70.92	2.25	0.14
W92.86	5.85	4.74	21.98	41.71	24.54	0.18
UGT/NAP	6.30	3.85	17.96	69.07	1.43	0.12

Table 3. Variation in oil lipid composition of the different flax cultivars (Łukaszewicz et al, 2004; Lorenc-Kukuła et al,2004; Lorenc-Kukuła et al, 2009)

There are many groups of compounds that can be partially responsible for flax bandage anti-inflammatory action, for example the previously mentioned groups of antioxidants, directly regulating the oxidation processes connected to inflammation. Among the different types of molecules, we chose the terpenophenols for further investigation, as some very interesting ones have recently been found in flax extracts. The new compound identification is based on UPLC retention time, UV spectra and GC-MS analysis in comparison to some terpenophenolic standards. The identification is still of a preliminary nature, but all the methods used confirm the presence of cannabinoid-like compounds in the examined extracts (results not published). Cannabinoids have never previously been discovered in any plants other than cannabis plants, so these results are very intriguing and interesting. Cannabinoids are a group of terpenophenolics that accumulate in considerable amounts in the glandular trichomes of *Cannabis sativa* (Cannabaceae). In cannabis plants, the biosynthesis of these terpenoids involves a common isoprenoid building block, isopentenyl diphosphate, while the biosynthesis of the phenyl part of the cannabinoid, olivetolic acid is connected to the polyketide pathway. Further alkylation of olivetolic acid with geranyl pyrophosphate leads to the formation of cannabigerolic acid (CBGA), the central precursor of various cannabinoids like tetrahydrocannabinol (THC), cannabidiol (CBD) or cannabichromene (CBC) (Sirikantaramas et al., 2007). The synthesis pathway of cannabinoids in cannabis plants is presented in Figure 11. All the precursors for the biosynthesis are present at relatively high levels in flax plants, so a similar pathway of synthesis is possible. Investigations of the activity of such a biosynthesis pathway are in progress, but there is still no evidence of its existence in flax.

The special properties of cannabinoids have been known and exploited for thousands of years for medical purposes, mainly as anti-inflammatory and pain- realising agents. There are many studies nowadays providing evidence for the biological activity of these compounds in pain relief and healing of many kinds of diseases, including neuropatic pain, multiple sclerosis, Alzheimer's disease, atherosclerosis, rheumatoid arthritis, asthma, many allergies and other inflammatory diseases including AIDS (Pacher et al., 2006). The inflammation state plays a crucial role in all the mentioned health issues and cannabinoids have been proven to have an influence on this process. Activation of specific cannabinoid receptors (CB1 and/or CB2) and the downstream signaling cascade inhibits the production

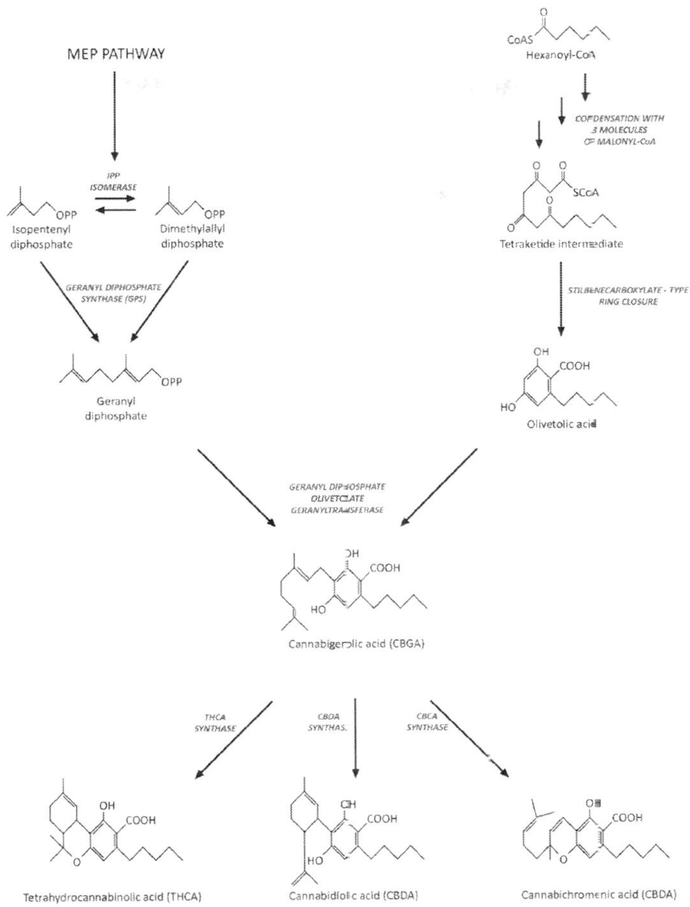

Fig. 11. The synthesis pathway of cannabinoids in cannabis plants

of cytokines and activates anti-inflammatory protein expression (Klein et al., 2000). The process of inflammation inhibition is presented in Fig. 12. This system, as the main target in new flax application, was the focus of examinations of the biological activity of the flax extracts containing cannabinoid-like compounds.

Real-Time PCR expression measurements of common cytokines level in both mouse and human fibroblast cell line experiments showed the inhibition of pro-inflammatory gene expression after flax cannabinoid-like extract treatments (results not published). Biological activity assays of the newly discovered compounds still need to be confirmed in many aspects, but the first results are very promising.

The existence, nature, biosynthesis pathway and activity of cannabinoids in flax requires much further investigation, but the discovered compounds give great new possibilities for flax product applications. The experiments in this field will give the opportunity for manipulations of the type and level of the compounds produced, which would be of great significance in the medical application of the natural non-psychoactive anti-inflammatory and pain-relieving products derived from flax.

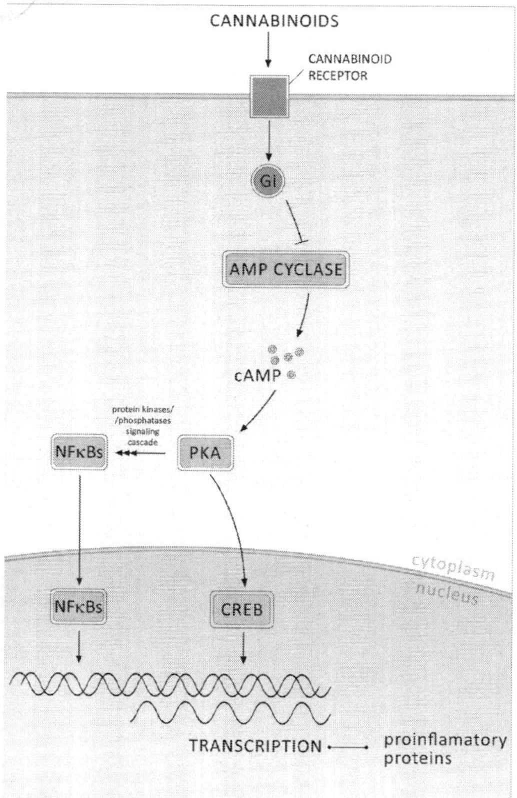

Fig. 12. The process of inflammation inhibition by cannabinoids through CB receptor

4. Conclusion

The interest in the medicinal, nutraceutical and industrial value of flax is still growing. The utility of this crop plant is not only restricted to edible oil and textile fibre production. Genetic manipulation enabled its use to be broadened in many fields, but mainly in medicine and human health. The research is not only focused on unsaturated fatty acids but also on precious antioxidants such as phenylopropanoids, lignans and terpenoids. Many new transgenic lines of flax characterized by better properties of fibre and oil have been generated. Genetic engineering methods allow the manipulation of the desired genes to improve the traits of flax. As the transformation protocol of flax is well established and the results are very promising, it is clear that genetically modified flax has a future in medical applications.

5. Acknowledgment

This paper was supported by grant nos. N R12 0009 06, NN 302061834, NN302 101136, and NN310 079038 from the Polish Ministry of Science and Higher Education.

6. References

Abbade, L.P. & Lastória, S. (2005). Venous ulcer: epidemiology, physiopathology, diagnosis and treatment. *Int J Dermatol*, 44: 449-456.

Abbadi, A.; Domergue, F.; Bauer, J.; Napier, J.A.; Welti, R.; Zähringer, U.; Cirpus, P. & Heinz, E. (2004). Biosynthesis of Very-Long-Chain Polyunsaturated Fatty Acids in Transgenic Oilseeds: Constraints on Their Accumulation. The Plant Cell, Vol.16, 2734–2748, 1040-4651.

Adlercreutz, H. &, Herman, S. (2002). Phytoestrogens and cancer. Lancet Oncol., 3, : 364–373.

Adolphe, JL.; Whiting, SJ.; Juurlink, BH.; Thorpe, LU. & Alcorn J. (2010). Health effects with consumption of the flax lignan secoisolariciresinol diglucoside. *Br J Nutr.*, Apr, 103(7):929-38.

Afaq, F.; Syed, DN.; Malik, A.; Hadi, N.; Sarfaraz, S.; Kweon, MH.; Khan, N.; Zaid, MA. & Mukhtar H. (2007). Delphinidin, an anthocyanidin in pigmented fruits and vegetables, protects human HaCaT keratinocytes and mouse skin against UVB-mediated oxidative stress and apoptosis. *J Invest Dermatol*, 127:222–32.

Amthor, JS. (2003). Efficiency of lignin biosynthesis: a quantitative analysis. Annals of Botany, 91:673–95.

Antonov, V.; Marek, J.; Bjelkova, M.; Smirous, P. & Fischer, H. (2007). Easily available enzymes as natural retting agents. *Biotechnology Journal*, 2:342–5.

Bae, JY.; Lim. SS.; Kim. SJ.; Choi, JS.; Park. J.; Ju, SM.; Han, SJ.; Kang, I. & Kang YH. (2009). Bog blueberry anthocyanins alleviate photoaging in ultraviolet-B irradiation-induced human dermal fibroblasts. *Mol Nutr Food Res*; 53: 726–38.

Barakat, A.; Bagniewska-Zadworna, A.; Choi. A.; Plakkat, U.; DiLoreto, D.S.; Yellanki, P. & Carlson, J.E. (2009). The cinnamyl alcohol dehydrogenase gene family in Populus: phylogeny, organization, and expression. *BMC Plant Biology*, 9 26.

Barceló-Coblijn, G.; Murphy, E.J.; Othman, R.; Moghadasian, M.H.; Kashour, T. & Friel, J.K. (2008). Flaxseed oil and fish-oil capsule consumption alters human red blood cell n–3 fatty acid composition: a multiple-dosing trial comparing 2 sources of n–3fatty acid. *American Journal of Clinical Nutrition*, Vol. 88, No. 3, 801-809, 0002-9165.

Bax, B. & Müssig, J. (2008). Impact and tensile properties of PLA/Cordenka and PLA/flax composites *Composites Science and Technology*, 68, 7-8, 1601-1607.

Bledzki, AK.; Faruk, O. & Sperber, VE. (2006) Cars from bio-fibers. *Macromolecular Materials and Engineering*, 291:449–57.

Brusselmans, K.; Vrolix, R.; Verhoeven, G. & Swinnen, JV. (2005). Induction of cancer cell apoptosis by flavonoids is associated with their ability to inhibit fatty acid synthase activity. *J Biol Chem*, Feb 18;280(7):5636-45.

Chen, J.; Stavro, PM. & Thompson, LU. (2002). Dietary flaxseed inhibits human breast cancer growth and metastasis and downregulates expression of insulin-like growth factor and epidermal growth factor receptor. *Nutr Cancer*, 43:187–192.

Chen, J-H.; Stoeber, K.; Kingsbury, S.; Ozanne, SE.; Williams, GH. & Hales, CN. (2004). Loss of proliferative capacity and induction of senescence in oxidatively stressed human fibroblasts. *J Biol Chem*, 279: 49439–4.

Chenga, Sh.; Chena, GQ.; Leski, M.; Zoua, B.; Wanga, Y. & Wua, Q. (2006). The effect of D,L-b-hydroxybutyric acid on cell death and proliferation in L929 cells. *Biomaterials*, 27 3758–3765.

Chiang, YM.; Lo, CP.; Chen, YP.; Wang, SY.; Yang, NS.; Kuo, YH. & Shyur LF.(2005). Ethyl caffeate suppresses NF-kappa B activation and its downstream inflammatory mediators, iNOS, COX-2, and PGE2 in vitro or in mouse skin. *Br J Pharmacol*, 146: 352–63.

Choi, Ch.; Kim, S. C.; Hwang, S. S.; Choi, B. K.; Ahn, H. J.; Lee, M. Y.; Park, S. H. & Kim, S. K. (2002). Antioxidant activity and free radical scavenging capacity between. Korean medicinal plants and flavonoids by assay-guided comparison. *Plant Sci.* 163, 1161-1168.

Fujisawa,M.; Watanabe, M.; Choi, S-K.; Teramoto, M.; Ohyama, K. & Misawa, N. (2008). Enrichment of carotenoids in flaxseed (Linum usitatissimum) by metabolic engineering with introduction of bacterial phytoene synthase gene *crtB*. *Journal Of Bioscience And Bioengineering*, Vol. 105, No. 6, 636–641, 1389-1723.

Gershenzon, J. & Dudareva N. (2007). The function of terpene natural products in the natural world. *Nat Chem Biol*, 3(7): 408-14.

Grassmann J. (2005). Terpenoids as plant antioxidants, *Vitam Horm*, 72: 505-35.

Gredes, T.; Kunert-Keil, C.; Wróbel-Kwiatkowska, M.; Heinemann, F.; Dominiak, M.; Gedrange, T. & Szopa J. (2010). The survival and proliferation of fibroblasts on biocomposites contained genetically modified flax fibers: an in vitro study. *Ann. Anat.*, submitted.

Gredes, T.; Dominiak, M.; Gedrange, T.; Kunert-Keil, C.; Wróbel-Kwiatkowska, M. & Szopa J. (2010). The influence of biocomposites containing genetically modified flax fibers on gene expression in rat skeletal muscle. *Biomed Eng*, submitted.

Huang, Y.S.; & Ziboch, V.A. (2001). Gamma-linolenic acid: An Introduction. In: Gamma-Linolenic Acid: Recent Advances in Biotechnology and Clinical Applications, Ed.Y.-S. Huang and V.A. Ziboh, 1-5, AOCS Press, Champaign, IL.

Ilvessalo-Pfaffli, M-S. (1995). Fiber Atlas: Identification of Papermaking Fibers, Springer-Verlag, Berlin, p. 292–337.

Johnson EJ. (2002). The Role of Carotenoids in Human Health, *Nutr Clin Care*, 5(2).

Jones, V.; Grey, J.E. & Harding K.G. (2006). Wound dressings. *BMJ*, 332, 777-780.

K. Saikhun, T. Faisaikarm, Z. Ming, K. H. Lu and Y. Kitiyanant a-Tocopherol and L-ascorbic acid increase the in vitro development of IVM/IVF swamp buffalo (Bubalus bubalis) embryos Animal (2008), 2:10, pp 1486–1490

Kapelusiak-Pielok, M.; Adamczewska-Goncerzewicz, Z.; Dorszewska, J & A. Grochowalska The protective action of alpha-tocopherol on the white matter lipids during moderate hypoxia in rats Folia Neuropathol 2005; 43 (2): 103-108

Kedar N. Prasad, PhD, Bipin Kumar, MD, Xiang-Dong Yan, MD, Amy J. Hanson, MS, William C. Cole, PhD-Tocopheryl Succinate, the Most Effective Form of Vitamin E for Adjuvant Cancer Treatment: A Review Journal of the American College of Nutrition, Vol. 22, No. 2, 108–117 (2003)

Kelly, GS. (1999). Squalene and its potential clinical uses. *Altern Med Rev*, Feb;4(1):29-36.

Klein, TW.; Lane, B.; Newton, CA. & Friedman, H. (2000). The cannabinoid system and cytokine network. *Proc Soc Exp Biol Med*, 225:1-8.

Kulma, A. Skorkowska- Telichowska, K.; Skała, J., Drulis- Kawa, J., Kostyn, K. & Szopa J. (2010). Comparative study of a use of a two fabrics made from transgenic flax for a chronic wound treatment. Submitted.

Lim, EK. &Bowles, DJ.(2004). A class of plant glycosyltransferases involved in cellular homeostasis. *The EMBO Journal*, 23, 2915–2922.

Lorenc- Kukuła, K.; Oszmiański, J.; Doermann, P.; Starzyki, M.; Skała, J.; Żuk, M.; Kulma, A. & Szopa J. (2005). Pleiotropic Effect of Phenolic Compounds Content Increases in Transgenic Flax Plant. *J. Agric. Food Chem*,. 53: p. 3685-3692.

Lorenc-Kukuła, K.; Wróbel-Kwiatkowska, M., Starzycki, M. & Szopa J. (2007). Engineering flax with increased flavonoid content and thus Fusarium resistance. *Physiological and Molecular Plant Pathology*, Vo. 70, Issue 1-3, 38–48, 0885-5765

Lorenc-Kukuła, K.; Żuk, M.; Kulma, A.; Czemplik, M.; Kostyn, K.; Skala, J.; Starzycki, M. & Szopa J. (2009). Enginiering flax with the GT Family I Solanum sogerandinum Gycosyltransferase SsGT1 Confers Increased Resistance to Fusarium Infection. *Agric.Food Chem*, 57(15):6698-705.

Łukaszewicz, M.; Szopa, J. & Krasowska, A. (2004). Susceptibility of lipids from diferent flax cultivars to peroxidation and its lowering by added antioxidants. *Food chemistry*, Vol. 88, 225-23, 0308-8146.

Misra, S.K.; Valappil, S. P.; Roy, I. & Boccaccini, A.R. (2006). Polyhydroxyalkanoate (PHA)/Inorganic Phase Composites for Tissue Enginiering Applications. *Biomacromolecules*, 7, 2249-2258.

Muir, A.D. & Westcott, N.D. (2003). *Flax: The genus Linum*. Taylor & Francis Inc, 0-415-30807-0, New York.

Munné-Bosch S The role of alpha-tocopherol in plant stress tolerance. J Plant Physiol. 2005 Jul;162(7):743-8.

Musialak, M.; Wróbel-Kwiatkowska, M.; Kulma, A.; Starzycka, E. & Szopa, J. (2008). Improving retting of fibre through genetic modification of flax to express pectinases. *Transgenic Research*, 17, 133-147, DOI: 10.1007/s11248-007-9080-4.

Pacher, P.; Batkai, S. & Kunos, G. (2006). The endocannabinoid system as an emerging target of pharmacotherapy. *Pharmacol Rev*, 58:389–462.

Peijs, T. (2002). Composites turn green! *E-Polymers*, available at http://www.e-polymers.org

Pellizzon, MA.; Billheimer, JT.; Bloedon, LT.; Szapary, PO. & Rader, DJ. (2007). Flaxseed reduces plasma cholesterol levels in hypercholesterolemic mouse models. Journal of the American College of Nutrition, 26(1):66–75.

Peltier, S.; Oger, JM.; Lagarce, F.; Couet, W. & Benoît JP. (2006). Enhanced Oral Paclitaxel Bioavailability After Administration of Paclitaxel-Loaded Lipid Nanocapsules. *Pharm Res.*, 23(6): 1243-50.

Prescha, A.; Siger, A.; Lorenc-Kukuła, K.; Biernat,J.; Nogala-Kałucka, M. & Szopa J. (2008). Badania nad składem i podatnością na utlenianie oleju z nasion lnu modyfikowanego genetycznie. *Bromat. Chem. Toksykol*, - XLI, 2008, 3, 286–292.

Ramakrishna, S.; Huang, Z.M.; Kumar, G.V.; Batchelor, A.W. & Mayer J. (2004). An introduction to biocomposites, Series on Biomaterials and Bioengineering, Vol.1. Imperial College Press, London.

Reddy, LH. & Couvreur ,P. (2009). Squalene: A natural triterpene for use in disease management and therapy *Adv Drug Deliv Rev.*, 2009 Dec 17;61(15):1412-26.

Rezwan, K.; Chen, Q.Z.; Blaker, J.J. & Boccaccini, A.R. (2006). Biodegradable and bioactive porous polymer/inorganic composite scaffolds for bone tissue engineering. *Biomaterials*, 27, 3413–3431.

Ross, JA. & Kasum, CM. (2002). Dietary flavonoids: bioavailability, metabolic effects, and safety. Annu Rev Nutr., 22:19-34.

Rowland, G. G. (1991) An EMS-induced low-linolenic-acid mutant in McGregor flax (Linum usitatissimum L.). *Canadian Journal of Plant Science*, Vol. 71, 2, 393-396, 0008-4220.

Saffron, A. (2008). Whitehead, Suman Rice. Phytoestrogens oestrogen synthesis and breast cancer. Journal of Steroid Biochemistry & Molecular Biology, 108, :186–195.

Saravanan, P.; Davidson, NC.; Schmidt, EB. & Calder PC. (2010). Cardiovascular effects of marine omega-3 fatty acids. The Lancet, 376, 9740, 540 – 550.

Saremi A, Arora R.Vitamin E and Cardiovascular Disease. Am J Ther. 2009 May 15

Siemieniuk, E. & Skrzydlewska, E. (2005). Coenzyme Q10: its biosynthesis and biological signifi cance in animal organisms and in humans. Postepy Hig Med Dosw. (online in polish), 59: 150-159.

Simopoulos, A.P. (2002). The importance of the ratio of omega-6/ omega-3 essential fatty acids. *Biomedicine and Pharmacotheraphy*, 56, 365-379.

Singh U, Jialal I.Anti-inflammatory effects of alpha-tocopherol. Ann N Y Acad Sci. 2004 Dec;1031:195-203.

Sirikantaramas, S.; Taura, F.; Morimoto, S. & Shoyama, Y. (2007). Recent advances in Cannabis sativa research: biosynthetic studies and its potential in biotechnology. *Curr Pharm Biotechnol*, 8(4), August, 237-43.

Skorkowska- Telichowska, K A.; Bugajska-Prusak, P.; Plucinski, Z.; Rybak, & Szopa, J. (2009). Physiology and pathology of a chronic wounds and its local treatment according to current medical knowledge (review in polish). *Dermatologia Praktyczna*, 5, 15-29.

Skorkowska- Telichowska, K.; Żuk, M.; Kulma, A.; Bugajska- Prusak, A.; Ratajczak, K. Gasiorowski, K.; Kostyn, K. & Szopa J. (2010). New dressing material derived from transgenic flax product to tread long-standig venous ulcers- a pilot study. *Woud Repair and Reg*, 18, 168-179.

Steinbüchel, A. & Füchtenbusch, B. (1998). Bacterial and other biological systems for polyester production. *Trends in Biotechnology* 16, 419-427.

Suddel, BC. & Evans, WJ. (2003). The increasing use and application of natural fiber Composite materials within the automotive industry, *Seventh Composite Conference on Woodfiber–Plastic Composites*, 7–14, Madison, WI, USA, 19–20 May, 2003.

Szopa, J.; Wróbel-Kwiatkowska, M.; Kulma, A.; Żuk, M., Skórkowska-Telichowska, K.; Dymińska, L.; Mączka, M.; Hanuza, J.; Żebrowski, J. & Preisner, M. (2009). Chemical composition and molecular structure of fibers from transgenic flax producing polyhydroxybutyrate, and mechanical properties and platelet aggregation of composite materials containing these fibers. Composites Science and Technology, 69, 2438–2446.

Thompson, LU.; Robb, P.; Serraino, M. & Cheung F. (1991). Mammalian lignan production from various foods. *Nutr Cancer*, 16:43–52.

Thompson, LU,.; Rickard, SE.; Orcheson, LJ. & Seidl, MM. (1996). Flaxseed and its lignan and oil components reduce mammary tumor growth at a late stage of carcinogenesis. *Carcinogenesis* 17:1373–1376.

Thompson, LU. (1998). Experimental studies on lignans and cancer. *Baillieres Clin Endocrinol Metab*, 12:691–705.

Thompson, LU & Ward, WE. (2002). Flaxseed lignans: health benefits, bioavailability, and safety. In: Gilani GS, Anderson JB, Eds. *Phytoestrogens and Health*. Champaign, IL: AOCS Press, 405–426,.

Tobias, CM. & Chow, EK. (2005). Structure of the cinnamyl alcohol dehydrogenase gene family in rice and promoter activity of a member associated with lignification. *Planta*, 220:678–88.

Wahle, K.W.J.; Heys S.D. & Rotondo D. (2004) Conjugated linoleic acids: are they beneficial or detrimental to health? *Progress in Lipid Research*, Vol. 43, Issue 6, 553-587, 0163-7827.

Wall, I.B.; M.R.; Baird D.M.; Kipling, D.; Giles, P.; Laffafian, I.; Price, P.E.; Thomas, D.W. & Stephens P. (2008). Fibroblast dysfunction is a key factor in the non-healing of chronic venous leg ulcers. *J.Invest.Dermatol.* Oct;128(10):2526-40.

Wang, L.; Chen, J. & Thompson LU. (2005). The inhibitory effect of flaxseed on the growth and metastasis of estrogen receptor negative human breast cancer xenograftsis attributed to both its lignan and oil components. *International Journal of Cancer*, 116(5):793–8.

Wong, S.; Shanks, R. & Hodzic A. (2004). Interfacial improvements in poly(3-hydroxybutyrate)-flax fibre composites with hydrogen bonding additives. *Compos Sci Technol*, 64:1321–30.

Wróbel, M.; Żebrowki, J. & Szopa J. (2004). Polyhydroxybutyrate synthesis in transgenic flax. J.Biotechnol, 107, 41-54.

Wróbel-Kwiatkowska, M.; Starzycki, M.; Zebrowski, J.; Oszmiannski, J. & Szopa J. (2006). Lignin deficiency in transgenic flax resulted in plants with improved mechanical properties. *Journal of Biotechnology* ,128:919–34.

Wróbel-Kwiatkowska, M.; Starzycki, M.; Żebrowski, J.; Oszmiański, J. & Szopa J. (2007). Engineering of PHB synthesis causes improved elastic properties of flax fibers. *Biotechnol.Prog.*, 23 269-277.

Wróbel-Kwiatkowska, M.; Skórkowska-Telichowska, K.; Dymińska, L.; Mączka, M.; Hanuza, J. & Szopa, J. (2009). Biochemical, mechanical, and spectroscopic analyses of genetically engineered flax fibers producing bioplastic (poly-β-hydroxybutyrate). *Biotechnol Prog*, Sep-Oct;25(5):1489-98.

Yamamoto K, Niki E. Interaction of alpha-tocopherol with iron: antioxidant and prooxidant effects of alpha-tocopherol in the oxidation of lipids in aqueous dispersions in the presence of iron. Biochim Biophys Acta. 1988 Jan 19;958(1):19-23.

Yan, J.; Xiao-Tao, L. & Guo-Qiang, Ch. (2008). Interactions between a poly(3-hydroxybutyrate-co-3-hydroxyvalerate-co-3-hydroxyhexanoate) terpolyester and human keratinocytes. *Biomaterials*, 29, 3807–3814.

Zhang, J.; Henriksson, G. & Johansson, G. (2000). Polygalacturonase is the key component in enzymatic retting of flax. *Journal of Biotechnology*, 81(1):85–9.

18

Characterization of Hydroxyapatite Blocks for Biomedical Applications

Masoume Haghbin Nazarpak[1],
Mehran Solati-Hashjin[2] and Fatollah Moztarzadeh[2]
[1]*New Technologies Research Center, Amirkabir University of Technology,*
[2]*Department of Biomedical Engineering, Amirkabir University of Technology,*
Iran

1. Introduction

There is an increasing demand for materials to be used in biomedical and dental applications. These materials are currently implemented in different forms, depending on the part of the body which needs repair. Biocompatibility, biofunctionality, and availability are three significant factors in selecting materials (L.L. Hench, 1998).

Historically, ceramics are the oldest materials in medical applications. Tricalcium phosphate (TCP) was used for repairing bone defects in the early 20th century (M. Bohner, 2000; T. Cuneyt, et al. 1997; J.G.J. Peelen, et al. 1987). Although, ceramics are brittle by nature, they have excellent compressive strength and a high wear resistance. Calcium phosphate compounds such as hydroxyapatite (HA), tricalcium phosphate (TCP), dicalcium phosphate dihydrate (DCPD), dicalcium phosphate anhydrous (DCPA), and tetracalcium phosphate (TTCP) (L.L. Hench, 1998; M. Bohner, 2000; T. Cuneyt, et al. 1997; J.G.J. Peelen, et al. 1987; C. Laverinia & J.M. Schoenung, 1991; M. Komath, et al. 2000; S.Takagi, et al. 1998) have almost the same chemical compositions as bone minerals. When these compounds are implanted into the living body (*in vivo*) for a period of time, they create a strong chemical bond with bone tissue (P. Luo, et al. 1998; H.H. Pham, et al. 1999).

In replacing bone defects, besides all compatibility parameters, the material should possess the same porosity as the bone. Bone has a complex structure with macro- and micro-pores. Pores are mostly interconnected to allow body fluids to carry nutrients and provide a medium where interfacial reactions between hard tissue and soft tissue can occur. An implant material should generally present similar properties to that of the bone. However, mechanical requirements dictate a high strength for implants which is associated with the elimination of some pores from them. As a result, reducing the porosity should result in an increase on the mechanical properties of HA as with any other ceramics. It is therefore important to find an optimum porosity to maintain the mechanical strength while pores provide the bone implant with an acceptable channel for nutrition to obtain the best implant properties (M. Jarcho, 1981; J.C. Le Hiec, et al. 1995).

The aim of the present work was to find the effect of sintering temperature on the microstructure, phase composition and the mechanical properties of hydroxyapatite ceramics.

2. Materials and methods

Medical grade hydroxyapatite powder was obtained from Sigma-Aldrich Chemical Company. The density of the powder was measured as 2.91 g/cm^3 using ACCU-PYC 1330 (Micromeritics Gemini 2375). In order to determine the sintering temperature, a dilatometry test was performed. Also, the X-ray diffraction technique was employed using a Siemens, D500 diffractometer at each sintering temperature to estimate the probable phase transformations and the upper limit of the decomposition temperature. The particle size distribution was measured using a Fritsch Analysette22 system. The starting powder was uniaxially compacted at 86 MPa to form cylindrical shaped samples 55* 13 mm. The sintering was performed in air at 700-1300 °C with 1 hour soaking time. The rate of temperature increase was 10 °Kh^{-1} while the cooling was carried out in the furnace. The mechanical properties of sintered bodies were examined by 3 and 4 point bending techniques using an Instron Universal Testing Machine 1196 was used with a cross head speed of 0.5 mm/min and maximum load application of 5 kN. Vickers hardness of specimens was measured using Vickers hardness testing device (Hardness Tester Akashi AVK cll) under 300 g loading at 20 seconds. Fracture toughness also was determined using Evans & Charles equation. The microstructures of the samples were studied under different sintering conditions using a Cambridge Stereosacn 360 scanning electron microscope.

3. Results and discussion

Figure 1 shows the particle size distribution. It is evident that the average size of the powder was around 4 micrometre. The particle size and specific surface area of the starting powder are the most important parameters affecting the sintering behavior of ceramics. By reducing the particle size and increasing the specific surface area, the same degree of sintering can be achieved at much lower temperatures.

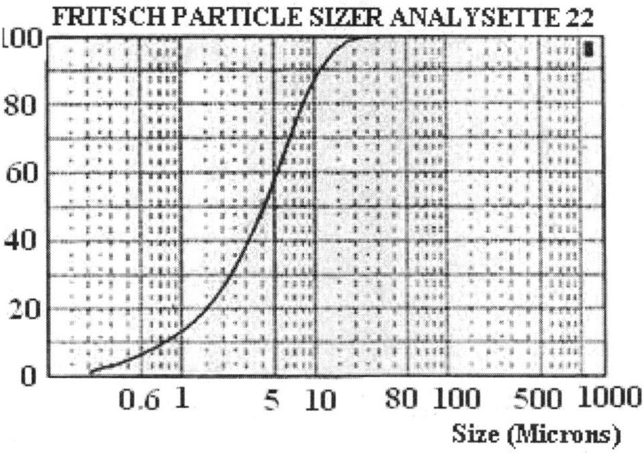

Fig. 1. Particle size distribution of the hydroxyapatite powder

The specific surface area of the starting powder was measured as 52.3 m^2/g which compared with other commercial powders can be considered as an active powder. The

molar ratio of Ca/P is another important parameter which is 1.5 in tricalcium phosphate, 2 in tetra calcium phosphate, and 1.67 in stoichiometric hydroxyapatite (A. Siddharthan, et al. 2005). The molar ratio of the Ca/P in the present powder was measured with the ICP technique at around 1.62. A ratio less than 1.64 will be interpreted as the creation of pores and voids in a sintered body. A ratio higher than 1.67 means that the rate of absorption in vivo will be increased (P. Vincenzini, 1986).
In order to gain insights into the sintering behavior of hydroxyapatite, dilatometric tests were carried out. Figure 2 shows a typical curve which indicates the shrinkage starts at about 700 °C and the sintering temperature is estimated to be between 900 and 1300 °C (K.A. Hing, et al. 2000; A.J. Ruys, et al. 1995; B.J. Meenan, et al. 2000; L.L. Hench, 1991; M. Jarcho, et al. 1976; M.K. Sinha, et al. 2000; A.J. Ruys, et al. 1995; G. De With, et al. 1981; P. Landuyt, et al. 1995; M.Y. Shareef et al. 1993; J. Zhou, et al. 1993).

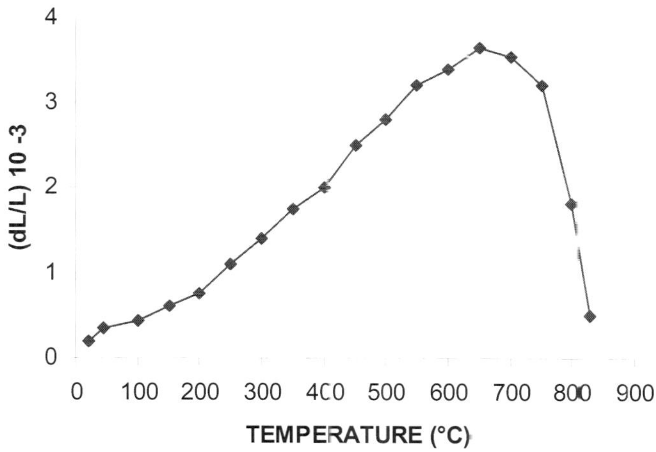

Fig. 2. Dilatometry measurement for a hydroxyapatite sample.

XRD results of the sintered samples are shown in figure 3a to 3d. As it is evident from these patterns, within the sintering range of 700-1300 °C, no other phases could be detected by XRD and the results confirmed formation of hydroxyapatite phase. Also, the CaO phase was checked for in particular to be absent since this phase has been shown to have negative effects on the growth of bone cells (K.A. Hing, et al. 2000).
The Vickers hardness of specimens was measured through indentation method. The results showed rising hardness from 1.5 to 6.1 GPa with increasing sintering temperature from 1100 ° C to 1300 ° C that is shown in Figure 4. Fracture toughness of samples was also calculated from Evans & Charles equation was approximately between 0.5 and 0.85 $MPam^{1/2}$ at sintering temperature about 1200° C.
In order to make microscopic studies, samples were etched in 1% phosphoric acid and gold sputtered prior to study by SEM studies. Figure 5 shows scanning electron microscope images of hydroxyapatite sintered at different temperatures. In all cases, the sintered samples were highly polished with different grades of polish; the last one being 1 micrometre of diamond paste.

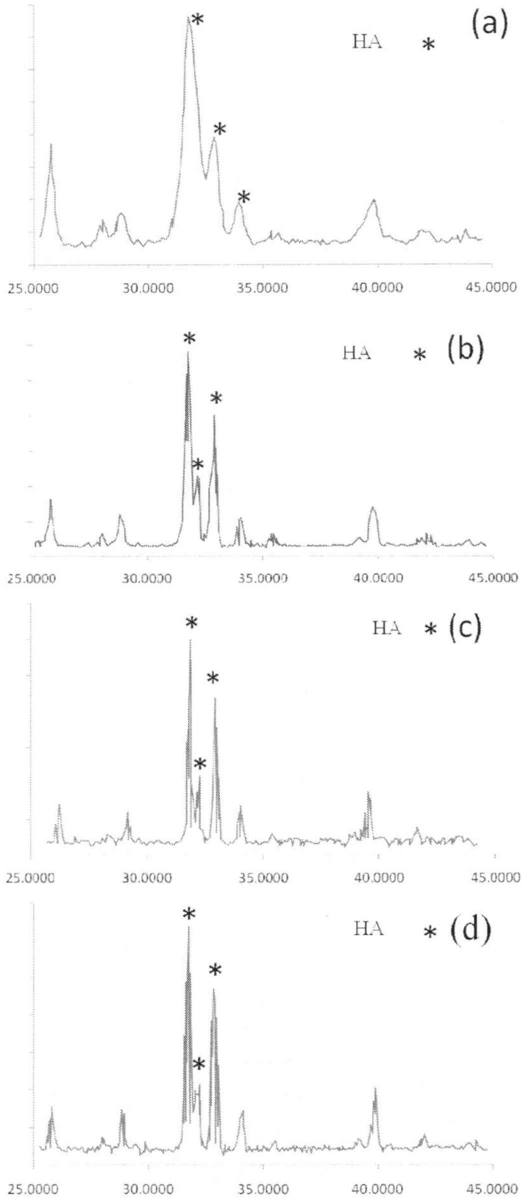

Fig. 3. X-ray diffraction pattern of: a) starting powder, b) fired at 900 °C for 1 hour, c) fired at 1100 °C for 1 hour, d) fired at 1300 °C for 1 hour.

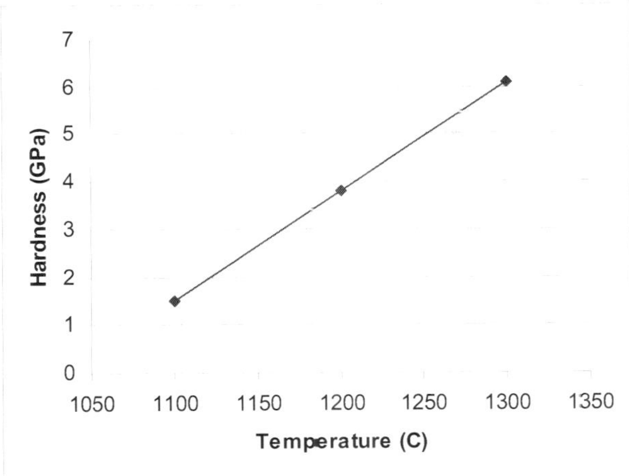

Fig. 4. Vickers hardness changes with increasing temperature

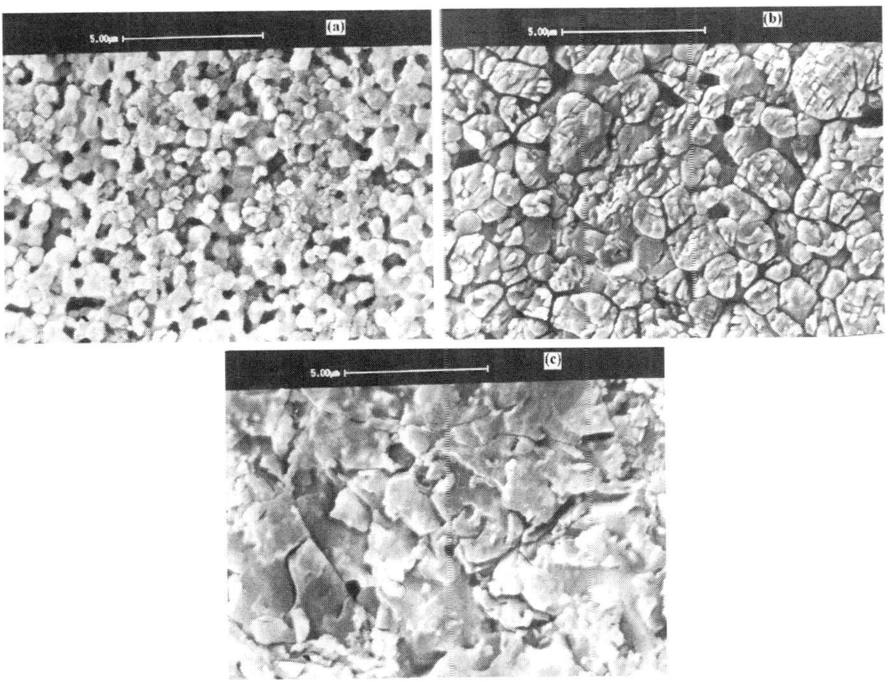

Fig. 5. Scanning electron micrographs of hydroxyapatite sintered for one hour at a) 1100 °C b) 1200 °C and c) 1300 °C.

As is evident from figure 5(a), when the samples were fired at 1100 °C, hardly any changes in grain size could be observed. Sintering at 1200 °C results in grain growth in the microstructure of samples as is shown in figure 5(b). The grain growth is also associated with a reduction in the apparent porosity which is a favorable condition as far as the mechanical strength of the part is concerned

Figure 5(c) shows an electron micrograph of a sample sintered at 1300 °C. Further grain growth is evident and a higher mechanical strength is expected for this sample which is in accordance with bending strength results.

The mechanical properties of sintered bodies were examined by 3 and 4 point bending techniques after samples polished with emery paper and diamond paste. An Instron Universal Testing Machine 1196 was used with a cross head speed of 0.5 mm/minute and maximum load application of 5 kN. In fact, in many cases, the mechanical properties of the samples were improved when they were fired at higher temperatures as is demonstrated in figures 6 a and b.

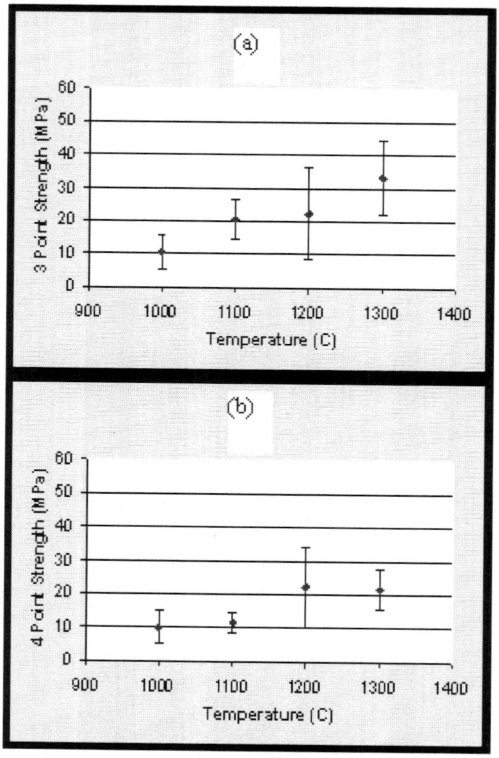

Fig. 6. Bending strength against sintering temperature a) 3 point and b) 4 point.

4. Conclusions

The present study revealed that the sintering of hydroxyapatite at 1100- 1300 °C results in an essentially porous body which can be used as an implant. XRD diffraction patterns of the sintered ceramics proved that no additional phase formation takes place even at elevated temperatures.

Mechanical measurements proved that the bending strength of the sintered bodies were between 7-44 MPa which improved proportional with sintering temperature. Microstructural studies showed that while the grain size of the bodies sintered at 1100 °C remained basically comparable to the particle size of the starting powder, ceramics fired at 1200 to 1300 °C showed an increase in grain size in line with the increased temperature.

5. References

Bohner M., *Injury Int. J. Care Injured.* 31 (2000): S-D37-47.

Cuneyt T., Korkusuz F., Timucin M. and Akkas N., *J. Mater. Sci.: Med.* 8 (1997) 91-96.

De With G., Van Dijk H.J.A., Hattu U., and Prijs K., *J. Mater. Sci.* 16 (1981) 1592-1598.

Hench L.L., *J. Am. Ceram. Soc.* 74 [7] (1991) 1487–1510.

Hench L.L., Bioceramics. *J. Am. Ceram. Soc.* 81[7] (1998)1705-1728.

Hing K.A., Gibson I.R., Revell P.A., Best S.M. and Bonfield W., *Key Eng. Mater.* 192-1 (2000) 373-376.

Jarcho M., Bolen C.H., Thomas M.B., Bobick J., Kay J.F. and Doremus R. H., *J. Mater. Sci.* 11 (1976) 2027-2035.

Jarcho M., *Clin Orthop* (1981) 259–78.

Komath M., Varma H. K. and Sivakumar R., *Bull. Mater. Sci.*, Vol. 23, No. 2 (2000) 135–140.

Landuyt P., Li F., Keustermans J. P., Streydio J. M., Delannay F. and Munting E., *J. Mater. Sci. Mat. Med* 16 (1995) 8-13.

Laverinia C. and Schoenung J.M., *Ceramic Bulletin;* Vol. 70, No.1 (1991) 95-100.

Le Hiec J.C., Schaeverbeke T., Clement D., Faber J. and Le Rebeller A., *Biomaterials* 16 (1995) 113-118.

Luo P., Liu N. and Thelen M., Proc. *24th Annual Meeting of the Society for Biomaterials,* Vol. 21 (1998) 278.

Meenan B.J., Boyd A., Love E. and Akay M., *Key Eng Mater* 192/196 (2000) 15–18.

Peelen J.G.J., Rejda B.V. and De Groot K., *Ceramurgia Int.* 4 (1987) 71-74.

Pham H.H., Luo P., Genin F. and Dash A.K., AAPS *Pharm Sci. 1999;1(suppl):S-373.*

Ruys A.J., Brandwood A., Milthorpe B.K., Dickson M.R., Zeigler K.A. and Sorrell C.C., *J. Mater. Sci: Mat. Med.* 6 (1995) 297-301.

Ruys A.J., Wei M., Sorrell C.C., Dickson M.R., Brandwood A. and Milthorpe B.K., *Biomaierials* 16 (1995) 409-415.

Shareef M.Y., Messer P.F. and van Noort R., *Biomaterials* 14 (1993) 69-75.

Siddharthan A., Seshadri S. K. and Sampath Kumar T. S., *Trends Biomater. Artif. Organs,* Vol 18 (2) (2005) 110-113.

Sinha M.K., Basu D., Sen P.S., *Interceram,* Vol. 49, No.2 (2000) 102-105.

Takagi S., chow L.C. and Ishikawa K., *Biomaterials,* 19 (1998) 1593-9.

Vincenzini P. (Ed.), *Proceedings of the International Symposium on Bioceramics (BIOTEC)*, Milan, Italy Vol. 39 (1986) Elsevier.

Zhou J., Zhang X., Chen J., Zeng S. and Groot K., *J. Mater. Sci: Mat. Med* 4 (1993) 83-85.

Part 6

Advances in Diagnostics

19

The Use of Phages and Aptamers as Alternatives to Antibodies in Medical and Food Diagnostics

Jaytry Mehta[1,2], Bieke Van Dorst[1,2], Lisa Devriese[2]
Elsa Rouah-Martin[1,2], Karen Bekaert[2], Klaartje Somers[3],
Veerle Somers[3], Marie-Louise Scippo[4],
Ronny Blust[1] and Johan Robbens[1,2]

[1]*University of Antwerp, Department of Biology, Laboratory of Ecophysiology, Biochemistry and Toxicology, Groenenborgerlaan 171, 2020 Antwerp*
[2]*Institute for Agricultural and Fisheries research (ILVO), Ankerstraat 1, 8400 Oostende*
[3]*Hasselt University, Biomedical Research Institute, B-3590 Diepenbeek*
[4]*University of Liège, Food Sciences Department, B-4000 Liège*
Belgium

1. Introduction

In the post-genomic and proteomic era, there is a better understanding of important physiological components such as DNA, RNA, proteins and small biological molecules, all of which have proven to be the mediums of disease progression Identification and investigation of disease-specific biomarkers in the initial stage of a disease can greatly increase accuracy in diagnosis, treatment and even prevention. This approach offers great potential to significantly reduce disease-related mortality rates. There is an increasing need in the medical field for rapid, cheap and reliable diagnostic systems in order to detect all the well-known and recently identified biomarkers for different diseases. This identification is not a trivial exercise because these disease biomarkers are present in minute quantities in physiological conditions such as the bloodstream or body fluids, which are often contaminated with many other compounds that can hinder detection. Apart from biomarker diagnosis, another area of concern for human health has been food contamination. Trading of contaminated food between countries and high population mobility increases the potential for outbreaks and health risks posed by microbial pathogens and toxins in food. Food safety has become a global health goal. Periodic toxin and microbiological analyses of food samples are important to diagnose and prevent problems related to health and food safety. However, food-borne pathogens are mostly present in very low numbers among various other microorganisms, making their detection difficult. To be able to detect these disease carriers and biomarkers in their natural conditions, highly sensitive as well as specific recognition elements are required. It is necessary to develop detection techniques that are reliable, fast, easy, sensitive, selective, cost-effective and also suitable for real time, *in situ* monitoring. Such techniques to detect pathogens and biomarkers would not only improve clinical success rates but also offer a great commercial advantage to the medical field and the food industry.

Conventional techniques for the detection of disease biomarkers, pathogens and toxins are immunology-based methods, polymerase chain reaction (PCR) based methods and culture and colony counting methods. Though these standard detection methods are sensitive, they lag behind in terms of detection time, taking from several hours to days to yield a response (Velusamy et al. 2010). Conventional analytical techniques like optical, chromatographic and electrochemical detection are faster, but have some limitations of equipment and cost. Furthermore, they are complicated and require highly trained personnel and extensive sample preparation. These constraints do not always allow frequent, real time or *in situ* monitoring of food or clinical samples. Thus, demands of high sensitivity, specificity, cost-effective, portable and rapid analyses have propelled the development of biosensors as novel diagnostic tools in the medical and food sectors.

Many diagnostic tools still rely on immunoassays and especially enzyme-linked immunosorbent assay (ELISA). Besides these classical tests, several phage and aptamer based sensors have also been proposed for a broad range of disease biomarkers or carriers such as antibodies, viruses, disease-related proteins, tumour cells, toxins and pathogens, among several others. The precise detection of these biomarkers or carriers before the onset of a disease can significantly revolutionise the medical field by providing cheap, fast, simple and easily produced diagnostic tests using phages and aptamers as their recognition elements. The wide range of assays that employ phages or aptamers to detect important clinical molecules, highlights the potential of these new receptors in clinical diagnostic tests and in food biosensors.

This chapter will define phages and aptamers and discuss their use as novel biorecognition elements in biosensors. We discuss two relevant cases in the field of biosensors: the use of diagnostics for clinical testing and the use of biosensors for food-related testing.

2. Biosensors

A biosensor is defined by the IUPAC as a self-contained integrated device that is capable of providing specific quantitative or semi-quantitative analytical information using a biological recognition element (biochemical receptor), which is retained in direct spatial contact with a transduction element.

Biosensors can be categorised by the type of recognition element used, such as enzymatic, whole cell or affinity-based biosensors. Enzymes are proteins that catalyse specific chemical reactions and were the first molecular recognition elements to be included in biosensors. They are attractive sensor recognition elements because their use can convert the analyte into a sensor-detectable product, evaluate the modification of enzyme properties upon interaction with the analyte or detect an analyte that acts as the enzyme inhibitor or activator. In fact, the most widely studied and acclaimed sensor success story is that of the glucose biosensor, an enzymatic sensor (Newman & Turner 2005; Wang 2007). Whole-cell biosensors, the next classification of biosensors, often use a genetically engineered cell of either eukaryotic or prokaryotic origin, containing responsive transcriptional promoter elements as the biological component. These whole cell biosensors are used for the profiling of the toxicological effects of compounds and for risk assessment of chemical contaminants or of new compounds (Robbens et al. 2010). The third type of biosensors which are of higher relevance for diagnostics, are affinity-based biosensors. In these, the affinity-based receptor molecule binds the analyte irreversibly and non-catalytically. The binding event between the target molecule and the bioreceptor, triggers a physicochemical change that can be measured by a transducer. In order to 'visualise' the binding event, the different transduction methods that are frequently used in these biosensors are optical, electrochemical or mass-based.

When the detection system requires a biomolecular recognition event, antibody-based detection methodologies are considered the standard assays in clinical analysis (Aizawa 1994; Stefan et al. 2000). These assays are well established and have been demonstrated to reach the required sensitivity and selectivity. However, the use of antibodies *in situ* detection methods and in the analysis of very complex samples could encounter some limitations mainly deriving from the nature and synthesis of these protein receptors. Antibodies are relatively cheap, but their production relies on the immune response of an animal. Besides the ethical problems related to the use of animals, it is also difficult to generate antibodies for toxic compounds or small compounds that cannot elicit an immune response. In order to avoid some of these drawbacks, recent advances in biotechnology, nanotechnology and surface chemistry offer the possibility of developing other novel, affinity-based recognition molecules that have been explored as alternatives to the traditionally used antibodies. This is a domain in which phages and aptamers can play a successful role. They have emerged as viable options thanks to their high selectivity and affinity towards their targets, comparable to that of antibodies. The high affinity and hence high sensitivity, high specificity, robustness, animal-friendly production and ease of modification are some of the defining properties that make the use of aptamers and phages advantageous in diagnostic and biosensing tools (Van Dorst et al. 2010b).

3. Phages

Phages are viruses that use their host bacterial cells as factories for their own replication and have the ability to display peptides or proteins on their surfaces. This technology is called phage display. Phage display can be used as a powerful tool to screen for affinity reagents for all kind of targets, ranging from small molecules to proteins and even cells. This selection can be performed by using phage libraries consisting of a high number of different phages (10^8 - 10^{10}), each displaying a different peptide or protein on its surface. Among the huge number of phages in these phage libraries, the ones with high affinity and specificity for a target can be isolated in an affinity selection procedure (Fig. 1). Moreover, the proteins and peptides displayed on these selected phages can be identified by sequencing the gene coding for the displayed protein or peptide. This coding gene can be found in the single-stranded DNA (ssDNA) inside the selected phage. The target specific phages can be used as affinity reagents in diagnostic tests. Besides the target specific phages, the soluble peptides or proteins, released from the phage coat, can also be used as affinity reagents. These peptides or proteins are then produced synthetically or by recombinant expression in bacterial cells.

Different types of phage libraries exist, displaying different types of peptides or proteins: peptides, cellular proteins (from cDNA libraries) or antibody fragments, like single chain variable fragments (scFv) and antigen binding fragment (Fab). **Antibody fragment phage libraries** are used commonly in immunology (Hoogenboom et al. 1998). Their wide diversity enables them to imitate the natural immune system. Phage display enables the production of sizeable amounts of the affinity reagents, avoiding the batch to batch

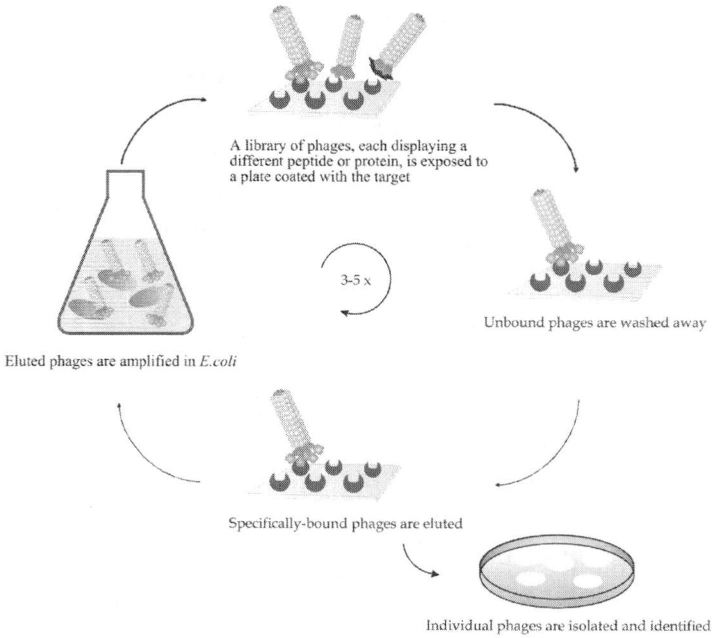

Fig. 1. Schematic representation of the phage affinity selection procedure (Van Dorst et al. 2010a)

variations which occur with classical antibodies. Moreover, there is no immune response required to produce affinity reagents for a target, making the selection of affinity reagents for poorly immunogenic targets possible. **Peptide phage libraries** can also be used to select affinity reagents, since the binding site, or epitope, only involves a few amino acids. Besides the monovalent phages that display one peptide on the phage surface, so-called landscape phages are also used as affinity reagents. These landscape phages display thousands of copies of peptides in a dense, repeating pattern around the tubular capsid (Petrenko & Smith 2000). The display of these thousands of peptides gives the phage surface different characteristics. The binding affinity of the landscape phages for the target is not determined by the affinity of one of these peptides alone, but by the whole structure. In **cDNA phage libraries**, cellular proteins are displayed on the surface of the phages. These cDNA phage libraries are frequently used for protein interaction studies (Crameri & Kodzius 2001; Pelletier & Sidhu 2001; Li & Caberoy 2010; Van Dorst et al. 2010c). Furthermore, they can be used as affinity reagents in diagnostic tests to detect antibodies for cellular proteins and to diagnose autoimmune diseases.

4. Aptamers

Aptamers are small sequences of nucleic acids, RNA or DNA, and more rarely peptide chains, able to specifically recognise a given target, ranging from small molecules to entire organisms (bacteria). The term *aptamer* derives from the Latin word *aptus* meaning *fitted* or *suitable,* and the Greek word *meros* meaning *part* or *portion,* referring to the folding properties of single-stranded nucleic acids, responsible for their specific tridimensional structure. This hairpin structure can bind targets so tightly that some aptamers can even differentiate between two isomers, or closely related molecules. For instance, an aptamer selected for theophylline has shown that its binding affinity was 10,000-fold more important for theophylline than caffeine, only differing in structure by a methyl-group (Jenison et al. 1994). In this application of nucleic acids in biotechnology, the recognition is based on the tridimensional structure of the aptamer, more than its sequence. Aptamers undergo significant conformational changes upon target binding, thus offering great flexibility in design of novel biosensors; for instance, being formatted into molecular beacon structures (Yamamoto et al. 2000a).

Aptamers are selected from synthetic nucleic acid libraries which can contain more than 10^{15} different sequences, by an *in vitro* selection procedure commonly called SELEX, an acronym for Systematic Evolution of Ligands by EXponential enrichment (Stoltenburg et al. 2007). This iterative process consists of binding and elution steps of aptamers in contact with the molecule or organism of interest, copying the resulting aptamers by using PCR and finally separating the two strands obtained after the polymerisation (Fig. 2). After each cycle, the pool is enriched and used for the next selection cycle, until the amount of eluted aptamers reaches 80 to 90% of the initial amount of the pool. Usually, eight to fifteen selection cycles are needed to isolate aptamers with a high binding potential. Once a specific aptamer is selected for a target, this recognition element can be integrated into a transducing structure or device, in order to construct a biosensor.

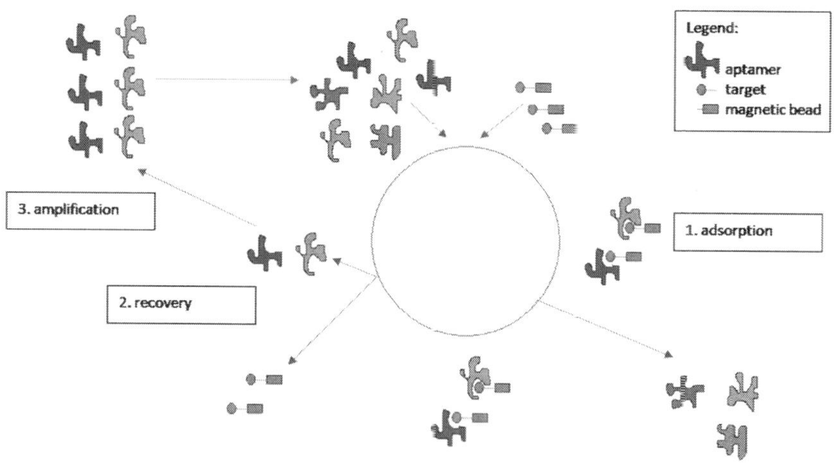

Fig. 2. Selection of aptamers via SELEX procedure (Van Dorst et al. 2010b)

5. Advantages and limitations of phages and aptamers

The use of both, phages and aptamers, as affinity reagents in diagnostic tests have some distinct advantages:

- High sensitivity and specificity for targets

Phages and aptamers are selected from their respective libraries which have a very wide diversity, even higher than that of antibody repertoires screened with the hybridoma technique. Strong selection conditions and counter selections with related targets result in specific binding phages and aptamers with high affinity. Moreover, the sensitivity and specificity of the selected phages can be increased with genetic modification (Sheedy et al. 2007). On the other hand, the selection process for aptamers can be directed to recognise specific structural or chemical motifs of the target, which is not always possible with antibodies. Phages and aptamers can both recognise their targets in ranges below nanomolar amounts, sometimes even down to picomolar ranges (Collett et al. 2005; Zhu et al. 2008).

- Fast, inexpensive and animal-friendly production

Phages are produced by infecting bacteria, a process which takes only a few hours and no animals need to be immunised; nucleic acid production is completely animal-free too, as it is chemically synthesised on a large scale. Thus both techniques avoid batch-to-batch variations, are very cost-effective and are reproducible.

- Stability

Phages are stable in a wide variety of conditions: at high temperatures (Brigati & Petrenko 2005) and in a wide pH range from 3 to 11 (Jepson & March 2004; Verma et al. 2009). Moreover, phages can even resist nucleases or proteases (Schwind et al. 1992). Their high degree of stability not only offers technical, but also economic advantages. The degree of stability extends the lifetime of diagnostic tests and reduces transport costs by avoiding the need for cooled shipment and storage.

Nucleic acids allow the use of a wide variety of buffers and organic solvents, which can be interesting for monitoring organic compounds. Indeed, nucleic acids remain stable in hydrogen bond forming solvents such as ethylene glycol, methanol, formamide, dimethyl sulfoxide or acetamide (Bonner & Klibanov 2000). As opposed to their protein counterparts, aptamers can be selected under nonphysiological conditions or real matrix conditions, which is particularly useful for biosensing clinical and food samples.

- Ease of modification

Phages are easily modified, because of the accessible amine groups on the phage coat protein VIII. Via these amine groups, phages can be immobilised or conjugated to labelling molecules (Jin et al. 2009).

Aptamers can easily bear labels at each end of the strand. For instance, reporter molecules such as enzymes or fluorophores, were used in the development of aptamer biosensors (Tombelli et al. 2005b). A wide variety of labels can also be used with nucleic acid to be immobilised onto different surfaces. Nucleic acid biotinylation is a technique widely spread in biotechnologies, based on the strong bond between biotin and avidin (or streptavidin). This allows nucleic acids to be fixed to almost any type of streptavidin-modified surfaces, which are in many cases commercially available. Alternatively, nucleic acid can be labelled with phosphate, amine or thiol moieties enabling a covalent immobilisation of the nucleic acid probe.

- Reusability

This is an advantage unique to aptamers. Unlike antibodies, aptamers can undergo several cycles of denaturation and regeneration. This allows aptasensor platforms to be recyclable and reusable.

Though phage and aptamer technology hold great promise, there are limitations:

- Unavailability of standardised protocols: For each new target, specific modifications are usually necessary. Moreover, protocols have to be adjusted and parameters often have to be optimised before the selection technique offers significant results, for both phages and aptamers.
- Immobilisation of targets: A requirement for phage and aptamer selections is that the targets need to be immobilised on a solid support; this is easily achieved for proteins and whole cells but is more complex for smaller molecules where specific functionalisations are necessary to enable efficient immobilisations.
- Nuclease sensitivity: Nucleic acids can be degraded in real matrices by the action of nucleases. This concern can be overcome by chemical modification of the ribose ring at the 2′ position with fluorine or amino groups. Another technique consists in using mirror-image analogues, called spiegelmers, which are nuclease resistant (Eulberg & Klussmann 2003)

6. Applications of phages

6.1 Medical diagnostics

6.1.1 Autoantibody detection in diseases characterised by deviations of the immune system

cDNA and peptide phage display are applicable for epitope mapping of monoclonal or polyclonal antibodies. In medical practice, this epitope mapping approach has potential value in the profiling of circulating antibodies in diseases characterised by immune system deviations, such as cancer and autoimmune disorders; the analysis of circulating antibodies allows the identification of immune-targeted tumour antigens in cancer and auto-antigens in autoimmunity. Depending on the affinity selection approach employed, disease-specific circulating antibody reactions can be used as diagnostic markers, as markers for prognosis and therapeutic outcome, and as markers for therapeutic responsiveness. The selected peptide or protein displaying phages can be used in diagnostic tests to detect disease-associated or disease-specific antibodies. Moreover, the identified antibodies and associated antibody-targets can be important for the discovery of novel therapeutic targets in cancer and autoimmunity research.

Serological antigen selection (SAS) is a phage display-based autoantibody profiling approach in which a cDNA expression library from diseased tissue or cell-lines is displayed at the surface of phage particles, followed by affinity-selection with pooled patient antibodies (Fig. 3). This procedure has recently been successfully applied for colorectal cancer (CRC) (Somers et al. 2002), atherosclerotic lesion rupture (Cleutjens et al. 2008), and multiple sclerosis (MS) (Somers et al. 2008; Govarts et al. 2009).

The SAS procedure entails subsequent rounds of affinity selection of a cDNA phage display library with patient immunoglobulins. An affinity selection round is initiated by incubating phage displaying the cDNA library with pooled patient body fluids (1). During this incubation step, antigen-antibody complexes are formed between the antibodies present in the patient body fluids and their respective target antigens at the surface of the phage (2).

These complexes are captured on a solid support by anti-human IgG capture antibody (3) while non-bound phages are washed away (4). Bound phages are eluted (5), amplified through infection of host bacteria (6) and used as input in a subsequent affinity selection procedure (7). The succession of affinity selection and amplification of selected phages results in enrichment op phage displayed antigens targeted by patient IgG.

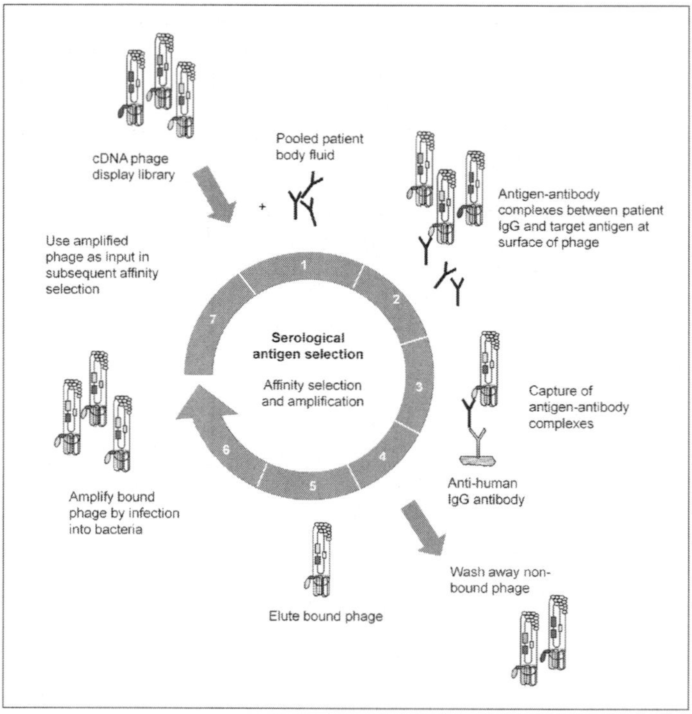

Fig. 3. Overview of the serological antigen selection (SAS) procedure

The SAS technology was initially developed to discover novel candidate tumour-antigens for CRC. In this study, the procedure was applied on a cDNA expression library from CRC cell line HT-29 using pooled CRC patient serum. Six phage clones with a CRC-related serological profile were identified, making excellent candidates for tumour vaccination and sero-diagnosis of cancer (Somers et al. 2002).

For the identification of novel markers for ruptured atherosclerotic lesions, SAS was performed on a cDNA expression library prepared from mRNA preferentially expressed in ruptured human atherosclerotic plaques. Sera from patients with ruptured atherosclerotic plaques were used for selection of phages expressing immunoreactive fusion proteins resulting in the identification of two phage clones. The presence of antibodies against the peptides displayed by these clones could discriminate between patients with peripheral ruptured lesions and patients with peripheral stable plaques with 100% specificity and 76% sensitivity. A positive serum response against a set of two novel identified cDNA phage clones thus showed a strong association with the presence of ruptured peripheral atherosclerotic lesions, allowing a promising novel approach for non-invasive diagnosis of atherosclerotic lesions (Cleutjens et al. 2008).

In another study, the use of the SAS procedure on a cDNA expression library from MS brain tissue and selection on pooled cerebrospinal fluid (CSF) of MS patients has led to the discovery of eight novel phage clones and associated autoantibody reactions with 45%

sensitivity and 86% specificity for the disease. As currently the diagnosis of MS is largely based on clinical symptoms, the implementation of objective laboratory tests that can measure the serological presence of the markers can be of great value to MS diagnostics. Moreover, the analysis of the MS-associated immune deviations through autoantibody profiling is also valid to provide the urgently needed clues regarding disease-associated autoantibody-targets and the underlying autoimmune aetiology (Somers et al. 2008; Govarts et al. 2009).

Phage-based biosensor platforms that incorporate the novel identified cDNA phage clones can be developed for serological screening of patients, resulting in clinical application of these phage clones in medical diagnostics.

6.1.2 Serum diagnosis of infectious disease by detection of antibodies with a phage-particle gel immunoassay (PPaGIA)

Infectious diseases are a matter of national security and may have a great impact on public health and the world economy, especially due to rapid dissemination and adaptation of pathogens. Proper diagnosis of infectious diseases with reliable, robust and sensitive tests is very important for individual health, but is also crucial for surveillance and control of infectious diseases worldwide. One possible diagnosis of infectious diseases is the detection of pathogen-specific antibodies in the blood or serum of patients. Phages are very appropriate for the development of these antibody detection tests. Peptide phages displaying a peptide that mimics the antigen (mimitope) and binds to antigen-specific antibodies, can be selected. Peptide phage display is already widely used for epitope mapping of poly- and monoclonal antibodies (Irving et al. 2001). However, the selected peptide phages that bind to pathogen specific antibodies in these studies can also be used in diagnostic tests to detect these pathogen-specific antibodies. Goulart et al. (2008) developed a phage-particle gel immunoassay (PPaGIA), which uses polystyrene beads conjugated with peptide phages with affinity for pathogen-specific antibodies. When pathogen-specific antibodies are present in blood or serum of infected patients they will bind to the beads conjugated with these peptide phages. These antibody-bead complexes can be separated by size from the beads that do not interact with the antibodies, by centrifuging through a gel matrix of chromatographic microcolumns. When antibody-bead complexes are formed, they are captured at the top of the column, in contrast with plain beads that will be detected at the bottom of the column after centrifuging. An example of leismaniasis diagnosis with PPaGIA is visualised in Fig. 4.

6.1.3 Metastatic cell detection

Metastasis is the spread of cancer from the place at which it starts as a primary tumour to other tissues in the body. An early detection of metastasis is important for early treatment of cancer, which increases the chances of a cure. The current diagnosis of metastasis is only possible by a series of biopsies in different tissues. However, biopsy is an invasive approach, which is not applicable in the early stage of metastasis and less applicable if patients do not have a clearly defined pathological site (Aggarwal et al. 2005). A promising alternative for metastasis diagnosis is the measurement of tumour cells in the blood, because the metastatic tumour cells are loosened and released into the blood or lymph. For the development of diagnostic approaches to detect metastatic tumour cells in blood, affinity reagents selective for metastatic markers, unique to tumours are required. Here, phage display can be used. A number of peptides that bind specific metastatic tumour cells are identified by differential

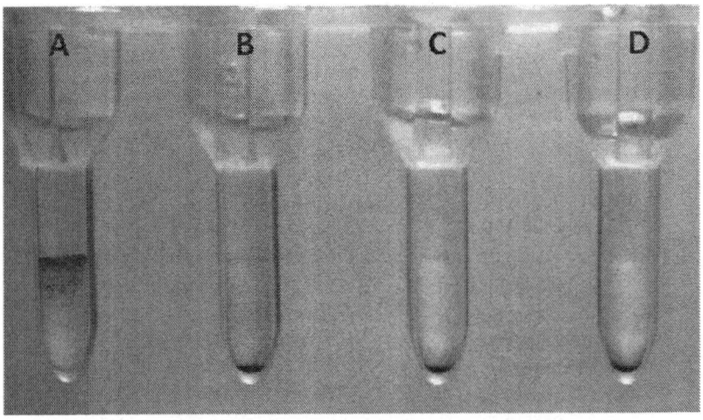

Fig. 4. Digital image of the PPaGIA. Circulating antibodies from leismaniasis patients were detected with peptide phages that specifically recognise antibodies for visceral leismaniasis (VL). A: positive serum from a patient with VL detected with specific phages (agglutination at the top); B: positive serum from a patient with cutaneous leismaniasis (CL) probed with specific phages (no reaction); C: positive serum from a patient with VL probed with nonspecific phages (no reaction); D: negative serum probed with specific phages (no reaction). (Goulart et al. 2010)

screening with phage display (Rasmussen et al. 2002; Jia et al. 2007; Rittner et al. 2007; Zhang et al. 2009). The selected metastatic specific peptide phages can be used to develop a diagnostic approach to detect metastatic cells in blood samples. Zhang et al. (2009) developed a light-addressable potentiometric sensor (LAPS), that measures the surface potential of an illuminated sensor chip. The metastatic-specific peptide phages are covalently coated on the sensor chip of this LAPS, as visualised in Fig. 5.
The blood sample is injected in the microchamber and metastatic cells are captured by the immobilised phages. This capturing of metastatic cells causes changes in surface potential, which is measured and translated in an output voltage with the lock-in amplifier. With this LAPS modified with metastatic-specific peptide phages, it was possible to distinguish between metastatic cells and non-metastatic cells and detect as few as 100 metastatic cells per ml. This approach shows the potential of peptide phage display to develop diagnostic approaches for metastatic cancer.

6.2 Food biosensors

6.2.1 Salmonella typhimurium detection

S. typhimurium is one of the leading sources of human gastroenteritis, causing mainly diarrhoea, vomiting and abdominal cramps 12 to 72 hours after infection and possibly lasting for up to seven days. Humans are usually infected with *Salmonella* by ingesting contaminated food such as raw meat, fish, unpasteurised dairy products and eggs. A conventional, accurate way to detect *S. typhimurium* in food samples can be carried out by means of microbiological culture growth techniques. The problem, however, is that the results are only obtained within three to five days. For this reason, several rapid DNA-based (McGuinness et al. 2009), biochemical, immuno-assay (Beumer et al. 1991) and immuno-latex agglutination methods have been developed. Mostly, they obtain results within 48 hours. Still, faster detection of *S. typhimurium* is necessary to avoid outbreaks by preventing infected food from being distributed and consumed. Biosensor technology can provide such rapid results.

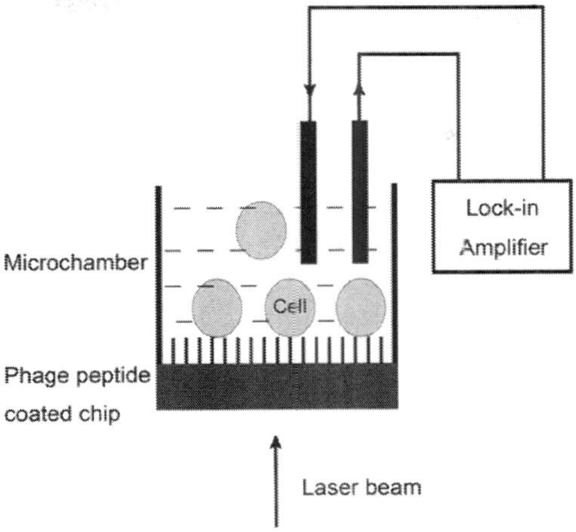

Fig. 5. Schematic representation of LAPS modified with metastasis specific peptide phages (Zhang et al. 2009)

A Magnetostrictive Microcantilever (MSMC) was developed as a transducer for the development of a biosensor for *S. typhimurium* by Fu et al (2007). The technology is based on applying a time-varying magnetic field, on the cantilever (Fig. 6). A filamentous peptide-displaying phage against *S. typhimurium* was used as a biorecognition element, which was immobilised on the surface of the cantilever by direct physical absorption. The resonance frequency, registered by two pick-up coils connected to a lock-in amplifier to measure the electric potential, shifts with time as the target bacterium binds on the sensor surface. The resonance characteristics of the MSMC in liquid were studied and the device proved to function well in water.

A similar sensor, based on the application of a magnetic field was built by (Lakshmanan et al. 2007) for the detection of *S. typhimurium*. The phage was derived from a landscape phage library. Instead of using a cantilever, a piece of ribbon on which the phages were immobilised, was utilised (Fig. 7) and the analyte was passed over the sample using a peristaltic pump. A detection limit of 103 cfu/ml was obtained for the sensor. The main advantages of these sensors are the sensitive and real-time detection.

The same approach of detection with magnetoelastic biosensors was used by different authors (Wan et al. 2007; Huang et al. 2008; Johnson et al. 2008) for *Bacillus anthracis*. Olsen et al (2006) developed a Quartz Crystal Microbalance (QCM) biosensor for the detection of *S. typhimurium*. QCM sensors are based on the resonation of the quartz crystals on application of an external alternation electric field. The frequency of the resulting oscillation is a function of the mass of the crystal. When the target binds to the phages, which are immobilised on the metallic electrodes on both sides of the piezoelectric quartz crystal, a shift in resonance frequency of the quartz crystal occurs. The sensor delivered a rapid response (< 180 s) and had a low-detection limit of 102 cells/ml.

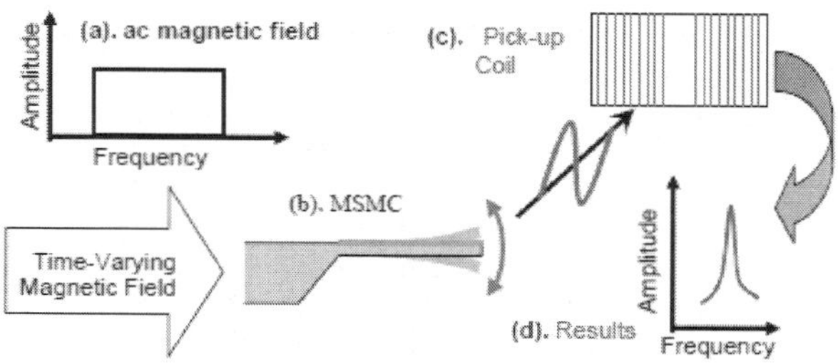

Fig. 6. Schematic illustration of the principle of MSMC as a transducer for biosensors. (Fu et al, 2007)

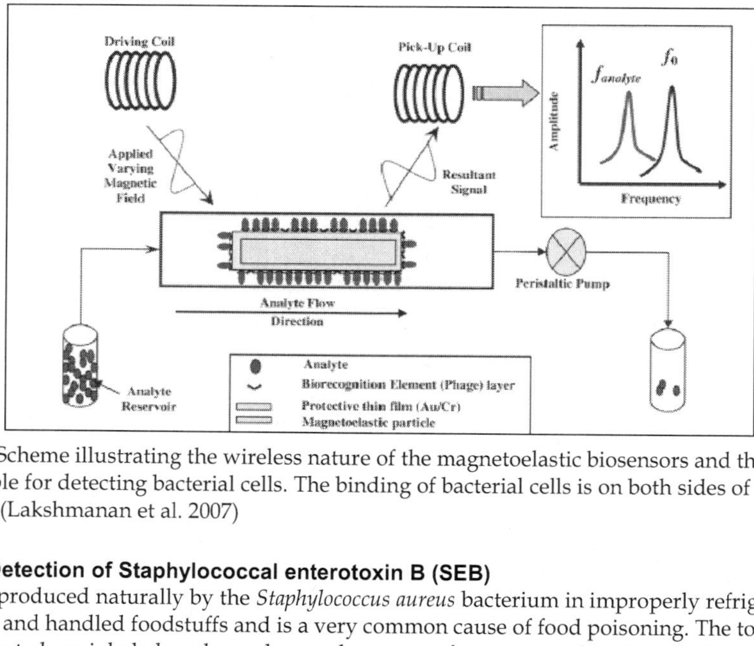

Fig. 7. Scheme illustrating the wireless nature of the magnetoelastic biosensors and the basic principle for detecting bacterial cells. The binding of bacterial cells is on both sides of the sensor (Lakshmanan et al. 2007)

6.2.2 Detection of Staphylococcal enterotoxin B (SEB)

SEB is produced naturally by the *Staphylococcus aureus* bacterium in improperly refrigerated, stored, and handled foodstuffs and is a very common cause of food poisoning. The toxin can be ingested or inhaled and can be used as a warfare agent. The clinical signs include symptoms such as headache, fever and chills. Depending on the route of exposure, additional symptoms can be observed. Ingestion results in nausea, vomiting and diarrhoea while inhalation provokes non-productive cough, chest pain and dyspnea. Classical ways of detection are mainly based on multiplex PCR (McLauchlin et al. 2000; Mehrotra et al. 2000) and immunoassays (Freed et al. 1982; Wieneke 1991), which allow quantitative or qualitative measurements in less than 24 hours.

A peptide displaying-phage for the optical detection of SEB with biosensor technology was developed by Goldman et al (2000). The SEB binding phage was selected from a random peptide library and was fluorescently labelled with Cy5 dye to allow detection. The labelled phages were among other methods tested in a portable fibre optic biosensor (RAPTOR) (Fig. 8). Four optical probes, placed in a disposable chamber were coated with SEB or streptavidin, and the labelled phage was loaded onto the chamber. The complex formation could be monitored by the surface-bound fluorophores with a diode laser. The optical probe captures a portion of the emitted fluorescence, which travels back up the fibre to the photodiode detector (Anderson et al. 2000). Different laser readings were taken at different moments of the one-hour assay. The phage did generate a robust signal however it gave a lower signal than that generated by a labelled antibody and the detection of small amounts of SEB was problematic. Nevertheless, in optimised forms, this approach has the potential to perform at levels comparable to their antibody counterparts.

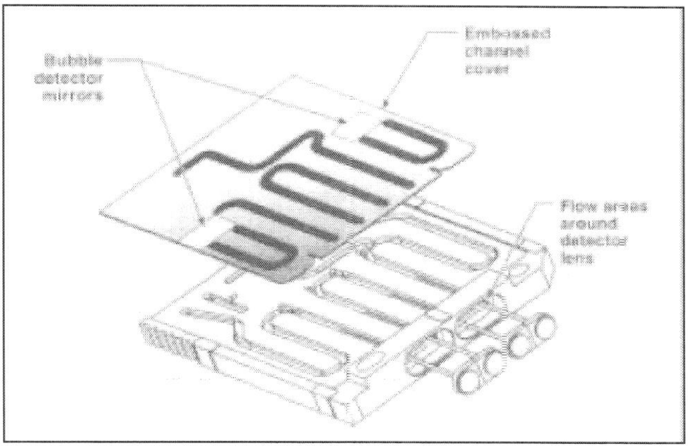

Fig. 8. Schematic of the RAPTOR showing four fibre optic probes, adhesive channel cover and bubble detector mirrors (Anderson et al. 2000)

7. Applications of aptamers

7.1 Medical diagnostics

7.1.1 Electrochemical detection of Platelet-derived growth factor (PDGF)

PDGF is a protein that regulates cell growth and division (Degefa & Kwak 2008) and is believed to be differentially expressed in human cancer (Polanski & Anderson 2006). Tumour cell lines produce and secrete PDGF (Famulok & Mayer 1999), thus making it a plasma biomarker that could be useful in early cancer detection and monitoring. This growth factor also participates in other proliferative disorders such as glomerulonephritis (Iida et al. 1991) and arteriosclerosis (Lindner et al. 1995; Lindner and Reidy 1995). Green et al (1996) identified DNA aptamers binding to PDGF (AB and BB variants) with subnanomolar affinity and which inhibit the mitogenic effects of PDGF. Using the highest binding aptamer, Lai et al. (2006) fabricated and characterised an electrochemical, aptamer-based (E-AB) sensor for the detection of PDGF directly in blood serum. The E-AB approach uses alternating current voltammetry to monitor target induced folding in a methylene blue (MB)-modified, PDGF binding aptamer. The E-AB sensor is constructed by attaching a MB-modified, PDGF-binding aptamer to a gold electrode via self-assembled monolayer chemistry. In the absence of its target (Fig. 9, left), the aptamer is thought to be highly dynamic and partially unfolded, retaining only one of the three stems intact. This reduces electron transfer between the electrode and the MB. Upon target binding (Fig. 9, right), the aptamer folds into a configuration, forming a stable three-way junction, forcing the MB label into close proximity with the electrode, leading to improved electron-transfer efficiency.

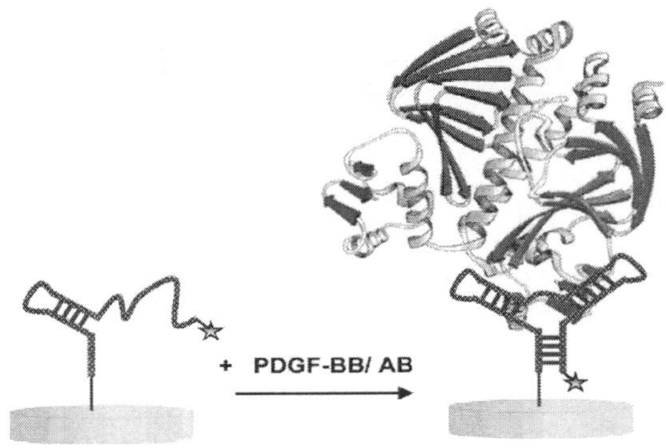

Fig. 9. E-AB-based PDGF sensor fabricated by a MB-labelled aptamer on a gold electrode surface (Lai et al. 2006)

This E-AB sensor combines the unprecedented sensitivity, selectivity and reusability of aptamers in a single approach, enabling it to detect physiologically relevant PDGF levels directly in largely unprocessed clinical samples, for the first time. It readily detects the BB variant of PDGF till 1 nM directly in undiluted blood serum and at 50 pM in serum-diluted two-fold with aqueous buffer. The detection limit attained in 50% serum is achieved against a >25 million-fold excess of contaminating blood proteins and represents a four order of magnitude improvement over the most sensitive optical PDGF aptasensor reported to date (Fang et al. 2001). This detection limit enables the sensor to easily measure 400-700 pM serum PDGF concentrations, from low levels found in healthy individuals to higher concentrations in cancer patients (Leitzel et al. 1991). The E-AB sensor's selectivity was studied using two control sequences sharing similar sequence identity and similar structure to the PDGF binding aptamer, respectively. However, both these sequences exhibited an insignificant signal increase (< 1%) under the same experimental conditions. Furthermore, the E-AB sensor is reusable and could be used and regenerated up to five times before unacceptable degradation was observed. Additionally, as an electrochemical sensor, the E-AB platform does not require light sources, high-voltage power supplies, or other heavy, cumbersome equipment. Given these advantages, E-AB sensors appear well suited for implementation in portable convenient point-of-care diagnostics, enabling direct detection of proteins and small molecules in complex, unprocessed clinical samples.

7.1.2 HIV -1 Tat protein detection using molecular beacon aptamer

Transcription of human immunodeficiency virus type-1 (HIV-1) is enabled via cellular factors and viral proteins (Gaynor 1992). Trans-Activator of Transcription (Tat) is an HIV-1 RNA-binding protein that exhibits an inherent affinity against the Trans-Activating

Response Element (TAR) of the virus and regulates viral transcription (Tombelli et al. 2005a). For HIV-1, oligonucleotides have been isolated that can efficiently interrupt essential steps in the viral life cycle, opening up the potential of treating viral diseases with aptamers (Famulok & Mayer 1999). A novel RNA motif that binds efficiently and specifically to the HIV-1 Tat protein and inhibits the trans-activation by Tat of transcription *in vitro* and *in vivo*, has been selected (Yamamoto et al. 2000b). This aptamer featured a similar structure to TAR and exhibited a 133-fold increased affinity for Tat, compared to TAR. Moreover, the aptamer does not require a cellular protein for efficient binding to the Tat, unlike the TAR of HIV-1. Hence the aptamer is not only useful for inhibiting the Tat function *in vivo* but also serves as a diagnostic reagent for the detection of Tat.

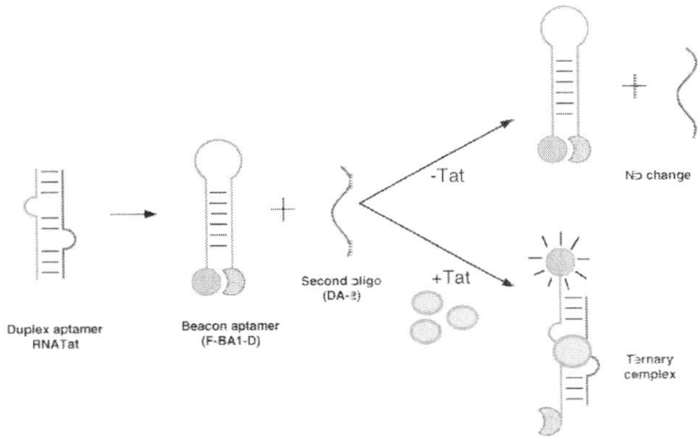

Fig. 10. Schematic representation of molecular beacon aptamer strategy for analysing the viral protein (Tat). (Yamamoto et al. 2000a)

To make a diagnostic test using a new molecular beacon aptamer, Yamamoto et al. (2000a) split the duplex aptamer into two RNA oligomers (Fig. 10). One of the split RNA oligomers (F-BA1-D), was designed to form a hairpin structure containing a fluorophore (fluorescein) and quencher (DABSYL) one at each end of the RNA strand and the other, DA-2, was a non-structured oligomer. It was observed that in the presence of Tat or its peptides (100 nM), the two oligomers underwent a conformational change to form a duplex that lead to relieving of fluorophore from the quencher, and thus a significant enhancement of the fluorescence of fluorescein, followed by the stabilisation of the ternary complex (Fig. 10). These results suggest that splitting of the aptamer into two oligomers does not affect the affinity of the oligomers to the Tat, as long as they possess the core binding sequence.

The molecular beacon aptamer (F-BA1-D) described here does not depend on the target sequence (DA-2) alone, but also depends on the target molecule (Tat protein of HIV) other than the nucleic acid.

As a specificity check, other RNA binding proteins were tested, but none of them enhanced the fluorescein intensity of the beacon aptamer. Thus the beacon aptamer responds specifically to the Tat protein or its peptides and is indeed suitable for specific detection of Tat protein, derived from either HIV-1 or HIV-2. Such a molecular beacon aptamer could find applications as an analytical tool for monitoring viral protein levels, both *in vitro* and in infected cells (such as HIV infected cells).

7.1.3 Mass based detection of Human IgE

An application of aptamers in biosensors was reported by Yao et al. (2009) to quantify immunoglobulin E (IgE), an antibody produced by the immune system under allergic reactions. A person who has an allergy usually has an elevated level of IgE in blood, therefore the quantification of IgE can considerably ease the clinical diagnosis of allergy-mediated disorders (Gokulrangan et al. 2005). Although the detection of IgE was already possible thanks to methods such as radioimmunoassay (RIA) or enzyme-linked immunosorbent assay (ELISA) (Peuravuori & Korpela 1993; Ollert et al. 2005), this aptasensor offers a fast and cheap detection method requiring less serum sample and reagents. The use of this aptamer as a recognition element of the sensor enables detection of concentrations as low as 2.5 μg/L of IgE in buffer and serum

In this sensor, a 5′-biotin modified nucleic acid aptamer has been fixed to an avidin modified gold layer of a quartz crystal microbalance device (QCM), providing a strong immobilisation of the recognition element. The piezoelectric sensor generates a frequency shift during the formation of the complex made by IgE and the aptamer. A linear relationship between the frequency (Hz) and the concentration of IgE has been observed, following the regression equation:

$$y = 1.03x - 0.06 \quad (1)$$

with x, the frequency, and y, the concentration of IgE in the range of 2.5-200 μg/l, the equation having a correlation coefficient of 0.996.

After the analysis of a sample, this piezoelectric aptasensor could be regenerated with 30 mmol ethylenediaminetetraacetic acid (EDTA) and reused ten times with the same chip without loss of function.

Finally, this piezoelectric biosensor showed a high specificity when tested with interfering proteins such as IgG or bovine serum albumin (BSA), which generated an insignificant frequency shift lower than 5% of the signal obtained for IgE.

7.1.4 Detection of insulin

Another example of application of nucleic acid aptamers in biosensors can be represented by the sensing of insulin by an aptameric enzyme subunit (AES) (Yoshida et al. 2009). Insulin is a key molecule in the regulation of glucose in blood (Khan & Pessin 2002). The concentration of insulin is lowered in patients suffering from type-1 diabetes because of a reduced production of this hormone. Therefore, sensing the concentration of insulin in blood or serum can help the detection of type-1 diabetes.

The AES is constructed by connecting an enzyme-inhibitor aptamer to a target molecule-binding aptamer, where thrombin is the enzyme (Fig. 11). In the presence of insulin, a structural change of the aptamer occurs, preventing the hybridisation to the enzyme-inhibitor aptamer. This results in activating the enzymatic activity of thrombin to degrade fibrinogen, present in the chip. The presence of insulin generates clotting of fibrinogen and can be monitored by this sensor.

7.2 Food biosensors

7.2.1 Detecting Campylobacter jejuni using fluorescent assays

An infection by *C. jejuni* is the most commonly reported cause of acute bacterial-mediated food poisoning. The disease is generally mild, but complications such as the Guillain Barré

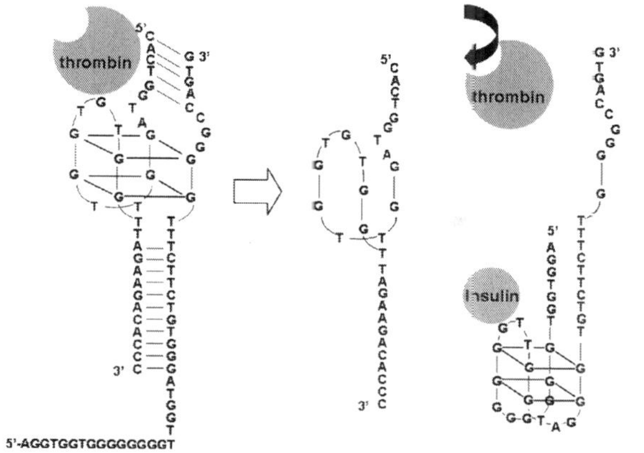

Fig. 11. Scheme of the AES-based insulin sensing. The target molecule-binding aptamer and a portion of its complementary strand were attached to the split thrombin-inhibiting aptamer. The nucleic acid aptamers are separated in the presence of insulin (Yoshida et al. 2009)

syndrome can occur. Remarkably, *C. jejuni* does not express a large number of so-called classical virulence factors. Additionaly, the role of the only verified *Campylobacter* toxin identified (cytolethal distending toxin) in *C. jejuni* has not been determined yet. The conventional culture detection method is time-consuming, while the more recent real-time PCR methods allow rapid and more reliable detection of the *Campylobacter* species. Bonjoch et al. (2010) used the gene encoding the ATP-binding protein CJE0832 to detect *C. jejuni* in a real-time PCR approach. Generally, even PCR-based methods need enrichment culturing to reach the desired detection limits.

Stratis-Cullum et al. (2009b) used the entire heat-killed *C. jejuni* cells as the selection target. A capillary electrophoretic assay was developed to investigate the relative binding affinity of *C. jejuni* aptamers. Fig. 12 illustrates the separation of the aptamer-bacterial cell complex, monitored by the emission of fluorescent labelled analytes at 520 nm. Migration depends on separation medium, size and shape of species, net charge on species and strength of electric field. The aptamer probe investigated, exhibited a pronounced mobility shift upon binding to the *C. jejuni* target, while a minimal response was obtained for two other food pathogen targets.

Bruno et al. (2009) developed DNA aptamers against the surface proteins of *C. jejuni*. The aptamers were used in a magnetic bead (MB) and red quantum dot (QD)-based sandwich assay, and the reactivity with bacterial species was evaluated with a spectrofluorimeter (Fig. 13). In this application the use of plastic cuvette-adherent technology improves detection of pathogens.

7.2.2 Electrochemical detection of Botulinum Neurotoxins (BoNTs)

Neurotoxins produced by *Clostridium botulinum* are among the most poisonous substances known. Food-borne botulism is the most common intoxication form due to the ingestion of pre-formed *Bo*NT in food. The gold standard method to confirm the presence of *Bo*NT consists of immunoassays, which are expensive, labour-intensive and slow. Recently, alternative rapid methods, such as quantitative real-time PCR assays, have been developed for the detection of *C. botulinum* (Kirchner et al. 2010; Satterfield et al. 2010). Brunt et al. (2010) developed a sensitive and rapid immunochromatography column-based test for the detection of *Bo*NTs.

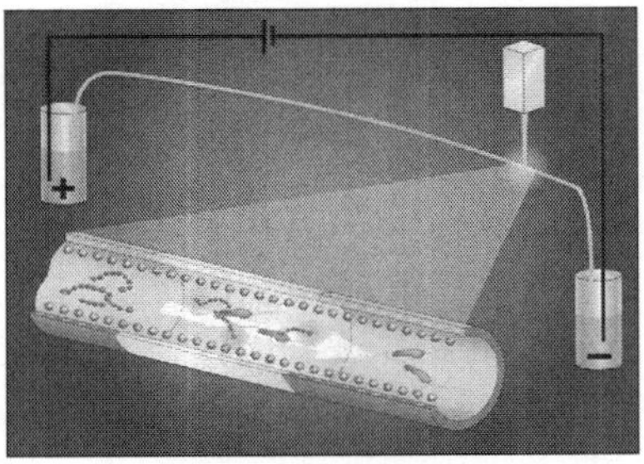

Fig. 12. Schematic representation of the capillary electrophoretic analysis of aptamer: bacterial cell complexes using laser-induced fluorescence detection

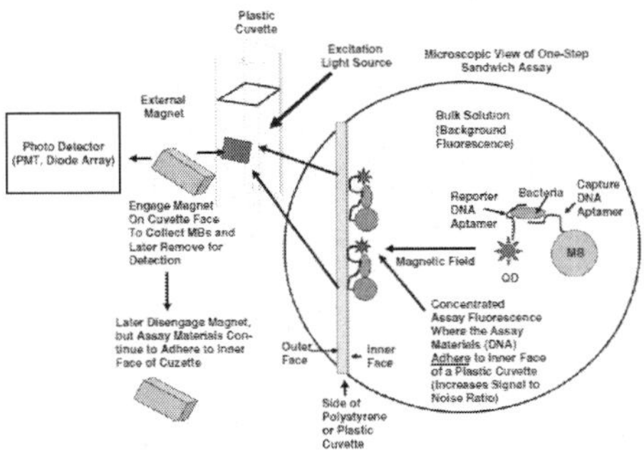

Fig. 13. Illustration of the self-assembling plastic-adherent aptamer-MB and aptamer-QD sandwich assay and magnetic collection system (Bruno et al. 2009)

Recently, Wei and Ho (2009) reported an electrochemical biosensor using an aptamer, which could measure *Bo*NT with a limit of detection of 40 pg/ml. The nucleic acid aptamers were selected via micro-bead SELEX procedure and their dissociation constants were determined to range between 3 nM and 50 nM, representing a quite good affinity towards *Bo*NT. When binding to *Bo*NT, a conformational change of the chosen aptamer was used for *Bo*NT monitoring (Fig. 14). A fluorescein label has been attached to one end of the aptamer in such a way that the label is hidden by the aptamer in the absence of the target. When *Bo*Nt is present in the sample, the aptamer unfolds and exhibits the fluorescein label, which can bind to an anti-fluorescein antibody linked to an enzyme, horseradish peroxidase (HRP), reducing hydrogen peroxide and oxidising tetramethylbenzidine (TMB); thus generating an electrochemical current signal due to the redox cycles between TMB, HRP and hydrogen peroxide. The specificity of the sensor has been proved by testing interfering proteins, which did not generate any electrochemical current, showing that the aptamer remained folded in the absence of *Bo*NT.

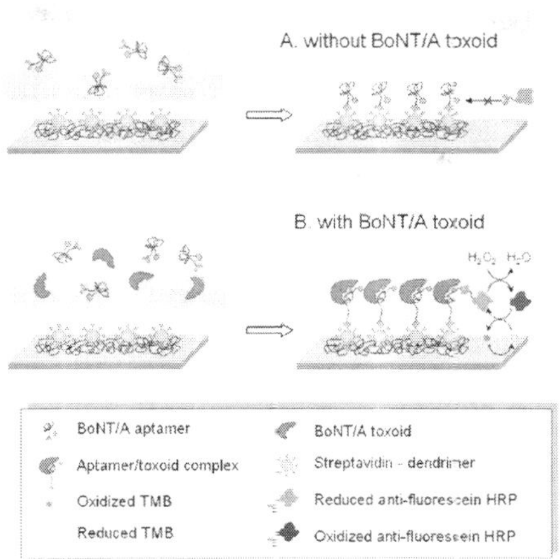

Fig. 14. Scheme of aptamer-based electrochemical detection of *Botulinum* neurotoxin (*Bo*NT) (Wei and Ho 2009)

8. Conclusions

Phages and aptamers have great potential as specific recognition elements in various biomedical and food applications. Their function as sensing receptors offers advantages over methods that are based on antibodies: their efficient immobilisation, the possibility of using different detection methods due to easy labelling and the easy regeneration of their functionality after immobilisation. Additionally, they can be modified, thus enhancing their stability, affinity and specificity and facilitating the functionalisation of nanoparticles and surfaces. These advantages enable the phage and aptamer biosensors to meet the requirements of sensitivity and stability that are necessary for the detection of disease biomarkers and food contaminants in their natural matrices.

The full potential of these novel biomolecules has not yet been realised completely and there are certain challenges that need to be overcome. However, proof-of-concept experiments demonstrating that aptamers and phages can specifically bind and regulate the function of various biomedically relevant targets, hold promise for the development of innovative diagnostics. The ability to develop affinity-based detection systems consisting of tailor-made characteristics, which can be applied to the analyses of disease biomarkers or carriers which are unlimited by size, complexity, toxicity and matrix effects, offers the field of biosensing the opportunity to explore new and dynamic routes of diagnostic sensor development. Overall, the potential of aptasensors and phage sensors is vast, and this exciting area of investigation is on the verge of exponential growth.

9. Acknowledgements

This work was funded by the Federal Public Service of Health, Food Chain Safety and Environment (contract RT 07/11 INVITRAB and RF6204 ERGOT). The authors would like to express their gratitude to Mandira Banerji for editorial assistance.

10. References

Aggarwal, S., S. Janssen, R. M. Wadkins, J. L. Harden and S. R. Denmeade (2005). A combinatorial approach to the selective capture of circulating malignant epithelial cells by peptide ligands. *Biomaterials* 26(30): 6077-6086.

Aizawa, M. (1994). Immunosensors for clinical analysis. Advances in clinical chemistry, vol 31. San Diego, Academic Press Inc. 31: 247-275.

Anderson, G. P., C. A. Rowe-Taitt and F. S. Ligler (2000). Raptor: A portable, automated biosensor. *Proceedings of the First Conference on Point Detection for Chemical and Biological Defense*, Williamsburg, Virginia

Beumer, R. R., E. Brinkman and F. M. Rombouts (1991). Enzyme-linked immunoassays for the detection of salmonella-spp - a comparison with other methods. *International Journal of Food Microbiology* 12(4): 363-374.

Bonjoch, X., L. Calvo, M. Soler, O. Ruiz-Rueda and L. J. Garcia-Gil (2010). A new multiplexed real-time pcr assay to detect campylobacter jejuni, c. Coli, c. Lari, and c. Upsaliensis. *Food Analytical Methods* 3(1): 40-46.

Bonner, G. and A. M. Klibanov (2000). Structural stability of DNA in nonaqueous solvents. *Biotechnology and Bioengineering* 68(3): 339-344.

Brigati, J. R. and V. A. Petrenko (2005). Thermostability of landscape phage probes. *Analytical and Bioanalytical Chemistry* 382(6): 1346-1350.

Bruno, J. G., T. Phillips, M. P. Carrillo and R. Crowell (2009). Plastic-adherent DNA aptamer-magnetic bead and quantum dot sandwich assay for campylobacter detection. *Journal of Fluorescence* 19(3): 427-435.

Brunt, J., M. D. Webb and M. W. Peck (2010). Rapid affinity immunochromatography column-based tests for sensitive detection of clostridium botulinum neurotoxins and escherichia coli o157. *Applied and Environmental Microbiology* 76(13): 4143-4150.

Cleutjens, K., B. C. G. Faber, M. Rousch, R. van Doorn, T. M. Hackeng, C. Vink, P. Geusens, H. ten Cate, J. Waltenberger, V. Tchaikovski, M. Lobbes, V. Somers, A. Sijbers, D. Black, P. Kitslaar and M. Daemen (2008). Noninvasive diagnosis of ruptured peripheral atherosclerotic lesions and myocardial infarction by antibody profiling. *Journal of Clinical Investigation* 118(8): 2979-2985.

Collett, J. R., E. J. Cho, J. F. Lee, M. Levy, A. J. Hood, C. Wan and A. D. Ellington (2005). Functional rna microarrays for high-throughput screening of antiprotein aptamers. *Analytical Biochemistry* 338(1): 113-123.

Crameri, R. and R. Kodzius (2001). The powerful combination of phage surface display of cdna libraries and high throughput screening. *Combinatorial Chemistry & High Throughput Screening* 4(2): 145-155.

Degefa, T. H. and J. Kwak (2008). Label-free aptasensor for platelet-derived growth factor (pdgf) protein. *Analytica Chimica Acta* 613(2): 163-168.

Eulberg, D. and S. Klussmann (2003). Spiegelmers: Biostable aptamers. *Chembiochem* 4(10): 979-983.

Famulok, M. and G. Mayer (1999). Aptamers as tools in molecular biology and immunology. *Current topics in microbiology and immunology* 243: 123-136.

Fang, X. H., Z. H. Cao, T. Beck and W. H. Tan (2001). Molecular aptamer for real-time oncoprotein platelet-derived growth factor monitoring by fluorescence anisotropy. *Analytical Chemistry* 73(23): 5752-5757.

Freed, R. C., M. L. Evenson, R. F. Reiser and M. S. Bergdoll (1982). Enzyme-linked immunosorbent-assay for detection of staphylococcal enterotoxins in foods. *Applied and Environmental Microbiology* 44(6): 1349-1355.

Fu, L. L., S. Q. Li, K. W. Zhang, I. H. Chen, V. A. Petrenko and Z. Y. Cheng (2007). Magnetostrictive microcantilever as an advanced transducer for biosensors. *Sensors* 7(11): 2929-2941.

Gaynor, R. (1992). Cellular transcription factors involved in the regulation of hiv-1 gene-expression. *Aids* 6(4): 347-363.

Gokulrangan, G., J. R. Unruh, D. F. Holub, B. Ingram, C. K. Johnson and G. S. Wilson (2005). DNA aptamer-based bioanalysis of ige by fluorescence anisotropy. *Analytical Chemistry* 77(7): 1963-1970.

Goldman, E. R., M. P. Pazirandeh, J. M. Mauro, K. D. King, J. C. Frey and G. P. Anderson (2000). Phage-displayed peptides as biosensor reagents. *Journal of Molecular Recognition* 13(6): 382-387.

Goulart, L. R., A. P. P. Freschi, J. M. Madurro, R Cardoso, F. E. Capparelli, J. F. Almeida, R. R. Gatti, C. R. Prudêncio and G. R. L. Souza (2008). Métodos para imunoaglutinação em micro e nanoesferas de poliestireno.

Goulart, L. R., C. U. Vieira, A. P. P. Freschi, F. E. Capparelli, P. T. Fujimura, J. F. Almeida, L. F. Ferreira, I. M. B. Goulart, A. G. Brito-Madurro and J. M. Madurro (2010). Biomarkers for serum diagnosis of infectious diseases and their potential application in novel sensor platforms. *Critical Reviews in Immunology* 30(2): 201-222.

Govarts, C., K. Somers, R. Hupperts, P. Stinissen and V. Somers (2009). Analysis of antibody reactivity in paired cerebrospinal fluid and serum of a relapsing remitting multiple sclerosis patient. *Autoimmunity* 42(8): 699-704.

Green, L. S., D. Jellinek, R. Jenison, A. Ostman, C.-H. Heldin and N. Janjic (1996). Inhibitory DNA ligands to platelet-derived growth factor b-chain. *Biochemistry* 35(45): 14413-14424.

Hoogenboom, H. R., A. P. de Bruine, S. E. Hufton, R. M. Hoet, J. W. Arends and R. C. Roovers (1998). Antibody phage display technology and its applications. *Immunotechnology* 4(1): 1-20.

Huang, S., H. Yang, R. S. Lakshmanan, M. L. Johnson, I. Chen, J. Wan, H. C. Wikle, V. A. Petrenko, J. M. Barbaree, Z. Y. Cheng and B. A. Chin (2008). The effect of salt and phage concentrations on the binding sensitivity of magnetoelastic biosensors for bacillus anthracis detection. *Biotechnology and Bioengineering* 101(5): 1014-1021.

Iida, H., R. Seifert, C. E. Alpers, R. G. Gronwald, P. E. Phillips, P. Pritzl, K. Gordon, A. M. Gown, R. Ross and D. F. Bowen-Pope (1991). Platelet-derived growth factor (pdgf) and pdgf receptor are induced in mesangial proliferative nephritis in the rat. *Proceedings of the National Academy of Sciences of the United States of America* 88(15): 6560-6564.

Irving, M. B., O. Pan and J. K. Scott (2001). Random-peptide libraries and antigen-fragment libraries for epitope mapping and the development of vaccines and diagnostics. *Current Opinion in Chemical Biology* 5(3): 314-324.

Jenison, R. D., S. C. Gill, A. Pardi and B. Polisky (1994). High-resolution molecular discrimination by rna. *Science* 263(5152): 1425-1429.

Jepson, C. D. and J. B. March (2004). Bacteriophage lambda is a highly stable DNA vaccine delivery vehicle. *Vaccine* 22(19): 2413-2419.

Jia, W. D., H. C. Sun, J. B. Zhang, Y. Xu, Y. B. Qian, J. Z. Pang, L. Wang, L. X Qin, Y. K. Liu and Z. Y. Tang (2007). A novel peptide that selectively binds highly metastatic hepatocellular carcinoma cell surface is related to invasion and metastasis. *Cancer Letters* 247(2): 234-242.

Jin, X. F., J. R. Newton, S. Montgomery-Smith and G. P. Smith (2009). A generalized kinetic model for amine modification of proteins with application to phage display. *Biotechniques* 46(3): 175-+.

Johnson, M. L., J. H. Wan, S. C. Huang, Z. Y. Cheng, V. A. Petrenko, D. J. Kim, I. H. Chen, J. M. Barbaree, J. W. Hong and B. A. Chin (2008). A wireless biosensor using microfabricated phage-interfaced magnetoelastic particles. *Sensors and Actuators a-Physical* 144(1): 38-47.

Khan, A. H. and J. E. Pessin (2002). Insulin regulation of glucose uptake: A complex interplay of intracellular signalling pathways. *Diabetologia* 45(11): 1475-1483.

Kirchner, S., K. M. Kramer, M. Schulze, D. Pauly, D. Jacob, F. Gessler, A. Nitsche, B. G. Dorner and M. B. Dorner (2010). Pentaplexed quantitative real-time pcr assay for the simultaneous detection and quantification of botulinum neurotoxin-producing clostridia in food and clinical samples. *Applied and Environmental Microbiology* 76(13): 4387-4395.

Lai, R. Y., K. W. Plaxco and A. J. Heeger (2006). Aptamer-based electrochemical detection of picomolar platelet-derived growth factor directly in blood serum. *Analytical Chemistry* 79(1): 229-233.

Lakshmanan, R. S., R. Guntupalli, J. Hu, D. J. Kim, V. A. Petrenko, J. M. Barbaree and B. A. Chin (2007). Phage immobilized magnetoelastic sensor for the detection of salmonella typhimurium. *Journal of Microbiological Methods* 71(1): 55-60.

Leitzel, K., W. Bryce, J. Tomita, G. Manderino, I. Tribby, A. Thomason, M. Billingsley, E. Podczaski, H. Harvey, M. Bartholomew and A. Lipton (1991). Elevated plasma platelet-derived growth-factor-b-chain levels in cancer-patients. *Cancer Research* 51(16): 4149-4154.

Li, W. and N. B. Caberoy (2010). New perspective for phage display as an efficient and versatile technology of functional proteomics. *Applied Microbiology and Biotechnology* 85(4): 909-919.

Lindner, V., C. M. Giachelli, S. M. Schwartz and M. A. Reidy (1995). A subpopulation of smooth muscle cells in injured rat arteries expresses platelet-derived growth factor–b chain mrna. *Circ Res* 76(6): 951-957.

Lindner, V. and M. A. Reidy (1995). Platelet-derived growth factor ligand and receptor expression by large vessel endothelium in vivo. *The American Journal of Pathology* 146(6): 1488–1497.

McGuinness, S., E. McCabe, E. O'Regan, A. Dolan, G. Duffy, C. Burgess, S. Fanning, T. Barry and J. O'Grady (2009). Development and validation of a rapid real-time pcr based method for the specific detection of salmonella on fresh meat. *Meat Science* 83(3): 555-562.

McLauchlin, J., G. L. Narayanan, V. Mithani and G. O'Neill (2000). The detection of enterotoxins and toxic shock syndrome toxin genes in staphylococcus aureus by polymerase chain reaction. *Journal of Food Protection* 63(4): 479-488.

Mehrotra, M., G. Wang and W. M. Johnson (2000). Multiplex pcr for detection of genes for staphylococcus aureus enterotoxins, exfoliative toxins, toxic shock syndrome toxin 1, and methicillin resistance. *Journal of Clinical Microbiology* 38(3): 1032-1035.

Newman, J. D. and A. P. F. Turner (2005). Home blood glucose biosensors: A commercial perspective. *Biosensors and Bioelectronics* 20(12): 2435-2453.

Ollert, M., S. Weissenbacher, J. Rakoski and J. Ring (2005). Allergen-specific ige measured by a continuous random-access immunoanalyzer: Interassay comparison and agreement with skin testing. *Clinical Chemistry* 51(7): 1241-1249.

Olsen, E. V., I. B. Sorokulova, V. A. Petrenko, I. H. Chen, J. M. Barbaree and V. J. Vodyanoy (2006). Affinity-selected filamentous bacteriophage as a probe for acoustic wave biodetectors of salmonella typhimurium. *Biosensors & Bioelectronics* 21(8): 1434-1442.

Pelletier, J. and S. Sidhu (2001). Mapping protein-protein interactions with combinatorial biology methods. *Current Opinion in Biotechnology* 12(4): 340-347.

Petrenko, V. A. and G. P. Smith (2000). Phages from landscape libraries as substitute antibodies. *Protein Engineering* 13(8): 589-592.

Peuravuori, H. and T. Korpela (1993). Pyrophosphatase-based enzyme-linked-immunosorbent-assay of total ige in serum. *Clinical Chemistry* 39(5): 846-851.

Polanski, M. and N. L. Anderson (2006). A list of candidate cancer biomarkersfor targeted proteomics. *Biomarker Insights* 1: 1-48.

Rasmussen, U. B., V. Schreiber, H. Schultz, F. Mischler and K. Schughart (2002). Tumor cell-targeting by phage-displayed peptides *Cancer Gene Therapy* 9(7): 606-612.

Rittner, K., V. Schreiber, P. Erbs and M. Lusky (2007). Targeting of adenovirus vectors carrying a tumor cell-specific peptide: In vitro and in vivo studies. *Cancer Gene Therapy* 14(5): 509-518.

Robbens, J., F. Dardenne, L. Devriese, W. De Coen and R. Blust (2010). *Escherichia coli* as a bioreporter in ecotoxicology. *Applied Microbiology and Biotechnology*: 1-19.

Satterfield, B. A., A. F. Stewart, C. S. Lew, D. O. Pickett, M. N. Cohen, E. A. Moore, P. F. Luedtke, K. L. O'Neill and R. A. Robison (2010). A quadruplex real-time pcr assay for rapid detection and differentiation of the clostridium botulinum toxin genes a, b, e and f. *Journal of Medical Microbiology* 59(1): 55-64.

Schwind, P., H. Kramer, A. Kremser, U. Ramsberger and I. Rasched (1992). Subtilisin removes the surface-layer of the phage-fd coat. *European Journal of Biochemistry* 210(2): 431-436.

Sheedy, C., C. R. MacKenzie and J. C. Hall (2007). Isolation and affinity maturation of hapten-specific antibodies. *Biotechnology Advances* 25(4): 333-352.

Somers, V., C. Govarts, K. Somers, R. Hupperts, R. Medaer and P. Stinissen (2008). Autoantibody profiling in multiple sclerosis reveals novel antigenic candidates. *Journal of Immunology* 180(6): 3957-3963.

Somers, V. A., R. J. Brandwijk, B. Joosten, P. T. Moerkerk, J. W. Arends, P. Menheere, W. O. Pieterse, A. Claessen, R. J. Scheper, H. R. Hoogenboom and S. E. Hufton (2002). A panel of candidate tumor antigens in colorectal cancer revealed by the serological selection of a phage displayed cdna expression library. *Journal of Immunology* 169: 2772-2780.

Stefan, R. I., J. F. van Staden and H. Y. Aboul-Enein (2000). Immunosensors in clinical analysis. *Fresenius Journal of Analytical Chemistry* 366(6-7): 659-668.

Stoltenburg, R., C. Reinemann and B. Strehlitz (2007). Selex--a (r)evolutionary method to generate high-affinity nucleic acid ligands. *Biomolecular Engineering* 24(4): 381-403.

Stratis-Cullum, D. N., S. McMasters and P. M. Pellegrino (2009a). Affinity probe capillary electrophoresis evaluation of aptamer binding to *campylobacter jejuni* bacteria. *Army Research Laboratory Report.*

Stratis-Cullum, D. N., S. McMasters and P. M. Pellegrino (2009b). Evaluation of relative aptamer binding to campylobacter jejuni bacteria using affinity probe capillary electrophoresis. *Analytical Letters* 42(15): 2389-2402.

Tombelli, S., A. Minunni, E. Luzi and M. Mascini (2005a). Aptamer-based biosensors for the detection of hiv-1 tat protein. *Bioelectrochemistry* 67(2): 135-141.

Tombelli, S., M. Minunni and M. Mascini (2005b). Analytical applications of aptamers. *Biosensors and Bioelectronics* 20(12): 2424-2434.

Van Dorst, B., W. De Coen, R. Blust and J. Robbens (2010a). Phage display as a novel screening tool for primary toxicological targets. *Environmental Toxicology and Chemistry* 29(2): 250-255.

Van Dorst, B., J. Mehta, K. Bekaert, E. Rouah-Martin, W. De Coen, P. Dubruel, R. Blust and J. Robbens (2010b). Recent advances in recognition elements of food and environmental biosensors: A review. *Biosensors and Bioelectronics* In Press, Corrected Proof.

Van Dorst, B., J. Mehta, E. Rouah-Martin, V. Somers, W. De Coen, R. Blust and J. Robbens (2010c). Cdna phage display as a novel tool to screen for cellular targets of chemical compounds. *Toxicology in Vitro* 24(5): 1435-1440.

Velusamy, V., K. Arshak, O. Korostynska, K. Oliwa and C. Adley (2010). An overview of foodborne pathogen detection: In the perspective of biosensors. *Biotechnology Advances* 28(2): 232-254.

Verma, V., K. Harjai and S. Chhibber (2009). Characterization of a t7-like lytic bacteriophage of klebsiella pneumoniae b5055: A potential therapeutic agent. *Current Microbiology* 59(3): 274-281.

Wan, J. H., M. L. Johnson, R. Guntupalli, V. A. Petrenko and B. A. Chin (2007). Detection of bacillus anthracis spores in liquid using phage-based magnetoelastic micro-resonators. *Sensors and Actuators B-Chemical* 127(2): 559-566.

Wang, J. (2007). Electrochemical glucose biosensors. *Chemical Reviews* 108(2): 814-825.

Wei, F. and C. M. Ho (2009). Aptamer-based electrochemical biosensor for botulinum neurotoxin. *Analytical and Bioanalytical Chemistry* 393(8): 1943-1948.

Wieneke, A. A. (1991). Comparison of 4 kits for the detection of staphylococcal-enterotoxin in foods from outbreaks of food poisoning. *International Journal of Food Microbiology* 14(3-4): 305-312.

Yamamoto, R., T. Baba and P. K. R. Kumar (2000a). Molecular beacon aptamer fluoresces in the presence of tat protein of hiv-1. (vol 5, pg 389, 2000). *Genes to Cells* 5(6): 523-523.

Yamamoto, R., M. Katahira, S. Nishikawa, T. Baba, K. Taira and P. K. R. Kumar (2000b). A novel rna motif that binds efficiently and specifically to the tat protein of hiv and inhibits the trans-activation by tat of transcription in vitro and in vivo. *Genes to Cells* 5(5): 371-388.

Yao, C. Y., Y. Z. Qi, Y. H. Zhao, Y. Xiang, Q. H. Chen and W. L. Fu (2009). Aptamer-based piezoelectric quartz crystal microbalance biosensor array for the quantification of ige. *Biosensors & Bioelectronics* 24(8): 2499-2503.

Yoshida, W., E. Mochizuki, M. Takase, H. Hasegawa, Y. Morita, H. Yamazaki, K. Sode and K. Ikebukuro (2009). Selection of DNA aptamers against insulin and construction of an aptameric enzyme subunit for insulin sensing. *Biosensors & Bioelectronics* 24(5): 1116-1120.

Zhang, H. K., X. Li, Y. P. Bai, R. F. Niu, Y. F. Jia, C. Z. Zhang, L. Zhang, X. Z. Feng and Y. J. Cao (2009). Metastatic cell detection using a phage-peptide-modified light-addressable potentiometric sensor. *Biotechnology and Applied Biochemistry* 53: 185-192.

Zhu, H., I. M. White, J. D. Suter and X. Fan (2008). Phage-based label-free biomolecule detection in an opto-fluidic ring resonator. *Biosensors and Bioelectronics* 24(3): 461-466.

20

Low Scaling Exponent during Arrhythmia: Detrended Fluctuation Analysis is a Beneficial Biomedical Computation Tool

Toru Yazawa[1] and Yukio Shimoda[2]
[1]Tokyo Metropolitan University,
[2]Tokyo Women's Medical University,
Japan

1. Introduction

Cardiovascular disease is one of the major social health problems. Heart attacks, in particular, are a major social concern because of the unpredictable and silent way they develop. Recently, it was reported that the incidence of myocardial infarction has decreased significantly (Yeh et al., 2010). However, some unlucky patients are unaware that they are at risk for the life threatening disease. We must acknowledge that while the default setting is good health, there is always an onset to a disease and never to a return to good health. This onset results in "silent" angina, and finally a "silent" attack can happen. In fact, Dutch researchers estimated that 43% of heart attacks went unrecognized (de Torbal et al., 2006). Our ultimate aim was to predict a heart attack, or at least to quantitatively analyze the heart condition, based on the belief that it is possible to predict a heart attack by observing fluctuations in heartbeat intervals. Fluctuation analysis first appeared in the physical literature a long time ago (Peng et al., 1995). However, strong empirical evidence of its accuracy and usefulness must still be collected.

Traditionally, cardiac studies have employed heart rate variability (HRV) to detect the onset of cardiac problems, including disorders of the autonomic nervous system. Problems arise, however, when patients are previously assumed to be healthy before the appearance of symptoms associated with HRV. An earlier marker is necessary because the early identification of symptoms aids in the prevention of the onset of chronic diseases. Detrended fluctuation analysis (DFA) (Peng et al., 1995) was proposed as a potentially useful method for detecting the signs of cardiovascular disease (See Stanley et al., 1999); although DFA has not yet been developed as a practical medical tool, such as the electrocardiogram (EKG). (We prefer the abbreviation "EKG" to "ECG," with due respect to the inventor, Dutch physiologist, Nobel laureate, Willem Einthoven.)

We recently tested the practical usefulness of DFA by using the heart of crustacean-animal models. In the test, we successfully showed that DFA could distinguish between intact and isolated hearts (Yazawa et al., 2004). In that study, we found out that the scaling exponent of the isolated hearts shifted and approached to 0.5 without exception. In turn, the scaling exponent of the intact hearts showed a value of about 1.0 without exception. As a result, we realized that DFA was reliable and useful because DFA was likely able to accurately reflect physiology. Unlike other methods like HRV, the value of DFA was that it has a baseline value of one (1), like a standard body temperature (37), a standard blood pH (7.4), and so on. Thus, we thought DFA was a simple tool. One (1) is nonlinearly determined a "healthy" outcome resulting from complex interactions between the structure and function of molecules, cells, and organs. Thereby, we hoped that DFA could determine the state of health "numerically." DFA seemed to not only reflect the state of the heart itself but also the (cardiac) nervous system. We considered that DFA might be used to detect the onset of cardiac problems, including disorders of the autonomic nervous system.

In this chapter, we provide empirical evidence of the practical usefulness of DFA and a new EKG amplification device that facilitates automatic DFA computation in practical use. The fluctuation analysis (i.e., DFA) was a potentially helpful early detection tool, as it revealed information that was not provided by EKG data.

2. Materials and methods

2.1 Peak detection of the heartbeat

Interval analysis requires detection of the precise timing of the heartbeat. A consecutive and perfect detection without miscounting is desirable. According to our preliminary test, approximately 2,000 consecutive heartbeats are required to obtain a reliable scaling exponent computation. We thought that the longer recording time resulted in a more accurate diagnosis. However, we found out that recording for longer than 2,000 beats was not helpful. We first reached this conclusion in model animal experiments. The ideal number of about 2,000 consecutive heartbeats is also applicable in human subjects.

To detect the timing of the heartbeats, both EKG recording and blood flow pulse recording are useful. Figure 1 shows an example of the premature ventricular contraction registered by both EKG and finger pulse recordings. Note the difference between Figure 1 A and B. Electrical excitation of the ventricle did not produce an observable pulse at the finger (see Figure 1A); in turn, an electrical excitation of the ventricle of the identical heart sent a small pressure pulse to the finger, which is indicated by an arrowhead (see Figure 1B). No matter what recording method was used, difficulty first arose when recording the timing of the heartbeats. The baseline drift of the commercial recording system presented the primary obstacle. When we saw the drift and contaminated the electric power-line noise, we were totally unable to detect 2,000 consecutive beats.

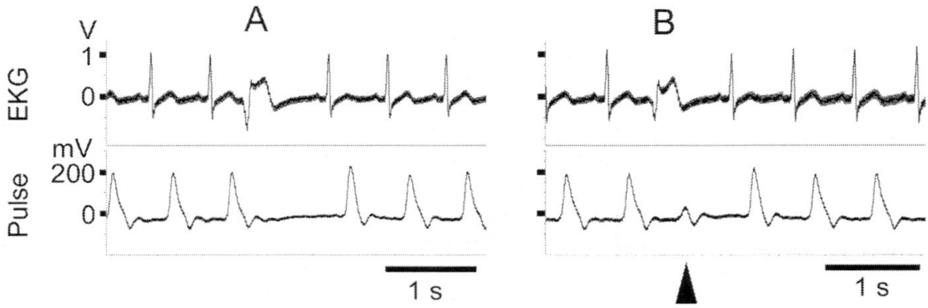

Fig. 1. Extrasystolic heartbeats in a 55-year-old man.

There was another obstacle: premature ventricular contraction (PVC). Among the "normal" subjects (age over 40 years old), about 60% of the subjects had arrhythmic heartbeats, such as PVC (Figures 1 & 2). Normally, PVC is believed to be benign arrhythmia, and, in fact, many healthy-looking people have exhibited this arrhythmia in our own experience. However, this PVC was an obstacle to the perfect detection of the timing of the heartbeat because the height of the signal was sometime very small (see Figure 1). If the baseline of the EKG recording was extremely stable, the heartbeats were automatically detectable even when irregular beats appeared sporadically (see Figure 2). However, in commercial EKG recording devices, the baseline of the recording was not as stable as shown in Figure 2.
Figure 2 shows an example of peak identification. In Figure 2A, the heartbeats were not detected by visual observation but by our peak-identification program. Heartbeats No. 5 and No. 8 show PVC spikes. In Figure 2B, after the peak identification, the interval time series is constructed automatically. This is comparable to the so-called R-R interval time series in medicine. The two arrows indicate the correlation between the heartbeats in A and B.

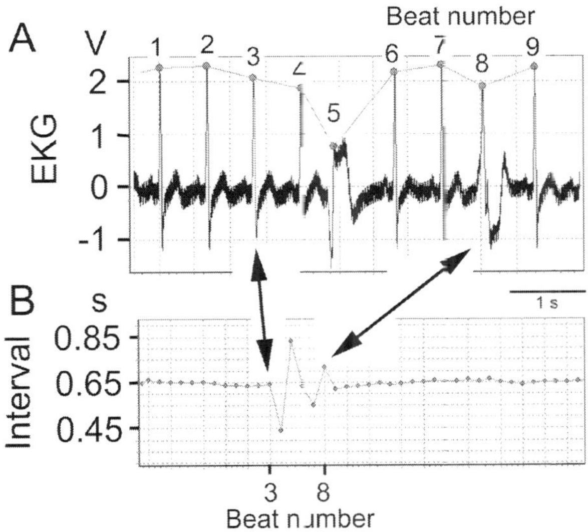

Fig. 2. An example of peak identification in a 55-year-old man.

2.2 EKG recording with stable baseline

To capture peaks without misdetection, we first needed to know how noise disturbs general EKG recordings. Figure 3 shows how false peak identifications occur. Here, 3 EKG electrodes (+, -, and ground (Nihonkoden Co. Ltd.; disposable Model Vitrode V) were placed on the chest of the subject. The subject was asked to hit his chest with his hands during the middle of the recording. Artificial noise-like spikes (4 arrowheads) appeared by hitting. They were automatically captured as the "false" heartbeats in this figure.
We made an EKG amplifier that enabled us to perform stable baseline recordings (see Figures 4, 5, & 6). An example set is shown in Figure 4. In the photograph, AC- and DC-EKG amplifiers, a 100-times amplifier, an analogue digital converter, and a USB connector can be

seen. Nothing was special with respect to the arrangement of the parts, but the important issue was that we found out that the time constant for the input stage of the recording must be adjusted to <0.22 s (Yazawa et al., 2010a; 2010b, Yazawa & Shimoda, 2010a; 2010b).

Figure 5 shows how our amplifier works for correct peak observation. The EKG trace is very stable. Body movements appeared on the record of the Piezo-electric pressure pulse (Finger p. trace), but the movements did not disturb the stable EKG recording (EKG trace).

Figure 6 shows an example of the long-period recording needed to perform instantaneous DFA computation. Here, a 15-year-old girl sat on a chair and engaged in fun conversation for a period of about 25 min. We used the amplifiers and a small time constant for the present study. This facilitated our DFA research. However, in some cases, inevitable noises contaminated the recordings, like the data shown in Figure 3. In such case, we removed the noises by eye observation on the PC screen in making a heartbeat interval time series. However, we have already identified how this problem occurred. It was due to the electrodes partially separating from the skin caused by sweating. We can overcome this problem by ensuring low smear clean skin.

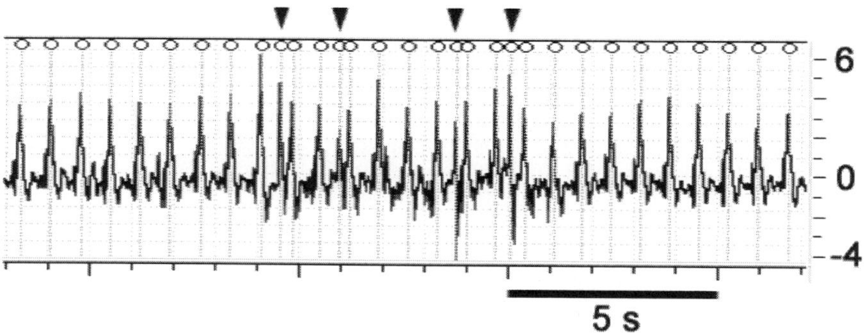

Fig. 3. False peaks incorporated into EKG in a 63-year-old man.

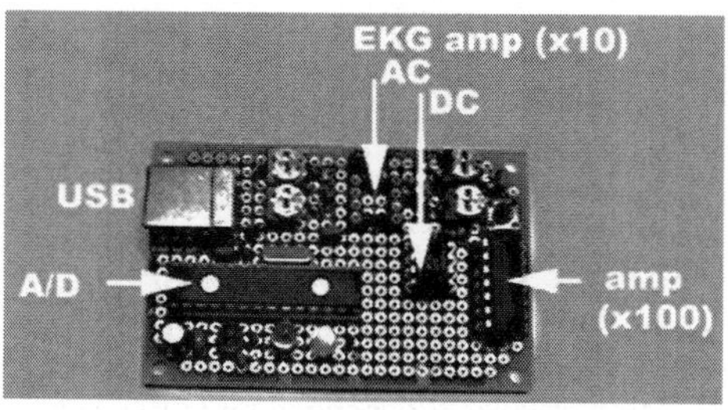

Fig. 4. An EKG amplifier.

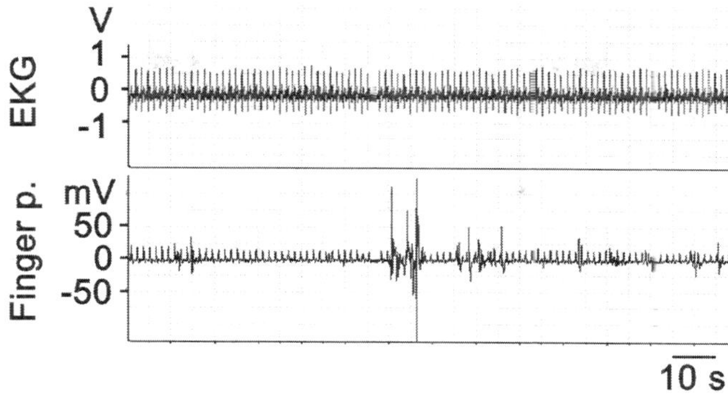

Fig. 5. Steady EKG recording during bodily movements in a 59-year-old man.

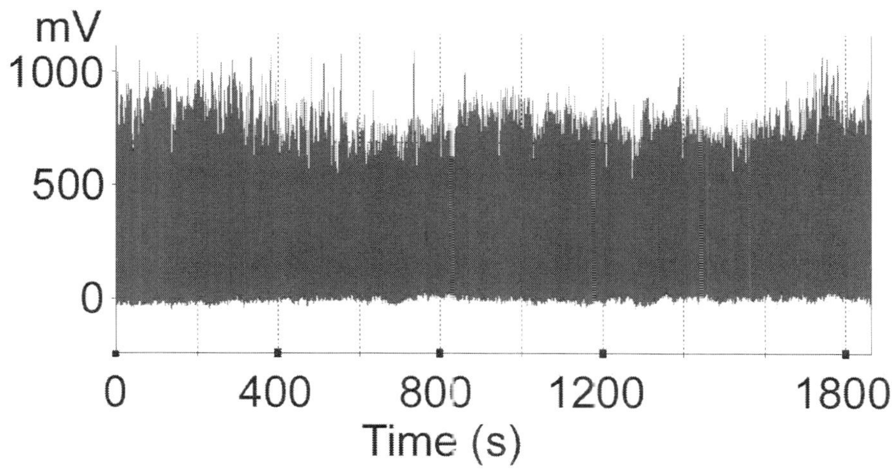

Fig. 6. A long-term EKG recording without obstacle noise in a 15-year-old girl.

2.3 DFA: Background

DFA is based on the concepts of "scaling" and "self-similarity" (Stanley, 1995). It can identify "critical" phenomena because systems near critical points exhibit self-similar fluctuations (Stanley, 1995, Peng et al., 1995, Goldberger et al., 2002), which means that recorded signals and their magnified/contracted copies are statistically similar. Self-similarity is defined as follows. In general, the statistical quantities, such as "average" and "variance," of a fluctuating signal can be calculated by taking the average of the signal through a certain section; however, the average is not necessarily a simple average. In this study, we took an average of the data squared. The statistical quantity calculated depended on the section size. The signal was self-similar when the statistical quantity was λ^{α} times for a section size magnified by λ. Here, "α" is the "scaling exponent" and characterizes the self-similarity.

Stanley and colleagues consider that the scaling property can be detected in biological data because most biological systems are strongly nonlinear and resemble the systems in nature that exhibit critical phenomena. They applied DFA to DNA arrangement and EKG data in the late 80s and early 90s, identified the scaling property (Peng et al., 1995, Goldberger et al., 2002), and emphasized the potential utility of DFA in the life sciences (Goldberger et al., 2002). Although DFA technology has not progressed to a great extent, nonlinear technology is now widely accepted, and rapid advances are being made in this technology.

2.4 DFA: Technique

DFA computation methods have been explained elsewhere (Katsuyama et al., 2003). In brief, DFA is performed as follows:

i. The heartbeat is recorded for 30–50 minutes in a single test because approximately 2,000 beats are required for determination of the scaling exponent. We recorded heartbeats using an EKG or finger pressure pulses.
ii. Pulse-peak time series $\{t_i\}$ (i = 1, 2, ... , N + 1) are captured from the record by using an algorithm based on the peak-detection method. To avoid false detection, we visually identified all peaks on the PC screen. Experience in neurobiology and cardiac animal physiology is occasionally necessary when determining whether a pulse-peak is a cardiac signal or noise.
iii. Heartbeat-interval time series $\{I_i\}$, such as the R-R intervals on an EKG, are calculated as follows:

$$\{I_i\} = \{t_{i+1} - t_i\}, i = 1, 2, ..., N \tag{1}$$

iv. The series $\{B_k\}$, upon which we conduct the DFA, is calculated as follows:

$$\{B_k\} = \left\{\sum_{j=1}^{k} \left[I_j - <I>\right]\right\}, \tag{2}$$

where $<I>$ is the mean interval defined as:

$$<I> = \frac{\sum_{i=1}^{N} I_i}{N} \tag{3}$$

v. The series $\{B_k\}$ is divided into smaller sections of j beats each. The section size j can range from 1 to N. To ensure efficient and reliable calculation of the scaling exponent in our program, we confirmed by test analysis that the number N should ideally exceed 1,000.
vi. In each section, the series $\{B_k\}$ is approximated to a linear function. To find the function, we applied the least square method. This function expresses the "trend"—slow fluctuations such as increases/decreases in B_k throughout the section size. A "detrended" series $\{B'_k\}_j$ is then obtained by the subtraction of $\{B_k\}$ from the linear function.
vii. We calculated the variance, which was defined as:

$$F^2(j) = <\left\{B'^{\,2}_k\right\}_j> \tag{4}$$

viii. Steps (v) to (vii) are repeated for changing j from 1 to N. Finally, the variance is plotted against the section size j. The scaling exponent is then obtained by

$$F^2(j) \propto j^{\alpha} \tag{5}$$

Most of computations mentioned above, which are necessary to obtain the scaling exponent, are automated. The automatic program gives us a scaling exponent relatively quickly. The scaling exponent is approximately 1.0 for healthy hearts and is higher or lower for sick hearts. Although we cannot have a critical discussion regarding whether the exponent is precisely 1.0, our automatic program can reliably distinguish a healthy heart from a sick heart. In this article, we classified the scaling exponent into 3 types, normal, high, and low.

2.5 EKG and finger pulse

For human subjects, we used both finger pulse recordings and EKG recordings. For pulse recordings, we used a Piezo-crystal mechano-electric sensor connected to a Power Lab System (AD Instruments; Australia). For EKG, 3 AgAgCl electrodes (+, -, and ground, manufacturer mentioned above) were used. Wires from the EKG electrodes were connected to our newly made amplifier (For EKG amplifier, see above). These EKG signals were also connected to a Power Lab System.

2.6 Model animals

It is very important that animal models be healthy before an investigation. To confirm that all the animals used were healthy, we captured them from a natural habitat and examined them. We used crustacean hearts because we are familiar with the structure and function of the crustacean heart and nervous system. One of the main reasons for using invertebrates was that all these animals have a common genetic code (DNA information) for body systems such as the cardiovascular system (Gehring, 1998, Sabirzhanova et al., 2009). All animals have a pump (the heart) and a controller (the brain).

2.7 Volunteers and ethics

Subjects were selected from colleagues in our university laboratories, volunteers who willingly visited our exhibition booth and desired have their heart checked, and the staff at NOMS Co. Ltd. and Maru Hachi Co. Ltd. All subjects were treated as per the ethical control regulations of our universities, Tokyo Metropolitan University and Tokyo Women's Medical University.

3. Results

3.1 Extrasystole: PVC

Figure 7 shows an example recording of extrasystole. This recording was obtained by a finger pulse recording. Large peaks were marked (o). Two small pulses are shown (A and B), which are PVCs. Our volunteers said that a PVC is perceived as a "skipped beat" or felt as palpitations, although some experienced no special sensation. In a normal heartbeat, the ventricles contract after the atria. In a PVC, the ventricles contract first. Therefore, the ejection volume is inefficient (see Figure 7). Single beat PVC arrhythmias do not usually pose a danger and can be asymptomatic in "healthy" individuals according to physicians. However, there is no way to accurately determine if someone is a "healthy" individual, which is the problem. That is why we tested DFA as a tool.

In Figure 7, one can see that there is difference in the pulse configuration between A and B. The two beats originated from different sites (a myocardial cell or cluster of myocardial cells) inside the ventricle, or at different times from an identical site. This is a typical extrasystole arrhythmia, although we did not pay further attention to cardiac physiology like the ectopic beat characteristics. For DFA, we just needed to measure the intervals of the heartbeats. Theoretically, irregularity itself carries hidden information.

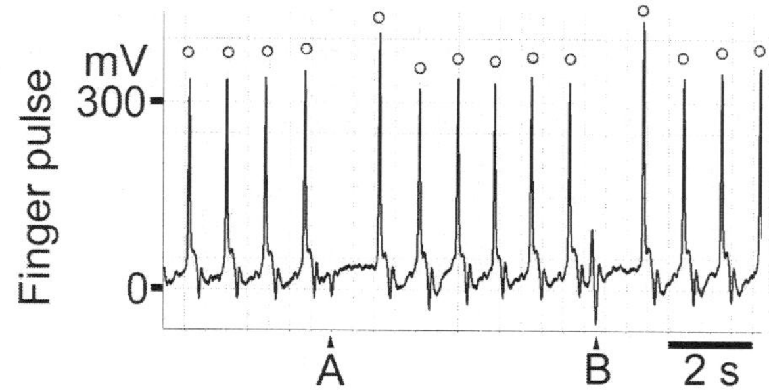

Fig. 7. An example of extrasystolic pulsations in a 65-year-old man.

During the past 4 years, we have encountered about 50 subjects who have extrasystole arrhythmia. Among all of our subjects (over 300) from age 2 to age 87, PVCs were not recorded in very young people (age < 19). One exception was a student (age 20); he showed benign PVCs. Most cases of PVCs were found in subjects over age 50 and about half were male.
Figure 8 shows the interval time series from the subject in Figure 7. Here, we recorded 1998 beats. Only 17 PVCs can be seen as downward swings.

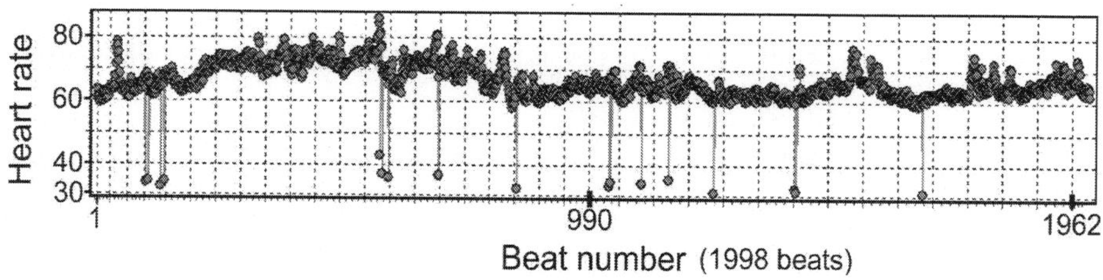

Fig. 8. A time series of the EKG with some PVCs. The same subject as in Figure 7.

We found that PVC hearts always exhibited a low scaling exponent (0.7–0.8). Figure 9 shows an example. The computation was worked out on the data of Figure 8. The slope in the graph shows a straight line, indicating that "scaling" is beautifully constituted over the entire range of the box size (10–1000). The scaling exponent for this subject was 0.8095 (see inset equation in Figure 9).
Most PVCs are benign according to physicians' assessments so long as the PVC does not exceed over 10 times per min. The subject (male 65 years old) shown in Figures. 7, 8, and 9 was a very active person. He told us he was working at a large electric company. He seemed to have no major health problems. He indicated he was not bothered by his PVC. In fact, it looked to be benign. However, on the basis of our DFA results, we do not agree that PVCs are always benign. His scaling exponent was 0.8, which is not perfect health in terms of fluctuation analysis. We would say the subject's health is dependant upon other factors. Therefore, we should treat individuals one by one. Everyone has a unique genomic blue print (DNA). The genetic code for the structure and function of life is never the same in any 2 individuals.
Another case study involves a volunteer we worked with for over 6 years. She has so-called benign PVCs. She is a German-American (age 58) living in Virginia, USA. She often told us that her palpitations (about 10 times per one hour) were uncomfortable when they occurred

(data not shown). Her scaling exponents were 0.7–0.8. She said that the PVCs were annoying. She was very nervous to have her PVCs compared to this male subject (Figures 7, 8, and 9). It is known that repetitive PVC leads to ventricular tachycardia. We so far do not have good solution for the problem of the low exponent.

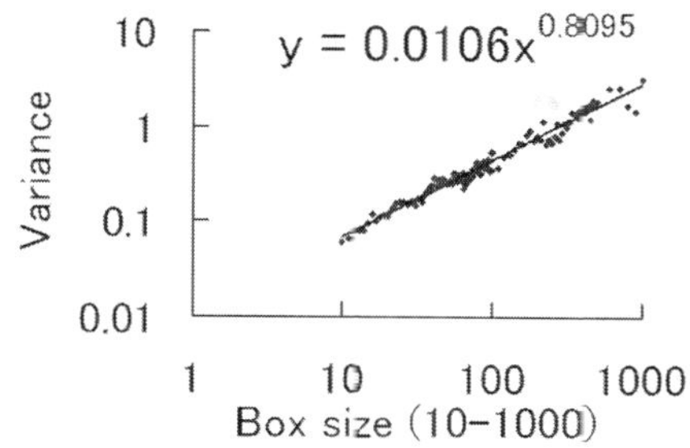

Fig. 9. DFA results for the subject shown in Figures 7 and 8.

3.2 Arrhythmia with dialysis

When we presented our work at an exhibition, Innovation Japan 2009, we met a representative from a company who had an interest in healthcare issues. According to his proposal, we recorded his EKGs and finger pulses (shown in Figures 1 & 2). We brought back his data to the university laboratory and started DFA analysis.

Figure 10 shows the results. In A, the time series data of 4265 heartbeats is shown. In B, the results of the calculation from the entire range of the box size, 10–1000, is shown. This box size is our normal calculation procedure. In C, the DFA results on a small box size of 30–110 are shown. The slope gives the scaling exponent, calculated by least mean square approximation, which was 1.1502. In D, the DFA results on a box size of 120–270 are shown. The scaling exponent was 0.6283.

We noticed that his heartbeat exhibited PVC-like arrhythmia (Figures 1, 2, & 10A). We were not 100% sure that his arrhythmia was PVC. We wondered how and why his arrhythmic beats were generated. After DFA computation was completed, we found that the slope was not a straight line (Figure 10B). The scaling exponent calculated from a small box size (30–110) was 1.15 (see Figure 10C). While 1.15 is within the normal value, we were concerned that it was a value higher than 1.0. In turn, his scaling exponent from a large box size (120–270) was extremely low, 0.6 (see Figure 10D). We could at least say that his health was not perfect; we wanted to recommend that he see a doctor.

Since he did not provide us with any personal health information about himself, we believed that he was normal when we took the recording. However, the results were not normal. It looked like PVC, but we were not sure. Then, we discussed his results in the laboratory, and decided to share our concerns about his heart. We made a telephone call to him, and stated: "I am not a physician. I am just a neurobiologist. However, I would like to suggest you visiting a cardiologist based on your data." He then replied that he already knew that he had skipped heartbeats, and he was regularly visiting a physician three times a week. He further explained that he has been on dialysis for about 20 years. The sickness started in his early 30s. He and his doctor always talked about the state of his heart. He thanked us for contacting him.

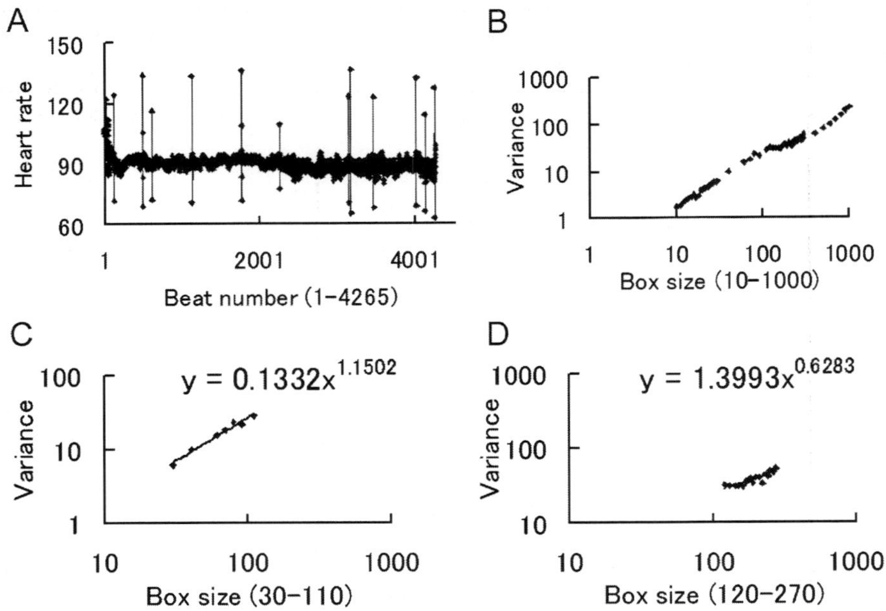

Fig. 10. DFA results from patient on dialysis. Male 55 years.

We felt that he was doubtful of our scientific skill. We passed his examination, which was set up without our knowledge. University and corporate collaboration was initiated thereafter.

3.3 PVC with smoking

Figure 11A shows that we recorded 2338 heartbeats from a subject (a friend of an author) when sitting on a chair in a coffee shop. His heartbeat showed PVCs as indicated by some short-interval beats (see downward swings in Figure 11A). Three long-interval heartbeats (Figure 11A) demonstrate a "skipped" heartbeat. These skipped beats and PVC beats were an extrasystolic phenomena. The occurrence of these arrhythmic beats did not exceed 10 per min (see Figure 11A). Therefore, we may conclude that his PVC was benign in terms of the physicians' guidelines. However, the scaling exponent was low, 0.7288 (see Figure 12A1 and 12A2) at a normal sitting state. We confirmed that the PVC exhibited a low scaling exponent. He loved smoking cigarettes very much, although a cardiac-scientist recommended that he quit. In Figure 11B, 2433 heartbeats were recorded in the coffee shop. When he started smoking, recording also began. Skipped beats increased in number during smoking (see under-bar periods in Figure 11B). During the smoking period (Figure 11B), the total number of PVCs increased. It seemed that the intake of tobacco-related chemicals (we did not determine whether it was the nicotine, tar, etc.) into the body quickly pushed the scaling exponent toward a much lower value, i.e., from a non-smoking value of 0.7288 (Figure 12A2) to smoking-value of 0.6195 (Figure 12B2). It was apparent that DFA monitors nervous system function as well as cardiovascular function.

DFA, therefore, can measure the wellness of the entire body system. However, DFA does not tell you in detail, for example, what is wrong with the body system or what local element is reacting to the environment.

Since the results of Figures 11 & 12 were so significant and intriguing, we wanted to examine other "smoking" subjects. We finally determined that smokers' heartbeats were not always susceptible to "smoking."

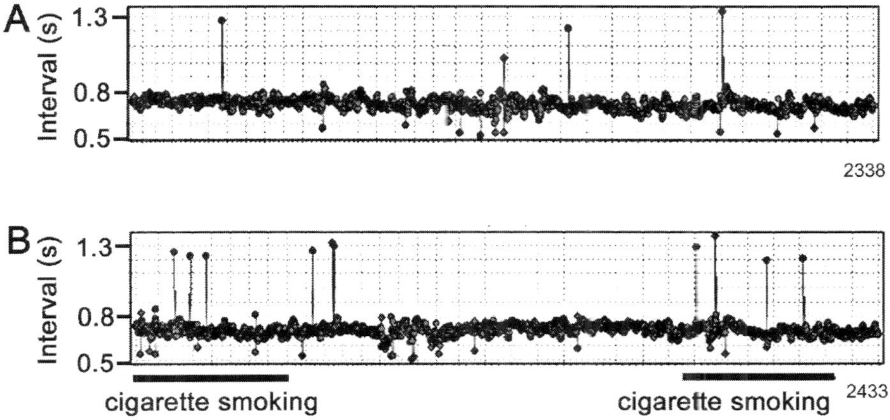

Fig. 11. Time series. A: Non smoking and B: Smoking 58-year-old man.

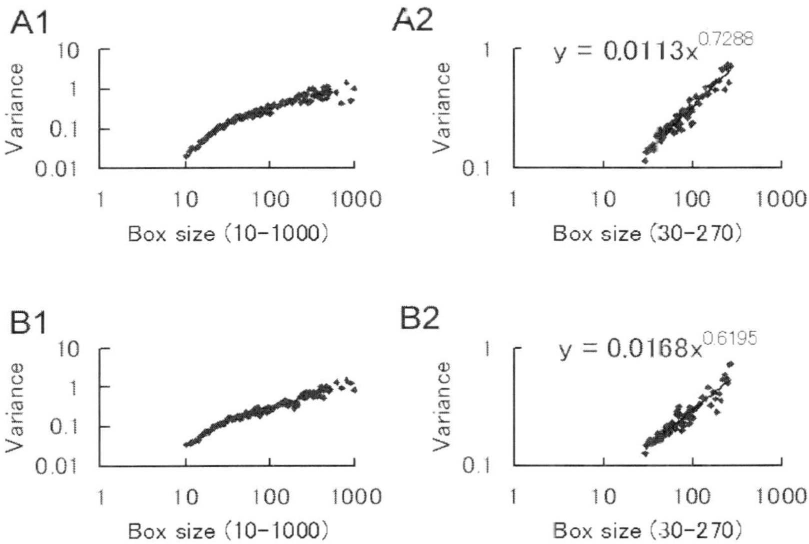

Fig. 12. DFA results on the data in Figure 11. A: Non-smoking. B: Smoking.

3.4 Alternans arrhythmia

Alternans (a period-2 rhythm) was first documented in 1872 by Traube. However, alternans did not receive particular attention from doctors until recently; in fact, alternans was previously referred to as the harbinger of death (Bragaa et al., 2004, Pieske & Kochskamper, 2002, Rosenbaum et al., 1994). The phenomenon of alternans is of continuing interest nowadays particularly because of its association with myocardial ischemia and cardiac arrhythmias. In animal models, we have already reported that the alternans heartbeat exhibits a low scaling exponent. This was measured on the heartbeats of crustacean animals such as crabs and lobsters (n = 13) (Yazawa et al., 2009). We also encountered human alternans subjects (n = 8, 5 Japanese and 3 Americans). Their scaling exponents were low (Yazawa et al., 2009).

Figure 13 shows an example of alternans in which the subject's heartbeats showed a period-2 rhythm (Figure 13A). We met him in 2007 at an exhibition called Innovation Japan 2007. At that time, he at first told us that he knew that his heart was not normal, and he regularly went to see a doctor. He visited us because we presented our DFA method at the exhibition. We recorded his heartbeat (Figure 13A). His scaling exponent in September 2007 was 0.6709 (see Figure 13B and 13C). We explained to him that he had alternans, and we explained the condition to the best of our knowledge.

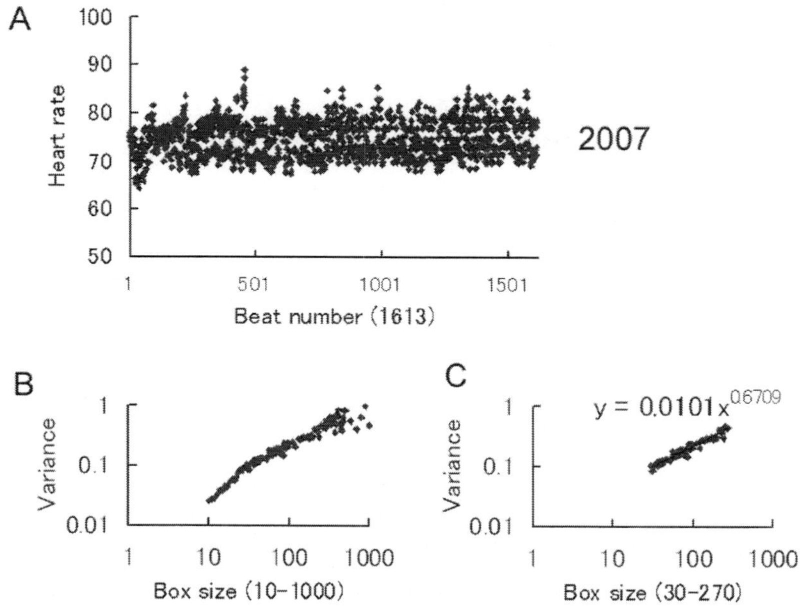

Fig. 13. DFA of alternans. Recorded in September 2007 in Tokyo. Subject was in his 60s.

Two years later, in September in 2009, we returned to the exhibition. We did not expect him to visit us again, but he came. We recorded his heartbeat and calculated his scaling exponent (Figure 14). To our surprise, the alternans was almost gone, and his scaling exponent was higher than in 2007 (see Figure 14A). In fact, there was a noticeable difference in the time series data between 2007 (Figure 13A) and 2009 (Figure 14A). He said that since learning the results shown in Figure 13A in 2007, he had been walking to work instead of driving.

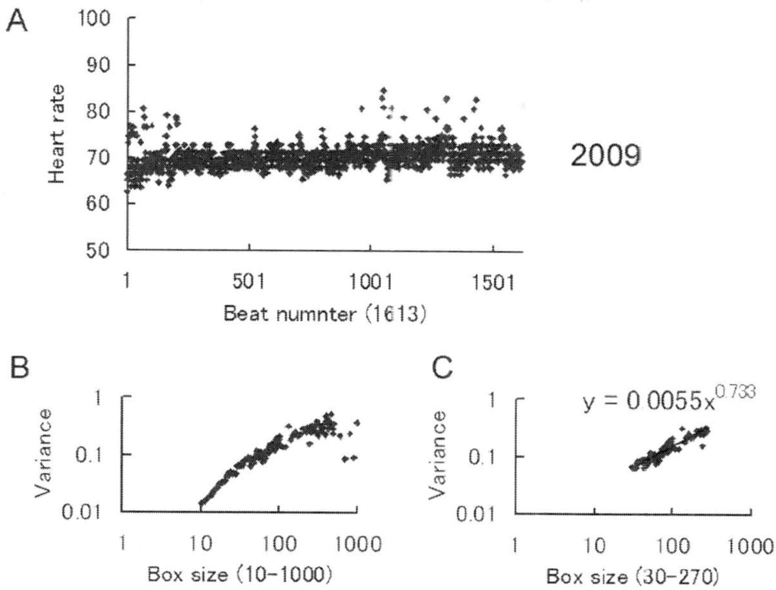

Fig. 14. DFA of alternans. Recorded again in September 2009 in Tokyo.

His scaling exponents are compared in Table 1. Three different DFA computations at different box sizes are shown. Years 2007 and 2009 are compared. The table shows that his scaling exponents were improved in all three areas. The exponents shifted toward the good health state, which is ultimately 1.0.

Box size	2007	2009
30-110	0.703	0.839
70-140	0.743	0.878
30-270	0.671	0.733

Table 1. Comparison of the scaling exponents at different box sizes. Computed from the data obtained from the subject shown in Figures 13 and 14.

Based on these results, we can conclude that DFA was useful in determining that his condition had improved.

3.5 Normal healthy rhythm

Several volunteers have helped conduct our follow-up test that has lasted for several years. The volunteers include the authors, their family members, and university colleagues. Figure 15 shows an example. A young woman, 26 years old in 2006, who was working in the

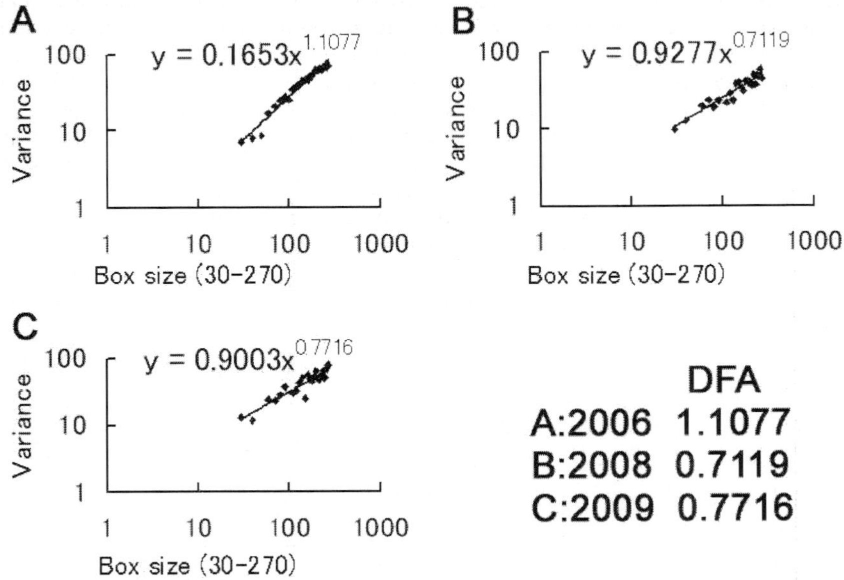

Fig. 15. DFA follow-up on a healthy subject. Female 27 years old in 2006.

university's intellectual property office, was willing to help us as a volunteer for long-range follow-up. Since we often worked together, we could obtain information about her everyday life if we needed.

Her scaling exponents have shifted toward a lower value over the course of 4 years. Herein, we have described our interpretation of why her scaling exponents gradually changed. This case study indicated how and why a once perfectly healthy subject gradually experienced stress.

In 2006, we submitted our patent regarding our DFA method from the university's intellectual property office. At that time, she was a newcomer. She supported us greatly. Her heartbeat exhibited a normal scaling exponent of 1.1077 (Figure 15A, in September 2006). One could argue that the value of 1.1 is higher than the normal perfect value 1.0. However, according to our preliminary guideline, 1.1 is normal. We recorded her heartbeat in September of 2006. She was pretty, active in her job, and she was thoughtful to colleagues. Most importantly, her exponent was fine.

In 2008, she lost a loved one. One day, she told us that her grandmother had become seriously ill. She returned to her hometown immediately. Her hometown was not located a short distance from Tokyo and, therefore, she could not commute back and forth. She stayed in her hometown for a while to take care of her grandmother. She only visited the workplace occasionally. We did not know the details about her life at that time. Therefore, we just took her heartbeat data as usual in September of 2008. Later, we leaned that her loved one had recently passed away.

In September 2009, we again recorded her heartbeat as usual. The Innovation Japan exhibition was held in September as well. During the 30 min period of recording of her heartbeat, we talked. While she had recovered from her grandmother's death, she found her present job to be boring. She wanted to be a skilful patent manager and wanted to quit her ordinary office job. At the end of the year 2009, she abruptly notified to us that she would be leaving since she had accepted another job. Although her salary would decrease, she would have the opportunity to perform much higher-level work involving the patent business.

When we measured her heartbeat in 2006, her exponents were always near 1.0. We believed for long time that she represented the perfect scaling exponent. Her EKG data from 2008 and 2009 were stored deep inside the PC and remained there without receiving attention. Recently, we accidentally analyzed her hidden data in August 2010. We discovered that her exponents correlated with a shift in her psychology.

The results are shown in Figure 15. We can trace back what has happened in her life, as mentioned above. We can interpret a correlation between the shift of her scaling exponent and the shift of her psychological states. In the year 2006, she was a fresh worker after finishing her master's degree, and she had a healthy scaling exponent (Figure 15A, see also inset of Figure 15). In the year 2008, she had hard days, and she had stress. In those days, her scaling exponent was the worst we hade measured (Figure 15B). In the year 2009, she seemed to be recovered although she did not tell us so. However, her scaling exponent was not fully recovered to 1.0 (Figure 15C). We now know that she was trying to get a promotion, although she never told us until she succeeded in getting a new job. In the spring of 2010, she disappeared and we lost contact with her. Nonetheless, her data can explain how and why her healthy scaling exponent has shifted.

This story suggests that DFA measurements might be helpful for monitoring the functioning of the entire body system function, including wellness, sickness, and psychology. It is apparent that we need to conduct further investigations with additional subjects before declaring DFA's power and ability are great and beyond what we have experienced before in the community of health care, medicine, biology, and physics. Biomedical computation is a growing field of science.

4. Discussion

Heart and skeletal muscle are structurally similar; both exhibit striations. However, unlike skeletal muscle, the heart muscle exhibits automaticity—the property of spontaneous contractions in the absence of nerve stimuli. Furthermore, the spontaneous contractions are generated regularly at their own rate like a clock, or so-called pacemaker. Spontaneity and regularity are the most advanced characteristics of myocardial cells, which have been achieved in evolution. To alter its robust rhythm, actions by the nerves and hormones to the pacemaker are necessary. The force of the action is determined by the number of demands coming from the cells in the body via nerves and hormones. Since the cell is the ultimate element composing the living body, interaction between cells is a key function in a multicellular organism. While all of the elements are nonlinearly connected to each other, the interaction is never the same in any 2 individuals because each individual has his/her own genome. For example, different cells (individual) respond differently to an antibiotic; thus, some are highly resistant, and some are less resistant (Lee et al., 2010). Here is another example showing that everybody has their own genetic code: It is believed that a medication, clopidogrel, reduces the rate of major vascular events among patients with acute coronary syndromes and atrial fibrillation. A recent study implied that the benefits of clopidogrel were attenuated in patients with genetic variants (Paré et al., 2010). Thus, everyone must be checked and considered independently when applying DFA. If we find a single exception, we should throw out our theory because it should not happen in terms of a nonlinear way of thinking. We so far have confirmed that PVC subjects have a low scaling exponent. There have been no cases where a PVC subject had a value higher than 1.0. We could not accept such a discrepancy. We have so far never found a paradox. We are able to explain all data under the criterion that 1.0 means wellness and a variation from 1.0 means sickness. However, there is a problem with the criterion: the border between wellness and sickness has not yet been established. Everlasting investigation is the only solution for confirming our theory is accurate.

What is wellness of life? Wellness is the state in which an individual can generate 1/f rhythm from the heartbeat (Kobayashi and Musha, 1993). The important point is whether the rhythm is 1/f or not. In this article, we showed that DFA works without exception. If you have a scaling exponent of 1.0, then you are healthy. If your scaling exponent is higher or lower than 1.0, something is wrong with you. The scaling exponent of 1.0 is the perfect state of life. To our surprise, only 10% of our subjects belonged to the perfect state (n = 300, human; the number was greater in animal models including lobsters, crabs, frogs, and insects).

Synchronous contractions of the cardiac muscles are a fundamental functional requirement for the heart to work as a pump. Further, this synchrony is established by electric coupling between the muscle cells. This synchronous and regular automaticity assures a constant flow of circulation and is widely observable throughout the animal kingdom, from invertebrates to vertebrates, i.e., from insects and lobsters to humans. This explains why our experiments on model animals were successful and useful for human physiology.

Our experiments on crustacean hearts (Yazawa et al., 2004) led us to the conclusion that DFA distinguished isolated hearts from intact hearts. From this conclusion, we deduced that DFA was useful for detecting the preliminary stage of sickness of the cardiovascular system. The present case studies verified this deduction.

The periodicity of contractions is a common and important characteristic of the heart. If regularity is disturbed for some reason, clotting/coagulation of the blood cells easily occurs. Thus, irregularity is a disadvantage for wellness. Rate change in the heartbeat normally occurs in a gradual manner in various time courses, either in a slow response or quick response. A mixture of the various time courses is required for wellness. In principle, DFA looks at the degree of mixture of the time courses. Skipping heartbeats (PVC) and alternans (2 beats) exhibited less dynamical changes in rate. This was well sensed by DFA as a low scaling exponent.

A gradually and dynamically changing heart rate is proof of wellness and a healthy scaling exponent of 1.0. Uncomfortable and adverse stimulation from the environment can interfere with the periodicity of cardiac contractions, e.g., stress-induced arrhythmic heartbeats. A typical example of stress-induced arrhythmia is a sudden reflexive slow-down in the rate of the heartbeat observed during a shadow stimulation (Mashimo et al., 1976, Yazawsa et al., 1977, see also Gwilliam, 1963 for shadow reflex). Changes in rate naturally reflect changes in external and internal environments. Dynamic change is itself normal. However, if interactions between the nerve signals (neurotransmitters/hormones) and muscle receptors are not normal, skipping beats, deficit beats, unstable intervals, and extremely fast beatings may occur. This is well sensed by DFA, and DFA will calculate a low scaling exponent as described in the present investigations.

We declare that DFA can distinguish wellness and sickness. If the scaling exponent is near 1.0, wellness is confirmed. If the scaling exponents are considerably higher or lower than 1.0, a masked condition is a possibility. Unfortunately, we must admit that DFA cannot tell what cells or what organ is the origin of that poor state. We cannot determine what is wrong with the subject. We admit that there is such a limit in DFA. However, DFA makes a "good" or "bad" judgement of health in a quantitative way.

Myocardial pacemaker cells produce the periodicity of cardiac contractions. The pace is determined by the rate of action potentials, which requires strictly controlled ionic flows. The ionic flows are controlled by ionic channels equipped on the myocardial cellular membrane. The millions of ionic channels work with quasi synchronously in the myocardial membrane. However, synchrony is not perfect among the millions of channels. Fundamentally, the ionic channels in the cells have electrical properties comprised of 2 states—open and closed. The consequences of modification/distortion of the open vs. closed states are arrhythmic heartbeats, i.e., heartbeat fluctuations. The fluctuation occurs within a millisecond in the time scale. From this consideration, we adopted a sampling rate of 1 kHz when we recorded heartbeat data. This was a key factor of the recording method, and it led us to a successful DFA analysis for determining whether or not subjects were healthy. The origin of arrhythmia, therefore, is the membrane of the ionic channels. Sodium (Na) and potassium (K) are the major ions that contribute to the rate of cardiac action potentials since these ions are present in the blood (and tissue fluid) at the highest concentrations. Other ions, such as calcium (Ca), are present in the blood at relatively low concentrations. Therefore, the rate of flow of Na/K ions is the key factor determining the heart rate. (We do not, however, ignore the contribution of Ca to heart rate.) The equilibrium potential of each ion and the membrane potential of the myocardium are important factors for determining heart rate. Without any changes in the equilibrium or membrane potentials, the heart rate cannot be changed in a constant temperature environment. The pace making mechanism is fundamentally robust in function because millions of channels work together in a quasi-synchronous way. To change this robust pacing function, chemicals (neurotransmitters and hormones) must act on receptor-ionic channels (complex molecules). Taken together, ionic balance and chemical balance (hormones and neurotransmitters) are the key variables for determining the heart rate. DFA indirectly examines this fundamental molecular mechanism. Ultimately, wellness and sickness are related to the ionic mechanism of nerves and muscles that receive influences from the chemical ingredients in the blood. We trust that the state of the blood and nerves plays a pivotal role in the state of wellness.

Gradual changes from wellness to sickness are invisible on ordinary EKG recordings. Nevertheless, pumping hearts may carry hidden information about wellness or sickness, and we can extract this information from the pattern of the heartbeats. Extremely irregular heartbeats may indicate sickness, the worst-case scenario being a heart attack.

Heart attacks do not recur with the precision of a timed life cycle, or have the signature of sudden psychological shock. However, we believe that they obey the laws of physics, which means that we should be able to predict their recurrence. For this purpose, we must employ physics and mathematics in addition to biology and medicine. In Chinese medicine, physicians feel the pulse of patients to make diagnoses. A skilled physician's nervous system seems to function like a computer and performs miraculous feats. This fact indicates that pulses and heartbeats carry hidden information about a patient's wellness or sickness. However, man-made machines have not been able to mimic this ability of physicians, even though more than a hundred years have elapsed since the inception of the industrial revolution. Despite the historical challenges, we hope to design a machine that can be used to detect irregularities in cardiac periodicity. Our new EKG amplifier belongs to such efforts. It is almost noise free so long as subjects do not make extremely hard movements of the body, the details of which were documented in the present article.

Based upon our preliminary guidelines, 0.9–1.19 indicates health, 1.2–1.5 indicates sudden death, and 0.5–0.89 indicates natural death. In our study, and in the study conducted by Peng et al., (1995), the "normal" state has been associated with a scaling exponent of 0.9–1.19 (our study) and 1.0 (Peng et al.). In the present article, we showed that PVC, a typical arrhythmia involving extrasystoles, exclusively lowered the scaling exponent; and alternans, an abnormal heart rhythm also known as the "harbinger of death," also exclusively lowered the scaling exponent of heartbeat fluctuation dynamics.

Moreover, we already found that transplanted human hearts (n = 3) exhibit a scaling exponent as high as 1.2 (Yazawa et al., 2006), and hearts with ischemic disease (n = 5) exhibit a scaling exponent of 1.2–1.4 (Yazawa et al., 2008, Yazawa and Tanaka, 2009). However, we have made some intriguing observations among our volunteers. We have met a volunteer subject (subject was in his late 60s, our colleague in Tokyo) who had received emergency medical care for ischemic heart disease. He received a stent placement. He had no myocardial cell damage according to his surgeon. We found that he had a normal scaling exponent (1.0). In this case, his wife was smart enough to notice her husband's sickness and made the quick decision to call an ambulance; in fact, she protected her husband from serious myocardial damage from coronary ischemia. Defibrillator implantation and continuous medication for atrial arrhythmia were also associated with a normal scaling exponent (subject in his 40s from in Nagoya City, subject in his 60s from Kawasaki City). Thus, the scaling exponent may indicate whether defibrillators and/or medications are working properly. Therefore, we consider that DFA will aid diagnostic decisions in patients with cardiovascular disorders. More case studies are required, although our guideline has thus far proved adequate, and we have found no exceptions to it, such as ischemic heart disease being associated with a high scaling exponent.

In this article, we have provided empirical proof of the practical usefulness of DFA. By presenting several case studies, we explained how the wellness of subjects could be evaluated using heartbeat recordings. Our purpose was to determine whether DFA is a useful method for the evaluation of the quality of a normal, healthy state. Our crucial target of this successive investigation was to discover the contradictions, if any, of our theory. Our preliminary guidelines for the interpretation of scaling exponents are as follows: 1, ideal state (wellness); >1, the heart is ready to stop any time; and <1, the heart is stressed, and its ionic balance and nerve activity are not ideal.

5. References

Bragaa, S. S., Vaninettib, R., Laportaa, A., Picozzia, A., & Pedrettia, R. F. E. (2004). T wave alternans is a predictor of death in patients with congestive heart failure. *Int. J. Cardiology*, Vol. 93, No. 1, pp. 31-38.

de Torbal, A., Boersma, E., Kors, J. A., van Herpen, G., Deckers, J. W., van der Kuip, D. A. M., Stricker, B. H., Hofman, A., & Witteman, J. C. M. (2006). Incidence of recognized and unrecognized myocardial infarction in men and women aged 55 and older, The Rotterdam Study. *European Heart Journal*, Vol. 27, No. 6, pp. 729-736.

Gehring, W. J., (1998). *Master Control Genes in Development and Evolution: The Homeobox Story*, Yale University Press, New Haven.

Goldberger, A. L., Amaral, L. A. N., Hausdorff, J. M., Ivancv, P. C., & Peng, C. -K. (2002). Fractal dynamics in physiology: Alterations with disease and aging. *PNAS*, Vol. 99, suppl. 1, pp. 2466-2472.

Gwilliam, G. F. (1963). The mechanism of the shadow reflex in Cirripedia. I. Electrical activity in the supraesophageal ganglion and ocellar nerve. *Biological Bulletin*, Vol. 125, No. 3, pp. 470-485.

Katsuyama, T., Yazawa, T., Kiyono, K., Tanaka, K., & Otokawa, M. (2003). Scaling analysis of heart-interval fluctuation in the in-situ and in-vivo heart of spiny lobster, *Panulirus japonicus. Bull. Housei Univ. Tama*, Vol. 18, pp. 97-108, (in Japanese).

Lee, H. H., Molla, M. N., Cantor, C. R., & Collins, J. J. (2010). Bacterial charity work leads to population-wide resistance. *Nature*, Vol 467, pp. 82-86.

Mashimo, K. Yazawa, T., & Kuwasawa, K. (1976). Effects of shadow reflex in crustacean hearts. *The Zoological Society of Japan, Doubutsugaku zasshi*, Vol. 85, No. 4, p. 380, (in Japanese).

Paré, G., Mehta, S. R., Yusuf, S., Anand, S. S., Connolly, S. J., Hirsh, J., Simonsen, K., Bhatt, D. L., Fox, K. A. A., & Eikelboom, J. W. (2010). Effects of CYP2C19 genotype on outcomes of clopidogrel treatment. *The New England Journal of Medicine*, August 29, 2010, Online First, 10.1056/NEJMoa1008410, pp. 1-11.

Peng, C. -K., Havlin, S., Stanley, H. E., & Goldberger, A. L. (1995). Quantification of scaling exponents and crossover phenomena in nonstationary heartbeat time series". *Chaos*, Vol. 5, pp. 82-87.

Pieske, B., & Kockskamper, K. (2002). Alternans goes subcellular. A "disease" of the ryanodine receptor? *Circulation Research*, Vol. 91, pp. 553-555.

Rosenbaum, D. S., Jackson, L. E., Smith, J. M., Garan, H., Ruskin, J. N., & Cohen, R. J. (1994). Electrical alternans and vulnerability to ventricular arrhythmias. *The New England J. of Medicine*, Vol. 330, pp. 235-241.

Sabirzhanova, I., Sabirzhanov, B., Bjordahl, J. Brandt, J., Jay, P. Y., & Clark, T. G. (2009). Activation of tolloid-like 1 gene expression by the cardiac specific homeobox gene Nkx2-5. *Develop. Growth. Differ.* 51, pp. 403-410.

Stanley, H. E. (1995). Phase transitions. Power laws and universality. *Nature*, Vol. 378, p. 554.

Stanley, H. E., Amarala, L. A. N., Goldberger, A. L., Havlina, S., Ivanov, P. C., & Peng, C.-K. (1999). Statistical physics and physiology: Monofractal and multifractal approaches. *Physica A*, Vol. 270, pp. 309-324.

Traube, L., E. (1872). Fall von Pulsus bigeminus nebst Bemerkungen uber die Leberschwellungen bet Klappenfehlern und uber acute Leberatrophie. *Berl kiln Wschr.* Vol. 9, pp. 185–221.

Yazawa, T., Asai, I., Shimoda, Y., & Katsuyama, T. (2010a). Evaluation of wellness in sleep by detrended fluctuation analysis of the heartbeats. *Proceeding WCECS 2010, The World Congress on Engineering and Computer Science 2010*, Vol. II, pp. 921-925. October, San Francisco, USA.

Yazawa, T., Kiyono, K., Tanaka, K., & Katsuyama, T. (2004). Neurodynamical control systems of the heart of Japanese spiny lobster, *Panulirus japonicus. Izvestiya VUZ · Applied Nonlinear Dynamics.* Vol.12, No. 1-2, pp. 114-121.

Yazawa, T., Kuwasawa, K., & Mashimo, K. (1977). Neural modifications of heart beat in the shadow reflex of crustacea. *The Zoological Society of Japan, Doubutsugaku zasshi.* Vol. 86, No. 4, p. 373, (in Japanese).

Yazawa, T. & Shimoda, Y., (2010a). EKG recording without obstructive noise due to physical movement: A terminal EKG-monitoring device for online communication in a public healthcare link *Proceeding IMCIC 2010, The International Multi-Conference on Complexity, Informatics and Cybernetics,* Vol. I, pp. 57-60. April, Orlando, USA,

Yazawa, T., & Shimoda, Y. (2010b). Health check performed by DFA of heartbeat. *Proceeding ASME BioMed2010, 5th Frontiers in Biomedical Devices Conference,* Paper No. BioMed2010-32026, pp. 1-2. September, Newport Beach, California, USA

Yazawa, T., Shimoda, Y., Suzuki, T., & Nakata, H. (2010b). Thermal therapy with heartbeat observation. *Proceeding i-CREATe 2010, International Convention on Rehabilitation,* pp. 34-37. July, Shanghai, China.

Yazawa, T., & Tanaka, K. (2009). Scaling exponent for the healthy and diseased heartbeat: Quantification of the heartbeat interval fluctuations. In, Advances in Computational Algorithms and Data Analysis. Chapter. 1, pp. 1-14. ed. Sio-long Ao. Springer, NY.

Yazawa, T., Tanaka, K., Kato, A., & Katsuyama, T. (2008). The scaling exponent calculated by the detrended fluctuation analysis, distinguishes the injured sick hearts against normal healthy hearts. *Proceeding IAING (WCECS08) International Conference on Computational Biology (ICCB),* Vol. 2, pp. 7-12. 22-24 October, San Francisco, USA,

Yazawa, T., Tanaka, K., & Katsuyama, T. (2009). Alternans lowers the scaling exponent of heartbeat fluctuation dynamics: A detrended fluctuation analysis in animal models and humans". *Proceeding CSIE2009, World Congress on Computer Science and Information Engineering. Computer Soc.* pp. 221-225, April, Los Angeles, CA, USA. IEEE DOI 10.1109/CSIE.2009.784,

Yazawa, T., Tanaka, K., Katuyama, T., MacField, V., & Otokawa, M. (2006). A nonlinear analysis of EKG on heart-transplanted subject. *Bulletin Hosei Univ. Tama,* Vol. 21, pp. 1-10.

Yeh, R. W., Sidney, S., Chandra, M., Sorel, M., Selby, J. V., & Go. A. S. (2010). Population trends in the incidence and outcomes of acute myocardial infarction. *New Engl. J. of Medicine,* Vol. 362, pp. 2155-2165.

21

Multi-Aspect Comparative Detection of Lesions in Medical Images

Juliusz Kulikowski and Malgorzata Przytulska
M. Nalecz Institute of Biocybernetics and Biomedical Engineering, PAS Warsaw, Poland

1. Introduction

Symmetry is an easily observable property of a normal human body. It also occurs in the anatomy of some of its organs: motion or sensory organs, brain, dentition, breasts, kidneys, etc. This property is often used as a basis of visual diagnosis of anatomical defects or of pathological lesions in the organs, expressed by local disparities between the (generally symmetric) pairs of compared images (Rogowska J., Preston K., Hunter G.J. & al., 1995). Such approach, based on an assumption that in most cases the defects or lesions have been caused by asymmetrically acting factors, leads to a simple algorithm of lesions detection by pixel-from-pixel subtraction of matched pairs of images. However, for several reasons this approach does not lead to satisfactory results: 1st a general symmetry of normal body organs does not mean that small anatomic differences in them cannot occur, 2nd small local differences in compared pixel values can also be caused by image acquisition defects, 3rd substantial differences may be hidden in specific subtle local morphological structure of analyzed organs. A comparative detection of lesions is thus a non-trivial problem needing advanced solution approach. This remark also concerns a comparison of acquired at distanced time-instants medical images of a given organ aimed at an assessment of the results of its medical treatment. A comparative lesions detection should consist not so much in a detection of any formal but rather of *medically significant* differences between the compared images. Medically significant image details may be manifested by occurrence of both simple differences between the local (monochromatic or multi-chromatic) pixel values as well as by occurrence of more subtle features characterizing local sub-areas in the examined images. This leads to a concept of comparative image analysis based on a *multi-aspect dissimilarity measure* (Kulikowski J. L., Przytulska M., 2009a). The notions of *similarity* and *dissimilarity* are evidently related: the more similar two objects are, the less they are dissimilar. In certain cases, when the objects can be considered as elements of a metric (e.g. Euclidean) space their dissimilarity can strongly be connected with a *distance* between them. However, not all objects of medical interest, usually described by combinations of their quantitative and qualitative features, as the elements of a formally defined metric space can be considered. That is why it seems more reasonable to define dissimilarity (as well as similarity) measure as a normalized dimensionless parameter. Using the notion of *multi-aspect dissimilarity* to comparative lesions detection seems not only to be intuitively justified but also more suitable to distinguish between the normal and pathological tissues than a distance notion.

The aim of this Chapter is presentation of an approach to computer-aided comparative analysis of medical images aimed at detection of lesions occurring in one of two symmetrically located body regions. In this approach the concept of *multi-aspect similarity measure* as well as of a based on it concept of *dissimilarity measure* presented in the mentioned paper (Kulikowski J. L., Przytulska M., 2009a) plays a basic role. Moreover, application of *morphological spectra,* originally presented in some former papers (Kulikowski J. L., Przytulska M., 2007a; Kulikowski J. L., Przytulska M, & Wierzbicka D., 2007b), is also presented in a context of multi-aspect similarity of biological tissues assessment. It will be shown how the above-mentioned concepts can be used to an iterative lesions detection process consisting in a step-wise reinforcing of the objects' discrimination criteria. The below-presented methods have been primarily tested on cerebral single photon emission tomography (*SPECT*) as well as on liver ultrasound elastography (*USE)* images and some results of those experiments will be shown below.

2. Formal model of lesions

A *lesion* can be defined as a *harmful change in the tissues of bodily organs, caused by injury or disease* (Hornby A.S., 1980). In computer-aided medical images analysis we are interested not only in a simple lesions detection but also in their localization (e.g. by contouring), size and form description, intensity assessment, etc. Of course, it is assumed that any lesion area is visually from the background distinguishable. However, 1st not all visual differences are for lesion detection substantial, and 2nd it may a priori be not known how a certain sort of lesion should visually be manifested. Lesion detection reminds thus detection of a pickpocket in a crowd of bus passengers: we know, that his behavior differs from this of other passengers, however, the face and wear differences for his reliable detection are not sufficient.

A comparative lesions detection is thus based on the following assumptions:

a. there is given a finite sequence of pairs of related images presenting symmetrically located organs or parts of a bodily organ available in different projections;
b. the lesion of interest in no more but one (and always the same) image of any pair is expected;
c. two types of local differences between the images of any pair are possible:
    1. substantial differences caused by occurring a lesion in one and lack in other one side of the examined organ;
    2. irrelevant differences caused by objects different positioning, secondary anatomical details existence, inaccurate pairs of images symmetry fixation, image distortions etc.;
d. the form, size and even the occurrence of lesion in different pairs of images within a given sequence may be different.

In Fig. 1 several examples of pairs of medical images prepared for comparative analysis are shown. In the images the pairs of symmetrical *regions of interest* (*ROIs*) on which the analysis is to be focused are marked by black rectangular contours. Note that not all differences for comparative analysis have been chosen there; their primary selection is usually done by an experienced medical specialist, the role of computer system is secondary, consisting in aiding the analysis: making its results more accurate and comparable if repeated several times.

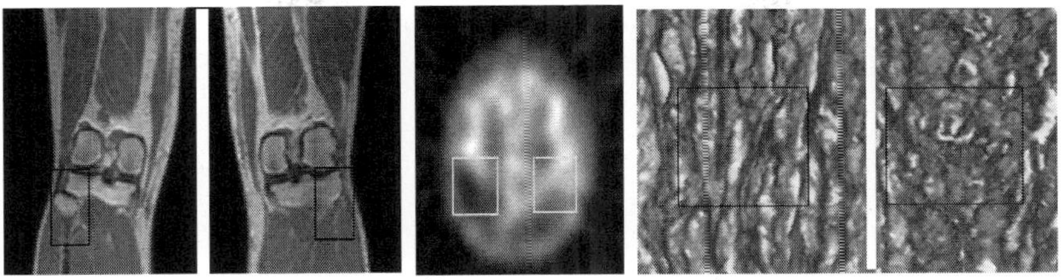

a) b) c)

Fig. 1. Pairs of medical images prepared for comparative analysis: a) radiological images of knees, b) *SPECT* image of brain, c) microscopic image of aorta tissue.

For comparative image analysis two basic types of image features can be used:

1. Primary, local features obtained by a direct point-to-point comparison of images:
   a. pixels' intensity levels,
   b. pixels' color components.
2. Secondary, environmental features defined and calculated as functions of pixel values in selected image fragments:
   a. spectral characteristics,
   b. statistical characteristics,
   c. fractal characteristics,
   d. micro-morphological characteristics,

etc. Local features neglect any spatial relationships between pixel values in the examined images. It can be observed in Fig. 2 where a *SPECT* image of a brain a) and its mirror-inversion b) have been subtracted in order to visualize the difference of respective pixel intensities c). The spots in Fig. 2.c) correspond to the regions of high brightness disparities in the compared brain hemispheres. However, no subtle differences of textures using this type of visualization can be detected.

Environmental features take into account spatial relationships within some regular (e.g. square or rectangular) sub-areas, called *basic windows*, covering the *ROIs*. The form of *ROI* is not obviously rectangular, as shown in Fig. 3. However, identical form and size of a pair of *ROIs* make their analysis easier. Black points in Fig. 3 represent image elements (pixels), adjacent basic windows of 4×4 pixels size are separated by dotted lines, the area under

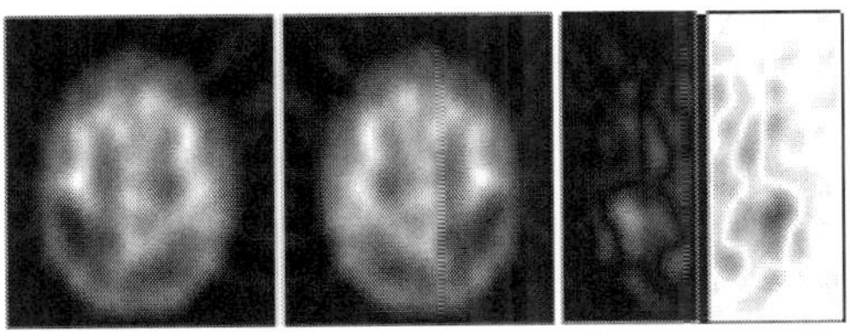

a) b) c)

Fig. 2. Result of subtraction of a *SPECT* brain image a) and its mirror-reflection b) visualizing the difference of respective pixel intensities c).

examination (*ROI*) consisting of a compact subset of basic windows has been contoured by a continuous line.

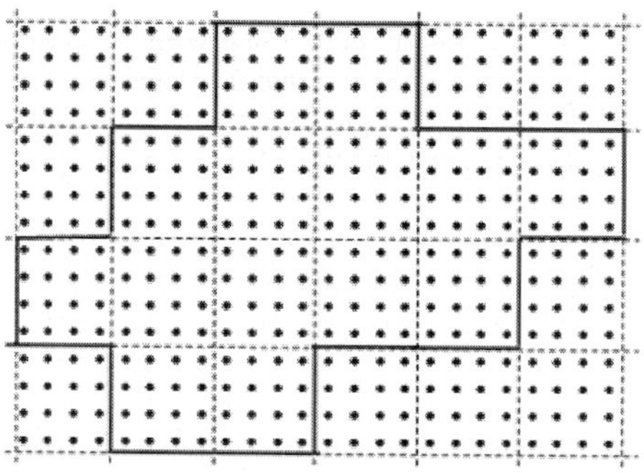

Fig. 3. Example of a region of interest (*ROI*) composed of basic windows.

An exact delineation of symmetrical pairs of *ROI*s needs taking both anatomical details and measurable geometrical image parameters into consideration. Before starting a computer-aided comparative lesions detection the images, if necessary, to a preliminary, symmetry correcting procedure should be subjected (Lester H., Arrige S.R., 1999). However, even in this case some remaining deficiencies of symmetry may affect the detection quality and this in design of lesions detection procedures should be taken into consideration.

Let us take into consideration a pair *A', A"* of *ROI*s selected for comparative analysis. There will be denoted by *M* the number of basic windows in a *ROI* and by *N* be the number of pixels in a basic window. In most medical imaging modalities, like *X*-ray, ultrasound (*USG*), computer tomography (*CT*), single photon emission computer tomography (*SPECT*), positron emission tomography (*PET*), nuclear magnetic resonance (*NMR*), monochromatic images are dealt with; otherwise, pixel values should be represented by triplets of numbers corresponding to basic, e.g. *RGB, HSV, CMY, YIQ* etc. color components (Foley J.D., Van Dan A., Feiner S.K. & al., 1994). Below, monochromatic images are considered; however, the methods presented on more general cases can easily be extended.

For comparative image analysis based on local features the contents of a pair of *ROI*s of identical form and size can be represented by two $M \times N$ matrices:

$$\mathbf{U'} = [u'_{\mu\nu}],\ \mathbf{U''} = [u''_{\mu\nu}],\ \mu \in [1,\ldots,M],\ \nu \in [1,\ldots,N], \tag{1}$$

where $u'_{\mu\nu}$, $u''_{\mu\nu}$ are pixel values belonging to a finite discrete space (brightness scale):

$$X = [0,1,\ldots,K\text{–}1] \tag{2}$$

value 0 being assigned to the maximum darkness. We also shall denote by

$$\mathbf{u'}_{\mu^*} = [u'_{\mu 1}, u'_{\mu 2},\ldots, u'_{\mu N}],\ \mathbf{u''}_{\mu^*} = [u''_{\mu 1}, u''_{\mu 2},\ldots, u''_{\mu N}],\quad \mu \in [1,\ldots,M], \tag{3}$$

the respective rows assigned to the basic windows, identically enumerated in both *ROI*s, and by

$$(\mathbf{u'}_{*\nu})^{tr} = [u'_{1\nu}, u'_{2\nu},\ldots, u'_{M\nu}],\ (\mathbf{u''}_{*\nu})^{tr} = [u''_{1\nu}, u''_{2\nu},\ldots, u''_{M\nu}],\ \nu \in [1,\ldots,N], \tag{4}$$

the (in transposed form presented here) columns of $\mathbf{U'}$ and $\mathbf{U''}$. Evidently, $\mathbf{u'}_{\mu^*}$ and $\mathbf{u''}_{\mu^*}$ represent the basic windows' contents while $\mathbf{u'}_{*\nu}$ and $\mathbf{u''}_{*\nu}$ collect the related components from the basic windows in the given *ROI*s.

We consider the vectors u'_{μ^*}, u''_{μ^*} as elements of a N-dimensional discrete vector space X^N. The M-row matrices $\mathbf{U'}$ and $\mathbf{U''}$ represent thus two M-element subsets in X^N. The subsets can geometrically be presented as sets of points surrounded by "clouds" (*similarity areas* denoted, respectively, by Ξ' and Ξ'') of other points (vectors) similar to those of U' and U'', as illustrated by Fig. 4.

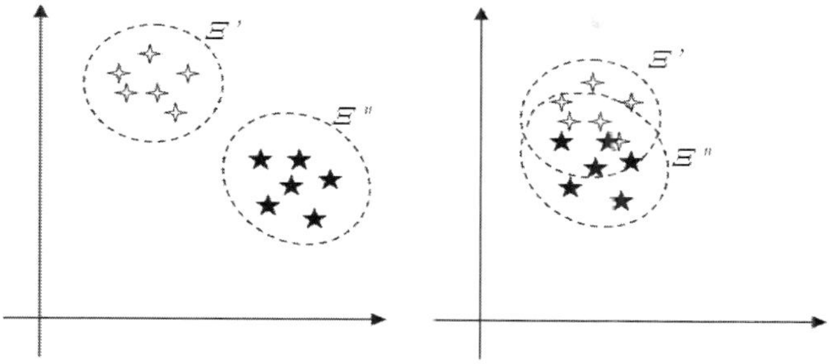

a) b)

Fig. 4. Geometrical illustration of the contents of two *ROIs* and their similarity areas Ξ', Ξ'': a) easily separable (dissimilar) subsets of vectors, b) similar subsets of vectors.

For comparative lesions detection not so much vectors representing basic windows but rather their differences $\xi_{\mu^*} = u'_{\mu^*} - u''_{\mu^*}$ are of particular interest. A condensation of difference vectors close to the initial point of coordinates, as it is shown in Fig. 5 below, corresponds to high similarity of basic windows contents.

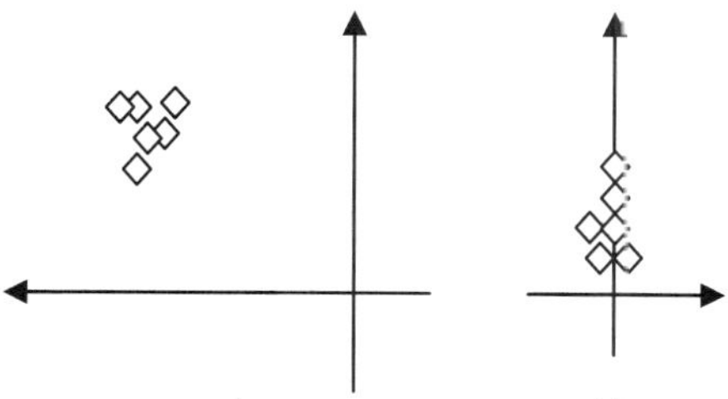

a) b)

Fig. 5. Differences of pairs of vectors corresponding to the sets Ξ' and Ξ''.

The notion of similarity area below will be more exactly defined. However, it follows from the above-made assumption c)-ii that even if significant disparities between the similarity areas Ξ' and Ξ'' (like those in Fig. 5 a) exist, they may be caused both by relevant as well as irrelevant factors. Some of them (e.g. those caused by small anatomical details) by a compensation technique can be removed. Removing other irrelevant differences needs more sophisticated methods using as it later on will be shown. Finally, at each step of an iterative lesions detection process it is assumed that the dissimilarities between objects within similarity areas Ξ' and Ξ'' are mostly irrelevant while those between Ξ' and Ξ'' are mostly relevant to the diagnostic purposes. The comparative lesions detection problem can thus roughly be formulated as follows:

Assume that Ξ' and Ξ'' are two subsets in X^N containing vectors in a certain sense *similar*, respectively, to those of U' and U''; check belonging of a significant part of vectors of U' and U'' to the intersection $\Xi' \cap \Xi''$.

Positive checking results mean that no significant differences between the vectors of U' and U'' have been detected; hence, A' and A'' are covered by non-distinguishable types of texture. Taking into account the above formulated assumption b) of comparative image analysis this leads to a conclusion that no lesion in the given pair of *ROI*s has been detected. Otherwise, a detected *dissimilarity* between U' and U'' suggests that a lesion in one of *ROI*s can be suspected. Is it a real lesion, depends on the relevance of the differences to medical expectations, as it has been mentioned. However, in the above formulated problem some notions should be explained; what do they: *similar, similarity area, significant part* or *dissimilarity*, exactly mean? This will be explained below.

3. Similarity and dissimilarity measures

The terms: *similar* and *dissimilar* as commonly used seem to be intuitively clear. In a formal sense they correspond to a relation between some objects satisfying the following conditions:

1. Each object is similar to itself (*reciprocity of similarity*);
2. If object ω' is similar to ω'' then ω'' is similar to ω' (*symmetry of similarity*).

Similarity is thus a sort of *neighborhood relation*. In *dissimilarity* relation symmetry holds as well; however, this relation is not reciprocal. In both cases a question of their *transitivity* arises: if an object ω' is similar to ω'' and ω'' is similar to ω''', does it mean that ω' is similar to ω'''? Undoubtedly, it is so in the case of similarity of triangles (among all possible triangles on an Euclidean plain) or similarity of all animals included into a given biological species. On the other hand, it may be not true if visual similarity of some objects is considered. E.g., if A (a son) is similar to B – his father (and vice versa, B is similar to A) as well as C (a sister of A) is similar to A, then not obviously C is similar to B (for example, because A and C were born by the same mother but have different fathers). The problem of a limited transitivity of similarity is illustrated in Fig. 6; the closer are any two patterns the higher is their similarity, external patterns a) and h) being totally dissimilar.

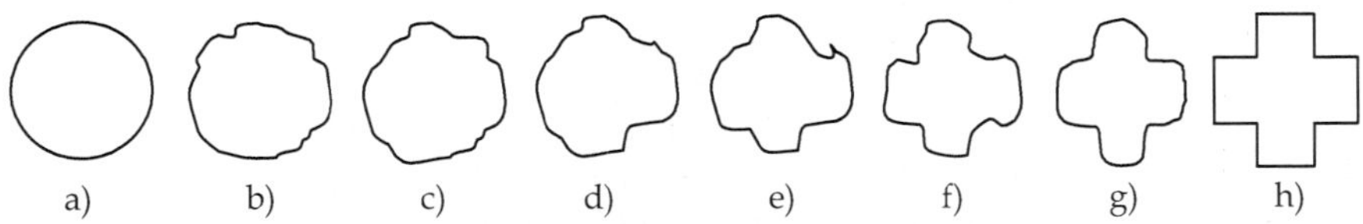

Fig. 6. A sequence of geometrical patterns whose similarity depends decreasingly on their distance in the row.

Evidently, it is reasonable to distinguish a *strong similarity* satisfying the transitivity condition and a *weak similarity* where transitivity is not satisfied or is satisfied within some limits only. Non-transitivity of similarity may also be caused by the fact that similarity of objects can be assessed in practice from different points of view when different pairs of objects are taken into consideration. This is illustrated in Fig. 7. The position, color and form of triangles have been taken into consideration as different aspects of similarity of triangular patterns.

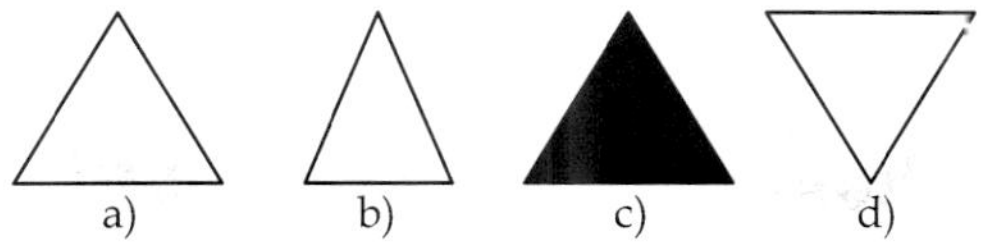

Fig. 7. Different aspects of similarity of triangular patterns: 1⁰ a), b) and c) – from their position point of view, 2⁰ a), b) and d) – from their color point of view, 3⁰ a), c) and d) – from their form point of view.

Therefore, it arises a problem of a general, multi-aspect objects' similarity definition. This will be done below by definition of a *similarity measure*. Many proposals of definition of this notion can be found in literature (Gotlieb C. C., Kumar S., 1968; Bonner R. E., 1954). However, not all of them are flexible enough to take into account the multi-aspect nature of similarity into consideration. The below-given definition, as it has been shown in (Kulikowski J. L., 2001) makes it possible.

Definition 1.

Let Ω denote any set consisting of more than 2 elements (objects). We call *similarity measure* a function σ described on a Cartesian product Ω^2 satisfying the conditions:

$$\left.\begin{array}{l} a/\ 0 \le \sigma(\omega',\omega'') \le 1, \\ b/\ \sigma(\omega',\omega') = 1, \\ c/\ \sigma(\omega',\omega'') = \sigma(\omega'',\omega') \\ d/\ \sigma(\omega',\omega'')\cdot\sigma(\omega'',\omega''') \le \sigma(\omega',\omega''') \end{array}\right\} \quad (5)$$

for any $\omega',\omega''\ \omega''' \in \Omega$.

Condition b/ corresponds to a reciprocity while c/ to a symmetry of similarity; a/ and b/ show also that 0 is the minimal and 1 is the maximal similarity measure of any two objects. Condition d/ reminds a so called *triangle inequality* in a distance measure definition (Rasiowa H., Sikorski R., 1968) and it really is connected with it as it will be shown later on. Moreover, it explains the sense of the *limited transitivity of similarity* notion.

A complementary to the similarity measure is the *dissimilarity measure.*

Definition 2

If $\sigma(\omega',\omega'')$ is a similarity measure satisfying the Definition 1 then

$$\delta(\omega',\omega'') = 1 - \sigma(\omega',\omega'') \quad (6)$$

is called a *dissimilarity measure* described on the same Cartesian product Ω^2.

There are many possibilities to define a similarity measure satisfying the above-given definition as well as the corresponding dissimilarity measures. Three of them are presented below.

Similarity based on a distance measure. If Ω is a metric space where a distance measure r between pairs of its elements has been established then similarity measure can be defined as

$$\sigma(\omega',\omega'') = exp[-\beta \cdot r(\omega',\omega'')] \quad (7)$$

where β is a scaling parameter. It is clear that the conditions a/, b/ and c/ of Definition 1 are satisfied due to the distance measure properties. Moreover, condition d/ due to the triangular inequality of distance measure is also satisfied. Distance measure may here mean an Euclidean, absolute, Chebyshevian, or any other of non-limited distance measures used in applications (Jain A.K., Murthy M.N., Flynn P.J., 1999).

Similarity based on angular distance. If Ω^+ is a positive sector of a linear vector space and $\angle(\omega',\omega'')$ denotes an angular measure between a pair of vectors in Ω^+ then a similarity measure can be defined as

$$\sigma(\omega',\omega'') = 1 - |\sin[\angle(\omega',\omega'')]| \tag{8}$$

The reciprocity and symmetry of this similarity measure is evident. For proving the inequality (5 d) we shall denote $\alpha = \angle(\omega',\omega'')$, $\beta = \angle(\omega'',\omega''')$, $\gamma = \angle(\omega',\omega''')$ and remark that a) the angles between any vectors consisting of non-negative components cannot exceed $\pi/2$, b) for any $\omega', \omega'', \omega''' \in \Omega^+$ it is $|\alpha-\beta| \leq \gamma \leq \alpha+\beta$. Hence, assuming that $\alpha \geq \beta$ (this being a problem of denotation only) it follows from (7) that $\sigma(\alpha-\beta) \geq \sigma(\gamma) \geq \sigma(\alpha+\beta)$. However, from the convexity of $\sigma(\omega',\omega'')$ it also follows that
$\frac{\sigma(\beta)}{1} < \frac{\sigma(\alpha+\beta)}{\sigma(\alpha)}$ (see Fig. 6) what leads to the inequality $\sigma(\alpha)\cdot\sigma(\beta) < \sigma(\alpha+\beta) \leq \sigma(\gamma)$ as it was to be shown •

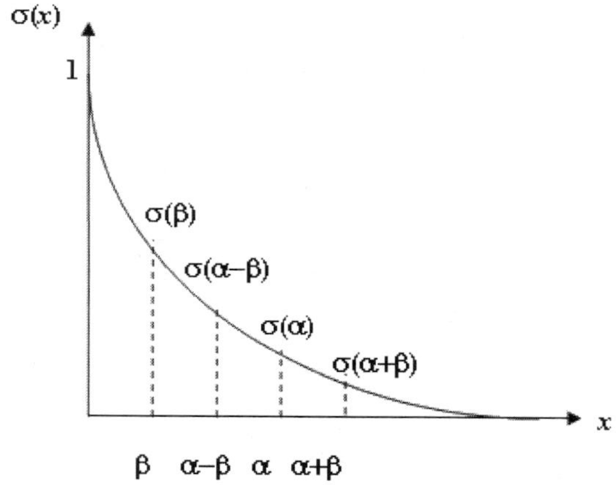

Fig. 6. Convexity of similarity measure based on angular distance.

Similarity based on logical tests. This type of similarity measure is particularly useful if some qualitative criteria to objects' similarity assessment are used. Such criteria may state, for example, that some external factors (noise, side anatomical details, lack of careful image preprocessing, etc.) could disturb the images and influence increasing the disparities. They also may state that difference of a qualitative feature characterizing the images is negligible. Let it will be defined a set of N *testing functions* (tests) of a general form

$$t_n: \Omega^2 \to \{0,1\}, \quad n = 1,2,\ldots,N, \tag{9}$$

assigning value 1 to a $t_n(\omega',\omega'')$ if (ω', ω'') satisfy a given condition confirming supposition of their similarity and value 0 otherwise. For the given series of tests $T = [t_1, t_2,\ldots, t_N]$, we denote by H the number of tests to which value 0 has been assigned. Then the similarity measure can be defined as

$$\sigma(\omega',\omega'') = \frac{N - H}{N + H} \tag{10}$$

Reciprocity and symmetry of the above-defined similarity measure is evident. The property (5d) follows, like before, from its convexity which for several values of N is shown in Fig. 7. Similarity measures satisfying the conditions of Definition 1 have an important property making possible creation of multi-aspect similarity measures:

Theorem 1

Let $\sigma_1(\omega',\omega'')$, $\sigma_2(\omega',\omega'')$,…, $\sigma_k(\omega',\omega'')$ be similarity measures satisfying the conditions of Definition 1. Then

$$\sigma(\omega', \omega'') = \prod_{\kappa=1}^{k} \sigma_{\kappa}(\omega', \omega') \tag{11}$$

is also a similarity measure in the sense of Definition 1.
Proof of this theorem is very simple, following directly from the Definition 1 •

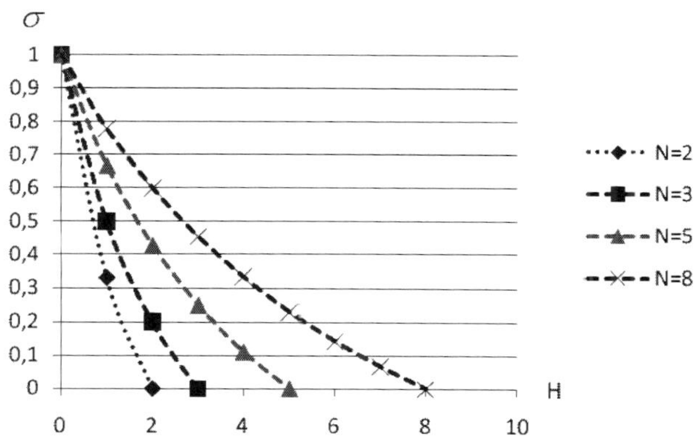

Fig. 7. Behavior of similarity measure based on logical tests.

It follows from this Theorem that if $\sigma(\omega',\omega'')$ is a similarity measure then $\sigma^{\nu}(\omega',\omega'')$ for any real $\nu > 1$ is a similarity measure as well. However, due to the inequality $\sigma^{\nu}(\omega',\omega'') \leq \sigma(\omega',\omega'')$ such a similarity measure is more rigid than $\sigma(\omega',\omega'')$. Using $\sigma^{\nu}(\omega',\omega'')$ instead of $\sigma(\omega',\omega'')$ for $0 < \nu < 1$ leads to a reciprocal effect of similarity measure weakening. However, it cautiously can be used because for ν close to 0 convexity of $\sigma^{\nu}(\omega',\omega'')$ may be lost.
Using dissimilarity instead of similarity measure in comparative image analysis may be more convenient. Basic dissimilarity measure properties follow directly from the expression (6) and the corresponding similarity measure properties. In particular:

Theorem 3

If $\delta(\omega',\omega'')$ is a dissimilarity measure described on Ω^2 according to the Definition 2 then for any $\omega',\omega'', \omega''' \in \Omega^2$ the following inequality holds:

$$\delta(\omega',\omega''') \leq \delta(\omega',\omega'') + \delta(\omega'',\omega''') - \delta(\omega',\omega'')\cdot\delta(\omega'',\omega'''). \tag{12}$$

Theorem 4

If $\delta_1(\omega',\omega'')$, $\delta_2(\omega',\omega'')$,… , $\delta_k(\omega',\omega'')$ are some dissimilarity measures described on Ω^2 then

$$\delta(\omega',\omega'') = \prod_{\kappa=1}^{k} [1 - \delta_{\kappa}(\omega',\omega'')] \qquad (13)$$

is also a dissimilarity measure in the sense of Definition 2.
Proving validity of (12) and (13) consists in substitution of $1-\delta(\,)$ instead of $\sigma(\,)$, respectively, in (5 d) and (11) •

4. Description of textures by morphological spectra

4.1 Morphological spectra.

In Sec. 1 several possibilities of features selection for comparative image analysis have been mentioned. It also was remarked that environmental features better suit to a deep texture analysis than a point-to-point comparison of pixel values. The main difficulty in texture analysis lies in the randomness and multi-level morphological textures' structure. In most cases a texture is given as an instance of a random field whose statistical properties are not exactly known. Detection of textures dissimilarity is in fact a heuristic attempt to prove a hypothesis that the given two fragments of textures belong (or do not belong) to the same statistical population. For proving this hypothesis spatial relationships between pixel values visually observed as morphological texture features should be taken into consideration. One of possible ways to do it consists in using 2-dimensional spectral texture description. For this purpose, in principle, any complete system of bi-variable orthogonal functions can be used. However, any system of this type better or worse suits to morphological structures characterization and needs less or more sophisticated calculations. Morphological spectra seem to offer a compromise between calculation complexity and accuracy of textures description including their ability to describe them on several morphological organization levels.

We call morphological spectra a system of discrete bi-variable Walsh functions arranged in a hierarchical tree (Kulikowski J. L., Przytulska M. & Wierzbicka D. (2007a). For image description by morphological spectra selected *ROI*s are divided into square basic windows of $2^n \times 2^n$ size (see Fig. 2), n being a natural number called *spectrum level*. Each n-th level morphological spectrum is represented by 4^n spectral components. For the sake of presentation consistency, original image (U' or U'' defined by (1)) is considered as its 0-th level morphological spectrum. However, morphological spectrum of any fixed level contains full information about morphological spectra of any other level and into them can easily be transformed.

For calculation of morphological spectra special vectors called *spectral component masks* will be used.

Let us take into consideration the contents of μ-th basic window in a *ROI* represented by the vector $u_{\mu^*} = [u_{\mu 1}, u_{\mu 2}, \ldots, u_{\mu N}]$ (see (3)). Then, its four 1st level morphological spectrum components are given by the formulae:

$$\left.\begin{aligned} S &= [1,1,1,1]\cdot(u_{\mu^*})^{tr} = u_{\mu 1} + u_{\mu 2} + u_{\mu 3} + u_{\mu 4}, \\ V &= [-1,1,-1,1]\cdot(u_{\mu^*})^{tr} = -u_{\mu 1} + u_{\mu 2} - u_{\mu 3} + u_{\mu 4}, \\ H &= [-1,-1,1,1]\cdot(u_{\mu^*})^{tr} = -u_{\mu 1} - u_{\mu 2} + u_{\mu 3} + u_{\mu 4}, \\ X &= [-1,1,1,-1]\cdot(u_{\mu^*})^{tr} = -u_{\mu 1} + u_{\mu 2} + u_{\mu 3} - u_{\mu 4}, \end{aligned}\right\} \qquad (14)$$

The same can graphically be presented as four *component masks* shown below:

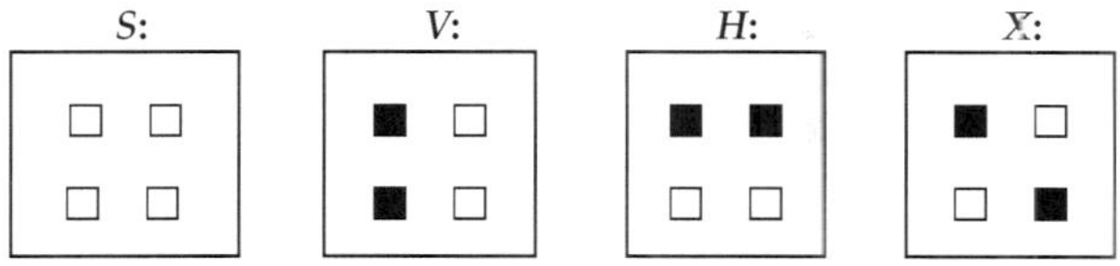

Fig. 8. Graphical masks of 1st level morphological spectrum components.

White marks denote the pixels in the basic window whose values should be taken with positive, while black - with negative sign in calculation of a sum corresponding to a given spectral component. A 1st level morphological spectrum of a given *ROI* consisting of *N* basic windows arranged into an $I \times J$ rectangular array ($I \times J = N$) will be given by four $I \times J$ real matrices collecting spectral components' values and denoted, respectively, by *S, V, H* and *X*. For calculation of the components of the next (i.e. 2nd) spectral level the matrices *S, V, H* and *X* are once more handled as original images: they are divided into 2×2 basic windows for which the spectral components *S*, V, *H* and X are calculated. Therefore, from the spectral matrix *S* next, 2nd level spectral matrices denoted by *SS, VS, HS* and *XS* are obtained, their seize being reduced to $\frac{1}{2}I \times \frac{1}{2}J$. Similarly, the spectral matrices *V, H* and *X* respectively generate the 2nd level spectral matrices *SV, VV, HV, XV, SH, VH, HH, XH, SX, VX, HX* and *XX*. This, iterative procedure can be used for higher-level spectral components. The components of morphological spectra can thus be presented in the form of a hierarchical tree shown in Fig. 9.

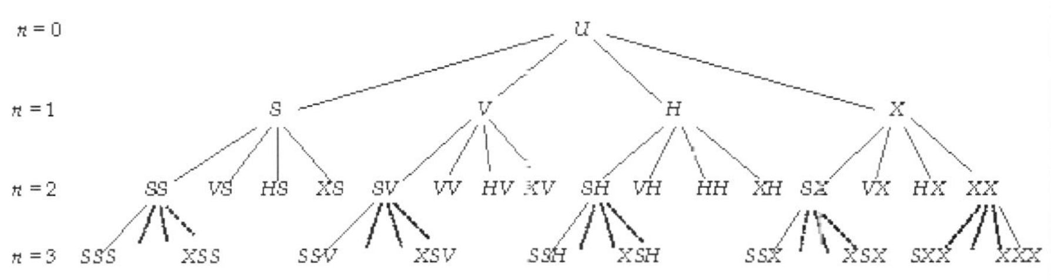

Fig. 9. Hierarchical tree of morphological spectral components.

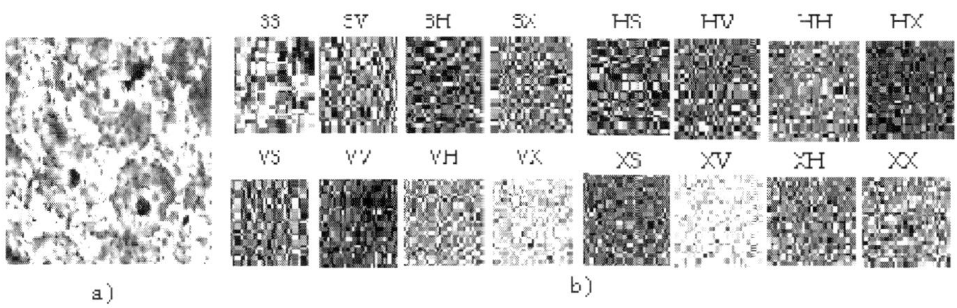

Fig. 10. Original image a) and its morphological spectral components b) of a bone section.

In Fig. 10 a 128×128 pixels-size *ROI* presenting texture of a bone section and 16 its 2nd level morphological spectral components are shown. It can be noticed that intensities of different components are different due to the fact that different micro-morphological details are by them represented.

4.2 Statistical analysis of morphological spectra.

Symbolic denotations of spectral components can also be interpreted as linear transformations which should be performed (from the right to left) on the image in order to get the corresponding component value. Transformation *S* (see (14)) plays a role of details smoothing operation: standing on the right side of the component's name it averages pixel values and reduces the image resolution power, while standing on the left side it averages on larger areas the former transformations results as it can be observed in Fig. 11.

Like the original image of a texture, its spectral components can be considered as instances of some random fields. Their direct interpretation is rather difficult; however, for comparative lesions detection they can be subjected to a statistical data processing. It should be remarked that spectral components of a given image are in general not statistically independent. Their cross-correlations thus can be used to a reduction of data necessary to aneffective lesions detection (Kulikowski J. L., Przytulska M. (2009b). However, for the sake of simplicity of lesions detection procedures statistical dependence of spectral components can in practice be neglected. Moreover, in order to avoid an effect of parallel image shift sensitivity of the results of spectral texture analysis using absolute spectral components instead of their original, real magnitudes is reasonable. For basic parameters characterizing statistical properties of the spectral components calculation, first, *histograms* (experimental probability densities) of their intensity in the given *ROI* should be calculated. For this purpose, instead of single matrices *U'*, *U"* (see (1)-(4)) used to contents of selected *ROI*s presentation sets of spectral matrices can be used. Let us denote by $\Lambda^{(n)}$ the set of symbolic names of n-th level spectral components and let λ be a shortly denoted symbolic name of a spectral component. We denote by $v_{\mu *} = [v_{\mu\lambda}]$, $\lambda \in \Lambda^{(n)}$, a vector of spectral components of μ-th basic window of the considered *ROI*, $\mu \in [1,2,\ldots,M^{(n)}]$, ($M^{(n)}$ being 4^n times reduced with respect to the number M of pixels in the original *ROI*). Then, the spectral *ROI* representation will be given by a matrix $V^{(n)}$ composed of $M^{(n)}$ rows $v_{\mu *}$ describing the spectra of basic windows. A λ-th column $v_{*\lambda}$ of $V^{(n)}$ consists of the λ -component values in the basic windows of the *ROI*. Any statistical parameters of spectral components should be thus calculated on the corresponding $V^{(n)}$ columns considered as random vector's instances. For a $v_{*\lambda}$ component's histogram $h_\lambda(\delta)$ calculation the minimal $v_{\lambda\, min}$ and maximal $v_{\lambda\, max}$ values in the column $v_{*\lambda}$ first should be found.

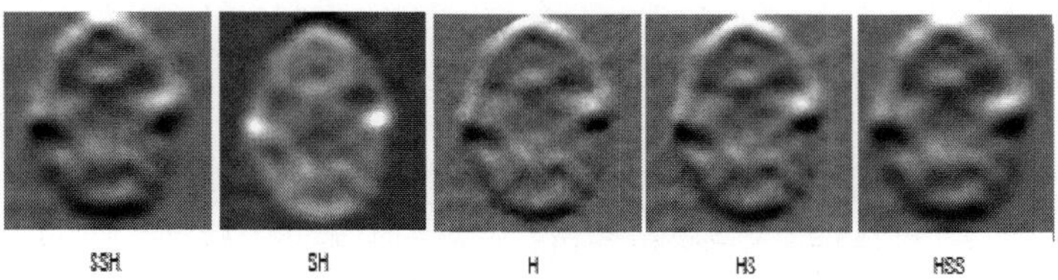

Fig. 11. Effects of image details smoothing by the *S* operation used after (*SH, SSH*) and before (*HS, HSS*) the basic operation *H* performed on a *SPECT* image of a brain.

Then, according to the desired statistical parameters estimation accuracy, an interval length

$$\beta = \frac{v\lambda\ \max - v\lambda\ \min}{\Delta - 1} \tag{15}$$

where $\Delta > 1$ is a fixed natural number, should be calculated. On the abscissa axis Δ left-open right-closed intervals:

$$b_\delta = (v_{\lambda\, min} + (\delta - 1 - ½)\beta,\ v_{\lambda\, min} + (\delta - 1 + ½)\beta],\quad \delta \in [1,2,\ldots,\Delta] \tag{16}$$

of δ length should be chosen and for each b_δ the number n_δ of the elements of $v_{*\lambda}$ whose values fall into b_δ should be evaluated. The histogram is then defined as a vector $h_\lambda(\delta) = [h_1, h_2,\ldots,h_\Delta]$ whose components are given by the frequency rates:

$$h\,\delta = \frac{n\,\delta}{M^{(n)}} \tag{17}$$

Of course, it should be $\sum_{\delta=1}^{\Delta} n\delta = M^{(n)}$. In Fig. 12 several histograms of morphological spectra components are shown. For comparison, the 1st level, *S* and *X* components of ultrasound liver imaging in a normal and liver fibrosis diagnosed patients have been chosen. The visual differences between the diagrams seem rather small. However, the beside shown estimated parameters of the histograms exhibit non-negligible differences: the histograms in ill patients are shifted to the right. This becomes evident if the minimal and mean values of the corresponding spectral components in normal and ill patients are compared. This example illustrates the idea of using morphological spectra as source of parameters suitable to comparative lesions detection. For this purpose, the following widely used parameters can be calculated and used:

- *Minimal, $v_{\lambda\, min}$ and maximal, $v_{\lambda\, max}$ component values;*
- *Statistical mean*:

$$m\lambda = \sum_{\delta=1}^{\Delta} \delta\, h\delta \tag{18}$$

- *Median*:

$$med_\lambda = \delta^* \text{ such that } \sum_{\delta=1}^{\delta^*-1} n\delta < \frac{M^{(n)}}{2} \le \sum_{\delta=1}^{\delta^*} n\delta \tag{19}$$

- *Standard deviation*:

$$sdev\lambda = \sqrt{\frac{1}{(M^{(n)}-1)} \sum_{\delta=1}^{\Delta} (\delta - m\lambda)^2 n\delta} \tag{20}$$

- *Skewness*:

$$sk\lambda = \frac{1}{\Delta} \frac{\sum_{\delta=1}^{\Delta} (\delta - m\lambda)^3}{(sdev\lambda)^3} \tag{21}$$

- *Kurtosis*:

$$kurt_{\lambda} = \frac{\Delta}{(\Delta - 2)(\Delta} \sum_{\delta=1}^{\Delta} \frac{(\delta - m_{\lambda})^4}{(sdev_{\lambda})^4} - \frac{3(\Delta - 1)^2}{(\Delta - 2)(\Delta - 3)} \tag{22}$$

- *Entropy*:

$$H_{\lambda} = - \sum_{\delta=1}^{\Delta} h_{\delta} \ln(h_{\delta}) \tag{23}$$

etc.

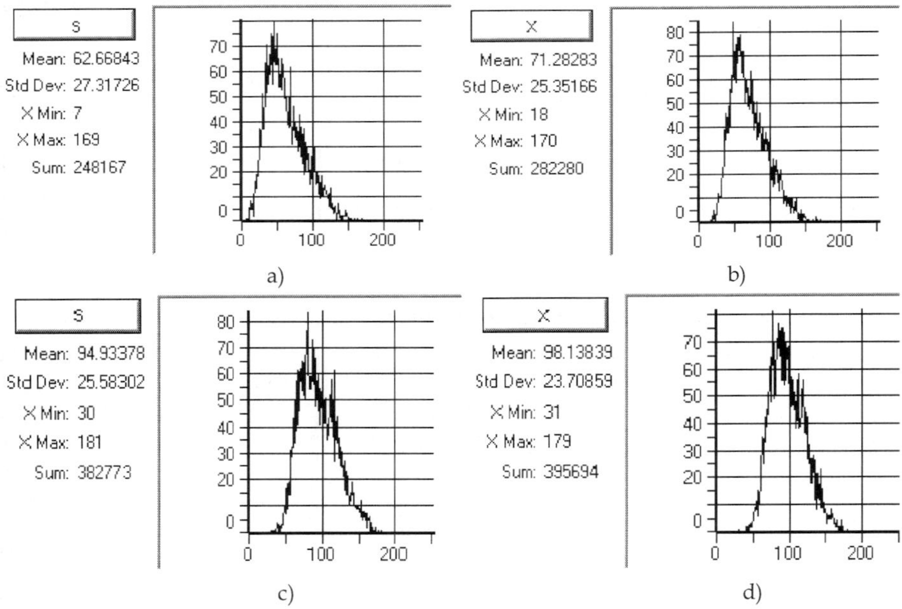

Fig. 12. Histograms of selected liver tissue morphological spectra components:
a) *S* component in a normal patient, b) *X* component in the normal patient,
c) *S* component in an ill (liver fibrosis diagnosed) patient, d) *X* components in the ill patient.

Finally, for each λ-th spectral component we get a sequence of *F* estimated parameters $w_{*\lambda} = [w_{1\lambda}, w_{2\lambda}, \ldots, w_{F\lambda}]^{tr}$ (for the sake of convenience presented here in transposed, horizontal form). For further considerations, the contents of compared *ROI*s instead of their original images *U'*, *U''* will thus be presented by two matrices *W'*, *W''* of $F \times L$ size, *L* denoting the number of spectral components selected for image analysis ($L \leq 4^n$), composed of the corresponding column-vectors $w'_{*\lambda}$, $w''_{*\lambda}$.

4.3 Statistical aspects of textures' similarity.

On the basis of morphological spectra the notion of textures' similarity can be formulated so that the randomness of textures is taken into consideration.

Definition 3

A set of objects $\Xi = \{u_{\mu^*}\}$ described by their morphological spectra v'_{μ^*} is called a *fuzzy e-similarity class* if for a given real non-negative vector $e = [e_\lambda]$, $\lambda \in \Lambda^{(n)}$, standard deviations $sdev_\lambda$ of its spectral components satisfy the inequalities

$$sdev_\lambda \leq e_\lambda \,. \tag{24}$$

Taking into account that various spectral components in textures similarity establishment may be of different importance, the inequalities (24) can be used as basis of a multi-aspect similarity measure based on logical tests. For different spectral components or their algebraic combinations different tests and final similarity criterion, according to Theorem 1, as their product can be established. In similar way, a dissimilarity of a pair Ξ', Ξ'' of objects can be defined.

Definition 4

For a given dissimilarity measure δ and a fixed d, $0 \leq d \leq 1$, two texture instances u'_{μ^*}, u''_{μ^*} are called *fuzzy d-dissimilar* if their morphological spectra v'_{μ^*}, v''_{μ^*} satisfy the condition

$$\delta(v'_{\mu^*}, v''_{\mu^*}) \geq d. \tag{25}$$

In this case, the dissimilarity measure can also be defined as multi-aspect, constructed according the Theorems 3 and 4, based on all estimated statistical parameters of morphological spectra.

5. General remarks on multi-aspect comparative detection of lesions

To the above-defined notions of fuzzy *e*-similarity and fuzzy *d*-dissimilarity in application to lesions detection a medical interpretation can also be assigned. A notion of medical diagnostic test's *sensitivity* is related to its ability to detect with high accuracy existence of a pathological factor. In comparative lesions detection this property is connected with ability to assign high dissimilarity measure to the textures of a normal and a pathological tissue. On the other hand, a diagnostic test's *specificity* means its ability to neglect seemingly pathological factors. In comparative lesions detection this means that high similarity measure is assigned to the basic windows within the same (normal or pathological) *ROI*. It might seem that both, high sensitivity and high specificity of lesions detection can easily be reached by choosing the (in Definitions 3 and 4 mentioned) threshold levels *e* and *d* as low as possible. However, it is not so. Low *d* means high that highly similar textures could be decided different. Moreover, it might happen in this case that certain objects are decided both, *e*-similar and *d*-dissimilar to a given set Ξ. In order to avoid this situation *d* should be chosen so that an intersection of the fuzzy *e*-similarity and (1− *d*)-similarity classes is reduced. However, this situation may on the other hand lead to existence of objects *e*-similar neither to Ξ' nor to Ξ''. The effect of strengthening the dissimilarity criterion by threshold *d* is illustrated in Fig. 13. For a 128×128 size *SPECT* image of brain (compare Fig. 2) absolute value of spectral component *SX*, as most sensible to fine local texture granularity, was calculated. Then, a difference of this component between the right and left cerebral hemisphere was taken into consideration as a parameter characterizing the disparities between the corresponding 4×4 basic windows in the two *ROI*s covering the hemispheres. The spectral images b), c) and d) are presented in artificially increased scale, compensating the effect of their size reduction caused by basic windows increasing. Logical dissimilarity test consisted in checking the difference value exceeding a threshold level d_{SX} . Higher threshold level brings to a reduction of detected local disparities.

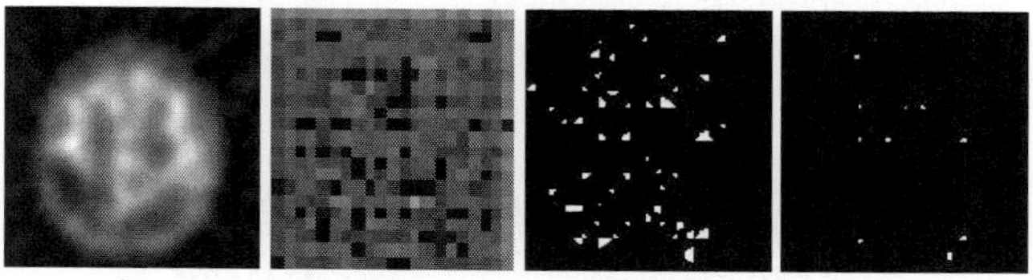

a) b) c) d)

Fig. 13. Disparities detection in cerebral *SPECT* image: a) original image, b) its morphological *X* component, c) disparities on low dissimilarity level, d) disparities on high dissimilarity level.

Hence, it follows from the analysis and example that **reaching simultaneously a detection rule of high sensitivity and high specificity is impossible**. Taking this basic constraint into account one can formulate the comparative lesions detection problem as follows:

Assume that Ξ' and Ξ'' are two subsets of objects in X^N considered as instances of two statistical populations. Let there be given criteria of fuzzy similarity of objects within the separately taken populations and fuzzy dissimilarity of objects belonging to different populations, based on estimated statistical parameters of the populations. Check: a) the fuzzy similarity requirement being satisfied by Ξ' and Ξ'', b) in positive case - the requirement of fuzzy dissimilarity of Ξ' and Ξ''.

This problem formulation does not settle the necessity of using morphological spectra to textures description. The concepts of multi-aspect similarity measure and dissimilarity measure admits using combinations of various types of objects description. However, statistical nature of textures forces preferring fuzzy similarity and dissimilarity concepts with respect to their deterministic versions. It also should be remarked that if fuzzy similarity of Ξ' and Ξ'' is not satisfied, checking their dissimilarity is pointless; such situation may arise if *ROI*s have been delineated on the borders between different textures.

Statistical nature of textures leads also to another type of limitation. Fuzzy similarity and dissimilarity of sets of instances of random objects can be the more accurately established the larger are the populations. This leads to a necessity of *ROI*s containing large number of basic windows delineation. However, this means that small-area lesions are poorly detectable. Therefore, **the requirements of high lesions detection sensitivity and of high accuracy of small lesions localization can not be together satisfied**. This can be considered as a sort of *uncertainty principle* in lesions detection.

A general scheme of comparative lesions detection realizing the above-presented concept based on morphological spectra application is shown in Fig. 14. In reaching high effectiveness of lesions detection selection of spectral components, choosing their statistical parameters and construction of similarity and dissimilarity measures play a crucial role. This can be reached by experiments rather than by solving a typical mathematical optimization problem. Moreover, experiments performed on different types of textures usually lead to different recommendations for choosing satisfactory solutions. In particular, it is necessary to distinguish isotropic and anisotropic biological tissues and to chose adequate to this combinations of spectral components for texture analysis. The *S*- and *X*-type operations are insensible to the anisotropy of texture, *V*-type operation is sensible to vertical, while *H*-type to horizontal structures. Therefore, in anisotropic textures analysis combinations of spectral components containing *V*- and *H*-operators (e.g. *SH* and *SV*, *XVH* and *XHV*, etc.) equally should used.

7. Conclusion

Comparative lesions detection is a well known technique used in medical diagnosis. It is based on an assumption that even if not only the existence, but also the form, size, location in patient's body, etc. of a lesion are not a priori known, nevertheless, it can be assumed that they exhibit differences with respect to a normal body. To detection of such differences

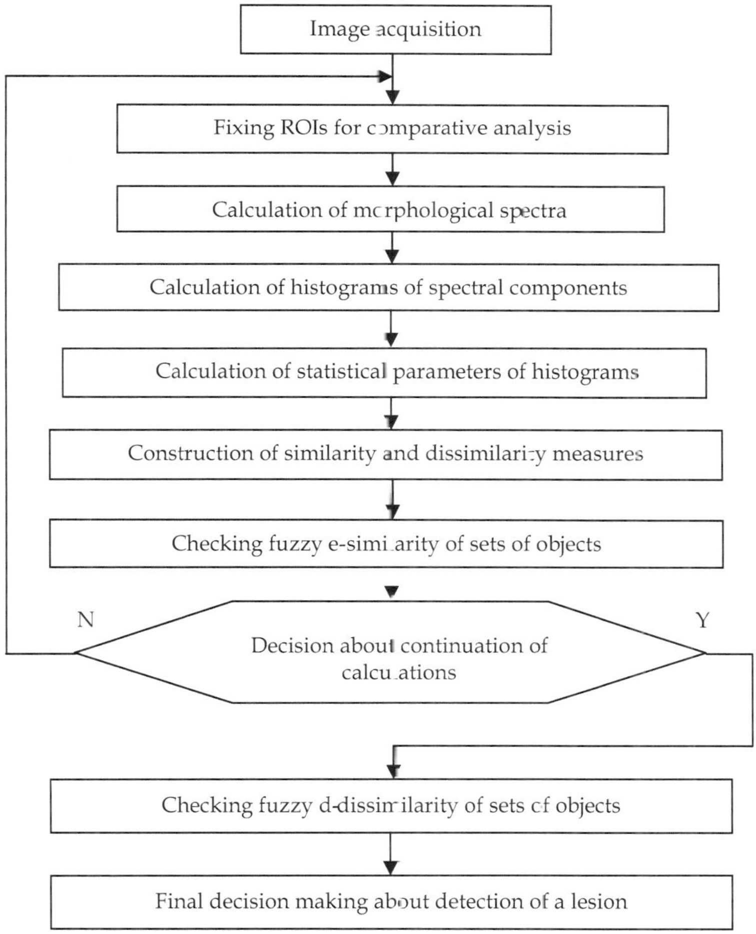

Fig. 14. Scheme of comparative lesions detection algorithm based on morphological spectra.

various approaches can be used. All they should satisfy the requirement of high sensitivity and specificity of lesions detection. Unfortunately, the requirements are in a sort of contradiction leading to the necessity of choosing a compromise between them. Moreover, a simultaneous reaching high detection effectiveness and high accuracy of lesion's localization in the body is also limited. The above-mentioned difficulties inspire looking for advanced lesions detection methods based on new concepts and effective mathematical tools.
The above-presented concept of multi-aspect similarity measures based on strongly defined assumptions, in combination with this of morphological spectra and on some standard statistical methods seems generally to satisfy those expectations. Nevertheless, at a present state it still needs more experiments to be verified on large and more diversified sets of clinical data.

8. References

Bonner R.E., (1954). On some clustering techniques. *IBM Journal Research and Development*, No 8, 22-32.

Foley J.D., Van Dan A., Feiner S.K. & al. (1994). *Introduction to Computer Graphics*. Addison-Wesley Publishing Comp. Inc., ISBN 83-204-1840-2, Reading Massachusetts.

Gotlieb C.C., Kumar S., (1968). Semantic clustering of index terms. *Journal of the ACM*, Vol.15, No 4, 493-513.

Hornby A.S. (1980). *Oxford Advanced Learner's Dictionary of Current English*. University Press, ISBN 83-01-02448-8, Oxford.

Jain A.K., Murthy M.N., Flynn P.J. (1999). Data clustering: a review. *ACM Computing Surveys*, Vol. 31, No 3, 264-323.

Kulikowski J. L. (2001). Pattern Recognition Based on Ambiguous Indications of Experts. In: *Computer Recognition Systems, KOSYR'2001*. Kurzynski M. & al. (Ed.), 15-22,.OW Politechniki Wrocławskiej, Wrocław.

Kulikowski J.L., Przytulska M. & Wierzbicka D. (2007a). Recognition of Textures Based on Analysis of Multilevel Morphological Spectra. *GESTS International Transactions on Computer Science and Engineering* Vol. 38, No 1, March, 99-107, ISSN 1738-6438.

Kulikowski J.L., Przytulska M, & Wierzbicka D., (2007b). Morphological Spectra as Tools for Texture Analysis. In: *Computer Recognition Systems 2*, Kurzyński M. & al. (Ed.), 510-517, Springer-Verlag, ISBN-13*978-3-540-75174-8, Berlin Heidelberg New York.

Kulikowski J.L., Przytulska M. & Kuraszkiewicz B. (2009a). Segmentation of Radiological Images Based on Dissimilarity Measure, In: *Image Processing & Communications Challenges*, Choras R.S., Zabludowski A. (Ed.), 326-333, APH EXIT, Warsaw.

Kulikowski J.L., Przytulska M. (2009b). Biomedical Image Segmentation Based on Aggregated Morphological Spectra. In: *Computers in Medical Activity*. Kacki E. (Ed.), 101-112, Springer, Berlin.

Rasiowa H., Sikorski R. (1968). *The mathematics of metamathematics*. PWN - Polish Scientific Publishers, Warsaw.

Rogowska J., Preston K., Hunter G.J. & al., (1995). Application of similarity mapping in dynamic MRI. *IEEE Tran. Med. Imaging*, vol. 14, 480-486.

Lester H., Arrige S.R., (1999). A survey of hierarchical non-linear medical image registration. *Pattern Recognition*, vol. 32, 129-149.

Part 7

Bioinformatics and Telemedicine

22

Biomedical Adaptive Educational Hypermedia System: a Theoretical Model for Adaptive Navigation Support

Maria Aparecida Fernandes Almeida and Fernando Mendes de Azevedo
Federal University of Santa Catarina, Brazil

1. Introduction

The first Adaptive Hypermedia System (AHS) was presented in the early nineties (Furuta & Scotts, 1990), (Ginderen, 1990). However, this model was not based in World Wide Web (WWW). The first use in WWW appeared in 1996 (Brusilovsky, 1996). Currently, AHS are used for information recovery; interface adaptation, user assistance, learning support, dialogue, cooperation support and others applications. The AHS have become an alternative to traditional static hypermedia systems with the incorporation of dynamics in Web applications that need to adapt according users.

Brusilovsky (1996) defines an AHS as hypertext and hypermedia system that reflect some user characteristic in a model and can adapt several visible aspects to the system for final user. In other words, the system should satisfy three main criteria: it should be hypertext or hypermedia, it should have an user model and it should be able to adapt using the user model.

Brad Campbell and Joseph Goodman (1987) developed a model known as Hypertext Abstract Machine (HAM). The Dexter Hypertext Reference Model was originated from NIST Hypertext Standardization Workshop (Halasz & Schwartz, 1994). These models served as a formal reference and informal to the abstractions found in a wide range of hypertexts systems. The Trellis Model, developed by Stotts and Furuta (1990) was based on three elements: information content, navigation structures and application dynamics control. In 1992, the Tower Model was presented in the Workshop of National Institute of Standard and Technology. It was an object-oriented model, based on HAM model (Campbell & Goodman, 1987). The Amsterdam Hypermedia Model (AHM) developed by Hardman (1994) was based on Dexter Model. This model introduced the concept of time necessary to the complex relationships in hypermedia modelling. The AHM Model included temporal and space relationships among the elements and paid attention in behavior definition of links among the dynamic media groups.

The work of Pagano (1992) presented a theoretical definition of hypertext. This model was extended by Almeida (Almeida, 2002) for educational hypermedia applications. The hypertexts and hypermedia systems that were mentioned previously are not adaptive. One the first efforts towards to put adaptivity of hypertexts / hypermedia systems was due to Benyon (1993) that proposed a model of AHS with modules composed User Model, Domain

Model and Interaction Model. Brusilovsky (1996) also proposed a model that contained User Model warehoused in a User Model Base and Adaptive Interface. The Adaptive Hypermedia Application Model (AHAM), proposed by DeBra (1993) it is a variant from Dexter Model, including the teaching model composed by pedagogic rules that are used by an adaptive engine to generate the features specifications. The AHAM uses the relationship concept among the components. The Adaptive Hypermedia Architecture (AHA), also developed by DeBra (1993) was considered as an AHS architecture but it contains an authorship tool that uses client-server technology. Today, the growth of distance education has led to the growth of Adaptive Educational Hypermedia Systems (AEHS).

The Web-based Education led to the development of Adaptive Educational Hypermedia Systems (AEHS). The AEHS are highly configurable systems that necessarily involve the user modelling. AEHS must to represent and to support the dynamic environment and user interaction. The AEHS become complex systems with many mechanisms of adaptation and several ways to presentation the interface. In these systems must be guaranteed a proper construction and that the system has a proper behaviour.

Many adaptive hypermedia systems were developed without use of modeling techniques; the developers have not followed the implementation methodology. Due to the countless applications of the AHS and the hypermedia technology development its is necessary to represent arbitrary references and mechanisms combination for specification these systems. A model is a theoretic referential to formalizes all the characteristics and essential functions that can be included in any hypertext application. The model should represent the static and dynamics structure of hypertext system. On Reference Models (Halasz & Schwartz, 1994) the conceptual abstracts of hypertext / hypermedia systems were created to establish standards to interchange different hyperdocuments among systems. The Design Method models (Rossi, 2010) brought a solid and systematic set of phases that helps the development of hypermedia systems. The hypermedia systems can be built obeying the phases of the development process: analysis, project, implementation and maintenance.

The growing AEHS complexity, whose operation is highly dependent of the users behaviors and of the own system, it turned a construction need of reliable systems whose ambiguities can be reduced by formal specifications in development process. In the AEHS specification, it is necessary to consider the state transitions, the functional behavior, the time relationships between the components and the multiple media integration to effectiveness from its usage.

This work presents a formal model of AEHS in the Biomedical Engineering based on the Category Theory (CT) (Arbib, 1975), (Adamek, 2004) in way to contribute with the development of these systems. The categorical approach in the Adaptive Educational Hypermedia System on Medical Education was proposed by Almeida and Azevedo (2008). The formal model was denominated of Biomedical Adaptive Educational Hypermedia System (B-AEHS). The components of an AEHS were modelled as objects and sub-objects of categories. The system parts were treated as categorical objects and their common aspects were explored to generate universal properties.

The CT is known as the "theory of structure" and has been applied to deal with the formalization of computer systems (Adamek, 2004), (Awodey, 2006), (Barrett & Mackaay, 2006). The categorical principles have been used to formalize different mathematical models of behaviour of systems, its specifications and its logical outputs (Fiadeiro, 2005).

The categorization of AEHS can be defined in several levels, in different structures. The categorical language simplifies the abstraction facilitating the uniform conception of these systems. The CT is a formal method useful in the definition of objects that have a universal property because it reveals how structures of different characteristics are related. The notion of abstraction is essential in the application of a formal method. The first step is to produce an abstract specification that characterizes the essential properties of the problem, to declare what is necessary to describe the problem and how this can be achieved (Gunawardena, 1996).

At some level of generalization an AEHS consists of a set of nodes or hyper documents connected by links. Each node contains some local information and links related to other nodes. The AEHS may also include an index or map with links to all available nodes. In this situation, the adjustment may occur at the level of content of the nodes or at the level of links, indexes and maps.

The adaptivity in AEHS is the ability to change dynamically the system according to the needs of users. All student interaction with the system is made by the adaptive interface. The adaptive interface is built from information about the user. There are two distinct areas of adaptation: adaptive presentation (content level adaptation) and adaptive navigation support (link level adaptation) (Brusilovsky, 2001). Adaptive presentation is concerned with the adaptations of text and multimedia. Adaptive navigation support is related into direct guidance, link hiding, sorting, annotation and hypermedia map adaptation. The adaptive navigation techniques are used to handle links and nodes for adapt the dynamic navigation features according to the state of the user model (Brusilovsky, 2002).

The chapter was structured as follows. In the next Section we present the basic concepts of the Category Theory. In Section 3 we present the formal method for the description of the structure of the adaptive navigation in the B-AEHS. In Section 4 we present a categorical model of an educational support system in Neuroanatomy. In a concluding Section 5, we give some final remarks.

2. Category theory

The CT (Arbib, 1975) was introduced as programs specification language in end of sixties. The categories can be:

- **Real**: are categories that exist in real world and can be represented by abstract categories.
- **Abstract**: are mathematical entities that can have several interpretations.

To characterize an abstract category it is necessary to identify the objects and morphism.

Definition 1. A category C consists of the following data (Adamek, 2004):

- Objects: $Ob_1, Ob_2, Ob_3, \ldots$
- Arrows, called morphisms: $f, g, h, \ldots$
- For each arrow f there are given objects:

$$dom(f),\ cod(f) \tag{1}$$

These objects are called the domain and codomain of f. We write:

$$f : Ob_1 \rightarrow Ob_2 \tag{2}$$

to indicate that $Ob_1 = dom(f)$ and $Ob_2 = cod(f)$.

Given arrows $f : Ob_1 \rightarrow Ob_2$ and $g : Ob_2 \rightarrow Ob_3$, i.e. with:

$$cod(f) = dom(g) \tag{3}$$

there is given an arrow:

$$g \circ f: Ob_1 \rightarrow Ob_3 \qquad (4)$$

called the composite of f and g.
To each object Ob_1 there is given an arrow:

$$1_{Ob1}: Ob_1 \rightarrow Ob_1 \qquad (5)$$

called the identity arrow of Ob_1.
Then, for all pair of arrows in the which the object origin is target of another is possible combine an in agreement more long arrow shown in the diagram of the Figure 1.

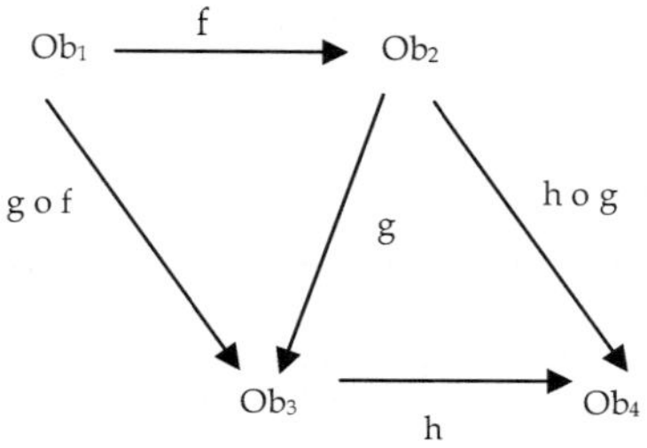

Fig. 1. Morphism of the category C

These data are required to satisfy the following laws:

- Associativity:

$$h \circ (g \circ f) = (h \circ g) \circ f, \text{ for all } f: Ob_1 \rightarrow Ob_2,\ g: Ob_2 \rightarrow Ob_3,\ h: Ob_3 \rightarrow Ob_4 \qquad (6)$$

- Unit:

$$f \circ 1_{Ob1} = f = 1_{Ob2} \circ f, \quad \text{for all } f: Ob_1 \rightarrow Ob_2 \qquad (7)$$

Definition 2: *Category* is equal (*Ob, Mor*) where *Ob* is the *object* of category and *Mor* is the *morphism*, satisfying:

- The morphism associates pairs of objects. A morphism should exist as $Mor(Ob_1, Ob_2)$;
- The morphism composition is morphism;
- The morphism composition is associative;
- The identity morphism exists.

Definition 3: If the composition of the morphism f with the morphism g is equal the composition of the morphism f with the morphism h:

$$f \circ g = f \circ h \rightarrow g = h \qquad (8)$$

Then f is a *monomorphism*:

$$Ob_1 \underset{h}{\overset{g}{\rightrightarrows}} Ob_2 \xrightarrow{f} Ob_3 \qquad (9)$$

Definition 4: If the diagram is commutative, the composition of the morphism g with the morphism f is equal the composition of the morphism h with the morphism f, that implies the morphism g is equal the morphism f:

If

$$g \circ f = h \circ f \tag{10}$$

Then, f is an epimorphism:

$$g \circ f = h \circ f \rightarrow g = f \tag{11}$$

$$Ob_1 \xrightarrow{f} Ob_2 \underset{h}{\overset{g}{\rightrightarrows}} Ob_3 \tag{12}$$

Definition 5: If the morphism g is equal the morphism h exists a monomorphism ($g = h$). In the same way, f is epimorphic if $f = k$. Therefore f is an *isomorphism* because it is monomorphic and epimorphic, as shown the equation 13:

$$Ob_1 \underset{h}{\overset{g}{\rightrightarrows}} Ob_2 \xrightarrow{f} Ob_3 \underset{k}{\overset{l}{\rightrightarrows}} Ob_4 \tag{13}$$

The correspondence of domain objects to another is produced by the morphism which preserves the defined characteristics in both domains (Barrett & Mackaay, 2006). An important concept in this work is the context change, in others words, the category change, this can be done by a functor (Lambek & Scott. 1986) that associates the category to the other categories.

Definition 6: A *Functor* it is the mathematical object that, given two categories, associates objects to objects and morphisms to morphisms, and that satisfy to the following conditions:

- The functors refer to pairs of categories. The properties of a specific AEHS can be associated other AEHS, for identification of objects and common properties of the both;
- An associative composition of functors that generates new functors exists. AEHS can be associated to compose connections that facilitate the reutilization of components;
- The *identity functor* that associates a category to it same exists. It allows defining exclusive characteristics of an AEHS for application in a specific domain that doesn't possess direct associations with other AEHS.

The functors, as well as the morphism, can be *monomorphic, epimorphic* and *isomorphic.*

3. The proposed formalism for B-AEHS

In general, the modeling of AEHS involves the student modeling, of the domain and adaptation. The letter (a) of Figure 2 shows an Educational Adaptive System composed by User Model, Domain Model and Interaction Model, similar to the classic system proposed by Benyon & Murray (1993).

The User Model represents the Student Model that contains the generic and psychological profile of the user. The student's model is used as the basis of adaptation of the feature content and it should assist their objectives. In the adaptation model, after the specification of the models of the domain and of the student, these are combined for the process of generation of appropriate feature content through an adaptive interface. In the student modeling, besides the student's preference the knowledge state of the same ones should be defined.

The students' preferences are not limited only for the feature aspects, but also related to the content. Usually, the system maintains user's individual model as a layer of the model of the

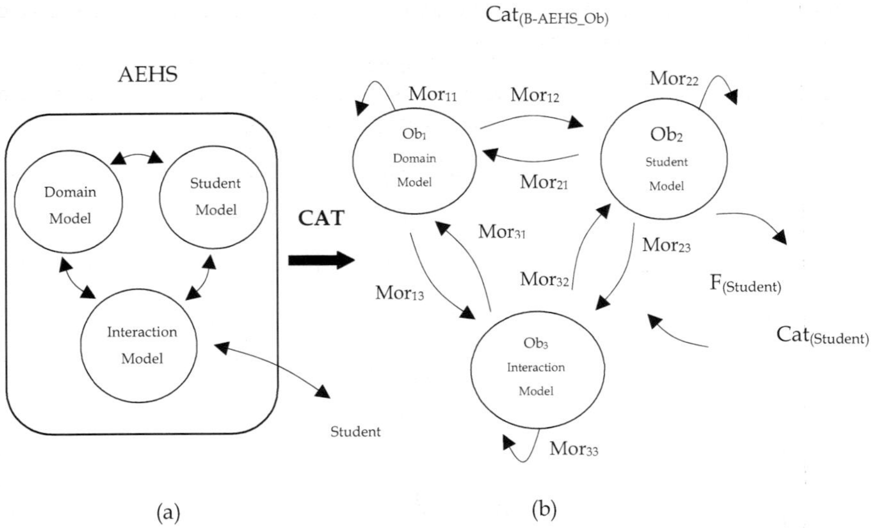

Fig. 2. The AEHS Model

domain to register the users related with the concepts of the domain current state. The Domain Model defines the main aspects of the system in the considered context to carry out the inferences. These aspects can be described in different levels such as Task Level, Physical Level and Logical Level (Benyon, 1993). Therefore, the domain model is the basis for all of the inferences and adaptations. The domain modeling that involves a specification of concepts and structure from crucial aspects of the system. The domain model is used to define which information will be processed in the application. The Interaction Model assures the dialogue between the user and application. It can register the precedent interactions in a Knowledge Base (Benyon, 1993). This model contains the mechanism to adaptation of the interface, inference of the user's properties and evaluation of the presented contents.

This AEHS model can be categorized considering each objects and their associations as morphisms of a category. A morphism allows specifying the courses and users' paths in AEHS. In a first abstraction, the modules AEHS are treated as objects that may or may not have associations with each other. The use of CT can facilitate the formal definition of these associations. We called the categorized model B-AEHS.

Given the three modules (student, domain and interaction), shown in section (a) of Figure 2. These modules can be categorized as objects Ob_1, Ob_2 and Ob_3, as shown in section (b) of Figure 2. The categorization of the model can be made, therefore they are satisfied the following conditions:

- The morphism refer to pairs of objects: the morphisms Mor_{12}, Mor_{21}, Mor_{23}, Mor_{32}, Mor_{13}, Mor_{31} may associate the objects Ob_1 (domain model), Ob_2 (student model) and Ob_3 (model of interaction) of AEHS;
- A composition of morphisms is morphism. The object Ob_1 can be associated to the object Ob_3 directly through the morphism Mor_{13} or Mor_{31}. These morphisms types allows identifying all of the paths traveled in AHS, in time of project, guaranteeing that

there is not break of the flow of information and the user does not loss in the space of information in run time of the system.

- The composition of morphisms is associative: the morphisms allow visual identification of nodes and links regardless of the authoring tool or implementation. An example of composition of morphisms involving AEHS objects is given below:

$$Mor_{12} \circ Mor_{23}=Mor_{31} \quad (14)$$

$$Mor_{23} \circ Mor_{31}=Mor_{12} \quad (15)$$

$$Mor_{31} \circ Mor_{12}=Mor_{23} \quad (16)$$

$$Mor_{32} \circ Mor_{12}=Mor_{13} \quad (17)$$

$$Mor_{13} \circ Mor_{32}=Mor_{21} \quad (18)$$

$$Mor_{21} \circ Mor_{13}=Mor_{32} \quad (19)$$

- The identity morphism must exist. The identity morphisms Mor_{11}, Mor_{22} and Mor_{33} allow associations of the objects themselves. The user can decide, for instance, not to change of page in B-AEHS, or the own system, given an access of the user can not change the method of adaptive presentation.
- The association can also be made by the composition of the morphisms Mor_{12} and Mor_{23} or Mor_{32} and Mor_{21}. The morphism allow the visual identification of links and nodes independently of the authorship tool or of the implementation.

Satisfied the categorical conditions, can be made formal representation:

- The properties of a specific B-AEHS can be associated to other for the identification of objects and common properties in both;
- B-AEHS can be associated to compose connections that facilitate the utilization of components;
- It is possible to define exclusive characteristics of a B-AEHS for application in a specific domain that does not have direct associations with other B-AEHS.

With this representation by morphisms and objects can be defined associations between the components of B-AEHS. For a model that involves a change of context or external for the object modeling system uses the concept of functors. In terms of domains transformations of domains, B-AEHS can be modeled categorically as:

$$Cat_{(B\text{-}AEHS)} = (Ob, F_t) \quad (20)$$

Where *Ob* are objects of the category *B-AEHS* and F_t are functors that associate the objects of the category $Cat_{(B\text{-}AEHS)}$ with it same or with other categories, as for instance, a category of users $Cat_{(Student)}$. This approach can be interesting to find universal properties of the systems, in different domains and applications.

In the case of specification of a B-AEHS, CT can be applied to define the user's models, of the domain and of the adaptation defining the associations among each module of the system. It is possible to use a functor forget (Almeida, 2002) that defines the unique characteristics of a system for application in a specific area that has no direct associations with other systems. Thus, on B-AEHS specification, the CT can be used at all levels. For example, it is possible to identify categories of B-AEHS, domain models, user models and

models of adaptation. It is possible also categorize only the objects and sub objects of different B-AEHS. This approach allows describe the relationships between systems and systems users and systems.
According the conceptual modeling, new objects can be defined and the conditions categories can be used to reduce the ambiguities of the system. The concepts presented here are extensible for any AEHS, because the categorical representation is independent of platform, number of objects and associations between them. The formal treatment can be given in any level of abstraction of the system.
For the design of an adaptive interface the Neuroanatomy system (B-AEHS) was divided into three modules (the user model, domain model and interaction model). The model of interaction was categorized so that each page was treated formally as an object and its components as sub-objects. Project-level navigation was chosen formalism more appropriate to simplify the specification as shown in the following sections of work.

3.1 The direct guidance

Direct guidance (Brusilovsky, 2004) is the simplest technology of adaptive navigation support. Direct guidance suggests the "next best" node for the user to visit according user's goals, knowledge, or/and other parameters represented in the user model. So that to provide direct guidance, an adaptive educational hypermedia system (AEHS) usually presents an additional dynamic link (Brusilovsky, 2004). From a given node, the system generates a link for more appropriate node, which is also given a link to another node most appropriate and so on. It is applied to decide which one is the next step the user must follow.
So that to categorize the Direct guidance is the use of the categorical concepts of the categorical Determination Problem (Lawvere & Schanuel,1997). The Figure 3 presents the categorical mapping for Direct guidance made by determination. If morphism f is given, each g can be obtained by $h=g \circ f$ composition. Therefore, given a set of known links Ob_1 for Direct guidance is possible to compose these links for association with another set of nodes Ob_2, to compose the path of the navigation. Assuming the existence of a morphism f that maps Ob_1 in Ob_2 $(Ob_1 \xrightarrow{f} Ob_2)$ and a set of links Ob_3 in the adaptive navigation. Then each morphism g of Ob_2 to the Ob_3 can be composed with f for generate the path for the user model by mapping $Ob_1 \rightarrow Ob_3$. Therefore, f maps Ob_2 in Ob_3, $(Ob_2 \rightarrow Ob_3)$ and also offers the mapping $Ob_1 \rightarrow Ob_3$.

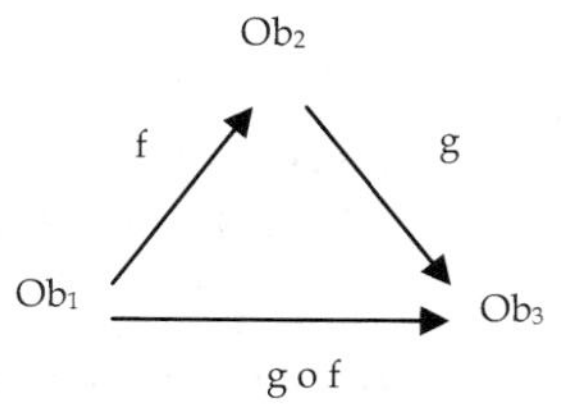

Fig. 3. Model of Direct Guidance by Determination Problem

Another way to categorize the Direct guidance is to use the constant morphism as showed in section 5.

3.2 Adaptive link sorting

Rather than provide the best link to the direct guidance, this technique offers a list of links in descending order of relevance for the user. Refers to the order in which the adaptive links are presented to the user according its relevance. The ordination may be a similarity, prerequisite, relevance, knowledge of the user, etc. The ordering of content is made in accordance with the user profile. From the node most important links are classified according to the user model, after being presented in descending order. In what order the links should be submitted? CT can be used to model the sort of links. Figure 4 presents a set of links that should be classified according the relevance R.

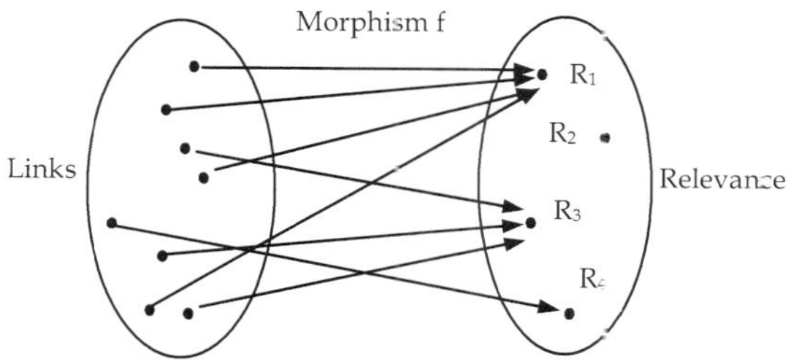

Fig. 4. Model of sort by relevance (adapted from Lawvere & Schanuel (1997)).

The classification can be made by a property (Lawvere & Schanuel,1997). As shown in Figure 5, assuming that Ob_2 has three elements that they represent different relevance assignments. Then, without change the morphism f is possible rearrange the elements of Ob_1 in three different classifications according to the user's model: ordering links for the user basic level, ordering of links for intermediary user level and ordering links for user advanced level. The classification consists of placing in the same group all the elements of Ob_1 that go to the same element of the Ob_2. The links are divided into fibers according to relevance R_1, R_2 and R_3. Therefore, a mapping $Ob_1 \rightarrow Ob_2$ produces a structure in Ob_1 domain and when we want to emphasize that the mapping effect is referred as the valuation property of the set of links Ob_2.

For a general mapping is possible to say that the morphism f ranks (or orders) Ob_1 in Ob_2 or that the morphism f is a classification of Ob_1 by Ob_2. This condition is valid if Ob_2 consists of numbers. Since f is given, each element ob_2 of Ob_2 determines which elements of the set of links Ob_1 are classified by ob_2.

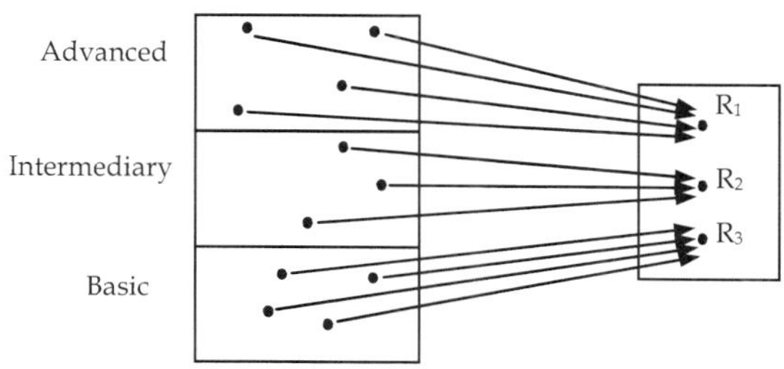

Fig. 5. Sort links by property (adapted from Lawvere & Scharuel (1997))

The categorization of the classification of links can be made by pullback of two morphisms, as shown in Figure 6.

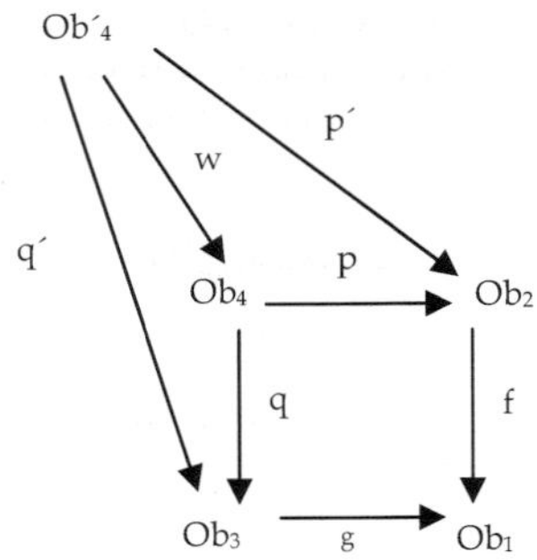

Fig. 6. Link classification by Pullback

Definition 7. The pullback is a limit of a diagram, constructed by two morphisms with the same target object (Lawvere & Schanuel,1997). Given two morphisms $f: Ob_2 \rightarrow Ob_1$ and $g: Ob_3 \rightarrow Ob_1$, the pullback Ob_4 is given by the pair of morphisms $p: Ob_4 \rightarrow Ob_2$ and $q: Ob_4 \rightarrow Ob_3$ such that the diagram commutes:

$$f \circ p = g \circ q \tag{21}$$

Since for all objects Ob_4' and all morphisms $p': Ob_4' \rightarrow Ob_2$ and $q': Ob_4' \rightarrow Ob_3$ such that: $p' \circ f = q \circ g$ exists a unique morphism $w: Ob_4' \rightarrow Ob_4$ such that $q \circ w = q'$ and $p \circ w = p'$. Each relevant R must be considered as a target.

3.3 Adaptive link generation

In order to generate new links of interest to the user on the information network that they had not been defined in the authorship. The link generation includes three cases: discovering new useful links between documents and adding them permanently to set existing links; generating links for similarity-based navigation between items; and dynamic recommendation of relevant links (Brusilovsky, 2004). How interesting links can be generated? The generation of links can be categorized by categorical product which is a structural generalization of the concept of Cartesian product.

Definition 8. The Cartesian product $Ob_1 \times Ob_2$ of the objects Ob_1 and Ob_2 consists of ordered pairs $< ob_1, ob_2 >$ where $ob_1 \in Ob_1, ob_2 \in Ob_2$ and there are projections $\pi: Ob_1 \times Ob_2 \rightarrow Ob_1$ and $\pi': Ob_1 \times Ob_2 \rightarrow Ob_2$.

3.4 Adaptive link hiding

The purpose of navigation support is hide and restrict the navigation space by hiding, removing, or disabling links that go to irrelevant pages. A page can be considered irrelevant for several reasons: for example, if it is not related to the user's current learning goal or if it presents materials which the user is not yet prepared to understand. Hiding protects users from the complexity of the whole hyperspace and reduces their cognitive overload (Brusilovsky, 2004). The categorial adaptive of the link hiding can be represented as a

Choice Problem (Lawvere & Schanuel,1997). The links that are hidden are chosen given a rule disabling a set of links selected as shown in Figure 7.
Considering that Ob_3 is a set of links are hidden in the adaptive presentation, Ob_1 is the set of all links and h the morphism of the Ob_1 to Ob_3 that determines the concealment of the links. Therefore taking Ob_2 as the set of all rules of deactivation, the problem is to find the morphism f that associates disabling link in accordance with its rule on the set Ob_3 by the morphism g.

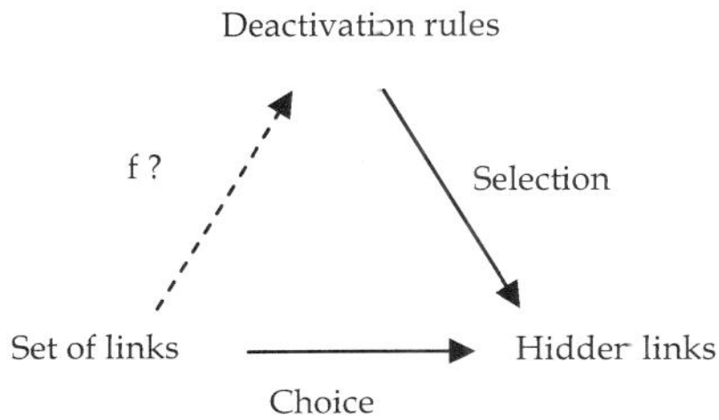

Fig. 7. Hiding links by deactivation rules

Figure 8 shows the categorization of hiding links. In order to find a morphism f such that $g \circ f = h$, must be chosen for each element ob_1 of Ob_1 an element ob_2 such that $g(ob_2) = h(ob_1)$.

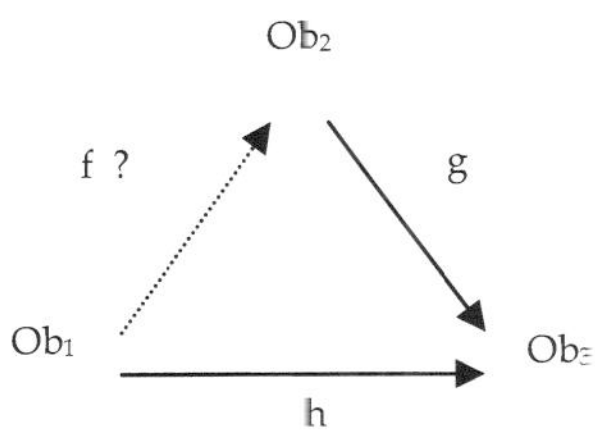

Fig. 8. Categorization of the hiding links

3.5 Map adaptation

This technique includes several forms of adaptation of maps to local and global hypermedia shown to the user, applied in a graphic display of the navigation structure (Brusilovsky, 2004). Maps (local and / or global) and indexes are presented for easy navigation. How to represent the maps and indexes? Map adaptation (Brusilovsky, 2002) can be modeled categorically defining sub-objects. The sub-object is the categorical version of subset in set theory (Lawvere & Schanuel,1997). Is defined as the subset of objects $Ob_1 \subseteq Ob_2$ as a monomorphism $f: Ob_3 \rightarrow Ob_2$.

Definition 9. If the composition of the morphism f with morphism g is equal to the composition of the morphism f with morphism h:

$$f \circ g = f \circ h \rightarrow g = h \tag{22}$$

Then f is a monomorphism.

Figure 9 shows a diagram of a monomorphism for mapping the routes driven by links. The paths (represented by the composition of morphisms) are equivalent when they lead to the same link, independently of the user navigation point.

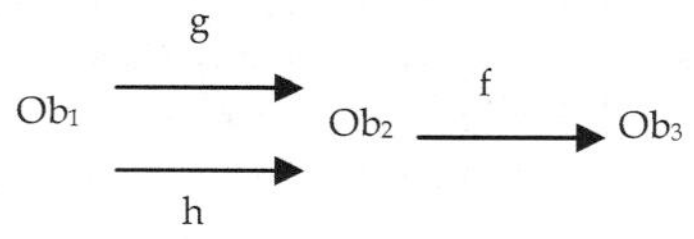

Fig. 9. Monomorphism

Figure 10 shows the equivalent diagram shown in Figure 9. The maps are produced as sub-objects of the category of nodes for guide the user in defined pathways.

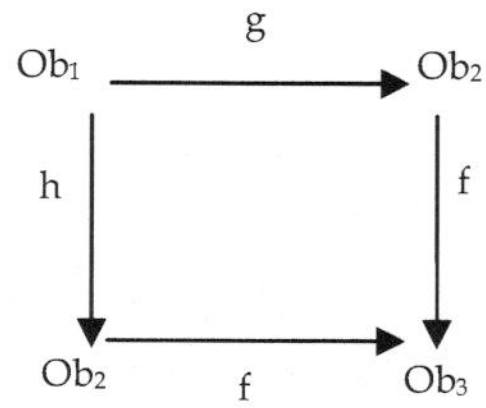

Fig. 10. Diagram equivalent mapping

Let C a category. If $f: b \rightarrow a$ and $g: c \rightarrow a$ are two arrows with a common target, then it is said that $f \leq g$ if and only if exists $h: b \rightarrow c$ such that $g \circ h = f$. If $f \leq g$ and $g \leq f$ then we say that $f \leftarrow g$ is an equivalence relation between monomorphisms which have a common target (Lawvere & Schanuel,1997). The indexes can be modeled as amalgamated sum (pushout) as shown in Figure 11.

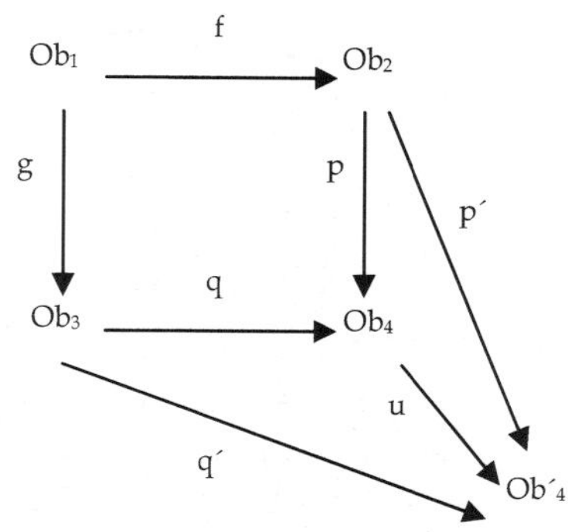

Fig. 11. Pushout of two morphisms f and g

Definition 10. The amalgamated sum (pushout) is the colimit of a diagram consisting of two morphisms with the same source object (Lawvere & Schanuel, 1997). Given the morphism $f: Ob_1 \rightarrow Ob_2$ and the morphism $g: Ob_1 \rightarrow Ob_3$, the pushout Ob_4 is obtained by the pair of morphisms $p: Ob_2 \rightarrow Ob_4$ and $q: Ob_3 \rightarrow Ob_4$ such that the diagram commutes.

$$p \circ f = q \circ g \tag{23}$$

Since for all objects Ob'_4 and all morphism $p' : Ob_2 \rightarrow Ob'_4$ and $q' : Ob_3 \rightarrow Ob'_4$ such that $p' \circ f = q' \circ g$ exists unique morphism $u : Ob_4 \rightarrow Ob'_4$ such that $u \circ q = q'$ and $u \circ p = p'$.
The amalgamated sum is dual concept of the fibered product (pullback) (Fiadeiro, 2005). Thus, an index is a point to which converge the various links of the system. In an adaptive interface, the categorization enhances the effect of construction of indexes according to the user model.

3.6 Adaptive link annotation

The links are commented to show its relevance, i.e., the anchors have a different aspect visible to show the relevance of the destination. Different modifications are performed in a link in order to increase their information, informing to the user what will come in the next nodes.
The aggregation of links to more information is given to providing more information about the target nodes of the links.
The annotations can be textual, visual (icons, colours or font size) (Brusilovsky, 2007). How to represent more information to the links? The adaptive annotation of links can be represented categorically with the sum as shown in Figure 12.

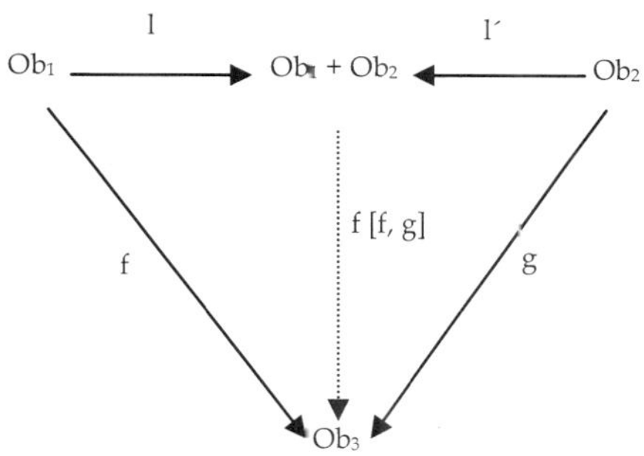

Fig. 12. Sum of objects

Definition 11. The sum or co-product is the dual concept of product. In sum concept the morphisms are called inclusions (Jay, 1993). Considering the objects Ob_1 and Ob_2 in a Category C. They have sum if the object formed by $Ob_1 + Ob_2$ is endowed with injections.

$$Ob_1 \overset{lOb_1.Ob_2}{\rightarrow} Ob_1 + Ob_2 \overset{l'Ob_1.Ob_2}{\leftarrow} Ob_2 \tag{24}$$

For each object Ob_3 and the pair of morphisms $f : Ob_1 \rightarrow Ob_3$ and $g : Ob_2 \rightarrow Ob_3$ exists a unique morphism $[f, g] : Ob_1 + Ob_2 \rightarrow Ob_3$ making the diagram commutative.
Figure 13 shows that considering on the link annotation modeling the pair of morphisms $Ob_1 \overset{a}{\rightarrow} Ob_3$, $Ob_2 \overset{b}{\rightarrow} Ob_3$ in a category is the sum of the Ob_3 and Ob_2, if each object of the Ob_4 and each pair $Ob_1 \overset{c}{\rightarrow} Ob_4$, $Ob_2 \overset{d}{\rightarrow} Ob_4$ is exactly an map $Ob_3 \overset{e}{\rightarrow} Ob_4$ to both

morphisms $c = e \circ a$ and $d = e \circ b$. The morphisms a and b are called morphisms injection of the sum representing the modeling will be presented to user through aggregations made in sets of links, represented by Ob_1 and Ob_2.

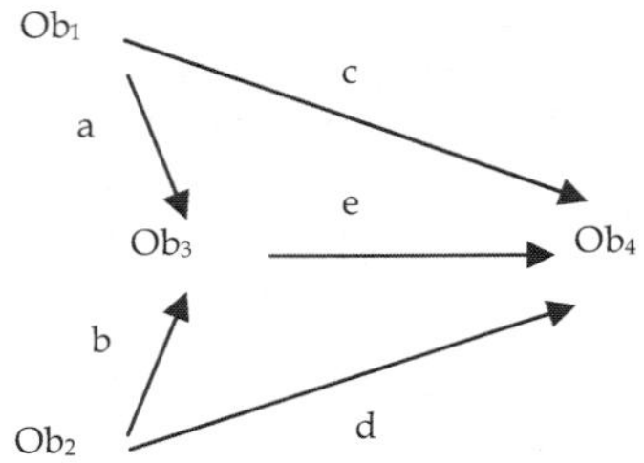

Fig. 13. Categorization of the adaptive link annotation

4. Formal modeling of a Neuroanatomy tutorial

The following sub-sections present the main techniques used in a project of a Neuroanatomy tutorial. Figure 14 shows the screen of an interactive system, called Virtual Laboratory of Neuroanatomy (VLN), developed at Pontifical Catholic University of Minas Gerais, Brazil.

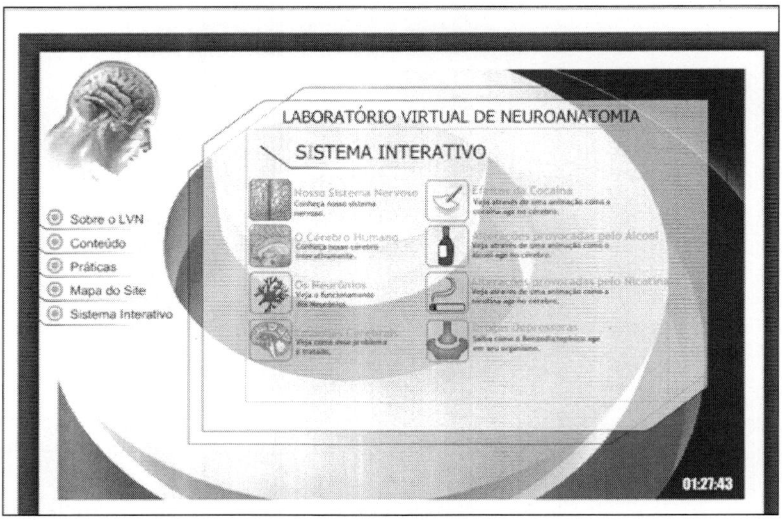

Fig. 14. Screen of the Neuroanatomy Educational System

The system formed the basis for the design of adaptive navigation treated in this work. The main pages of the system were treated as objects. The main parts of system structure were categorized into four distinct objects:

- Ob_1 - page presentation of the VLN,

- Ob_2 - Content
- Ob_3 - Practice
- Ob_4 - Site Map e;
- Ob_5 - Interactive System.

The goal of the study was to development the system parts using a formal method for abstraction in high level. The part projected consists of an agent (robot) that presents the drugs effect in nervous system and then presents a quiz to the student.

The chosen methodology was to project of the adaptive navigation support. The adaptive navigation helps users to follow the paths in hyperspace by adapting the form of presentation of the links in the hypermedia network.

The categorization is used in this work to model the actions related to adaptation of navigation, which is to change the navigation structure or in how this structure is presented to the user.

The adaptive navigation helps users to follow the paths in hyperspace by adapting the form of presentation of the links in the hypermedia network.

Figure 15 shows representations of direct guidance, sorting and generation of links in educational contexts in the VLN screen. For simplicity, we consider only the design of a single page (page 5) of an interactive system specified as the object Ob_5. This page presents a quiz to the student.

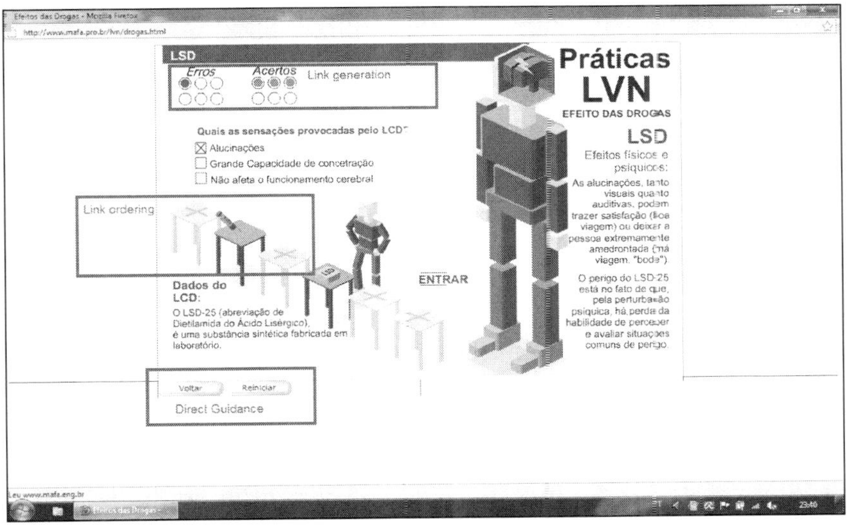

Fig. 15. Links of Adaptive navigation in VLN

Considering each page as an object of the category page and each object (links, images, actions) as sub objects of the category page is possible to refine the structure. The letter (a) of Figure 16 shows the direct guidance in modeling categorical one page of practice of a Virtual Laboratory of Neuroanatomy (VLN). In a first abstraction, formalization of direct guidance offered by the CT through the mapping done by a constant morphism. Considering Ob_3 as an only target node is equivalent to an only choice for user direct guidance in the AEHS, if exist a morphism g that maps Ob_2 to Ob_3 , the composition $h = g \circ f$ will send all of the elements of Ob_1 to Ob_3 to form the structure of the presentation of the links in the navigation.

Let is suppose that Ob_2 is a one-element set, so f is already known: it takes all elements of Ob_1 to the only element of Ob_2. A map h must send all elements of Ob_1 to the same element of Ob_3.

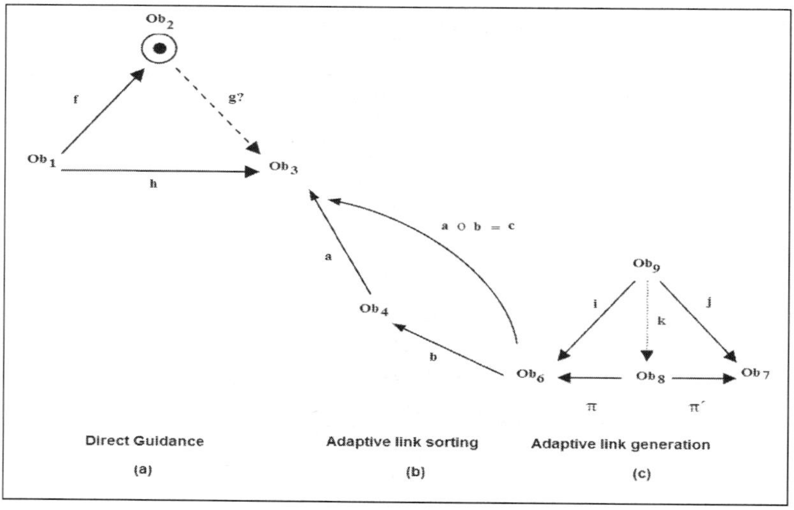

Fig. 16. Categorical denotation of navigation support in a VLN screen page

The letter (b) of Figure 16 shows the specification of the ordering of links in the page object of Practice Interactive System. The morphism classifies all links; each link determines the relevance and the relevant links are then sorted again to form the paths of adaptive navigation. If Ob_6 is the set of all links and Ob_4 is the set of all relevant values assigned in accordance with the user level. Then the morphism $(Ob_6 \xrightarrow{b} Ob_4)$ assigns each link with a relevance.

The letter (c) of Figure 16 shows the generation of new links of interest to the users that were not defined at the time of authorship in information network. The modeling to link generation was formalized by categorical product.

As shown in Figure 16 the object Ob_8 is considered as a new link (or set of links) generated. Considering that Ob_6 and Ob_7 are objects of the category *C ("Question and Answers")*, the product of Ob_1 and Ob_2 is given by an object Ob_4 and the pairs of morphisms $\pi : Ob_4 \rightarrow Ob_1$ and $\pi' : Ob_4 \rightarrow Ob_2$ called first and second projection, respectively. For each object Ob_9 and the pair of morphisms $i: Ob_9 \rightarrow Ob_6$ and $j: Ob_9 \rightarrow Ob_7$ there is a unique morphism $k: Ob_9 \rightarrow Ob_8$ such that the diagram is commutative. The object Ob_4 is considered as a new link (or set of links) generated.

The diagram commutes if each pair of paths through the diagram is such that they have the selfsame start and end points defining a same morphism. Therefore, the diagram in letter (c) of Figure 16 we have:

$$\pi \circ \kappa = i \tag{25}$$

$$\pi' \circ \kappa' = j \tag{26}$$

The CT showed to be a useful method for modeling the characteristics of the VLN adaptive navigation. The use of CT allowed more complex representations in topological space. To design the structure of links and of nodes, CT seemed a more natural approach.
Figure 17 presents the equivalent model of the Figure 16.

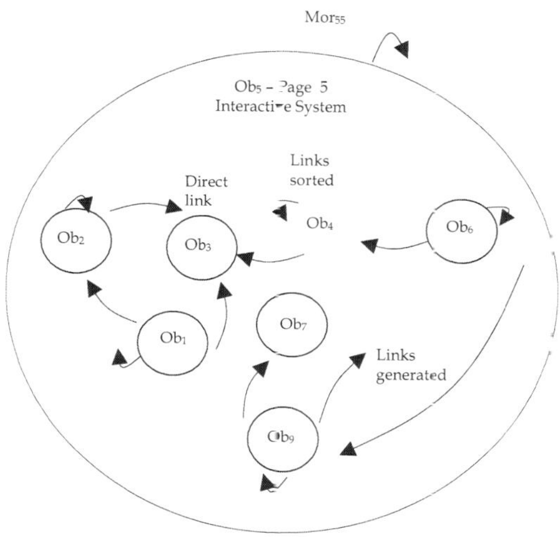

Fig. 17. A simple diagram equivalent for denotation of navigation support for page 5

A categorical model of AEHS aims to represent high-level connections that can be made between the components of an educational hypermedia system. For instance, the identity morphisms may represent, for example, the links that associate the page to themselves, the behavior of the user can decide not to change the page in the AEHS, the system behavior not changes the method of presentation adaptive to the student, etc.
The diagram of Figure 17 was used to describe the pathways of the B-AEHS for Neuroanatomy tutorial. It was possible to reduce the problems with navigation. The results showed that the great advantage of using CT was to provide a high degree of generalization to the conceptual representation of the system. The level of abstraction and generality offered by CT allows its use in the development of many different models AEHS. The decomposition of the system leads to breaking up large specifications into components that can be refined independently with the composition of combinations that must meet a higher specification.
The system was viewed as a whole however their parts were built separately. The formal model of adaptive navigation support simplified the structure of links reducing the problems of orientation while maintaining the degree of freedom in navigation.

5. Conclusion

In all architectures exists the general consensus that a model of AEHS should contain minimal a student model, a domain model, an adaptation model and interaction mechanisms with the user. AEHS can adapt its behavior for the user or the context of the considered domain. A construction of students' models usually requests that are made a lot of suppositions on the same ones: abilities, knowledge, needs, or preferences, as well as its behavior and interaction with the system. Besides, a consensus of the specialists exists, mainly, to that are devoted applied AEHS to the education area that the system should consider the user's cognitive aspects.

Many studies are dedicated to the study of quality of Health Education Systems. However, much of the literature studies are focused on teaching (Kosone, 2009), learning strategies (Patel et al, 2009), usability (Ng et al., 2002), etc. No importance is given to studies on the construction of educational programs in this area.

This work emphasizes that the use of categorical techniques can contribute to the quality of these systems because a great benefit of the use of formal methods is to reduce the number of errors in systems.

Several conventional systems and adaptive hypermedia have been developed without the use of modelling techniques, did not follow a formal methodology for implementations. Due to the numerous applications of these systems and the development of hypermedia technology models have emerged to represent references and arbitrary combination of mechanisms for specification of systems. There are few studies of adaptive navigation support in educational hypermedia systems in Biomedical Education. In modelling the characteristics of adaptive navigation the CT was applied to provide formalisms useful in defining the interconnections between the links. The adaptive navigation treats of the definition of the spatial layout and information related to the user interface (Brusilovsky, 2007). The use of CT allows more complex representations in topological space used to model adaptive navigation in AEHS context.

An important contribution of CT is to illustrate the formal mapping among different levels of the architecture of the program. In others words, there is the concept of the components generalization of low level in the programs architecture. Although any theory can be used for to define the objects of multiple levels of the B-AEHS architecture, compared with other theories, reduces the project complexity when different levels for schemata and diagrams are necessary.

Another advantage is that, as CT is based in diagrams, this primitive concept is most natural for definition of the dynamic and static aspects of B-AEHS model. This approach can be interesting to find universal properties of the systems, in different levels and modules.

The model design methods provide a systematic and consistent set of steps that assist the development of hypermedia systems. The use of CT can complement these methods simplify the modeling process. CT can offer a high level of abstraction for languages of description of AEHS architectures.

Finally, from our analysis, we concluded that CT has a rich symbolism that allows quickly visualize complicated facts and connections to model Adaptive Educational Hypermedia System by diagrams.

Future works can build CASE (Computer-Aided Software Engineering) tools to modeling B-AEHS in the several biomedical areas. The CT treats of objects and its associations, therefore the tool can incorporate the benefits of the object-orientation and the usage of visual diagrams easily.

6. References

Almeida, M. A. F. ; Azevedo, F. M. (2008). B-AEHS: a formal model for adaptive educational hypermedia system in a Biomedical Project evaluation, *4th European Conference of the International Federation for Medical and Biological Engineering*, pp. 2734-2737, ISBN 978-3-540-89207-6, November, Springer Berlin Heidelberg, Antwerp, Belgium.

Almeida, M. A. F. (2002). *Hipertômatos na Computação aplicada à Educação*, PhD thesis, Federal University of Santa Catarina, Florianopolis.

Adamek, J.; Herrlich, H. & Strecker, G.E. (2004). *Abstract and Concrete Category: the Joy of Cats*, John Wiley & Sons, ISBN 9780471609223, New York, USA.

Arbib, M.; Manes, E. (1975) *Arrows, Structures, and Functions - The Categorical Imperative*. Academic Press, Inc., ISBN 0-12-059060-3, New York, USA.

Awodey, S. (2006). *Category Theory*, Oxford University Press Inc, ISBN 0-19-856861-4, New York, USA.

Barrett, J. W. & Mackaay, M. (2006). Categorical representations of categorical groups, *Theory and Applications of Categories*, Vol. 16, No. 20, pp. 529–577, ISSN 1201-561X.

Benyon, D. ; Murray, D. (1993). Applying User Modelling to Human-Computer Interaction Design. *Artificial Intelligence Review*, Vol. 7, No. 3-4, pp. 199-225, ISSN 0269-2821.

Brusilovsky, P. (1996). Methods and Techniques of Adaptive Hypermedia, *Journal of User Modelling and User-Adapted Interaction* , Vol. 12, No. 6, pp. 87-129.

Brusilovsky, P. (2001). Adaptive hypermedia, *User Modelling and User Adapted Interaction*, Vol. 11, No. 1, pp. 87–110, ISSN 0924-1868.

Brusilovsky, P. (2002). Domain, task, and user models for an adaptive hypermedia performance support system, *Proceedings of the 7th international Conference on intelligent User interfaces (IUI02)*, pp. 23-30, ISBN 1-58113-459-2, January, ACM Press, San Francisco, USA.

Brusilovsky, P. (2004). Adaptive navigation support: from adaptive hypermedia to the adaptive web and beyond, *PsychNology Journal*, Vol.2, No. 1, pp. 7-23, ISSN 1720-7525.

Brusilovsky, P. & Millán, E. (2007). User models for adaptive hypermedia and adaptive educational systems, *The Adaptive Web Methods and Strategies of Web Personalization*, Vol. 4321, pp.3–53, Springer Berlin Heidelberg, ISSN 0302-9743.

Campbell, B. ; Goodman, J.M. (1987) HAM: A General-Purpose Hypertext Abstract Machine In: *Hypertext' 87 Proceedings*, ACM, 1987, pp. 21-32.

De Bra, P.; Houben, G & Kornatzky, Y (1993). Browsing Semantics in the Tower model. In: *Computing Science Notes*, Prentice-Hall.

Fiadeiro, J. L. (2005). *Categories for Software Engineering*, Springer Berlin Heidelberg, ISBN 3-540-20909-3, New York.

Furuta, R. & Scotts, P. (1990). The Trellis Hypertext Reference Model, In: *Proceedings NIST Hypertext Standardization Workshop*.

Ginderen, B. V. (1990). *An Object-oriented Hypertext System for Computer-Aided Learning*. Master's thesis, Eindhoven University Technology.

Gunawardena, J. (1996) *New Connections between Mathematics and Computer Science*, Technical Report 96002, Hewlett Packard Labs, Bristol, UK.

Halasz, F. ; Schwartz, M. (1994) The Dexter Hypertext Reference Model, *Communications of the ACM*, vol. 37.

Hardman, L. ; Bulterman, D. C.A & Van Rossum, G. (1994) The Amsterdam Hypermedia Model: adding time and context to the Dexter model, *Communications of the ACM*, vol. 37, pp. 50-52.

Jay, C. B. (1993). *An introduction to Categories in Computing*, University of Technology, Sidney, Australia.

Kosonen, A. L. ; Haapala, I.; Kuurala, S. ; Savonlinna, S. M.; Hanninen, O. ; Carvalho, G.S. (2009). Health knowledge construction and pedagogical style in Finnish health education textbooks, *Health Education*, vol. 109, no. 3, pp. 226-241.

Lawvere, F. W. & Schanuel, S. H. (1997). *Conceptual Mathematics: a first introduction to categories*, Cambridge University Press, ISBN 0-521-47249-0, New York, USA.

Lambek, J, Scott, P J (1986) *Introduction to higher order categorical logic*. Studies in Advanced Mathematics, Cambridge, Cambridge University Press.

Ng, M. H., Hall, W., Maier, P. and Armstrong, R. (2002) The Application and Evaluation of Adaptive Hypermedia Techniques in Web-based Medical Education. *Association for Learning Technology Journal*, 10 (3). pp. 19-40.

Pagano, R. L. (1992) *Computer Simulation as an Educational Tool*, PhD thesis, Faculty of Applied Sciences, University of Louvain la Neuve, Belgium.

Patel, V. L. ; Yoskowitz, N.A.; Arocha, J. F., Shortliffe, E. H. (2009) Cognitive and learning sciences in biomedical and health instructional design: a review with lessons for biomedical informatics education, *Journal of Biomedical Informatics*, ISSN: 1532-0464, vol. 42, pp. 176–197.

Rossi, G., Schwabe, D., Lyardet, F.(2010) Web Application Models Are More than Conceptual Models, *Advances in Conceptual Modelling Lecture Notes in Computer Science*, 2010, Volume 1727/2010, 239-252, DOI: 10.1007/3-540-48054-4_20.

23

eHealth Projects of the Microgravity Centre

Thais Russomano, Ricardo B Cardoso, Christopher R Jones,
Helena W Oliveira, Edison Hüttner and Maria Helena Itaqui Lopes
Pontifical Catholic University of Rio Grande do Sul
Brazil

1. Introduction

This Chapter aims to present the activities of the Telemedicine Laboratory of the Microgravity Centre/PUCRS (Brazil) and to discuss eHealth initiatives around the globe, emphasising the benefits of the use of telecommunication and computer technologies in remote and deprived areas, where specialised medical care is limited or non-existent. Based on the experience of this Lab in the areas of eResearch, eLearning and eHealth Assistance, a review of virtual tools used in academic activities and of telemedicine endeavours applied for the identification and treatment of a broad range of diseases worldwide is presented. Relevant eHealth terminology is also introduced to help the reader gain a better understanding of the concepts described in this text.

2. The Microgravity centre

Established in 1999, the Microgravity Laboratory emerged as a result of joint efforts between the Schools of Medicine, Aeronautical Sciences, and Engineering at the Pontifical Catholic University of Rio Grande do Sul (PUCRS) in Brazil. The Laboratory grew and expanded over the next few years with an ever increasing work output, and earned international acknowledgement for the pioneering and highly qualified research conducted there. In 2006, the Laboratory of Microgravity was transformed into the Centre of Microgravity (MicroG), and officially integrated the research of several academic departments of PUCRS. Today, the MicroG is, par excellence, a multidisciplinary research centre participating in both undergraduate and graduate courses in numerous areas of knowledge. The Centre currently comprises of seven unique research Laboratories, developing projects in different fields of aerospace sciences and in eHealth (www.pucrs.br/feng/microg).

The MicroG has established several partnerships with both national and international institutions, and with researchers prominent in their field. Consequently, two of the seven Laboratories at the MicroG Centre have been named after internationally recognised professionals who have made significant contributions to their development, and to the area of aerospace science: The John Ernsting Aerospace Physiology Laboratory, carrying out research into the behaviour and adaptation of human beings to aerospace environments, and the Joan Vernikos Aerospace Pharmacy Laboratory, dedicated to studying the effects of microgravity, hypogravity, and hypergravity conditions on pharmaceutical medications and their effects on humans. For the purposes of this Chapter, however, we will concentrate on one of the fastest growing and innovative research Laboratories currently at the MicroG Centre, working in the dynamic and fast-paced field that is Telemedicine.

3. The telemedicine laboratory of the MicroG centre

Telemedicine, an emerging area of health assistance, research, and education, aims to apply information and telecommunication technologies (ICT) to enable the remote assistance of communities who currently lack specialist healthcare or access to any type of medical assistance. Supported by the São Lucas Hospital of PUCRS, the School of Medicine, the German TEMOS (Telemedicine for a Mobile Society) Project and other Universities, the MicroG Centre established the Telemedicine Laboratory as a research environment for the development of eResearch, eLearning and eHealth Assistance projects and tools.

The establishment of a Telemedicine Laboratory in a developing country, however, is not always an easy task, and the creation of the Telemedicine Lab of the MicroG Centre was no exception. The first years of the Lab were dedicated to overcoming many difficulties that were encountered, such as a lack of ICT knowledge of professionals involved, the hostile environments encountered in sites for planned eHealth projects, a resistance to new technology, poor local infrastructure, and restricted funding.

The most common limiting factors can be summarized as:

- Weak ICT knowledge, strategic planning, and limited experience with complex ICT implementation;
- Inconsistent leadership, especially in remote and rural areas;
- Lack of human resources at all levels;
- Inadequate local funding;
- Resistance to change, poor computer literacy, and technophobia ;
- Lack of culture of data collection and interpretation;
- Weakness in the conceptualization of the eHealth framework.

The Telemedicine Lab of the MicroG Centre has been able to surpass the limiting factors inherent to the establishment of a new area of knowledge in a developing country. With less than half a decade of experience of projects, the Lab has become both nationally and internationally recognised for the excellence of its work. This Chapter will describe and discuss the eHealth activities of the MicroG Centre Telemedicine Laboratory, including originality, experiences, limitations faced, and future proposed researches.

Some important concepts, however, must be first defined for a better understanding of the terminology applied, since these terms will be used often when eHealth projects and activities are presented (eHealth Related Terminology, Glossary of Terms Commonly Used in Health Care; AcademyHealth, 2004)

4. Definition of terms and concepts

eHealth is considered to be comprised of health informatics, teleHealth, and eLearning activities. They include tools for health authorities and professionals, as well as personalised health systems for patients and citizens. Examples are health information networks, electronic health records, telemedicine services, personal wearable and portable communicable systems, health portals, and many other information and communication technology based tools assisting prevention, diagnosis, treatment, health monitoring, and lifestyle management.

TeleHealth is the use of information and communication technologies (ICT) to exchange health information and provide health care services across geographic, time, social, cultural, and political barriers.

mHealth or mobile health is the practice of medical and public health, supported by mobile devices. The term is most commonly applied in reference to using mobile communication devices, such as mobile phones and PDAs, for health services and information.

Health Informatics comprises of the systematic study of the identification, collection, storage, communication, retrieval, and analysis of data about medical care services that can be used to assist decision making by physicians and managers of healthcare organizations.

eLearning is the utilization of technology to deliver learning and training programmes through media, such as CD-ROM, Internet, intranet, wireless, and mobile learning.

Database Management System (DBMS) is a system or software designed to manage a database, and run operations on the data requested by multiple clients.

Clinical Decision Support System (CDSS) is a system or software application primarily used to consolidate, summarize, or transform transaction data; it is specifically designed to assist health care providers in making decisions on care options by using structured (rules-based) information on diagnoses, treatments, and medications.

Electronic Patient Record (EPR) is a patient-centred record with information from multiple institutions. It supports health care providers by offering complete and accurate data, practitioner reminders and alerts, links to bodies of medical knowledge, and other aids.

Electronic Medical Record (EMR) is the repository of electronically maintained information about an individual's health status and health care, stored such that it can serve the multiple legitimate users of the record.

Electronic Health Record (EHR) is a systematic collection of continuously updated and current information relating to the past, present, or future physical and mental health, or condition of a patient, which resides in computers that capture, transmit, receive, store, retrieve, link, and manipulate multimedia data for the primary purpose of providing healthcare and health-related services. Accessible from any location by any provider caring for a patient, it allows the collection of data for uses other than for direct patient care, such as quality improvement, outcome reporting, resource management, and public health communicable disease surveillance.

TeleHealth Site is a geographic location (healthcare facility or clinic) from which one or more teleHealth activities, applications, or services are provided or received. Within any single teleHealth site will be either, or both, teleHealth facilities and teleHealth units.

Receiving and Delivering Sites - the "delivering site" is the site at which the specialist or referred clinician is located, and the "receiving site" is the site at which the referring clinician and/or patient is located.

Store and Forward is a telecommunications technique in which information is sent to an intermediate station where it is kept and sent at a later time to the final destination or to another intermediate station. The intermediate station, or node in a networking context, verifies the integrity of the message before forwarding it. In general, this technique is used in networks with intermittent connectivity, especially in the wilderness or environments requiring high mobility. It may also be preferable in situations when there are long delays in transmission with variable and high error rates, or if a direct, end-to-end connection is not available.

TeleHealth Unit is a related group of elements (hardware and software, including peripheral devices) that comprises a distinct and functioning apparatus that can be used to perform a specific teleHealth activity, application, or service. A teleHealth unit may be static, mobile, or handheld, and includes units for off-site use.

TeleHealth Facility is a discrete and identifiable physical location (e.g. dedicated room, or dedicated space within a room) from which clinical, research, education, administration, or mixed teleHealth related pursuits are provided or received. A teleHealth site may have more than one teleHealth facility.

TeleHealth Activity is a teleHealth mediated pursuit, at the experimental, pilot, or formative evaluation stage.

TeleHealth Service is a specific and proven teleHealth application (clinical applications) offered routinely between teleHealth sites typically within a teleHealth programme e.g. forensic telemental health assessment; pre-catheterization teleassessment; home telemonitoring.

TeleHealth Program is a distinct, appropriately conceived, designed, staffed, managed, funded, and accredited set of teleHealth services orchestrated under a common theme and common administrative structure, such as a telemental health programme; a telecardiology programme; or a home teleHealth programme.

eHealth Policy is defined as a set of statements, directives, regulations, laws, and judicial interpretations that direct and manage the life cycle of eHealth. More generically, policy is a plan or course of action of a government, political party or business intended to influence and determine decisions and actions.

A still controversial and debatable area of eHealth is related to the **Ethical Issues** involved in delivering health care from a distance. This theme is evolving daily and still presents a huge variability of applications and definitions from place to place. In general terms, **Ethical Issues in eHealth** include the discussion of the topics described below:

Consent for care in eHealth: Laws differ in many areas of the globe on obtaining consent for care before transferring patient information online, or before arranging video-conferencing sessions, especially when open source softwares are used. Clear policies to guide such consent can benefit and legally protect healthcare institutions and providers.

Liability issues (also called **medical malpractice liability**) and **Medico-legal issues** are related to policies regarding medico-legal issues in eHealth, which are crucial, and must be developed before eHealth programs are implemented. Local laws and policies for healthcare services and providers must be respected, but also adapted to cover aspects related to eHealth issues.

Other **Ethical** topics to be considered are the policies that define the **patient's right** to access his or her own electronic information and database of medical history, diagnoses, exams and treatment history. These policies can constitute an important matter for eHealth decision makers, since it can help managers and providers to safely and legally share the requested information with the patients (WMA, 2007 & 2008).

Establishment of international **policies in eHealth** can be a huge challenge (Scott et al., 2002; Scott et al., 2004). eHealth expectations and requirements differ in the developed world when compared with the needs of the developing world. In a developed country, for example, eHealth programmes are designed to provide products like eCards and aim to decrease the healthcare costs of an aging population by introducing adequate and sustainable homecare services. The developing countries, on the other hand, are generally more concerned with issues such as finding ways of overcoming extreme shortages of healthcare workers, especially in remote areas, and improving rural healthcare, whist at the same time implementing electronic health information systems. Therefore, what seems perfectly acceptable in the developed world, in terms of data security and quality, patient confidentiality, and privacy, may be major impediments to the eHealth policy of a developing country. A good example is the eHealth roadmap of Europe. The 27 European Member States identified 36 policy targets, with the most common aims being: improved efficiency and quality of care in health system performance; healthcare system reform; citizen-oriented, patient-centred healthcare; quality of care; better data for system management and communication between stakeholders; efficiency; access to care; promoting quality of life; and improved economy via eHealth technology. They are undoubtedly very important goals to be achieved, but every single one is complex, requiring enormous political, social, and economic investments. Developing countries are perhaps those most in need of global assistance but for this to be successfully accomplished they need to have in place adequate and well defined eHealth policies, a difficult enough undertaking for the more structured countries of Europe to achieve, and therefore a far more problematic task for countries still struggling to attain sustainable development (Scott, RE, 2007).

5. Current issues in global health

Since the beginning of the new millennium there has been an increasing emphasis placed on global health, both in the political agenda and within the healthcare profession. In the year 2000, the United Nations outlined Eight Millennium Development Goals (MDG) with the aim of alleviating hunger and poverty by the year 2015 (UN General Assembly, 2000). Health forms a large part of these goals and there has subsequently been an increasing focus on both academic and clinical pursuits, from a national policy level right down to the level of the individual. There is an ever increasing amount of funding available and initiatives in place for the 'big three' infectious diseases - human immunodeficiency virus/acquired immune deficiency syndrome (HIV/AIDS), malaria, and tuberculosis. Furthermore, previously neglected tropical diseases, such as schistosomiasis, leishmaniasis, Chagas disease, and soil transmitted helminths are now beginning to receive some of the attention that they deserve, although there is still a lot more that needs to be done (Fenwick et al., 2009). Disease is a universal entity, not recognising political and continental boundaries, as evidenced by the rapid global spread of the pandemic influenza A(H1N1) virus in 2009. Therefore, a coordinated approach on a global scale with both intra- and intercontinental cooperation is warranted.

However, whilst there have been significant improvements in global health, large inequalities remain, particularly in low and middle income countries. A review by Beaglehole and Bonita (2008) has summarised the recent trends and agendas in global public health. People living in poorer nations have a shorter life expectancy and live more of their lives in bad health, as opposed to those in richer countries. The MDGs have experienced mixed fortunes; progress has been erratic and it is unlikely that any of the goals will be met by 2015 where they are needed the most, in sub-Saharan Africa. The balance between communicable and non-communicable disease has firmly shifted in favour of the latter. It is now cardiovascular disease, diabetes, cancer, chronic respiratory disease, mental disorders, and injuries that are the main threat to health throughout the world. Non-communicable diseases cause substantial morbidity and mortality; in 2005 they were responsible for 60% of all global deaths (WHO, 2005). It has been estimated that 80% of all deaths attributable to non-communicable diseases occur in low and middle income countries (WHO, 2008). Health gaps within and between countries are widening and efforts at socioeconomic development are impeded by the heavy burden of disease, highlighting the close association between poor health and poverty (Alwan & MacLean, 2009).

Unfortunately it is the people living in remote and resource-poor settings who bear a large proportion of the global disease burden. They commonly live far from health centres and may not have the physical or financial capacity to travel and seek attention. These rural health centres are frequently understaffed, underequipped, and underfunded; they are neglected by the health system and the international community. There is usually a shortage of trained physicians and those that remain within the country often avoid working in remote areas due to isolation caused by difficult access to and from cities, as well as the low availability of resources. Specialist care is hard to find outside of big cities and the healthcare staff working in remote areas often have gaps in their skills and knowledge due to a lack of opportunities and resources for further training. All of this means that when patients do eventually present to a healthcare professional, their condition is at a more advanced stage and therefore more complicated to manage, with a decreased likelihood of a successful outcome.

6. How can eHealth help?

Bashshur and Shannon (2009) present telemedicine as a cost-effective and clinically useful option for those planning healthcare interventions. They provide a comprehensive summary of how it can be applied and its potential benefits. Whilst the authors focus on a developed country, there are several principles that can be extracted and applied to developing countries also. Telemedicine can provide specialist healthcare in remote environments without the need for patient or physician to travel, saving money and time as well as making the patient's life more convenient. The reach of specialists at tertiary care centres is significantly extended. Telemedicine can link primary and tertiary care, providing access to specialist information and advice when required for general practitioners. It enables a sensible triaging of patients and can minimise the duplication of diagnostic tests and clinical services. As well as access to specialist information and opinions at initial appointments, it can also be used for ongoing follow-up care after previous treatment.

Telemedicine can:

- Stabilise rural providers and local economies;
- Facilitate the care of institutionalised populations;
- Integrate medical services across multiple delivery sites;
- Enhance chronic disease management, both in rural settings and in long-term care institutions;
- Put the patient at the centre of the focus of care;
- Decrease the difficulty of accessing healthcare due to socioeconomic, geographic, and cultural differences.

Emerging and re-emerging infectious diseases in Africa, such as cholera or viral haemorrhagic fevers, can be considered examples of how telemedicine can help. There are regular outbreaks of disease that cause many problems in the African continent because of complex environmental, economic, and political factors. Many countries in Africa have a decreased capacity to monitor disease trends and instigate appropriate public health action. This is because of a lack of laboratory facilities and poorly integrated disease surveillance systems. To be able to rapidly and efficiently tackle an emerging public health threat, the following are required: good local level disease surveillance; a network of reference laboratories on a national and international scale; and rapid collection and dissemination of data. Without the aforementioned features, outbreaks may reach epidemic proportions before they are detected at a local or national level. eHealth networks can bring together the activities of district laboratories, enable efficient data collection and transmission, and provide support through quality control and technical advice. This has the potential to improve disease surveillance and enable healthcare systems to react and get on top of disease outbreaks rapidly (Shears, 2000).

There are several factors that must be considered for a telemedicine initiative to be successful. It is important that the group of patients to be referred for a virtual outreach programme is selected carefully. The staff working in the receiving site must possess the correct skills and equipment to be able to undertake the appropriate history and examination, the results of which must be carefully documented (Rinde & Balteskard, 2002). Other aspects that must be addressed are the costs involved in any new project, limited internet connectivity, and unreliable power supplies, especially in sub-Saharan Africa. Telemedicine needs to be considered at a policy level to ensure that a sustainable budget is available. Ongoing training must be provided to receiving staff to ensure that computer literacy is sufficient and that technical support can be provided in the event of a system failure. The unpredictable nature of politics means that changing priorities or conflicts may disrupt local infrastructure and the healthcare system (Mars, 2009).

Furthermore, as previously discussed, there are ethical and legal considerations, which are of utmost importance when planning a telemedicine initiative. Rather than creating new ethical and legal considerations, telemedicine accentuates existing ones. Patient privacy, confidentiality, and consent must be comprehensively addressed, as it is frequently these issues that concern patients most. When storing, transmitting, receiving, or disposing of confidential information, it is the eHealth technical personnel that are responsible for ensuring the protection against improper disclosure (Stanberry, 2001).

7. The main areas of the telemedicine laboratory of the MicroG Centre

The Telemedicine Lab has three main areas of activity – **eResearch, eLearning and eHealth assistance.**

8. eResearch

Globalisation has allowed researchers to share information regarding projects and studies being developed around the world. eResearch, however, aims to foster greater national and international multidisciplinary collaboration, enabling researchers to actively participate in practical studies taking place in other countries, without the need to leave their own universities.

The Telemedicine Laboratory/MicroG Centre has successfully performed a series of eResearch activities. These are related to the development of software and hardware that have been used in eHealth projects and in the teletransmission to national and international partners of live surgeries, lectures, and data collection for several studies.

8.1 Virtual data collection

In order to facilitate greater international collaboration for aerospace physiological studies at the MicroG Centre, the Telemedicine Laboratory has used video-conferencing technology to allow virtual participation during data collection (Figure 1). This has allowed partner researchers from European institutions to take part in joint studies whilst remaining in their own laboratories. This technique has enabled new interactions between professors, researchers, and students from different countries during project development, with the benefit of reducing costs and avoiding the need to travel.

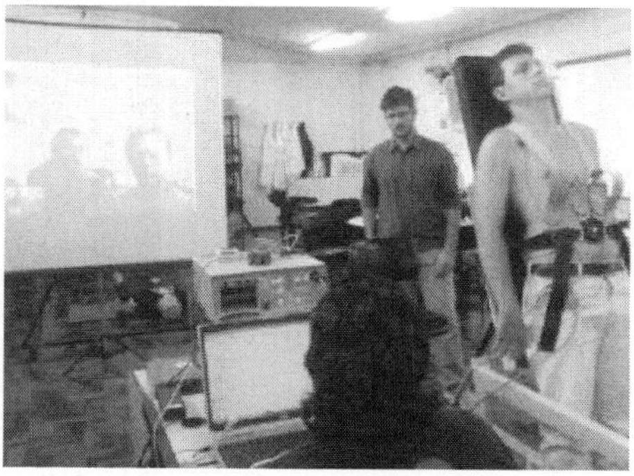

Fig. 1. Virtual participation of researchers from Lithuania during data collection at the MicroG Centre in Brazil

8.2 Research and development eHealth equipment – digital camera illuminator

Ensuring standard lighting conditions for the collection of image data is not possible in remote locations lacking in proper infrastructure, or in healthcare unit consultation rooms, without the proper equipment (Miot, 2006). Therefore, having learnt from the experience of several assistance missions to the Amazon region of Brazil, the Telemedicine Laboratory has developed a series of illuminator prototypes to provide a standard light intensity and colour contrast, during acquisition of skin and mouth lesion images (Figure 2). One of the main objectives of these missions was to enable remote second opinion of dermatological issues though the exchange of electronic patient records between teleHealth receiving and delivering sites (Cardoso, 2007).

Consequently, a research project was conceived to develop and validate an illumination device which would be adaptable for use with multiple brands of amateur and semi-professional digital cameras. This equipment, when employed together with electronic patient record systems, enables the implementation of teledermatology and teleodontology services, improving healthcare delivery in locations with no specialised health professionals. The development of these prototypes was accomplished through a series of studies conducted at the Telemedicine Laboratory, the dermatology clinic of PUCRS Academic Extension Unit for Health Care Services, and during the Amazon missions. The resultant images obtained permitted the identification of different problems in each project, allowing solutions to be suggested and improvements in prototype design and construction (Figure 3).

An image acquisition protocol was created to standardise the methodology utilised by users, preventing misplaced camera configuration, incorrect illuminator assembly, or equipment positioning difficulties when acquiring lesion pictures.

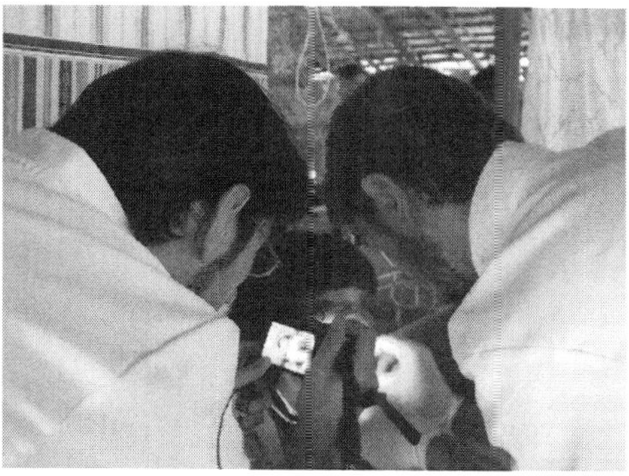

Fig. 2. Image acquisition of patient lesion using illuminator prototype attached to a Sony digital camera

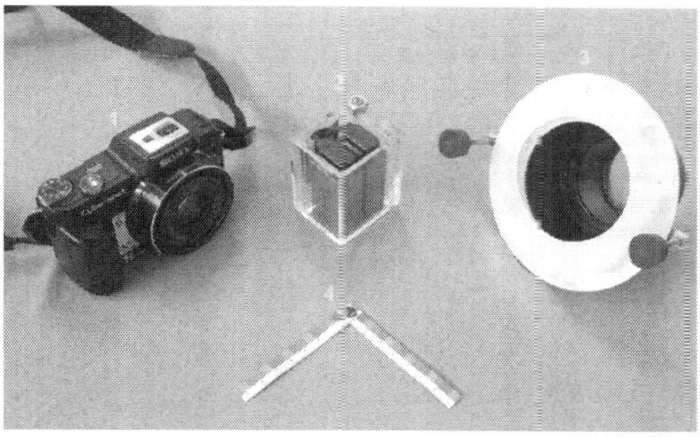

Fig. 3. Current Illuminator prototype. 1: Sony Digital Camera. 2: Illuminator power supply support. 3: Illuminator. 4: Colour ruler (size, colour and focus reference)

Electronic patient record

In order to allow the electronic patient record exchange between teleHealth receiving and delivering sites, the telemedicine laboratory has developed several asynchronous communication platforms, which can be divided into two groups:

Desktop applications

Due to the lack of internet access in remote locations, electronic patient record software in these areas requires local database management systems in order to employ "store and forward" methodology for data communication. A Delphi desktop application, associated with File Transfer Protocol (FTP) and MySql database servers, was considered most suitable for use in these conditions (Figure 4). As a result, data exchange between sites takes place upon internet availability, allowing a greater flexibility and mobility of the specialised virtual assistance service.

The tool data input is divided into general patient information and the specialised areas, such as dermatology, odontology, cardiology, pharmacy, and nutrition. Each area is used according to the need of the receiving physician for second opinion.

All patient data is secure and its access is protected by user login into the system.

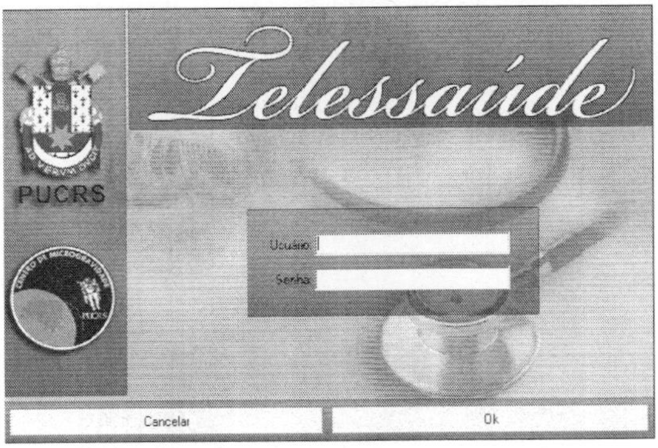

Fig. 4. Electronic patient record software developed by the telemedicine laboratory of the Microgravity Centre - FENG/PUCRS. User login window

Web application

The rapid change of modern technology demands a fast adaptation of computational tools and systems for the evolving requirements of its users. Cloud computing, well known for Google applications such as Google Docs, can provide cost-effectiveness, flexibility, and ease of access benefits leading to a wider scale of use of electronic patient record platforms by hospitals, health units, and remote locations. It allows users to access patient data in real time or from record, from any internet connection point via a web browser, without the need for software installation or update.

In order to provide such a service, the Telemedicine Laboratory developed a web portal (Figure 5), which enables receiving and delivering health professionals to communicate over geographical distances. Medical records and short messages can be securely exchanged over the internet, thus allowing physicians in remote teleHealth facilities to obtain expert second opinion.

Web technologies, such as Hypertext Preprocessor (PHP), Asynchronous Javascript (AJAX), Structured Query Language (SQL), Database Management System (DBMS) and File Transfer Protocol (FTP) were employed in the platform development, creating a dynamic display of stored clinical information.

8.3 Telesurgery system

eHealth education programs are becoming a reality in universities, providing the opportunity for students to have greater interaction at live surgery classes by means of virtual participation. Undergraduate students can be introduced to new concepts of medical care, remote second opinion delivery, and to telecommunication systems, whilst virtually experiencing surgical procedures and lectures. The improved access this provides to the operating theatre environment, the patient, and the surgeon, can improve the learning process for students.

At PUCRS, an analogical system was developed and used for transmitting video and audio from the surgery theatre to a lecture hall (Figure 6.A). The telesurgery lectures were also transmitted to other national and international partner universities by means of a video-conference system (Figure 6.B), featuring H.323 communication protocol, located in the São Lucas University Hospital. Telemedicine technology has proven to be an important

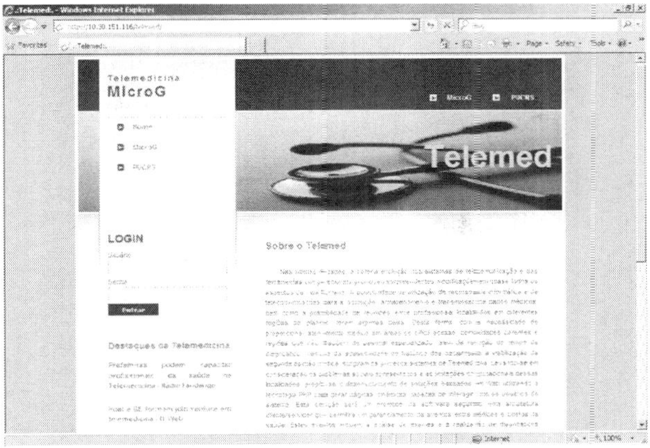

Fig. 5. Web portal developed by the Telemedicine Laboratory of the Microgravity Centre – FENG/PUCRS. User login window

instrument for the improvement of medical education and health care. This methodology allowed health professionals, professors, and students to have greater interaction during surgical procedures, thus enabling a greater opportunity for knowledge exchange.

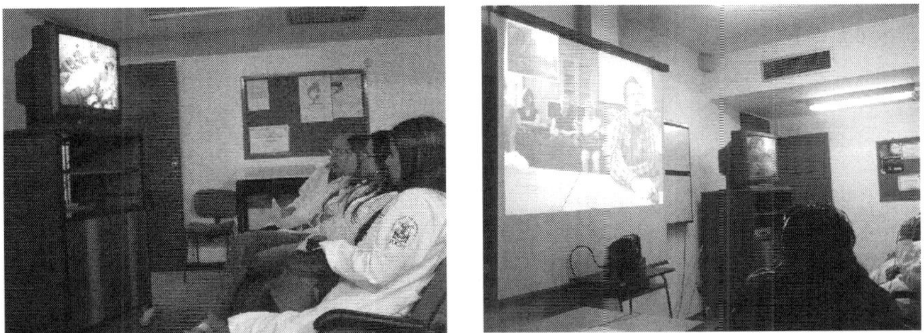

(a) PUCRS students and professors watching live transmission

(b) Live transmission from PUCRS to students and

Fig. 6. Telesurgery lecture. Image and audio transmission of surgery procedures from the surgery theatre and the lecture hall

8.4 3D virtual eye

The establishment of a partnership between the Telemedicine Laboratory of the Microgravity Centre, the School of Informatics at PUCRS, and the Telemedicine Centre of Kaunas University of Medicine, enabled researchers from both universities to develop successful joint projects in the area of telemedicine. The 3D Model Eye project, with a graphic design team of students and professors from the School of Informatics, PUCRS, aimed to develop a virtual tool for educational and medical proposes. As a result of knowledge exchange between the two universities, a 3D stereo animation of a healthy human eye was created using open source graphic modelling software. This model (Figure 7) was accepted by consultant ophthalmologists of both universities as a clear representation of a human eye.

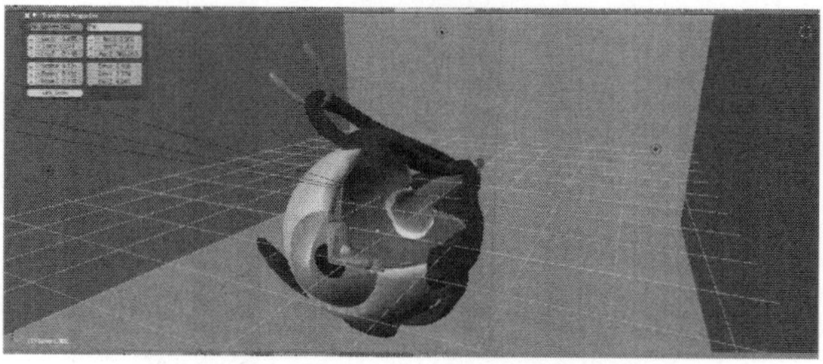

Fig. 7. 3D virtual eye model developed at PUCRS in partnership with the Kaunas University of Medicine.

9. eLearning

The recent development of numerous virtual and electronic communication systems and tools allows learning to be a real time process, which for students and professors is dynamic, challenging, and creative. It eliminates distance and walls in the classroom, giving participants greater motivation with multiple perspectives, promoting connections to be established with other cultures and nations.

In the health area, clinical case discussions and transmission of virtual live surgeries allow for the exchange of specialist medical opinion and treatment suggestion between different countries. Through the establishment of eHealth programs as educational tools, students can become involved in the process, thus making them more aware of the diversity or convergence of clinical conducts, enabling them to develop a more critical judgment, greater autonomy, and an enhanced competence to create and act in knowledge networks, therefore being better prepared for professional reality.

This new educational method has facilitated the diversification of teaching techniques and the development of new ways of interaction among students, professors, and the content, being defined as the use of electronic information and communication networks to disseminate health knowledge.

The MicroG Telemedicine Laboratory has developed multicentre, multidisciplinary virtual activities in order to encourage Brazilian students to experience contact with new telecommunication technologies, and to share educational experiences as an integral part of their learning process.

The Multipoint eHealth Education Programme was established in collaboration with PUCRS, the TEMOS project (Telemedicine for a Mobile Society) of the German Aerospace Centre (DLR), the Faculty of Medicine at the RWTH Aachen University (Germany), the Medical University of Warsaw (Poland) and the Medical University of Kaunas (Lithuania).

The activities of the Multipoint eHealth Education Programme aim to stimulate the interest of undergraduate and postgraduate students to different cultural and social realities and to enable the exchange of health knowledge through videoconferences, and to develop virtual medical education tools.

The eLearning activities comprise of several multipoint and point-to-point virtual lectures among different Brazilian universities and also between educational institutions from Brazil, Germany, Lithuania, Poland, England, Colombia, Mexico, USA, Panama, South Africa and Pakistan. Students from each university choose the topic to be covered and prepare a Microsoft PowerPoint presentation under the supervision of a designated professor. All the presentations and discussions occur in English.

Scientific themes selected were related to diseases, new available treatments, development of technology for medical exams, bioethics, local and international health politics, space life sciences, aerospace medicine, and physiology. In order to carry out the telelectures, different virtual communication systems via the internet were used, with the common characteristic of the capacity to employ H.323 protocol for the transmission of the information between participating universities. The institution in charge was responsible for making the link between the other members of the activity, using a video-conference system with a Multipoint Control Unit (MCU) able to hold a maximum of five connections at the same time. The speed connection between the participants, which varied between 768Kbps and 2Mbps, was configured by each taking into consideration equipment and internet bandwidth capability.

The set up of the virtual lecture room was intended to give all those present eye contact when speaking to each other directly, as this plays a large role in conversational turn-taking, perceived attention and intent, and other aspects of group communication. An important tool used to accomplish this task was Continuous Presence, a feature of MCUs, which enables multiple parties to be seen on-screen at once, allowing presenter and audience to interact in a more effective way (Figure 8). To show close up images of the participants during subject discussions, remote controlled cameras with zoom ability were used together with table microphones capable of efficient echo cancelation.

The Microsoft PowerPoint 2003 files containing presentations were sent in advance to all participants in order to ensure the quality of the display for the classes, allowing them to locally administer the slides. The presentations used multimedia content, including videos and animations, which provided a greater clarity for the explanation of the topic discussed.

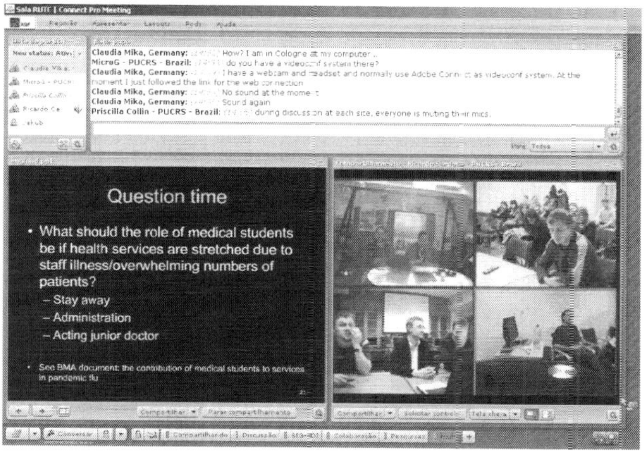

Fig. 8. Continuous Presence set up: Camera placed close to the projected image

10. eHealth assistance

Brazil is a country with continental dimensions, an uneven distribution of financial resources, and diverse social problems. Physicians often avoid working in remote areas due to the isolation caused by difficult access to and from cities, the low availability of resources, and a lack of local infrastructure and comfort. Consequently, these locations are often deprived of specialist care, which has proven to delay the diagnosis and adequate management of several medical conditions.

The Brazilian Amazon assistance projects conducted by PUCRS

eHealth Assistance initiatives, such as the eHealth Amazon Project developed by the Telemedicine Laboratory, are an example of the improvements in health service that can be provided by the use of telemedicine in isolated areas. This project aimed to make available specialised medical assistance to remote and deprived communities using telecommunication systems, software development, mobile technologies, and biomedical engineering. As a consequence of providing this assistance, the Telemedicine Laboratory could validate the tools and systems developed.

These projects were organized in partnership with the Nucleus of Research in Indigenous Culture and the schools of medicine, odontology, and pharmacy of PUCRS, and were divided into two distinct phases: system development and team training; and eHealth missions - validation.

10.1 System development and team training

- Technological tools
  - Data delivery system – *Store and Forward* technique
    - Data storage: Mysql database
    - File Storage: FTP server
    - Interface development: Delphi language
    - Software test and adjustments
  - Illuminator device
    - Improvement from previous developed systems
      - Better camera attachment
      - Stronger structure
      - Better light distribution
  - Multidisciplinary eHealth team training
    - Data delivery software and equipment familiarisation
    - Lectures regarding local cultures
    - Presentation of previous experiences

10.2 eHealth missions – validation

The validation activities were carried out by multidisciplinary eHealth teams, composed of PUCRS professors and students from technical and health areas, such as dentistry, pharmacy, engineering, nutrition, medicine, education, and nursing. Participating students were selected by curriculum analysis and interview or by their previous or present involvement in eHealth projects.

Remote areas of Brazil were chosen as receiving sites due to their lower population density and human development index (Table 1), in order to enable a greater impact on local health care. The sites were as follows:

Delivering site - Sao Lucas hospital of PUCRS

The São Lucas Hospital (HSL), a tertiary hospital, occupies an area of 57.700m² divided into the hospital area (49.000m²) and the clinic centre (8.700m²) in Porto Alegre, Rio Grande do Sul, Brazil. The hospital has a capacity of 603 beds, of which 495 are for conventional hospitalisation, 87 for intensive care (general, cardiovascular, paediatrics, and neonatal), and 21 for observation (emergency patients). 52 specialities are available in hospitalisation care and 31 in emergency and clinic care.

Receiving site - remote locations

The visited areas were characterised by the provision of primary care facilities, where a general practitioner would be responsible for all healthcare delivery. The availability of resources with which to work would typically range from a nurse's station in a healthcare centre to a more basic environment requiring a degree of improvisation to provide the comfort and privacy for patients and the eHealth team.

Local / Aspects	Area (Km²)	Population	Population Density (inh/Km²)	Human development index	GDP (R$) (thousand)	GDP per capita (R$)
Porto Alegre	497	1,436,123	2,890	0.865	33,434,026	23,534
Ji-Parana	6,897	111,010	16.2	0.753	1,121,152	10,412
Alto Xingu	10,000	2,907	0.2907	-	-	-

Table 1. Comparison between receiving sites and delivering site (Porto Alegre city)

The Telemedicine Laboratory successfully organised three missions to the Amazon region of Brazil, which are summarised in Tables 2 and 3:

Mission	Date	Local	Specialities (N° of health interviews)	Total of interviews	Total of patients
I	8th - 28th Jan 2007	Region of Ji-Parana City, Rondonia State	Dermatology (181)	181	181
II	5th - 23rd Jan 2008	Region of Ji-Parana City, Rondonia State	Dermatology (146) Odontotology (30)	176	167
III	18th Jul - 3rd Aug 2008	Xingu Area, Mato Grosso State	Dermatology (62) Odontotology (12) Cardiology (43)	117	112

Table 2. Summarised information from the missions

Mission	Main Findings
I	The main diagnoses made by the specialist were superficial mycosis (32.6%), eczema (8.84%), and keratoses (6.1%). Among interviewed cases, 11.6% were inconclusive. The high incidence of dermatological lesions of fungal origin in adults and children in villages is believed to be influenced by close contact with domestic (i.e. chickens, ducks, and pigs) and wild animals (i.e. birds and monkeys), often kept within the communities. This mission is illustrated in Figure 9.A
II	A second opinion was provided remotely by specialists in odontology and dermatology. From all dermatologic cases analysed, 21.2% were inconclusive and further medical information was required. This mission is illustrated in Figure 9.B
III	Expert opinion analysis verified that 62.7% of electrocardiogram (ECG) exams were normal, while 37.3% had alterations of some degree. In dermatology, the most common diagnoses were eczema (19.3%), Pityriasis Versicolor (14.5%), and Tinea (12.9%). In odontology, angular cheilitis (25%) and traumatic ulcer (25%) were the most frequent findings. Among all, 6 cases (5.12%) were inconclusive due to lack of available information.

Table 3. Main Findings of missions and second opinion data analysis

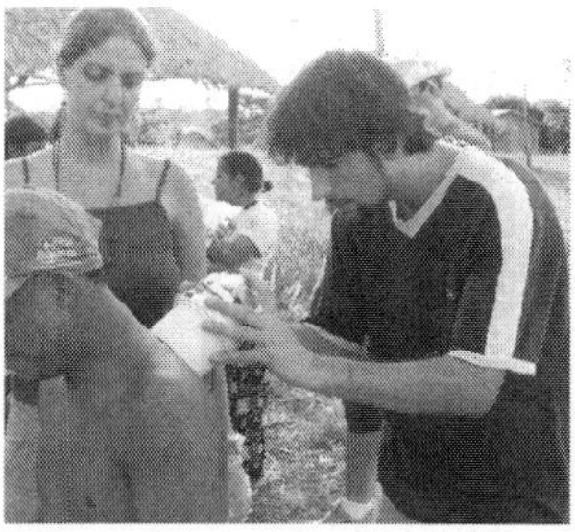

(a) Patient skin image acquisition near Ji-Parana city (Mission I)

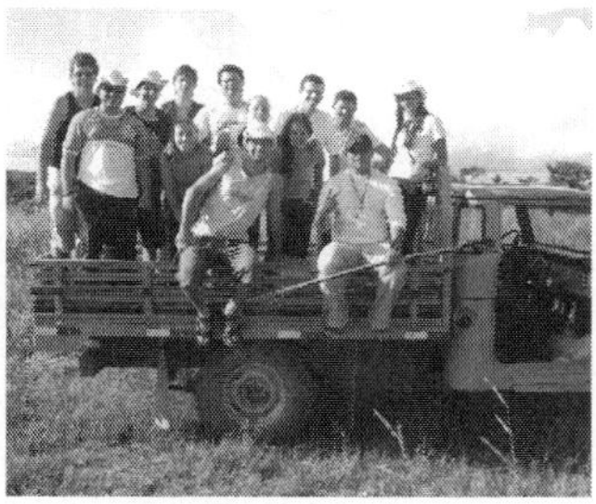

(b) Transportation vehicle of the multidisciplinary team in the Ji-Parana regions (Mission II)

Fig. 9. Amazon missions

During each mission, the activities were divided into the following steps:

1. Patient screening

Interviewed patients were pre-selected by the local health team (receiving site) for each location visited, taking into consideration patient ailments and family medical history. An initial interview was carried out by the PUCRS team to determine the health area to which each patient would be referred, and to create a record on the database.

2. Patient interview - electronic patient record information input

Once referred, each patient was interviewed regarding specific aspects related to their health condition. This information was uploaded to the electronic patient record together with skin/mouth images or electrocardiogram (ECG) exams, depending on the referred area.

2.1 Image acquisition

A Sony digital camera, together with the developed illuminator, was used to acquire images of mouth and skin lesions. Subsequently, pictures with the best quality were uploaded to the software;

2.2 ECG exam

A digital ECG machine was used to acquire electrical wave patterns from patient hearts. After each exam, a data file was generated and uploaded to the electronic patient record.
3. Data transmission - specialist access to patient information
Upon internet availability, the system was programmed to connect to the Microgravity Centre's main server and to synchronise all collected data Specialist health professionals had secure access to the electronic patient records via this server, through use of an application installed on personal computers.
4. Expert second opinion
Patient information, images, and exams were analysed by health specialists at the delivering site, and an opinion and treatment suggestion was offered. The inconclusive cases were due to lack of available information or need for further laboratory exams. The opinions were secured in an encrypted PDF envelop and sent back to the receiving site, where final diagnosis and treatment were the responsibility of the local health team.
The experience gained from organizing and conducting such activities highlighted important issues which should be addressed when developing assistance projects:

- Team training proved to be crucial for the success of the missions as it prepared the groups to: 1) deal with the local conditions of the Amazon region; 2) better interact with the local communities; 3) Solve equipment problems if required.
- The use of software capable of managing all patient data proved to be essential for avoiding information loss or misplacement during data collection. Importantly, the software also enabled users to operate from multiple workstations connected to the same database, allowing access to information uploaded by colleagues, and optimising an efficient team effort.
- The illumination system developed proved to be an essential tool to ensure standardisation of light conditions for all images. This procedure enabled the specialist to better compare and contrast patient skin colour lesions, an important characteristic for dermatological diagnosis.

Telemedicine tools and telecommunication systems proved to have a great applicability in remote regions for the diagnosis of dermatological skin and mouth lesions as well as cardiologic diseases. Each mission completed proved successful at making possible the remote diagnosis of patient ailments in a short period of time, at low cost, and without the need for patient transportation to another location. It is believed that the eHealth assistance model applied in this project can be transferred to any location having access to an internet connection.

11. How else has telemedicine been used around the world?

The scarcity of healthcare professionals in developing countries, particularly specialists, has long been recognised. SatelLife is a charitable organisation set up in Boston in 1987 with the aim of meeting the needs of healthcare providers in the developing world by bridging the digital and information divides. It was a pioneer for telemedicine in resource-poor settings. It provided E-mail access in more than 100 countries serving more than 10,000 healthcare workers, using a low earth orbit satellite and telephone lines. A store and forward technique was applied; E-mails containing the pertinent clinical details and image attachments were sent to specialists for advice on the management of difficult cases. This proved to be a cheap and rapid way of seeking a second opinion (Fraser & McGrath, 2000). SatelLife has since expanded its operations keeping in line with technological advances and continues to provide information and support services for healthcare professionals in resource-poor settings. In 2001, it began to explore the potential use of Personal Data Assistants (PDAs) in Africa (Lucas, 2008), which led to the development of the Uganda Health Information Project (UHIP) in 2003. Initially involving two districts in Uganda, more than 200 PDAs were distributed amongst healthcare workers, and these were linked to connection points at health facilities allowing data communication. This enabled the electronic compilation of Ministry of Health routine data forms, as well as the dissemination of information about planned Ministry of Health activities, and details of disease outbreaks. This venture significantly increased the rate of compliance on weekly disease surveillance reporting. Furthermore, this initiative proved popular with healthcare staff who displayed a strong demand for access to additional information over the network. This project has subsequently expanded and now involves more than 600 workers in five districts throughout Uganda. SatelLife also organise a similar project in Mozambique. This is a good example of how improvements in public health can be achieved through the rapid dissemination of vital information across a large area, in a resource-poor setting, using telemedicine.

Zolfo et al. (2006) describe a HIV/AIDS telemedicine initiative in a resource-poor setting. Doctors at the Institute of Tropical Medicine in Belgium created a hybrid E-mail/web support telemedicine service in order to support physicians in resource-poor settings, using remote consultations to provide expert advice on antiretroviral therapy (ART) and the management of opportunistic infections. The patient's history, examination findings, laboratory results, and questions to be answered were sent along with any relevant images to the telemedicine website, where an HIV/AIDS specialist from the institute in Belgium could assess the case remotely. The price of ART is reducing rapidly, thus opening up the market to more and more developing countries, however, for the treatment to be efficiently and safely used it is important that the healthcare staff have the appropriate knowledge and skills required. This telemedicine service provided an opportunity for clinicians from resource-poor settings to receive training and advice on difficult HIV/AIDS cases, as well as providing resources for their ongoing education.

Bagayoko et al. (2006) performed an evaluation of an internet-based telemedicine network in developing countries in Africa, using the Réseau Afrique Francophone de Télémédecine (RAFT) project as an example. The RAFT project was born out of a partnership between the Mali University Medical School and the University of Geneva. Its focus is sustainable development of an international network, enabled through low cost telemedicine and an appreciation of local necessities. It facilitates interaction between healthcare staff from both sites using teleeducation and teleconsultations. Similar initiatives were deployed in other countries in West Africa and by 2006 a total of nine countries were connected. The RAFT project contains an online database of weekly seminars; it broadcasts scientific conferences over the web; it provides specialist advice for physicians in countries where certain medical fields are under-represented or even absent; it allows European physicians to seek advice and education on tropical diseases that are usually rare in Europe; and it creates opportunities for healthcare staff to receive education or training at the partner institutions. The authors conclude that any telemedicine strategy must be adapted to local needs and realities. Whilst links between developed and developing countries are useful, there still exist vast differences in resources and sociocultural contexts, and as such, an intra-regional network with links to developed countries may be more beneficial. Finally, it is important to avoid a digital divide within a health system by involving the periphery in the development of any network.

Breslauer et al. (2009) combined light microscopy with mobile phones to enable the remote diagnosis of infectious diseases in resource-poor settings. Furthermore, the role of mobile phones in assisting the diagnosis of tuberculosis in developing countries was recently evaluated (Zimic et al., 2009). Tuberculosis is a highly infectious bacterial disease that causes substantial morbidity and mortality around the world, but predominantly in developing countries. Fortunately, it is curable and therefore timely detection and treatment of infected patients is vital to improve their health and prevent further spread. A new tool for the rapid diagnosis of tuberculosis (including multidrug resistant tuberculosis) and determination of drug susceptibility has been developed – the Microscopic Observation Drug Susceptibility (MODS) assay. This test uses inverted microscopy to visually recognise the characteristic pattern of growth of mycobacteria in liquid medium. Whilst it provides a rapid diagnosis and advice on the management of tuberculosis, it also requires specially trained personnel to assess the results in order to achieve the best sensitivity and specificity. This creates a problem for developing countries, where there is a shortage of staff, yet the test is arguably most needed. In this study, mobile phones were used to take and transmit an image of the MODS culture using a web server, with subsequent specialist analysis of the image online and return of the results back to the mobile phone. Concordance between readings directly from the microscope and from the mobile phone image was 98.7%. The authors concluded that this is a cheap and effective way of overcoming the limitation of a shortage of trained personnel.

In addition to its potential in developing countries, telemedicine also has an important role to play in remote areas within developed countries. Raza et al. (2009) report their experiences using videoconference telemedicine for providing outpatient pulmonary consultations in a remote area of the USA. Patient referrals from primary care to a pulmonary specialist were categorised as either urgent or non-urgent; the former went to a hospital whilst the latter were considered for remote teleconsultation. A nurse at the receiving site obtained a history and vital signs before the patient interacted with a specialist at the delivering site via live two-way videoconference. An electronic stethoscope was available for the specialist to perform a physical examination if required. The authors found that a definitive diagnosis was possible in 94% of cases and that a clinically significant alteration in management was achieved in almost 50%. Furthermore, more than 90% were able to receive care close to home, with the remaining few needing to travel for an in-person consultation. This approach made the lives of both patient and clinician more convenient and improved specialty coverage in remote areas, whilst at the same time maintaining a high quality of patient care.

Teledermatology has become one of the most successful and widely implemented areas of telemedicine in recent years. Schmid-Grendelmeier et al. (2000) report on one of the first teledermatologic connections in Sub-Saharan Africa. A link was formed between the Regional Dermatology Training Centre in Moshi, Tanzania and the University Hospital of Zürich, Switzerland. Both store-and-forward and real time approaches were taken, enabling the exchange of digital images and histopathology slides to facilitate diagnosis in challenging and interesting cases. Not only were the clinicians in Tanzania able to seek expert advice, they were also able to provide assistance to Swiss clinicians for tropical diseases in returning travellers.

Surgical telemonitoring has been used in Ecuador to guide inexperienced surgeons through advanced procedures in remote areas within a mobile theatre (Rosser Jr et al., 1999). The original initiative did not use telemedicine, meaning that surgeons needed to travel long distances across difficult terrain to reach the patients in order to perform preoperative and postoperative evaluation. This obstacle has now been overcome, decreasing costs, saving time, and increasing efficiency. Clinicians at the delivering site are able to effectively guide surgeons at the receiving site through procedures with which they may be inexperienced. Of course, with any application of telesurgery, patient safety and satisfaction are arguably of more importance due to the nature of the intervention, and this aspect must be considered when designing a programme.

This is just a selection of what has happened around the world recently and is designed to stimulate ideas and imagination. There are many initiatives occurring within and between countries, and the area is so vast that one could dedicate a book to this area alone. Throughout it all there is one very important consideration. The emphasis in modern medicine is on the biopsychosocial model of health and disease (Engel, 1977). There are many individual factors at play when considering why a particular illness has occurred in a particular patient. The temptation with telemedicine can be to focus purely on the biological aspects of disease, neglecting the equally important psychological and social factors. Therefore, any initiative should take care to incorporate a more rounded assessment of the patient to ensure that they are provided with the best level of care possible.

12. References

Alwan, A. & MacLean, DR. (2009). A review of non-communicable disease in low- and middle-income countries. *International Health,* Vol. 1, No. 1, (September 2009) 3-9, ISSN 18763413

Bagayoko, C.O., Mueller, H. & Geissbuhler, A. (2006). Assessment of internet-based telemedicine in Africa (the RAFT project). *Computerized Medical Imaging and Graphics,* Vol. 30, No. 6-7, (September-October 2006) 407-16, ISSN 08956111

Bashshur, R.L. & Shannon, G.W. (2009). National telemedicine initiatives: essential to healthcare reform. *Telemedicine and eHealth,* Vol. 15, No. 6, (July-August 2009) 600-10, ISSN 15305627

Beaglehole, R. & Bonita, R. (2008). Global public health: a scorecard. *Lancet,* Vol. 372, No. 9654 (December 2008) 1988-96, ISSN 01406736

Breslauer, D.N., Maamari, R.N., Switz, N.A., Lam, W.A. & Fletcher, D.A. (2009). Mobile phone based clinical microscopy for global health applications. *PLoS ONE,* Vol. 4, No. 7 (July 2009) e6320, ISSN 19326203

Cardoso, R.B., Huettner, E., Hoppe, A., Winter, C., Huettner, E., Celia, S., Duval, V., Fernandes, J., Sparenberg, A.L.F. & Russomano, T. (2007). A successful telemedicine experience in the Brazilian Amazon region. *Acta Informatica Medica,* Vol. 15, No. 4 (December 2007) 211-15, ISSN 03538109

Engel, G.L. (1977). The need for a new medical model: a challenge for biomedicine. *Science,* Vol. 196, No. 4286 (April 1977) 129-36, ISSN 00368075

Fenwick, A., Zhang, Y. & Stoever, K. (2009). Control of the neglected tropical diseases in Sub-Saharan Africa: the unmet needs. *International Health,* Vol. 1, No. 1 (September 2009) 61-70, ISSN 18763413

Fraser, H.S.F. & McGrath, J.D. (2000). Information technology and telemedicine in sub-Saharan Africa. *BMJ,* Vol. 321, No. 7259 (August 2000) 465-66, ISSN 00071447

Glossary of Terms Commonly Used in Health Care. AcademyHealth. 2004 www.academyhealth.org/files/publications/glossary.pdf (accessed on 28 August 2010)

Lucas, H. (2008). Information and communications technology for future health systems in developing countries. *Social Science and Medicine,* Vol. 66, No. 10 (May 2008) 2122-32, ISSN 02779536

Mars, M. (2009). Telemedicine in sub-Saharan Africa, In: *Telehealth in the developing world,* Wootton, R., Patil, N.G., Scott, R.E. & Ho, K., (Ed.), 232-41, The Royal Society of Medicine Press Ltd, ISBN 9781853157844, London

Microgravity Centre/PUCRS-Brazil. www.pucrs.br/feng/microg (accessed on 28 August 2010)

Raza, T., Joshi, M., Schapira, R.M. & Agha, Z. (2009). Pulmonary telemedicine - a model to access the subspecialist services in underserved rural areas. *International Journal of Medical Informatics,* Vol. 78, No. 1 (January 2009) 53-59, ISSN 13865056

Rinde, E. & Balteskard, L. (2002). Is there a future for telemedicine? *Lancet,* Vol. 359, No. 9322 (June 2002) 1957-58, ISSN 01406736

Rosser Jr, J.C., Bell, R.L., Harnett, B., Rodas, E., Murayama, M. & Merrell, R. (1999). Use of mobile low-bandwidth telemedical techniques for extreme telemedicine applications. *Journal of the American College of Surgeons,* Vol. 189, No. 4 (October 1999) 397-404, ISSN 10727515

Russomano, T., Cardoso, R.B., Duval, V., Lopes, M.H.I., Celia, S., Hutter, E. & Hutter, E. (2009). Space technology used to improve health care in remote areas. *Aviation Space And Environmental Medicine,* Vol. 80, No. 1 (January 2009) 61-63, ISSN 00956562

Schmid-Grendelmeier, P., Masenga, E.J., Haeffner, A. & Burg, G. (2000). Teledermatology as a new tool in sub-Saharan Africa: an experience from Tanzania. *Journal of the American Academy of Dermatology,* Vol. 42, No. 5 (May 2000) 833-35, ISSN 01909622

Scott R.E., Chowdhury, M.F.U. & Varghese, S. (2002). TeleHealth policy: looking for global complementarity. *Journal of Telemedicine and Telecare,* Vol. 8, No. 6, Supp. 2 (December 2002) 55-58, ISSN 17581109

Scott, R.E., Jennett, P.A. & Yeo, M. (2004). Access and authorisation in a glocal eHealth policy context. *International Journal of Medical Informatics,* Vol. 73, No. 3 (March 2004) 259-66, ISSN 13865056

Scott, R.E. (2007). Future proofing telehealth in developing countries. *Journal of Telemedicine and Telecare, Vol. 13, No. 8, Supp. 3 (December 2007)* 70-72, ISSN 17581109

Shears, P. (2000). Emerging and reemerging infections in Africa: the need for improved laboratory services and disease surveillance. *Microbes and Infection,* Vol. 2, No. 2 (February 2000) 489-95, ISSN 12864579

Stanberry, B. (2001). Legal ethical and risk issues in telemedicine. *Computer Methods and Programs in Biomedicine,* Vol. 64, No. 3 (March 2001) 225-33, ISSN 01692607

UN General Assembly, (2000). United Nations Millenium Declaration. http://www.un.org/millennium/declaration/ares552e.pdf (accessed 23 August 2010)

World Medical Association. World Medical Association statement on accountability, responsibilities and ethical guidelines in the practice of telemedicine 1999. 2008: http://www.wma.net/e/policy/a7.htm (accessed on 28 August 2010)

World Medical Association. World Medical Association statement on the ethics of telemedicine, October 2007. 2007: http://www.wma.net/e/policy/t3.htm (accessed on 28 August 2010)

World Health Organization (2005). *Preventing chronic diseases: a vital investment,* World Health Organisation, ISBN 9789241563000, Geneva

World Health Organization (2008). *World Health Statistics 2008,* World Health Organisation, ISBN 9789241563598, Geneva

Zimic, M., Coronel, J., Gilman, R.H., Luna, C.G., Curioso, W.H. & Moore, D.A.J. (2009). Can the power of mobile phones be used to improve tuberculosis diagnosis in developing countries? *Transactions of the Royal Society of Tropical Medicine and Hygiene,* Vol. 103, No. 6 (June 2009) 638-40, ISSN 00359203

Zolfo, M., Lynen, L., Dierckx, J. & Colebunders, R. (2006): Remote consultations and HIV/AIDS continuing education in low-resource settings. *International Journal of Medical Informatics* Vol. 75, No. 9 (September 2006) 633-37, ISSN 13865056

24

Social and Semantic Web Technologies for the Text-To-Knowledge Translation Process in Biomedicine

Carlos Cano[1], Alberto Labarga[1], Armando Blanco[1] and Leonid Peshkin[2]

[1]*Dept Computer Science and Artificial Intelligence. University of Granada. c/. Daniel Saucedo Aranda, s/n 18071, Granada,*
[2]*Dept of Systems Biology, Harvard Medical School. 200 Longwood Ave, Boston, MA 02115*
[1]*Spain*
[2]*USA*

1. Introduction

Currently, biomedical research critically depends on knowledge availability for flexible re-analysis and integrative post-processing. The voluminous biological data already stored in databases, put together with the abundant molecular data resulting from the rapid adoption of high-throughput techniques, have shown the potential to generate new biomedical discovery through integration with knowledge from the scientific literature.

Reliable information extraction applications have been a long-sought goal of the biomedical text mining community. Both named entity recognition and conceptual analysis are needed in order to map the objects and concepts represented by natural language texts into a rigorous encoding, with direct links to online resources that explicitly expose those concepts semantics (see Figure 1).

Naturally, automated methods work at a fraction of human accuracy, while expert curation has a small fraction of computer coverage. Hence, mining the wealth of knowledge in the published literature requires a hybrid approach which combines efficient automated methods with highly-accurate expert curation. This work reviews several efforts in both directions and contributes to advance the hybrid approach.

Since Life Sciences have turned into a very data-intensive domain, various sources of biological data must often be combined in order to build new knowledge. The Semantic Web offers a social and technological basis for assembling, integrating and making biomedical knowledge available at Web scale.

In this chapter we present an open-source, modular friendly system called BioNotate-2.0, which combines automated text annotation with distributed expert curation, and serves the resulting knowledge in a Semantic-Web-accessible format to be integrated into a wider bio-medical inference pipeline. While this has been an active area of research and development for a few years, we believe that this is an unique contribution which will be widely adopted to enable the community effort both in the area of further systems development and knowledge sharing.

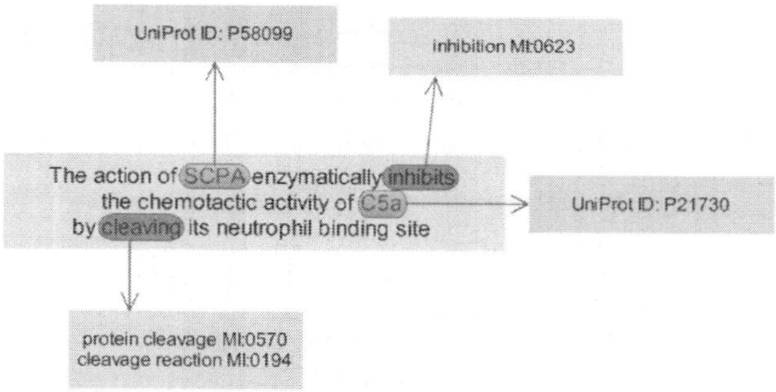

Fig. 1. Some annotations on a piece of biomedical text. Entities of interest and evidences of interaction are marked up in the text and mapped to external resources. In this case, genes and proteins are mapped to UniProt entries, and interaction keywords are linked to terms from the ontology PSI-Molecular Interactions (PSI-MI). Annotated snippets constitute a *corpus*. Large *corpora* are required to train Machine Learning systems.

Particularly, this chapter describes the design and implementation of BioNotate-2.0 for: 1) the creation and automatic annotation of biomedical corpora; 2) the distributed manual curation, annotation and normalization of extracts of text with biological facts of interest; 3) the publication of curated facts in semantically enriched formats, and their connection to other datasets and resources on the Semantic Web; 4) the access to curated facts with a Linked Data Browser.

Our aim is to provide the community with a modular and open-source annotation platform to harness the great collaborative power of the biomedical community over the Internet and allow the dissemination and sharing of semantically-enriched biomedical facts of interest. Specifically, we illustrate several cases of use of BioNotate 2.0 for the annotation of biomedical facts involving the identification of genes, protein-protein, and gene-disease relationships. By design, the provided tools are flexible and can implement a wide variety of annotation schemas.

1.1 Information extraction systems in biology

Efficient access to information contained in on-line scientific literature collections is essential for life science research, playing a crucial role from the initial stage of experiment planning to the final interpretation and communication of the results. The biological literature also constitutes the main information source for manual curation of biological databases and the development of ontologies (Krallinger, Valencia & Hirschman, 2008). However, biological databases alone cannot capture the richness of scientific information and argumentation contained in the literature (Krallinger, Valencia & Hirschman, 2008; Baumgartner Jr et al., 2007).

The biomedical literature can be seen as a large integrated, but unstructured data repository. It contains high quality and high-confidence information on genes that have been studied for decades, including the gene's relevance to a disease, its reaction mechanisms, structural information and well characterized interactions. However, an accurate and normalized representation of facts and the mapping of the information contained within papers onto existing databases, ontologies and online resources has traditionally been almost negligible.

Extracting facts from literature and making them accessible is approached from two directions: first, manual curation efforts develop ontologies and vocabularies to annotate gene products based on statements in papers; second, text mining aims to automatically identify entities and concepts in text using those controlled vocabularies and ontologies and employing information retrieval and natural language processing techniques (Winnenburg et al., 2008).

The best known community-wide effort for the evaluation of text-mining and information extraction systems in the biological domain is the BioCreative (Critical Assessment of Information Extraction systems in Biology) challenge (Krallinger, Morgan, Smith, Leitner, Tanabe, Wilbur, Hirschman & Valencia, 2008). The goal of BioCreative has been to present algorithmic challenges that would result in scalable systems targeted for the general community of biology researchers as well as for the more specialized end-users, such as annotation database curators. One special case is the Gene Mention recognition, which evaluates systems that find mentions of genes and proteins in sentences from PubMed abstracts. Another case is the Gene Normalization, focused on providing direct links between texts and actual gene and protein-focused records in biological databases. In contrast to these indexing challenges, the Interaction Article Subtask (IAS) addressed the first step in many biological literature review tasks, namely the retrieval/classification and ranking of relevant articles according to a given topic of interest. Particularly, in the second edition of the challenge, the goal was to classify a collection of PubMed titles and abstracts based on their relevance for the derivation of protein-protein interaction annotations. As a direct result of these competitive evaluations, a platform which integrates the participant's servers for detecting named entities and relationships has been released (Leitner et al., 2008). This platform, called BioCreative Meta-Server (`http://bcms.bioinfo.cnio.es/`), allows to simultaneously annotate a piece of biomedical text using different NLP tools and systems and visualize and compare their results. U-compare (`http://u-compare.org/`) is a similar platform which allows the user to design a customized text-mining annotation pipeline using different available tools and corpora (Kano et al., 2009).

Recently, the efforts have shifted from the localization and annotation of the character strings towards the identification of concepts (Hunter et al., 2008). Concepts differ from character strings in that they are grounded in well defined knowledge resources. Thus, concept recognition provides an unambiguous semantic representation of what the text denotes. A related initiative is the Collaborative Annotation of a Large Biomedical Corpus (CALBC, `http://www.calbc.eu`). CALBC is an European support action addressing the automatic generation of a very large, community-wide shared text corpus annotated with biomedical entities. Their aim is to create a broadly scoped and diversely annotated corpus (150,000 Medline immunology-related abstracts annotated with approximately a dozen semantic types) by automatically integrating the annotations from different named entity recognition systems. The CALBC challenge involves both Name Entity Recognition and Concept recognition tasks.

In theory, text mining is the perfect solution to transforming factual knowledge from publications into database entries. However, the field of computational linguistics have not yet developed tools that can accurately parse and analyse more than 30% of English sentences in order to transform them into a structured formal representation (Rebholz-Schuhmann et al., 2005).

On the other hand, manually curated data is precise, because a curator, trained to consult the literature and databases, is able to select only high-quality data, and reformat the facts according to the schema of the database. In addition, curators select quotes from the text as evidence supporting the identified fact, and those citations are also added to the database. Curators know how to define standards for data consistency, in particular, the most relevant terminology, which has led to the design of standardized ontologies and controlled vocabularies. The issue with curation of data is that it is time consuming and costly, and therefore has to focus on the most relevant facts. This undermines the completeness of the curated data, and curation teams are destined to stay behind the latest publications. Therefore, an environment where manual curation and text mining can effectively and efficiently work together is highly desirable (Rebholz-Schuhmann et al., 2005).

1.2 Social annotation and tagging in life sciences

Web resources such as Delicious (`http://delicious.com`), or Connotea (`http://connotea.org`) facilitate the tagging of online resources and bibliographic references. These online tools harness the collective knowledge that is modeled by the collective tagging. Collaboration is thus based on similarities in tags and tagged objects. The more annotations the system gets, the better the chances are for users to interact with researchers who share similar interests, such as elucidating the same pathway, methodology or gene function.

General-purpose annotation tools, such as Knowtator *Knowtator* (n.d.), WordFreak *WordFreak* (n.d.), SAFE-GATE (Cunningham et al., 2002) and iAnnotate *iAnnotate* (n.d.), can be adapted to the annotation of biomedical entities and relationships in scientific texts. Some BioNLP groups have also created customized annotation tools implementing their specific annotation schemas, such as the Xconc Suite's implementation for annotating events in the GENIA corpus (Kim et al., 2008). While these tools allow a restricted group of well-trained annotators to curate corpora, they are not intended for massive annotation efforts by the broad research community.

In contrast, our work is largely inspired by the recent distributed and collaborative annotation efforts that have emerged, such as those in the image analysis domain (*Google Image Labeler*, n.d.; Russell et al., 2008) or related to the Amazon Mechanical Turk (AMT) annotation web services (*Amazon's Mechanical Turk*, n.d.; Callison-Burch, 2009). These efforts have shown a great potential since they allow any interested user world-wide to contribute in the annotation task.

In a recent work, Snow *et al.* (Snow et al., 2008) show the effectiveness of collaborative non-expert annotation on some traditional NLP problems such as emotion recognition from text, word synonymy, hypothesis inference, chronological ordering of facts and ambiguity resolution. Particularly, this work demonstrates that the accuracy achieved by a Machine Learning system trained with annotations by a few non-expert curators equals the accuracy achieved by the same system trained with annotations made by experts. For example, for the emotion recognition from text task, 4 non-expert annotations (in average) per item are enough to emulate the results of one expert annotation, with significantly reduced costs (Snow et al., 2008). After this pioneer work, others have proposed and evaluated the effectiveness of using AMT for massive collaborative annotation of corpora to train machine learning systems (Raykar et al., 2009; Donmez et al., 2009; Callison-Burch, 2009; Carlson et al., 2010).

Within the biomedical field, the notion of community annotation has also recently started to be adopted. For instance, WikiProteins (Mons et al., 2008) or WikiGene (Maier et al., 2005) deliver appropriate environments in which it is possible to address the annotation of genes and proteins. Since 2007, GoPubMed also includes a collaborative curation tool for the annotation of concepts and Pubmed authors profiles. While these efforts allow the wider research community to directly benefit from the generation and peer-review of knowledge at minimal cost, they are not intended for the creation of corpora for training NLP tools. Such capabilities allow a feedback from the curation effort back to the automated processing in order to improve its accuracy, in turn enabling human curation to focus on more sophisticated instances.

Baral et al. (Baral et al., 2007), proposed a methodology where the community collaboratively contributes to the curation process. They used automatic information extraction methods as a starting point, and promote mass collaboration with the premise that if there are a lot of articles, then there must be a lot of readers and authors of these articles. Our approach is similar to that implemented by their system called CBioC. This system allows the user to annotate relationships between biomedical concepts while browsing PubMed records. The user is presented with potential relationships from the current record extracted by automated tools or suggested by other users. Registered users can add new relationships and vote for suggested relationships. For a given PubMed record, a relationship is defined by providing the literals of the two interacting entities and the keywords of the interaction. However, CBioC does not allow to highlight the exact mentions of these words in the text. Furthermore, the users can only access to the annotated facts from within CBioC. The whole corpus of annotations is not directly available until it is distributed by the CBioC team.

Within the publishing industry, there has also been a series of efforts in promoting community interaction by Social Networks. BioMedExperts (BME, `http://www.biomedexperts.com`) is a professional network in which literature references are used to support interaction. Although this system does not support tagging by users, it does support automatic tagging based on a reference terminology; thus allowing the identification of researchers with similar interests. Nature Network (`http://network.nature.com/`) works in a similar way; however it does not facilitate any controlled vocabulary for annotating the literature references.

1.3 The emerging role of the semantic web technologies in life sciences

Current research in biology heavily depends on the availability and efficient use of information. Life sciences have turned into a very data-intensive domain and, in order to build new knowledge, various sources of biological data must often be combined. Therefore, scientists in this domain are facing the same challenges as in many other disciplines dealing with highly distributed, heterogeneous and voluminous data sources.

The Semantic Web offers a social and technological basis for assembling, integrating and making biomedical knowledge available at Web scale. Its emphasis is on combining information using standard representation languages and allowing access to that information via standard web protocols and technologies to leverage computation such as in the form of inference and distributable query.

As the Semantic Web is being introduced into the Life Sciences, the basis for a distributed knowledge-base that can foster biological data analysis is laid. Biomedical ontologies provide essential domain knowledge to drive data integration, information retrieval, data annotation, natural-language processing and decision support, and so, new ontologies are being developed to formalize knowledge (Shah et al., 2009). Such major bioinformatics centers as the European Bioinformatics Institute or the National Center for Biotechnology Information provide access to over two hundred biological resources. Links between different databases are an important basis for data integration, but the lack of a common standard to represent and link information makes data integration an expensive business.

Recently, such key databases as Uniprot (Bairoch et al., 2005) began providing data access in RDF format. Resource Description Framework (`http://www.w3.org/RDF/`) is a core technology for the World Wide Web Consortium's Semantic Web activities (`http://www.w3.org/2001/sw/`) and is therefore well suited to work in a distributed and decentralized environment. The RDF data model represents arbitrary information as a set of simple statements of the form subject-predicate-object. To enable the linking of data on the Web, RDF requires that each resource must have a (globally) unique identifier. These identifiers allow everybody to make statements about a given resource and, together with the simple structure of the RDF data model, make it easy to combine the statements made by different people (or databases) to allow queries across different datasets. RDF is thus an industry standard that can make a major contribution to solve two important problems of bioinformatics: distributed annotation and data integration.

The Bio2RDF project has successfully applied these semantic web technologies to publicly available databases by creating a knowledge space of RDF documents linked together with normalized URIs and sharing a common ontology (Belleau et al., 2008). The benefits promised by the Semantic Web include aggregation of heterogeneous data using explicit semantics, simplified annotation and sharing of findings, the expression of rich and well-defined models for data aggregation and search, easier reuse of data in unanticipated ways, and the application of logic to infer additional insights. The Linking Open Drug Data (LODD) (Jentzsch et al., n.d.) task within the W3C's Semantic Web for Health Care and Life Sciences Interest Group is another related initiative that gathered a list of data sets that include information about drugs, and then determined how the publicly available data sets could be linked together. The project has recently won the first prize of the Linking Open Data Triplification Challenge, showing the importance of Linked Data to the health care and life sciences.

In addition, the concept of nanopublication (Mons & Velterop, 2009) has recently emerged to contribute to model and share Life Sciences discoveries using Semantic Web technologies. A nanopublication is defined as a core scientific statement (e.g. "malaria is transmitted by mosquitos") with associated annotations (i.e. evidence supporting this biological fact, references to the authors of this assertion, etc.) which can be represented as a Named Graph /RDF model. Such representation makes for efficient vehicle of knowledge dissemination and large-scale aggregation, due to its machine-readable characteristics.

2. Proposed approach

In this work we present an integrated approach to concept recognition in biomedical texts, which builds upon both the Semantic Web, which values the integration of well-structured data, and the Social Web, which aims to facilitate interaction amongst users by means of user-generated content. Our approach combines automated named entity recognition tools with manual collaborative curation and normalization of the entities and their relations for a more effective identification of biological facts of interest. Identified facts are converted to a standardized representation for making connections to other datasets and resources on the Semantic Web.

The system is composed of five basic modules which cover the different stages of the annotation pipeline: administration, search, automatic annotation, manual curation and publication. Figure 2 shows how these modules are interconnected.

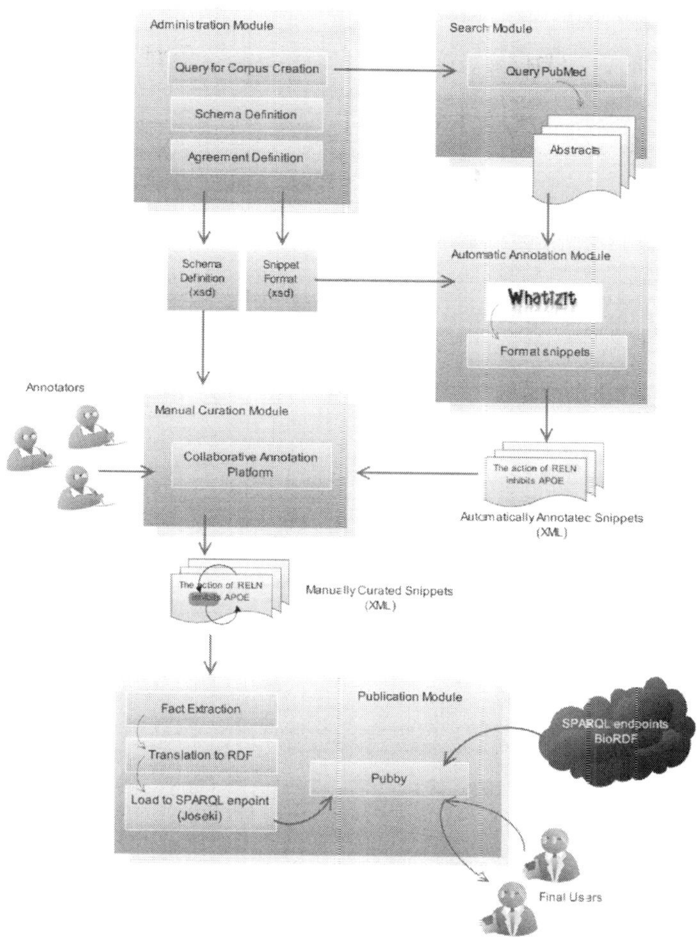

Fig. 2. System architecture of BioNotate-2.0 represents distinct modules and their interconnections.

2.1 Administration module

The administration module allows users to generate the problem definition, the annotation schema and the format for the snippets that will be employed in the annotation and curation tasks. It consists of an intuitive user interface in which administrators can define entities and relationships of interest for the annotation task and provide a function for determining whether two annotations made by different users significantly agree. As part of the problem definition, administrators can also provide the references to the bio-ontologies or terminological resources which will be used to normalize the entities of interest in the annotation task. Finally, they are also allowed to upload their own corpus or create it by providing query terms and making use of the automatic retrieval module.

2.2 Automatic retrieval and annotation module

To generate the base collection, users can start by sending a query to the system. This query is forwarded to Pubmed or Citexplore. Returned abstracts (and full texts, if available) are presented to the user, who can refine the query, remove non relevant articles and save the query for later updates.
This module also includes resources for carrying out an initial automatic annotation of the retrieved publications using Named Entity Recognition (NER) and automatic text-mining systems. This first annotation eases latter manual curation efforts by providing fast and moderately accurate results, and enables textual semantic markup to be undertaken efficiently over big collections. Our system uses Whatizit web services (Mcwilliam et al., 2009; Rebholz-Schuhmann et al., 2008) to annotate entities of interest and their relationships as defined by the administrator. Whatizit is a Java-powered NER system that searches for terms in the text that match those included in vast terminological resources, allowing morphological variations (Kirsch et al., 2006). Whatizit also considers syntactic features and POS tags obtained by TreeTagger (Schmid, 1994). Whatizit implements different modules depending on the NEs or relations to be identified. Our system includes the following:

- whatizitSwissprot: focuses on the identification and normalization of names of genes and proteins.
- whatizitChemical: focuses on the identification of chemical compounds based on the ChEBI terminology (Degtyarenko et al., 2008) and the OSCAR3 NER system (Corbett & Murray-Rust, 2006).
- whatizitDisease: focuses on the extraction of names of diseases based on MEDLINE terminology.
- whatizitDrugs: identifies drugs using DrugBank terminology (`http://redpoll.pharmacy.ualberta.ca/drugbank/`).
- whatizitGO: identifies GO terms.
- whatizitOrganism: identifies species and organisms based on NCBI taxonomy.
- whatizitProteinInteraction: identifies protein-protein (gene-gene) interactions using Protein Corral (`http://www.ebi.ac.uk/Rebholz-srv/pcorral`).
- whatizitSwissprotGo: detects protein-GO term relationships using UniProtKb/Swiss-Prot terminological resources.

For a complete list of available Whatizit modules, refer to `http://www.ebi.ac.uk/webservices/whatizit/info.jsf`.

2.3 Collaborative annotation tool

The central idea of our approach is to leverage annotations contributed by the users and utilize it as feedback to improve automatic classification. Annotation is generally a simple task for the user and may amount to a "yes/no" vote on whether the current annotation is correct when examining an individual entry. More sophisticated schemas may require specialized domain expertise on the problem addressed. The collaborative manual annotation tool is

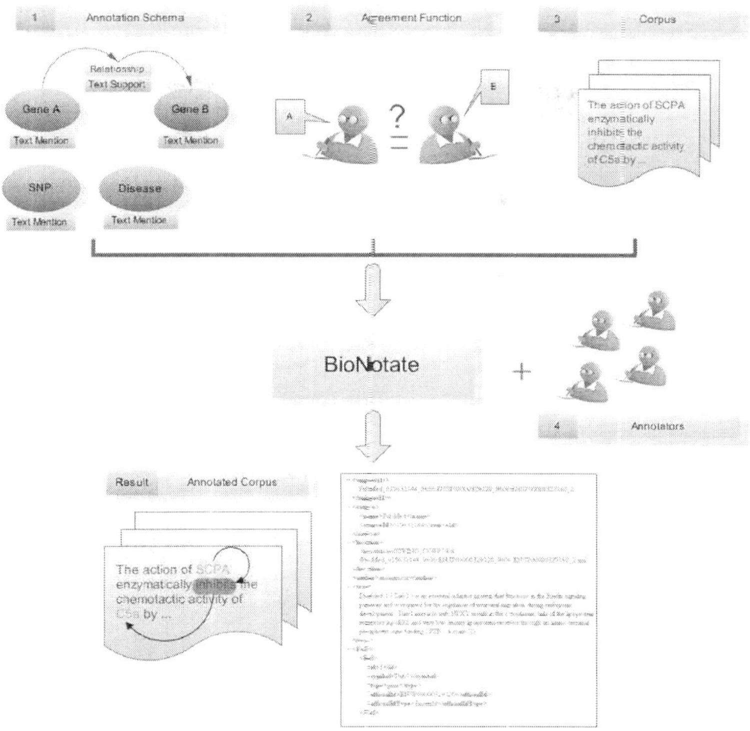

Fig. 3. Information workflow *in* and *out* of the collaborative annotation module. The annotation schema, function for agreement among annotators, and un-annotated corpora are provided as input. The collaborative annotation tool supports a distributed annotation effort with contributions from different users. Consensus annotations are provided as output.

based on BioNotate (Cano et al., 2009)– an open source platform for supporting distributed collaborative annotation efforts via a simple interface over a standard Internet browser-based client/server system.

2.3.1 Architecture of the annotation tool

Although BioNotate was originally designed for annotating gene-gene and gene-disease relationships, current releases of the tool allow users to define arbitrary annotation schemas. Figure 3 shows the information workflow *in* and *out* of the collaborative annotation module. The annotation schema, agreement function and corpora are provided by the administrator. BioNotate supports a distributed annotation effort with contributions from different users. Consensus annotations following the proposed schema are provided as output.

2.3.2 Technical features of the annotation tool

Here we provide some technical features of the annotation tool:

- Support for parallel and simultaneous annotations by different users.
- Annotator management. The system tracks all the annotations being made by every user.
- Distribution of annotating tasks among annotators. The system implements a k-blind annotation process. When an annotator logs in the system and requests a snippet to annotate, he is assigned a new one from the pool of documents pending annotation. The assigned document is picked at random from the documents not previously annotated by this user. Each snippet is annotated by at least k different annotators. If the k annotations of a snippet do not meet a minimum degree of agreement, the snippet is presented to another annotator at random. The process continues until at least k annotations performed on the snippet meet a minimum degree of agreement (See Figure 4).
- Access to the annotation system is available from any computer with Internet access and a modern web browser. Annotators do not need to install any extra software. Our browser-based system allows the annotators to log in the system from any machine and add new annotations at any time. On the client side, the application consists of an intuitive user interface where snippets are displayed and the user can perform annotations on the snippets by highlighting arbitrary chunks of text and assigning any of the available labels. On the server side, several Perl scripts serve on request snippets not yet annotated by the user, save the annotations and check the agreement with previous users (see Figure 5).
- Custom annotation schema. The tool is able to deploy arbitrary annotation schemas provided by the administrator in Extensible Markup Language (XML) format. The current version of BioNotate supports the definition of *entities* and *questions* in the annotation schema. *Entities* refer to the different types of named entities of interest and the relationships between them (i.e., each label available in the annotation interface is defined by an *entity* in the annotation schema). *Questions* define the questions to be asked to the annotator for each snippet (if any), with the set of available answers. The schema definition is rendered into the annotation interface by Extensible Stylesheet Transformations (XSLT).

2.3.3 Annotation schema and function for agreement between annotators

For the demo installation of BioNotate-2.0, we have customized the annotation schema for annotating protein-protein (gene-gene) interactions. Furthermore, we require that the interactors are normalized against Uniprot and the interaction keywords are associated to selected terms from the ontology PSI-Molecular Interactions (PSI-MI) (see Figure 6).

Description of the annotation process

The annotator will be shown a snippet and a pair of proteins (genes) of interest. All the mentions of these two proteins of interest detected by automated annotation tools will be highlighted in the text of the snippet in advance. For each snippet the annotator is asked to:

1. Indicate (Yes/No) whether the text implies that there is an interaction between the provided proteins.
2. Highlight the minimal and most important phrase in the text (if any) that supports his answer. This text is labeled as "interaction".
3. Locate and highlight the one mention of each of the entities of interest which is essential to the relation of interest. These are the mentions which, if altered, would result in a phrase which no longer conveyed the same relation. For example, in the snippet: "Protein A is

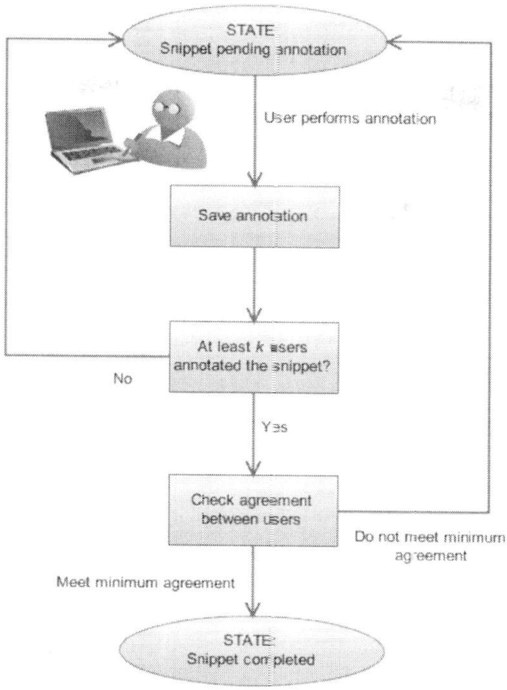

Fig. 4. State diagram representing the annotation of a snippet from state *pending annotation* to state *annotation completed*. The annotation of one snippet is completed when it has been annotated by at least k different users and their annotations meet a minimum agreement. Once the annotation of a snippet is completed, the snippet is not served again for annotation.

found in tissue T. Protein A interacts with protein B", only the second mention of "Protein A" should be highlighted.

4. Provide a PSI-MI term for the keywords highlighted in 2. and Uniprot identifiers for the two proteins highlighted in 3. Only one mention of every gene/disease of interest should be highlighted in each snippet. The annotator should check whether the highlighted regions comply with these guidelines, and correct annotations that do not.

The resulting sets of available tags for the annotation are the following:

- PROTEIN: for protein and gene mentions (e.g. RELN, GRM8, WNT2);
- INTERACTION: minimal, most relevant phrase that supports the Yes/No decision (e.g. "binds to", "inhibits", "phosphorylates").

Detailed annotation guidelines together with annotation examples are provided at the project site. However, disagreement among experts and nomenclature specific to different scientific fields make it non-trivial to create annotation guidelines. k given annotations are said to meet the minimum agreement if they satisfy the following three conditions:

- The Yes/No answer is the same.
- The token sequences highlighted with labels PROTEIN completely overlap and their provided Uniprot identifiers are the same.
- The token sequences highlighted with label INTERACTION overlap (up to 1 different token with respect to the shortest highlighting is allowed between every pair of the k annotations) and their provided PSI-MI ontology matching terms are the same.

Similar agreement requirements have been previously proven to provide good quality results with acceptable agreement rates (Cano et al., 2009). Community voting is another paradigm that we are planning to include in the future.

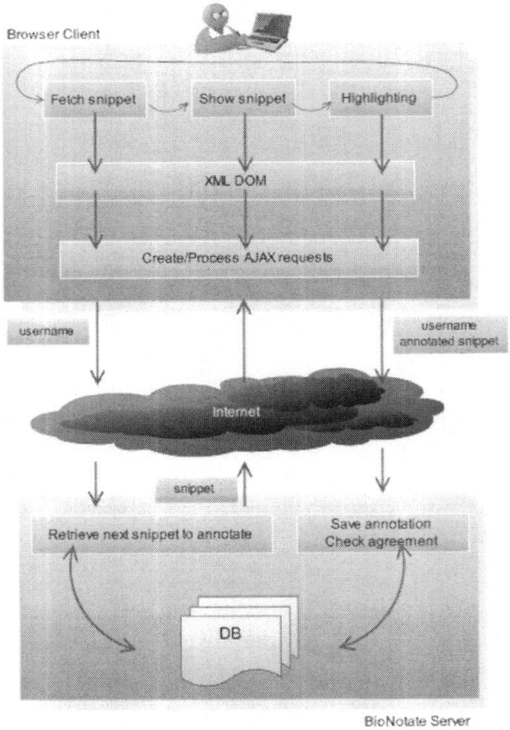

Fig. 5. Components and communications in the annotation tool. The client side iterates in the loop: Fetch the next snippet for the current annotator, present it to the user, allow him to add the annotations and save them. The process continues until the annotator closes the browser window. Each of these modules in the client side communicates with the server side. On the server side, one CGI Perl script serves snippets to the client browsers and another script attends requests for saving annotations.

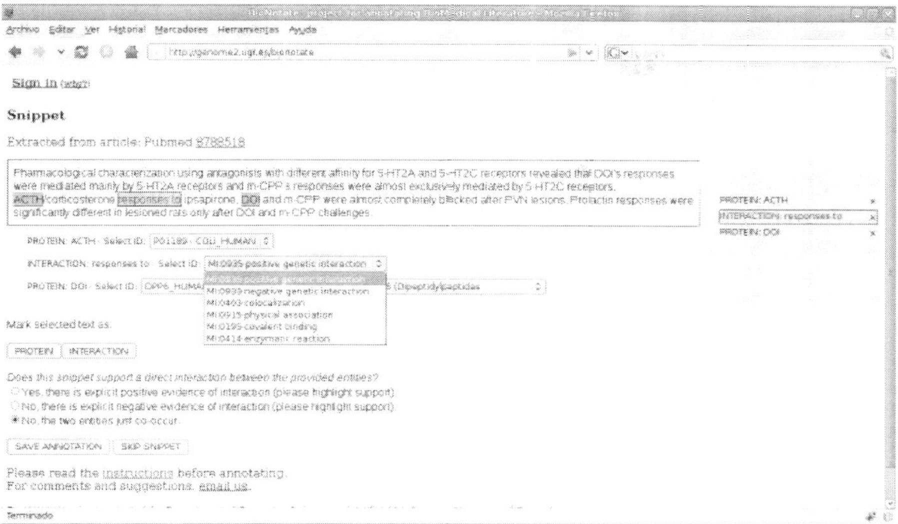

Fig. 6. Demo installation of BioNotate's annotation interface showing two proteins and an interaction keyword in a snippet. Entities may be normalized using bio-ontologies and other terminological resources. In the Figure, proteins are normalized against Uniprot, and interaction keywords are normalized against the ontology PSI-Molecular Interactions (PSI-MI).

2.4 Publication module

The overall goal of the Bionotate framework is to improve the quality and accessibility of life science research data on the Web by bringing together automatic annotation and manual curation. From the perspective of the life scientist, discovery is the final objective for the generation and use of the information generated by the system.

The dawn of the Semantic Web Era has brought a first wave of reduction of ambiguity in the Web structure, as terms and other tokens are increasingly mapped to shared identifiers for the concepts they denote. Linked Data is a style of publishing data on the Semantic Web that makes it easy to interlink, discover and consume data on the semantic web by making the connections between the datasets explicit in the form of data links. This connection should be done at the concept level rather than at the term level.

The connection at the concept level can be accomplished using RDF as a standardized data representation format, HTTP as a standardized access mechanism, and through the development of algorithms for discovering the links between data sets. Such explicit links allow scientists to navigate between data sets and discover connections they might not have been aware of previously. The standardized representation and access mechanisms allow generic tools, such as Semantic Web browsers and search engines, to be employed to access and process the data (Jentzsch et al., 2009).

But beyond the term to concept we need to go further, from concepts to statements and then to annotate these statements with context and provenance, treating richly annotated statements as nanopublications (Mons & Velterop, 2009).

In the context of Bionotate, we have made the resulting knowledge extracted after the

annotation process available as open linked data connected to the existing resources on the web like Bio2RDF or LODD. Particularly, the system allows to export the gathered information as RDF (actually using Notation3 language) or to publish it as a SPARQL endpoint. SPARQL is a query language able to retrieve and manipulate data stored in RDF.
The publication module allows to publish the RDF data to any available RDF server, such as Sesame or Joseki. The reference implementation uses Joseki (`http://www.joseki.org`), an HTTP engine that supports the SPARQL Protocol and the SPARQL RDF Query language. It is part of Jena, a Java framework for building Semantic Web applications developed at HP labs. In order to expose the data as Linked data, we use Pubby `http://www4.wiwiss.fu-berlin.de/pubby/`), a system developed by the Free University of Berlin that makes it easy to turn a SPARQL endpoint into a Linked Data server.

3. Discussion and conclusions

We have developed a framework where users can manage biological literature and related information, share their knowledge with their peers and discover hidden associations within the shared knowledge. Basically, it provides web based tools for: 1) the creation and automatic annotation of biomedical corpora 2) the distributed manual curation, annotation and normalization of extracts of text with biological facts of interest 3) the publication of curated facts in semantically enriched formats 4) the access to curated facts with a Linked Data Browser.
Our implementation is based on several open-source projects and allows disparate research groups to perform literature annotation to suit their individual research needs, while at the same time contributing to a large-scale annotation effort. There are multiple levels of integration built into the system. At one level, several annotators could collaborate on processing statements from a single corpus on their own server. At another level, multiple corpora could be created on different servers, and the resulting corpora could be integrated into a single overarching resource.
The system we propose uses BioNotate-1.0 as the collaborative annotation platform (Cano et al., 2009). BioNotate-1.0 was shown to be effective for the annotation of a small corpus on interacting genes related to autism, with averaged inter-annotator agreement rates over 75% (Cano et al., 2009). In this case, the annotation task involved providing spans of text for the interacting entities and the interaction keywords. Previous annotation efforts on gene identification and normalization reported agreement rates ranging from 91% to as low as 69% for certain contexts (Colosimo et al., 2005). BioNotate's agreement rates are thus similar to other annotation tasks, showing that the approach we propose is effective for collaborative annotation.
Our aim is to provide the community with a modular and open-source annotation platform to harness the great collaborative power of biomedical community over the Internet and create a substantially sized semantically-enriched corpus of biomedical facts of interest. Specifically, we focus on the annotation of genes and gene-disease and protein-protein relationships. However, the provided tools are flexible and can implement a variety of annotation schemas. Such versatility has already led to a wide interest in diverse user communities. One visible success story for BioNotate is the integration with the Autism Consortium research efforts (see Figure 7 or `http://bionotate.hms.harvard.edu/autism`). In that application, BioNotate is integrated with a Java-based tool kit for text processing using computational linguistics called LingPipe (Carpenter & Baldwin, 2008). Particularly, the gene-spotter class of LingPipe is used for pre-processing of autism-related abstracts. This exemplifies the flexibility

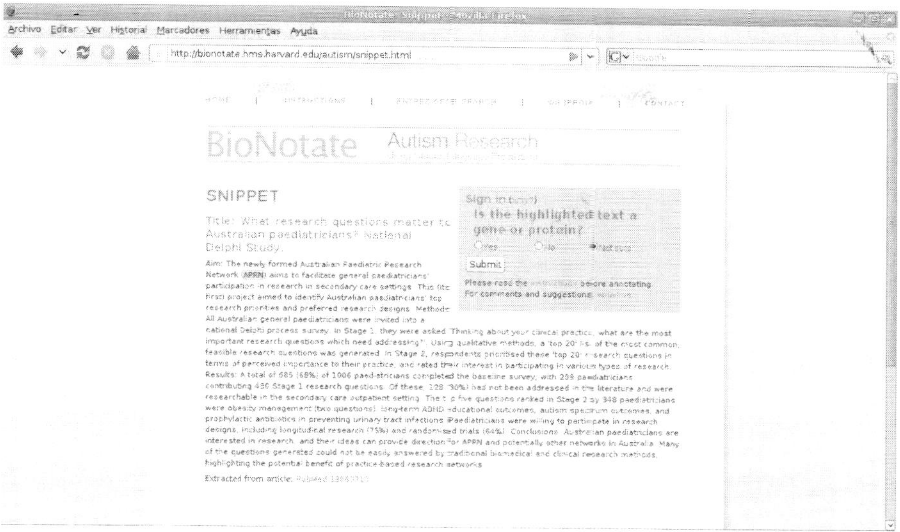

Fig. 7. Annotation interface for AutismNotate, a project for identifying autism-related genes based on BioNotate platform. `http://bionotate.hms.harvard.edu/autism`.

and modular structure of BioNotate-2.0.

In this chapter we have presented BioNotate-2.0, an open-source system which takes advantage of both manual and automated curation methods to generate reliable biological facts on protein relationships that are highly interconnected with other databases and resources. There are many directions in which this resource can be developed in both automated and manual aspect. We plan to add new Named Entity Recognition tools and incorporate new types of entities and relationships in the annotation process: diseases, drugs and SNPs. This platform is available to the community to download and integrate into diverse computational environments. In many cases, anyone with a web browser can contribute to the curation effort within a few minutes of studying the instructions.

BioNotate-2.0 extends our previous system, BioNotate-1.0, by providing several new modules for populating and automatically annotating a corpus before the current manual curation process is carried out. By assisting curators with automated annotations we expect their work to be considerably reduced in terms of time and complexity, since they have to correct previous annotations rather than create them from scratch. BioNotate-2.0 also includes a new publication module which allows curated facts to be published and shared with the community in RDF format, and conveniently accessed and browsed with the provided Linked Data front-end. All in all, we hope that the flexibility and functionality of BioNotate-2.0 will be well received by the community of bio-informatics developers and adopted for a multitude of versatile applications.

3.1 Availability

BioNotate-2.0 is available at `http://genome2.ugr.es/bionotate2/`. BioNotate-1.0 is available at `http://bionotate.sourceforge.net/`. The demo installation of BioNotate on protein-protein interactions is available at `http://genome2.ugr.es/bionotate/`.

The installation of BioNotate for assisting the Autism Consortium research efforts is available at `http://bionotate.hms.harvard.edu/autism/`.

4. Acknowledgements

C. Cano and A. Blanco are supported by the projects P08-TIC-4299 of J. A., Sevilla and TIN2009-13489 of DGICT, Madrid

5. References

Amazon's Mechanical Turk (n.d.). http://aws.amazon.com/.

Bairoch, A., Apweiler, R., Wu, C., Barker, W., Boeckmann, B., Ferro, S., Gasteiger, E., Huang, H., Lopez, R., Magrane, M. et al. (2005). The universal protein resource (UniProt), *Nucleic Acids Research* 33(Database Issue): D154.

Baral, C., Gonzalez, G., Gitter, A., Teegarden, C. & Zeigler, A. (2007). CBioC: beyond a prototype for collaborative annotation of molecular interactions from the literature, *Computational Systems Bioinformatics: CSB2007 Conference Proceedings, Volume 6: University of California, San Diego, USA, 13-17 August 2007*, Imperial College Pr, p. 381.

Baumgartner Jr, W., Cohen, K., Fox, L., Acquaah-Mensah, G. & Hunter, L. (2007). Manual curation is not sufficient for annotation of genomic databases, *Bioinformatics* 23(13): i41.

Belleau, F., Nolin, M., Tourigny, N., Rigault, P. & Morissette, J. (2008). Bio2RDF: Towards a mashup to build bioinformatics knowledge systems, *Journal of biomedical informatics* 41(5): 706–716.

Callison-Burch, C. (2009). Fast, Cheap, and Creative: Evaluating Translation Quality Using Amazon's Mechanical Turk, *Proceedings of EMNLP 2009* .

Cano, C., Monaghan, T., Blanco, A., Wall, D. & Peshkin, L. (2009). Collaborative text-annotation resource for disease-centered relation extraction from biomedical text, *Journal of Biomedical Informatics* 42(5): 967–977.

Carlson, A., Betteridge, J., Wang, R., Hruschka Jr, E. & Mitchell, T. (2010). Coupled Semi-Supervised Learning for Information Extraction, *Proceedings of the Third ACM International Conference on Web Search and Data Mining (WSDM)*, p. 110.

Carpenter, B. & Baldwin, B. (2008). Lingpipe. http://alias-i.com/lingpipe/.

Colosimo, M., Morgan, A., Yeh, A., Colombe, J. & Hirschman, L. (2005). Data preparation and interannotator agreement: BioCreAtIvE task 1B, *BMC bioinformatics* 6(Suppl 1): S12.

Corbett, P. & Murray-Rust, P. (2006). High-throughput identification of chemistry in life science texts, *Lecture Notes in Computer Science* 4216: 107.

Cunningham, D., Maynard, D., Bontcheva, D. & Tablan, M. (2002). GATE: A framework and graphical development environment for robust NLP tools and applications, *Proceedings of the 40th Anniversary Meeting of the Association for Computational Linguistics*. www.gate.ack.uk .

Degtyarenko, K., de Matos, P., Ennis, M., Hastings, J., Zbinden, M., McNaught, A., Alcantara, R., Darsow, M., Guedj, M. & Ashburner, M. (2008). ChEBI: a database and ontology for chemical entities of biological interest, *Nucleic acids research* 36(Database issue): D344.

Donmez, P., Carbonell, J. & Schneider, J. (2009). Efficiently learning the accuracy of labeling sources for selective sampling, *Proceedings of the 15th ACM SIGKDD international conference on Knowledge discovery and data mining*, ACM New York, NY, USA, pp. 259–268.

Google Image Labeler (n.d.). http://imagesgoogle.com/imagelabeler/.

Hunter, L., Lu, Z., Firby, J., Baumgartner, W., Johnson, H., Ogren, P. & Cohen, K. (2008). OpenDMAP: An open source, ontology-driven concept analysis engine, with applications to capturing knowledge regarding protein transport, protein interactions and cell-type-specific gene expression, *BMC bioinformatics* 9(1): 78.

iAnnotate (n.d.)Protege Plug-in. Available at: http://www.dbmi.columbia.edu/ cop7001/iAnnotateTab/iannotate.htm.

Jentzsch, A., Hassanzadeh, O., Bizer, C., Andersson, B. & Stephens, S. (2009). Enabling Tailored Therapeutics with Linked Data, *Proceedings of the 2nd Workshop about Linked Data on the Web.*

Jentzsch, A., Zhao, J., Hassanzadeh, O., Cheung, K., Samwald, M. & Andersson, B. (n.d.). Linking Open Drug Data.
http://triplify.org/files/challenge_2009/LODD.pdf

Kano, Y., Baumgartner, W., McCrohon, L., Ananiadou, S., Cohen, K., Hunter, L. & Tsujii, J. (2009). U-Compare: share and compare text mining tools with UIMA, *Bioinformatics* 25(15): 1997.

Kim, J., Ohta, T., Tsujii, J. et al. (2008). Corpus annotation for mining biomedical events from literature, *BMC bioinformatics* 9(1): 10. http://www-tsujii.is.s.u-tokyo.ac.jp/GENIA/home/wiki.cgi.

Kirsch, H., Gaudan, S. & Rebholz-Schuhmann, D. (2006). Distributed modules for text annotation and IE applied to the biomedical domain, *International journal of medical informatics* 75(6): 496–500.

Knowtator (n.d.). http://knowtator.sourceforge.net.

Krallinger, M., Morgan, A., Smith, L., Leitner, F., Tanabe, L., Wilbur, J., Hirschman, L. & Valencia, A. (2008). Evaluation of text-mining systems for biology: overview of the Second BioCreative community challenge, *Genome biology* 9(Suppl 2): S1.

Krallinger, M., Valencia, A. & Hirschman, L. (2008). Linking genes to literature: text mining, information extraction, and retrieval applications for biology, *Genome biology* 9(Suppl 2): S8.

Leitner, F., Krallinger, M., Rodriguez-Penagos, C., Hakenberg, J., Plake, C., Kuo, C., Hsu, C., Tsai, R., Hung, H., Lau, W. et al. (2008). Introducing meta-services for biomedical information extraction, *Genome Biology* 9(Suppl 2): S6.

Maier, H., Dohr, S., Grote, K., O'Keeffe, S., Werner, T., de Angelis, M. & Schneider, R. (2005). LitMiner and WikiGene: identifying problem-related key players of gene regulation using publication abstracts, *Nucleic acids research* 33(Web Server Issue): W779.

Mcwilliam, H., Valentin, F., Goujon, M., Li, W., Narayanasamy, M., Martin, J., Miyar, T. & Lopez, R. (2009). Web services at the European Bioinformatics Institute-2009, *Nucleic Acids Research* 37(Web Server issue): W6.

Mons, B., Ashburner, M., Chichester, C., van Mulligen, E., Weeber, M., den Dunnen, J., van Ommen, G., Musen, M., Cockerill, M., Hermjakob, H. et al. (2008). Calling on a million minds for community annotation in WikiProteins, *Genome biology* 9(5): R89.

Mons, B. & Velterop, J. (2009). Nano-Publication in the e-science era, *Workshop on Semantic Web Applications in Scientific Discourse (SWASD 2009).*

Raykar, V., Yu, S., Zhao, L., Jerebko, A., Florin, C., Valadez, G., Bogoni, L. & Moy, L. (2009). Supervised Learning from Multiple Experts: Whom to trust when everyone lies a bit, *Proceedings of the 26th Annual International Conference on Machine Learning*, ACM New

York, NY, USA.

Rebholz-Schuhmann, D., Arregui, M., Gaudan, S., Kirsch, H. & Jimeno, A. (2008). Text processing through Web services: calling Whatizit, *Bioinformatics* 24(2): 296.

Rebholz-Schuhmann, D., Kirsch, H. & Couto, F. (2005). Facts from text-is text mining ready to deliver?, *PLoS Biol* 3(2).

Russell, B., Torralba, A., Murphy, K. & Freeman, W. (2008). LabelMe: a database and web-based tool for image annotation, *International Journal of Computer Vision* 77(1): 157–173.

Schmid, H. (1994). Probabilistic part-of-speech tagging using decision trees, *Proceedings of International Conference on New Methods in Language Processing*, Vol. 12, Manchester, UK.

Shah, N., Jonquet, C., Chiang, A., Butte, A., Chen, R. & Musen, M. (2009). Ontology-driven indexing of public datasets for translational bioinformatics, *BMC bioinformatics* 10(Suppl 2): S1.

Snow, R., O'Connor, B., Jurafsky, D. & Ng, A. (2008). Cheap and fast—but is it good?: evaluating non-expert annotations for natural language tasks, *Proceedings of the Conference on Empirical Methods in Natural Language Processing*, Association for Computational Linguistics, pp. 254–263.

Winnenburg, R., Wachter, T., Plake, C., Doms, A. & Schroeder, M. (2008). Facts from text: can text mining help to scale-up high-quality manual curation of gene products with ontologies?, *Briefings in Bioinformatics* 9(6): 466.

WordFreak (n.d.). http://wordfreak.sourceforge.net.

25

Extract Protein-Protein Interactions From the Literature Using Support Vector Machines with Feature Selection

Yifei Chen, Feng Liu and Bernard Manderick
Vrije Universiteit Brussel
Belgium

1. Introduction

The objective of text mining is to automatically identify, extract, manage, integrate and exploit the information in texts (Ananiadou & McNaught, 2006). In order to understand biological texts, it is not enough to know what the extracted proteins are. Also the interactions between them should be extracted. Therefore, extracting relations between proteins is an important and more advanced text mining task in biological domain.
The study of the protein-protein interactions (PPI) is one of the most pressing problems. Characterizing protein interaction pairs is crucial to understand not only the functional role of individual proteins but also the organization of entire biological processes (Krallinger et al., 2007). Several approaches have been applied to PPI pair extraction including purely statistical co-occurrence approaches (De Bruijn & Martin, 2002; Craven, 1999), pattern-matching approaches (Baumgartner Jr. et al., 2007; Ray & Craven, 2001; Hakenberg et al., 2008) and machine learning approaches such as maximum entropy (Grover et al., 2007) and support vector machines (SVMs) (Airola et al., 2008; Bunescu et al., 2005; Zelenko et al., 2003).
In this chapter, we propose a *Protein-Protein Interaction Pair Extractor* (*PPIEor*) to extract PPI pairs from the biological literature. *PPIEor* is essentially a SVM for binary classification, which uses a linear kernel and a rich and informative set of features based on linguistic analysis, contextual words, interaction words, interaction patterns, specific domain information and so forth.

2. Methods

2.1 System description

Fig. 1 shows the overall architecture of *PPIEor* consisting of a number of components including a preprocessor, a feature extractor and feature selector, a SVM-based classifier and a post-processor.
PPIEor's input data are the biological articles annotated with protein names. Before extracting the features, the inputs have to go first through the *preprocessor* which includes a *clause parsing* module, a *coreference resolution* module and a *pair extraction* module. Then these processed articles and the extracted candidate PPI pairs together with external interaction databases

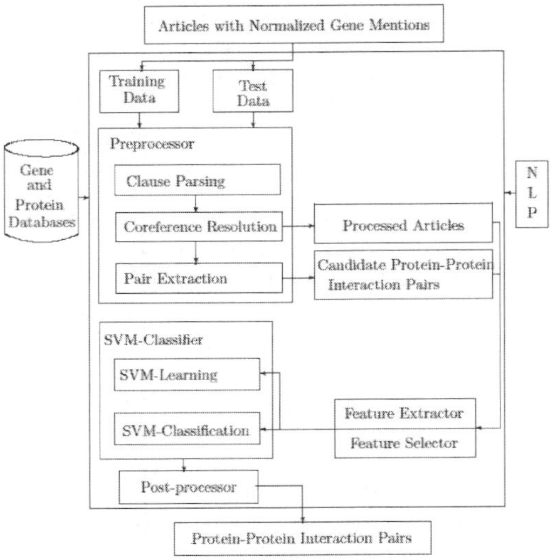

Fig. 1. The overall architecture of the Protein-Protein Interaction Pair Extractor (*PPIEor*)

like MINT[1] and IntAct[2] are used by the *feature extractor* and the *feature selector* to extract a rich and informative set of features. Next, the *binary SVM classifier*, the core component of *PPIEor*, is used to predict whether the candidate PPI pairs are correct or not. Finally, the output from the SVM classifier is combined with the self-interaction protein pairs generated by the *post-processor* to produce the final PPI pairs.

2.2 Data set

The data set used to train, tune and evaluate *PPIEor* consists of articles that have Structured Digital Abstracts (SDAs) (Ceol et al., 2008) from the journal, *FEBS Letters*[3]. More specifically, the total of 61 articles taken from DOI:10.1016/j.febslet.2008.01.064 to DOI:10.1016/j.febslet. 2008.11.009 are used as the training set. And the total of 39 articles with SDAs in FEBS Letters (from DOI:10.1016/j.febslet.2008.11.022 to DOI:10.1016/j.febslet .2009.03.013) are used as the test set. The SDA is an extension of the regular journal article abstract containing the PPI relations between the protein pairs mentioned in the article. Making use of these SDAs, we can obtain the PPI pairs of the articles in the data set. We denote this data set as $Data_{FEBS}$ and it contains 228 unique PPI pairs in the training set and 123 unique PPI pairs in the test set.

2.3 Protein name annotation

As it can be seen in Fig. 1, *PPIEor*'s input data are the articles annotated with *protein names*. Because the interactions only exist between proteins, protein names have to be recognized before we can extract the PPI pairs. Therefore, after building $Data_{FEBS}$, the next step is to annotate $Data_{FEBS}$ with protein names.

[1]http://mint.bio.uniroma2.it/mint/ [accessed on 20/03/2010]

[2]http://www.ebi.ac.uk/intact/ [accessed on 20/03/2010]

[3]http://www.febsletters.org/ [accessed on 20/03/2010]

In FEBS Letters, protein names are represented by database identifiers (database ID) of UniProt[4]. Therefore, we manually annotated articles with *golden standard* protein names which were obtained from the Structured Digital Abstracts (SDAs) of the selected articles. In this way we focus solely on the performance of *PPIEor* as a standalone system and avoid the errors derived from protein name recognition.

2.4 Preprocessor

Before passing on the input articles that have been annotated with the protein names to the SVM classifier in order to extract the features, they will first go through the preprocessor containing 1) a clause parsing module to split complex sentences into simpler units, 2) a coreference resolution module to find which protein a pronoun refers to, and 3) a pair extraction module to distill the candidate PPI pairs for the SVM classifier. These components are discussed in detail below. The sentence S_{FEBS}

> Our previous results revealed that *Q9HBI1* associates with PIX/ARHG EF6/Cool2 (*Q8K4I3*) at the tips of lamellipodia of motile cells and transmits integrin-*O55222* signals which activate *P60766* and *P63001*, small Rho GTPases.

taken from the input article DOI:10.1016/j.febslet.2008.01.064 in *FEBS Letters* and annotated with the UniProt identifiers *Q9HBI1*, *Q8K4I3*, *O55222*, *P60766* and *P63001* is used to illustrate the preprocessing steps.

2.4.1 Clause parsing

Sometimes compound sentences are too complex to analyze and may induce too much irrelevant and noisy information. Therefore instead of using the whole sentence, we separate it into several unit structures called *clauses* (Ejerbed, 1988). Based on these simpler structures, interaction relations can be extracted more easily and more efficiently because the candidate PPI pair extraction can be limited to the pairs appearing within the same clause rather than in the same whole sentence. Hence the amount of the false PPI pairs can be reduced a lot. So we propose to use the clause-based representation for the input articles in *PPIEor*.

We design the clause parsing module based on a widely used statistical syntactic parser, *nlparser* (Charniak & Johnson, 2005), to split each compound sentence into a main sentence and several clauses. Charniak & Johnson (2005) reported that the nlparser could obtain a $F_{\beta=1}$ measure of 91.0 on the sentences of length 100 or less and it could produce multiple-best parses. Here we use the first-best parses to decompose the sentences However, producing a full parse tree sometimes fails due to grammatical inaccuracies. Hence, when the nlparser fails to output a parse tree, we use the original sentence instead.

After this step, the sentence S_{FEBS} is split into 1 main sentence S_{MAIN} and 2 clauses $S_{CLAUSE1}$ and $S_{CLAUSE2}$:

- S_{MAIN}: Our previous results revealed that
- $S_{CLAUSE1}$: *Q9HBI1* associates with PIX/ARHGEF6/Cool2 (*Q8K4I3*) at the tips of lamellipodia of motile cells and transmits integrin-*O55222* signals
- $S_{CLAUSE2}$: which activate *P60766* and *P63001*, small Rho GTPases.

[4]http://www.uniprot.org/ [accessed on 20/03/2010]

2.4.2 Coreference resolution

After splitting the sentences into clauses another essential step needs to be done, i.e. coreference resolution. For example, in $S_{CLAUSE2}$ "which" refers to "O55222". Now suppose there are 2 PPI pairs in $S_{CLAUSE2}$: "O55222:P60766" and "O55222:P63001". Without using the coreference resolution module, these two pairs can never be retrieved. Unfortunately, because of the ambiguity of natural language in general, it is difficult to get full coreference resolution in practice. As a result, we restrict ourselves to a simple rule-based coreference resolution module that only resolves the Wh-pronominal coreference. Wh-pronouns refer to WHO, WHICH, THAT, WHAT and WHOSE. Detailed information about Wh-pronouns can be found in Santorini (1991).

Because the first word "which" in $S_{CLAUSE2}$ refers to "integrin-*O55222* signals", the coreference resolution module replaces "which" with "integrin-*O55222* signals". Hence, S_{MAIN} and $S_{CLAUSE1}$ remain unchanged and the clause $S_{CLAUSE2}$ becomes:

- $S_{CLAUSE2}$: integrin-*O55222* signals activate *P60766* and *P63001*, small Rho GTPases.

2.4.3 Candidate pair extraction

After preprocessing, we are ready to extract the candidate PPI pairs from the clause-based articles. First those clauses that do not contain any database ID or contain only 1 database ID are ignored. Then for each remaining clause, every two different database IDs are selected to compose one candidate PPI pair. If both database IDs occur only once in that clause, the choice of the candidate PPI pair is straightforward. However, in case one or both database IDs appear more than once in that clause, the nearest two database IDs are chosen to compose a candidate PPI pair.

Therefore, the input sentence S_{FEBS} is finally transformed into a set of *pair-based clauses* from which the SVM classifier will extract the features based on which it will predict whether the candidate PPI pairs are correct or not. For example, in $S_{CLAUSE1}$, the pair-based clauses are

- **Q9HBI1:Q8K4I3** *Q9HBI1* associates with PIX/ARHGEF6/Cool2 (*Q8K4I3*) at the tips of lamellipodia of motile cells and transmits integrin-*O55222* signals
- **Q9HBI1:O55222** *Q9HBI1* associates with PIX/ARHGEF6/Cool2 (*Q8K4I3*) at the tips of lamellipodia of motile cells and transmits integrin-*O55222* signals
- **Q8K4I3:O55222** *Q9HBI1* associates with PIX/ARHGEF6/Cool2 (*Q8K4I3*) at the tips of lamellipodia of motile cells and transmits integrin-*O55222* signals

2.5 Feature extractor

After extracting the candidate pairs, a list of candidate PPI pair-based clauses "(P_1:P_2) C" is obtained where P_1 and P_2 are the protein names (i.e. UniProt identifiers) and C is the clause where P_1 and P_2 are extracted. Then based on these pair-based clauses we derive a set of features including surface features and advanced features to train the SVM model. All the features used in *PPIEor* are listed below and we use the pair-based clause

> S_1 "**Q9HBI1:Q8K4I3** *Q9HBI1* associates with PIX/ARHGEF6/Cool2 (*Q8K4I3*) at the tips of lamellipodia of motile cells and transmits integrin-*O55222* signals"

to illustrate the feature extraction procedure.

2.5.1 Surface features

Surface features are derived from the pair-based clauses describing the explicit properties of candidate PPI pairs and their interactions. In the following feature extraction procedures, all punctuation marks are ignored when counting tokens.

- $Feature_{pair}$: The candidate PPI pair "P_1:P_2". For example, $Feature_{pair}(S_1)$ = ("Q9HBI1: Q8K4I3") in S_1.
- $Feature_{P_1}$: P_1 and the two tokens before and after it. Then $Feature_{P_1}(S_1)$ = ("-", "-", "Q9HBI1", "associates", "with") where"-" stands for the empty token.
- $Feature_{P_2}$: P_2 and the two tokens before and after it. $Feature_{P_2}(S_1)$ = ("ARHGEF6", "Cool2", "Q8K4I3", "at", "the").
- $Feature_{iWord}$: Usually interaction words are good indicators for the occurrence of interactions. We construct a lexicon called *iLexicon* that consists of interaction nouns and verbs similar to the ones proposed by Plake et al. (2005). Then we refine and extend *iLexicon* based on the training data of $Data_{FEBS}$. Due to the spacial limitation, we cannot present *iLexicon* here but it can be found in the PhD thesis of Chen (2009). Declensions of these nouns and conjugations of these verbs are also accepted. Every token in the given clause is matched against the entries of *iLexicon* to find the corresponding interaction words. If several interaction words exist, the one nearest to the proteins consisting of candidate PPI pairs is chosen while if no interaction word exists the value of this feature is NULL. In S_1, only the interaction word "associate" is found. So, $Feature_{iWord}(S_1)$ = ("associate").
- $Feature_{Location}$: Sometimes the importance of a clause is related to the location of that clause in the article. For example, the candidate PPI pairs appearing in the TITLE or the ABSTRACT have a higher probability to be correct than those appearing somewhere else. Usually, authors only write the most essential information in the TITLE or the ABSTRACT. We consider the following 5 categories for the location of the clauses: TITLE, ABSTRACT, FIGURE, TABLE and BODY. As a consequence, $Feature_{Location}(S_1)$ = ("BODY").
- $Feature_{P2Pdistance}$: The distance in tokens between the two proteins P_1 and P_2. So, $Feature_{P2Pdistance}(S_1)$ = (5).
- $Feature_{NP}$: This feature is the number of other identified proteins between the two proteins. $Feature_{NP}(S_1)$ = (0).
- $Feature_{iWordLocation}$: The relative location of iWord within candidate PPI pairs, which is whether iWord appears between, before or after the pairs. In S_1, $Feature_{iWordLocation}(S_1)$ = ("between"). The value of $Feature_{iWordLocation}$ is set to NULL if no iWord exists.
- $Feature_{iWord2P1distance}$: The distance in tokens between the iWord and P1, e.g. from S_1, $Feature_{iWord2P1distance}(S_1)$ = (0). If no iWord exists, the value of $Feature_{iWord2P1distance}$ is NULL.
- $Feature_{iWord2P2distance}$: The distance in tokens between the iWord and P2. For example $Feature_{iWord2P2distance}(S_1)$ = (4). In the same way, the value of $Feature_{iWord2P2distance}$ is NULL if no iWord exists.

2.5.2 Advanced features

As discussed before, surface features only use basic information. In order to improve the performance further, we also incorporate some more advanced features.

	Pattern
1:	$\mathbf{P_1}$ $W_{1.1}$ **iVerb** $W_{1.2}$ $\mathbf{P_2}$
2:	$\mathbf{P_1}$ $W_{2.1}$ **iVerb** $W_{2.2}$ by $W_{2.3}$ $\mathbf{P_2}$
3:	**iVerb** of $W_{3.1}$ $\mathbf{P_1}$ $W_{3.2}$ by $W_{3.3}$ $\mathbf{P_2}$
4:	**iVerb** of $W_{4.1}$ $\mathbf{P_1}$ $W_{4.2}$ to $W_{4.3}$ $\mathbf{P_2}$
5:	**iNoun** of $W_{5.1}$ $\mathbf{P_1}$ $W_{5.2}$ (by|through) $W_{5.3}$ $\mathbf{P_2}$
6:	**iNoun** of $W_{6.1}$ $\mathbf{P_1}$ $W_{6.2}$ (with|to|on) $W_{6.3}$ $\mathbf{P_2}$
7:	**iNoun** between $W_{7.1}$ $\mathbf{P_1}$ $W_{7.2}$ and $W_{7.3}$ $\mathbf{P_2}$
8:	complex between $W_{8.1}$ $\mathbf{P_1}$ $W_{8.2}$ and $W_{8.3}$ $\mathbf{P_2}$
9:	complex of $W_{9.1}$ $\mathbf{P_1}$ $W_{9.2}$ and $W_{9.3}$ $\mathbf{P_2}$
10:	$\mathbf{P_1}$ $W_{10.1}$ form $W_{10.2}$ complex with $W_{10.3}$ $\mathbf{P_2}$
11:	$\mathbf{P_1}$ $W_{11.1}$ $\mathbf{P_2}$ $W_{11.2}$ **iNoun**
12:	$\mathbf{P_1}$ $W_{12.1}$ $\mathbf{P_1}$ $W_{12.2}$ **iVerb** $W_{12.3}$ with each other
13:	$\mathbf{P_1}$ $W_{13.1}$ **iVerb** $W_{13.2}$ but not $W_{13.3}$ $\mathbf{P_2}$
14:	$\mathbf{P_1}$ $W_{14.1}$ cannot $W_{14.2}$ **iVerb** $W_{14.3}$ $\mathbf{P_2}$
15:	$\mathbf{P_1}$ $W_{15.1}$ (do|be) not $W_{15.2}$ **iVerb** $W_{15.3}$ $\mathbf{P_2}$
16:	$\mathbf{P_1}$ $W_{16.1}$ not $W_{16.2}$ **iVerb** $W_{16.3}$ by $W_{16.4}$ $\mathbf{P_2}$

Table 1. A set of 16 patterns for $Feature_{Pattern}$. Pattern 1−12 indicate the interactions between candidate PPI pairs while Pattern 13−16 indicate that no interaction exists. $W_{i.j}$ means the ith word gaps in Pattern j.

- *Pattern Matching Features ($Feature_{Pattern}$)*: Inspired by Plake et al. (2005), we designed a set of 16 syntactic patterns based on the training data. Each pattern is a syntactic description of sentence parts expressing protein locations, interaction nouns and verbs, and particular words. Two types of semantic information are integrated into these syntactic patterns, i.e. a protein-protein interaction exists or not. 12 patterns are designed to describe interactions between proteins and the remaining 4 patterns describe negations. Hence, in total 16 pattern matching features are designed: $Feature_{Pattern_1}, Feature_{Pattern_2}, \cdots, Feature_{Pattern_{16}}$. If a clause matches a pattern $Pattern_i$, the value of corresponding $Feature_{Pattern_i}$ is "1", otherwise it is "0". The 16 syntactic patterns are listed in Table 1 and they contain five different types of components:

  1. *P_1 and P_2*: P_1 and P_2 refer to the first and second proteins respectively in the PPI pair.
  2. *iNoun*: iNoun refers to the nouns indicating interactions taken from *iLexicon*.
  3. *iVerb*: iVerb refers to the verbs indicating interactions taken from *iLexicon*.
  4. *Fixed words*: Besides PPI pairs and iNouns/iVerbs, some patterns require that particular words occur in the clause. A pattern can require a fixed word like "by" in Pattern 2, or a word from a list, e.g. (with|to|on) in Pattern 6.
  5. *Word gaps*: Word gaps describe an optional sequence of words between the four components above. These gaps are limited in length but they do not require particular words. As recommend in Plake et al. (2005) we have set the maximum length of the gaps equal to 5.

- *Database Matching Features*: We match each candidate PPI pair with the entries of the protein interaction database used to see if this pair has already been recorded. Note that this feature will not be used by *PPIEor* until we have discussed the impact of the interaction databases in Section 3.5. For the moment, the most popular protein interaction databases are MINT and IntAct. Therefore we use the following two database matching features:

  1. $Feature_{MINT}$: Each candidate PPI pair is matched against all the entries in MINT. If matched, $Feature_{MINT} = 1$ otherwise $Feature_{MINT} = 0$. For instance, in S_1, the pair "Q9HBI1:Q8K4I3" can be found in MINT, hence $Feature_{MINT}(S_1) = (1)$.
  2. $Feature_{IntAct}$: Each candidate PPI pair is matched against all the entries in IntAct. If matched, $Feature_{IntAct} = 1$ otherwise $Feature_{IntAct} = 0$. For instance, in S_1, the pair "Q9HBI1:Q8K4I3" cannot be found in IntAct, hence $Feature_{IntAct}(S_1) = (0)$.

2.6 Feature selector

A feature selection method was used to select a subset of the most relevant features in order to build a robust machine learning model. By removing the most irrelevant and redundant features from the feature set, feature selection helps to improve the learning performance, to reduce the curse of dimensionality, to enhance the generalization ability, to accelerate the learning process and to boost the model interpretability.
The most straightforward method is subset selection with greedy forward search. This method is very simple to use but it has some drawbacks. It is more prone than other methods to get stuck in local optima and computationally it is very expensive (Saeys et al., 2007). Hence, for *PPIEor* we decided in favor of *SVM Recursive Feature Elimination (SVM RFE)* proposed by Guyon et al. (2002) to do the feature selection. SVM RFE interacts with the SVM classifier to search the optimal feature set and is less computationally intensive than the subset selection method. For a more detailed discussion about feature selection methods, the reader is referred to the review paper (Saeys et al., 2007).
In case of a linear kernel, SVM RFE uses the weights w_i appearing in the decision boundary to produce the feature ranks. The best subset of r features is the one that generates the largest margin between the two classes when the SVM classifier is using this subset. Stated in Guyon et al. (2002), the criteria $(w_i)^2$ estimates the effect on the objective function of removing one feature at a time. The feature with the smallest $(w_i)^2$ is removed first and as a result it has the lowest rank. In this way a corresponding feature ranking can be achieved. However, the features that are top ranked (eliminated last) are not necessarily the ones that are individually the most relevant. In some sense the features of a subset are optimal only when they are taken together. For computational reasons, it may be more efficient to remove several features at a time but at the expense of possible classification performance degradation.
In this chapter we use the toolbox *Java-ML* designed by Abeel et al. (2009) to implement the SVM RFE algorithm. Java-ML is a collection of machine learning and data mining algorithms and it has a usable and easily extensible API used by *PPIEor*. The library is written in Java and is available from http://java-ml.sourceforge.net/ under the GNU GPL license.

2.7 Classification model

After extracting features for the candidate PPI pair-based clauses $(P_1{:}P_2)C$, a binary classifier is needed to decide whether the candidate PPI pairs are correct or not. $Model_{SVM\_linear}$ is proposed using a linear kernel and the features described above. The toolbox LIBSVM (Chang & Lin, 2001) is used to train and tune $Model_{SVM\_linear}$ using 5-fold cross validation.

2.8 Post-processor

PPIEor makes an implicit assumption, i.e. the proteins in PPI pairs are different. This assumption leads to the problem that we cannot find self-interaction proteins. In the article DOI:10.1016/j.febslet.2008.12.036, the only correct PPI pair is "P64897:P64897", i.e. "P64897" interacts with itself. However, usually self-interactions are not stated explicitly in the articles. Therefore, we develop a post-processor to recover some self-interaction protein pairs and it consists of three steps:

- First, recall from Section 2.4.3 that the clauses that contain only 1 protein are ignored. Now we want to see if these proteins can interact with themselves. Therefore, for each article the proteins that do not consist of any candidate PPI pair are picked out.
- Second, for each protein obtained in the first step, search the MINT and IntAct databases to see if it can interact with itself.
- Finally, if the answer is yes, regard this protein as a self-interaction protein and add the corresponding pair to final PPI pair list.

Same as the database matching features discussed in Section 2.5.2, this component will not be used by *PPIEor* until the impact of the two databases on its performance is discussed in Section 3.5.

3. Results and discussion

3.1 Experimental purpose

Before discussing the experimental results, we would like to state the two purposes of *PPIEor*. The first purpose is to extract PPI pairs in the articles as accurately as possible to help the researchers avoid reading all the available articles. In this case, the performance of the system can be improved a lot by making use of interaction databases like MINT and IntAct. The second purpose is to help database curators who want to extract newly discovered PPI pairs from the articles that have not been recorded yet in databases. In this case it is not realistic to use existing interaction databases.
In the following we first focus on the second purpose, i.e. to build *PPIEor* without using any interaction database. First, in Section 3.2 we compare the fine-tuned *PPIEor* with other leading protein-protein interaction pair extraction systems built on similar data sets. Then in Sections 3.3 and 3.4 we show the impact of these components on *PPIEor* including the contribution of the preprocessor, the features and the feature selection method. Finally, in Section 3.5 we turn to the first purpose mentioned above and discuss the impacts of the databases, i.e. MINT and IntAct.

3.2 Results

PPIEor is developed and tuned on the training data of $Data_{FEBS}$ by doing 5-fold cross validation. After finding the optimal parameter value $C = 2^{-7}$ for the box constraint in the SVM the system is applied to the test data of $Data_{FEBS}$ and evaluated using the precision, the recall and the $F_{\beta=1}$ measure (Van Rijsbergen, 1979). The confidence intervals shown here are obtained by the *bootstrap resampling* method (Efron & Tibshirani, 1994) making use of 1,000 samples and for a confidence level of $\alpha = 0.05$.
The performance of *PPIEor* using $Model_{SVM\_linear}$ is compared with some of the leading protein-protein interaction extraction systems in Table 2. *PPIEor* is built by using the optimal feature set obtained by the SVM RFE feature selection method in Section 2.6. All systems

	Precision	Recall	$F_{\beta=1}$
PPIEor ($Model_{SVM\_linear}$)	72.66%	75.61%	74.10 ± 2.11
Syntax Pattern-based System	60.00%	46.00%	52.00
MDL-based System	79.80%	59.50%	68.17

Table 2. Evaluation results of *PPIEor* compared with other systems.

are evaluated on similar data sets, i.e. biological literature annotated with golden standard protein names.

Since we cannot reproduce the other systems, we compare the performance of *PPIEor* on the test set of $Data_{FEBS}$ with the ones reported in the literature by these competitors.

The *Syntax Pattern-based System* proposed by Plake et al. (2005) matched sentences against syntax patterns describing typical protein interactions. The syntax pattern set was refined and optimized on the training set using a genetic algorithm. This system was evaluated on the corpus of the BioCreAtIvE I challenge, Task 1A (Yeh et al , 2005) and got a $F_{\beta=1}$ measure of 52.00.

Another leading system, *MDL-based System*, proposed by Hao et al. (2005) used a minimum description length (MDL)-based pattern-optimization algorithm to extract protein-protein interactions and used a manually selected corpus from biological literature consisting of 963 sentences. This system got a $F_{\beta=1}$ measure of 68.17.

From Table 2, it can be seen that *PPIEor* using $Model_{SVM\_linear}$ gets a comparable $F_{\beta=1}$ measure with the above two leading systems, which is 74.10 ± 2.11. Therefore we can conclude that *PPIEor*'s performance is quite promising.

3.3 Contribution of preprocessor

First, we discuss the contribution of the preprocessor. It transforms the original sentences into a clause-based representation consisting of main sentences and a number of clauses followed by a coreference resolution module that resolves the Wh-pronominal coreference in order to facilitate the extraction of the candidate PPI pairs. Table 3 shows the performance of *PPIEor* without and with preprocessor. In the former case, the original sentences themselves are used as input data. It can be seen that with the preprocessor *PPIEor* performs much better, i.e the precision is increased by 4.08, the recall by 1.62 and the $F_{\beta=1}$ measure by 2.89. And the difference of the $F_{\beta=1}$ measures is significant for a confidence level $\alpha = 0.05$.

Another advantage of the preprocessor is that less candidate PPI pairs are extracted especially negative ones, which is illustrated in Example 3.1.

Example 3.1 *Consider that the sentence S consists of 2 clauses, C_1 and C_2. In C_1 2 proteins P_1 and P_2 are recognized and in C_2 also 2 proteins P_3 and P_4 are recognized. Only the PPI pair "P_1:P_2" are correct.*

$$S_1 : \underbrace{\cdots P_1 \cdots P_2 \cdots}_{C_1}, \underbrace{\cdots P_3 \cdots P_4 \cdots}_{C_2}.$$

With using the preprocessor, only 2 candidate PPI pairs are extracted: 1 positive PPI pair "P_1:P_2" and 1 negative PPI pair "P_3:P_4". However, without using the preprocessor, 6 candidate PPI pairs are extracted: 1 positive PPI pair "P_1:P_2" and 5 negative PPI pairs: "P_1:P_3", "P_1:P_4", "P_2:P_3", "P_2:P_4" and "P_3:P_4".

From Example 3.1, we see that on one hand, the preprocessor can handle the unbalance in the distribution of candidate positive and negative pairs to some extent and hence avoid the problems caused by such unbalance when building machine learning based models. On the

Data set	Precision	Recall	$F_{\beta=1}$
The sentence-based data set	50.51%	80.49%	62.69 ± 1.27
The clause-based data set	54.59%	82.11%	65.58 ± 1.31

Table 3. Comparison of the performance of *PPIEor* without (the data set consists of sentences) and with (the data set consists of clauses) preprocessor.

other hand, *PPIEor* becomes more efficient since less candidate PPI pairs has to be considered. Hence, it is better to use the preprocessor as a component of *PPIEor*.

3.4 Contribution of feature selection

The SVM Recursive Feature Elimination (SVM RFE) algorithm is designed specifically for SVMs and hence this feature selection method interacts directly with the SVM model. Since the core component of *PPIEor* is the SVM-based binary classifier $Model_{SVM\_linear}$, we think that the SVM RFE algorithm is to be prefered over other feature selection techniques like χ^2 (White & Liu, 1994), information gain (Quinlan, 1986) and gain ratio (Quinlan, 1993) which ignore interactions with the classifier. Hence the SVM RFE algorithm is applied to the original feature set (except the two database matching features $Feature_{MINT}$ and $Feature_{IntAct}$) discussed in Section 2.5 to select the optimal subset of features.

However, it is important to note that based on the specifications of the PPIE task, the performance of $Model_{SVM\_linear}$ is not exactly same as the performance of the final *PPIEor*. We will illustrate this in Example 3.2.

Example 3.2 *Consider the snippet of the input instances from the article DOI: 10.1016/j.febslet.200 8.01.064 shown below. The first item is the class label and the rest are the extracted features.*
1|O55222:Q9HBI1|DISTANCE:CLOSE|P2P:0|NULL|...
1|Q9ES28:Q9HBI1|DISTANCE:CLOSE|P2P:0|NULL|...
1|O55222:Q9HBI1|DISTANCE:CLOSE|P2P:0|LOC:BETWEEN|...
1|O55222:Q9HBI1|DISTANCE:MIDDLE|P2P:0|LOC:RIGHT|...

It is clear that there are two different candidate PPI pairs "O55222:Q9HBI1" and "Q9ES28:Q9HBI1". Because the candidate PPI pair "O55222:Q9HBI1" is discussed many times in the article DOI: 10.1016/j.febslet.2008.01.064, e.g. it appears in the figure, the title and the abstract, three instances are created, i.e the first, third and fourth instance above.

First, we use Example 3.2 to see the performance changes in $Model_{SVM\_linear}$:

- *Step 1*: $Model_{SVM\_linear}$ classifies all these 4 instances correctly, the recall is $4/(3+1) \times 100\% = 100\%$.
- *Step 2*: If $Model_{SVM\_linear}$ classifies the first instance incorrectly but the other three ones correctly, this gives 3 true positives and 1 false negative and hence the recall is $3/(3+1) \times 100\% = 75\%$.
- *Step 3*: If $Model_{SVM\_linear}$ classifies the first and second instances incorrectly but the other two ones correctly, the recall is $2/(3+1) \times 100\% = 50\%$.
- *Step 4*: If $Model_{SVM\_linear}$ only classifies correctly the fourth instance, the recall is $1/(3+1) \times 100\% = 25\%$.
- *Step 5*: If $Model_{SVM\_linear}$ misclassifies all the instances, this gives a recall of $0/(3+1) \times 100\% = 0\%$.

Hence it can be seen that as the number of misclassifications increases, the performance of $Model_{SVM\_linear}$ decreases.
However, the purpose of *PPIEor* is to find *distinct* PPI pairs in each article. For example, in the article DOI: 10.1016/j .febslet.2008.01.064, the correct PPI pairs are "O55222:Q9HBI1" and "Q9ES28:Q9HBI1". Again using Example 3.2, the performance of *PPIEor* changes as follows:

- *Step 1*: All these 4 instances are classified correctly, the recall is $2/2 \times 100\% = 100\%$.
- *Step 2*: If the first instance is misclassified but the other three ones are classified correctly, the recall is still $2/2 \times 100\% = 100\%$.
- *Step 3*: If the first and second instances are classified incorrectly but the other two ones correctly, the recall becomes $1/2 \times 100\% = 50\%$.
- *Step 4*: If only the fourth instance is classified correctly, the recall is $1/2 \times 100\% = 50\%$.
- *Step 5*: If all the instances are misclassified, this gives a recall of $0/2 \times 100\% = 0\%$.

As in the case of $Model_{SVM\_linear}$, as the number of misclassifications increases, the performance of *PPIEor* also decreases but differences are not the same. Therefore, we can conclude that the performances of $Model_{SVM\_linear}$ and *PPIEor* are *different* but *closely related*.
Since the performance of *PPIEor* is our final purpose, we decide to tune the feature selection based on the $F_{\beta=1}$ measure of *PPIEor*. Fig. 2 shows the contribution of the SVM RFE algorithm to the performances of both *PPIEor* and $Model_{SVM\_linear}$.
As explained above, $Model_{SVM\_linear}$ and *PPIEor* perform differently. In Fig. 2 one can see that their best $F_{\beta=1}$ measures are achieved for a different number of highest ranked features.
However, it can also be seen that the performances of $Model_{SVM\_linear}$ and *PPIEor* are closely related. Using the SVM RFE algorithm to rank the features by interacting with $Model_{SVM\_linear}$ also imposes the positive effect on the performance of *PPIEor*. The $F_{\beta=1}$ measure of *PPIEor* with all the features is 65.58 ± 1.31. When the top ranked 143 features (4.04%) are used, which are obtained by 5-fold cross validation on the training data, *PPIEor* achieves a $F_{\beta=1}$ measure of 74.10 ± 2.11. After applying the SVM RFE algorithm, the $F_{\beta=1}$ measure of *PPIEor* is increased by 8.52. This is significantly different for a confidence level $\alpha = 0.05$.
Finally, we look at types of the 143 best features. In Table 4, the types of the designed features are listed in a descending order according to their relative importance for *PPIEor*. Here importance means the more features are selected from a certain feature type, the more important that type is. It can be seen that the most important feature types are $Feature_{pair}$ and $Feature_{Pattern}$ with 122 and 9 features among the 143 best ones. In contrast, $Feature_{iWord}$, $Feature_{Location}$ and $Feature_{iWord2P1distance}$ are not important since no features of this type are selected.

3.5 Impact of the interaction databases

In this section we turn to the first purpose of *PPIEor*, i.e. to extract the PPI pairs in the articles as accurately as possible to help the researchers avoid reading all the available articles. For this situation, the interaction databases used by the database matching features and the post-processor give the positive contribution.
First, the two interaction databases, MINT and IntAct, are used to extract the database matching features, $Feature_{MINT}$ and $Feature_{IntAct}$. Second, based on MINT and IntAct, the post-processor will recover some self-interaction pairs. Table 5 shows the comparison of the performance of *PPIEor* without the interaction databases, with the database matching features and with the post-processor.

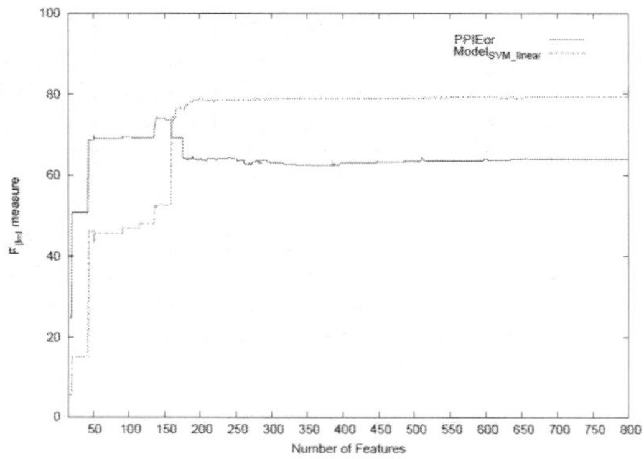

Fig. 2. Contributions of the SVM Recursive Feature Elimination (SVM RFE) algorithm to the performances of both *PPIEor* and $Model_{SVM\_linear}$. Note that x-axis is restricted to the range from 0 to 800 features since the performances do not change anymore when more features are added. The SVM RFE algorithm ranks the total of 3,543 features in a descending order according to their weights. The $F_{\beta=1}$ measure of *PPIEor* with all the features is 65.58 ± 1.31. When the optimal parameter values obtained by 5-fold cross validation on the training data are used, *PPIEor* achieves the $F_{\beta=1}$ measure of 74.10 ± 2.11 when the top 143 features (4.04%) are used. For $Model_{SVM\_linear}$, the best $F_{\beta=1}$ measure of 79.35 is obtained when the top 635 features are used while the $F_{\beta=1}$ measure for all the features is 79.17.

From the results shown in Table 5, it can be seen that the database matching features can greatly improve the performance. They increase the $F_{\beta=1}$ measures from 74.10 to 88.99. This makes sense because the PPI pairs that are recorded in MINT and IntAct have been verified by biological experiments and hence the matched candidate pairs have higher probabilities to be correct PPI pairs. The post-processor which has to recover some self-interaction pairs also contributes to the performance of *PPIEor*. It is clear that with post-processor the recall and the $F_{\beta=1}$ measure increase significantly although the precision drops slightly. Therefore we

Feature Type	Number of Selected Features after the feature selection
$Feature_{pair}$	122/290 (42.07%)
$Feature_{Pattern}$	9/37 (24.32%)
$Feature_{NP}$	3/6 (50.00%)
$Feature_{P1}$	3/1532 (0.20%)
$Feature_{P2Pdistance}$	2/3 (66.67%)
$Feature_{P2}$	2/1566 (0.13%)
$Feature_{iWordLocation}$	1/4 (25.00%)
$Feature_{iWord2P2distance}$	1/4 (25.00%)
$Feature_{iWord}$	0/92 (0.00%)
$Feature_{Location}$	0/5 (0.00%)
$Feature_{iWord2P1distance}$	0/4 (0.00%)

Table 4. Importance of the different types of features in descending order according to the number of selected features.

	Precision	Recall	$F_{\beta=1}$
Without Using Databases	72.66%	75.61%	74.10 ± 2.11
+Database Matching Features	97.12%	82.11%	88.99 ± 0.81
+Post-Processor	96.36%	86.18%	90.99 ± 0.81

Table 5. Contribution of the interaction databases to *PPIEor*.

conclude that the post-processor reduces to some extent the self-interaction problem. However it should be noted that using the interaction databases makes *PPIEor* hardly capture newly discovered PPI pairs that are not recorded in the databases yet. Hence it is better not to use the interaction databases when searching for new PPI pairs.

4. Conclusion

In this chapter we presented a protein-protein interaction pair extractor (*PPIEor*), which used a binary SVM classifier as the core component. Its purpose was to automatically extract protein-protein interaction pairs from biological literature. During the preprocessing phase, the original sentences from the articles were transformed into clause-based ones and the candidate PPI pairs were distilled. Then we derived a rich and informative set of features including surface features and advanced features. In order to improve the performance further, we used a feature selection method, the SVM Recursive Feature Elimination (SVM RFE) algorithm, to find the features most relevant for classification. Finally, the post-processor recovered some of the self-interaction proteins which could not be identified by our SVM model. The experimental results has proved that *PPIEor* can achieve the quite promising performance.

However, PPI pairs that appear in the figures, span different sentences or interact with themselves cannot be handled well for the moment. More advanced techniques need to be exploited in the future, like anaphora resolution used for semantic analysis to detect the inter-sentence PPI pairs, or specifically designed patterns to recover more self-interaction PPI pairs, etc.

5. References

Abeel T.; Van de Peer Y. & Saeys Y. (2009). Java-ML: A Machine Learning Library. *Journal of Machine Learning Research*, Vol.10, 931-934

Airola A.; Pyysalo S.; Björne J.; Pahikkala T.; Ginter F. & Salakoski T. (2008). A Graph Kernel for Protein-Protein Interaction Extraction. *Proceedings of the Workshop on Current Trends in Biomedical Natural Language Processing*, pp. 1-9

Ananiadou S. & McNaught J. (2006). *Text Mining for Biology and Biomedicine*, Artech House, Inc., ISBN:158053984X, London.

Baumgartner Jr. W.; Lu Z.; Johnson H.; Caporaso J.; Paquette J.; Lindemann A.; White E.; Medvedeva O.; Cohen K. & Hunter L. (2007). An integrated approach to concept recognition in biomedical text, *Proceedings of the Second BioCreative Challenge Evaluation Workshop*, pp. 257-271

Bunescu R. & Mooney R. (2005). Subsequence kernels for relation extraction, *Proceedings of the 19th Conference on Neural Information Processing Systems*, pp. 171-178

Ceol A.; Chatr-Aryamontri A.; Licata L. & Cesareni G. (2008). Linking entries in protein interaction database to structured text: the FEBS Letters experiment. *FEBS Letters*, Vol.582, No.8, 1171-1177

Chang C. & Lin C. (2001). LIBSVM : a library for support vector machines.

Charniak E. & Johnson M. (2005). Coarse-to-fine n-best parsing and MaxEnt discriminative reranking, *Proceedings of the 43rd Annual Meeting on Association for Computational Linguistics*, pp. 173-180

Chen Y. (2009). *Biological Literature Miner: Gene Mention Recognition and Protein-Protein Interaction Pair Extraction*, Vrije Universiteit Brussel.

Craven M. (1999). Learning to extract relations from MEDLINE, *Proceedings of the AAAI-99 Workshop on Machine Learning for Information Extraction*, pp. 25-30

De Bruijn B. & Martin J. (2002). Literature mining in molecular biology, *Proceedings of the EFMI Workshop Natural Language*, pp. 1-5

Efron B. & Tibshirani R. (1994). *An Introduction to the Bootstrap*, Chapman & Hall/CRC.

Ejerbed E. (1988). Finding Clauses In Unrestricted Text By Finitary And Stochastic Methods, *Proceedings of the second conference on Applied Natural Language Processing*, pp. 219-227

Grover C.; Haddow B.; Klein E.; Matthews M.; Neilsen L.; Tobin R. & Wang X. (2007). Adapting a Relation Extraction Pipeline for the BioCreAtIvE II Tasks, *Proceedings of the Second BioCreative Challenge Evaluation Workshop*, pp. 273-286

Guyon I.; Weston J.; Barnhill S. & Vapnik V. (2002). Gene Selection for Cancer Classification using Support Vector Machines. *Machine Learning*, Vol.46, No.1-3, 389-422

Hao Y.; Zhu X.; Huang M. & Li M. (2005). Discovering patterns to extract protein-protein interactions from the literature: Part II. *Bioinformatics*, Vol.21, No.15, 3294-3300

Hakenberg J.; Plake C.; Royer L.; Strobelt H.; Leser U. & Schroeder M. (2008). Gene mention normalization and interaction extraction with context models and sentence motifs, *Genome Biology*, Volume 9, Suppl 2, Article S14

Krallinger M.; Leitner F. & Valencia A. (2007). Assessment of the second BioCreative PPI task: Automatic Extraction of Protein-Protein Interactions, *Proceedings of the Second BioCreative Challenge Evaluation Workshop*, pp.41-54

Plake C.; Hakenberg J. & Leser U. (2005). Optimizing syntax patterns for discovering protein-protein interactions, *Proceedings of the 2005 ACM symposium on Applied computing*, pp. 195-201

Quinlan J. (1986). Induction of decision trees. *Machine Learning*, Vol.1, No.1, 81-106

Quinlan J. (1993). *C4.5: Programs for Machine Learning*, Morgan Kaufmann.

Ray S. & Craven M. (2001). Representing Sentence Structure in Hidden Markov Models for Information Extraction, *Proceedings of the 17th International Joint Conference on Artificial Intelligence*, pp. 1273-1279

Saeys Y.; Inza I. & Larrañaga P. (2007). A review of feature selection techniques in bioinformatics. *Bioinformatics*, Vol.23, No.19, 2507-2517

Santorini B. (1991). *Part-of-Speech Tagging Guidelines for the Penn Treebank Project*, Department of Computer and Information Science, University of Pennsylvania.

Van Rijsbergen C. (1979). *Information Retrieval*, Butterworth-Heinemann.

White A. & Liu W. (1994). Bias in Information-based measures in decision tree induction. *Machine Learning*, Vol.15, No.3, 321-329

Yeh A.; Morgan A.; Colosimo M. & Hirschman L. (2005). BioCreAtIvE Task 1A: gene mention finding evaluation. *BMC Bioinformatics*, Vol.6(Suppl 1), S2

Zelenko D.; Aone C. & Richardella A. (2003). Kernel methods for relation extraction. *The Journal of Machine Learning Research*, Vol.3, 1083-1106

26

Protein-Protein Interactions Extraction from Biomedical Literatures

Hongfei Lin, Zhihao Yang and Yanpeng Li
Dalian University of Technology
China

1. Introduction

Protein-protein interactions (PPI) play a key role in various aspects of the structural and functional organization of the cell. Knowledge about them unveils the molecular mechanisms of biological processes. A number of databases such as MINT (Zanzoni et al., 2002), BIND (Bader et al., 2003), and DIP (Xenarios et al., 2002) have been created to store protein interaction information in structured and standard formats. However, the amount of biomedical literature regarding protein interactions is increasing rapidly and it is difficult for interaction database curators to detect and curate protein interaction information manually. Thus, most of the protein interaction information remains hidden in the text of the papers in the literature. Therefore, automatic extraction of protein interaction information from biomedical literature has become an important research area.

Existing PPI works can be roughly divided into three categories: Manual pattern engineering approaches, Grammar engineering approaches and Machine learning approaches.

Manual pattern engineering approaches define a set of rules for possible textual relationships, called patterns, which encode similar structures in expressing relationships. The SUISEKI system uses regular expressions, with probabilities that reflect the experimental accuracy of each pattern to extract interactions into predefined frame structures (Blaschke & Valencia, 2002). Ono et al. manually defined a set of rules based on syntactic features to preprocess complex sentences, with negation structures considered as well (Ono et al., 2001). The BioRAT system uses manually engineered templates that combine lexical and semantic information to identify protein interactions (Corney et al., 2004). Such manual pattern engineering approaches for information extraction are very hard to scale up to large document collections since they require labor-intensive and skill-dependent pattern engineering.

Grammar engineering approaches use manually generated specialized grammar rules that perform a deep parse of the sentences. Sekimizu et al. used shallow parser, EngCG, to generate syntactic, morphological, and boundary tags (Sekimizu et al , 1998). Based on the tagging results, subjects and objects were recognized for the most frequently used verbs. Fundel et al. proposed RelEx based on the dependency parse trees to extract relations (Fundel et al., 2007).

Machine learning techniques for extracting protein interaction information have gained interest in the recent years. In most recent work on machine learning for PPI extraction, the PPI extraction task is casted as learning a decision function that determines for each unordered candidate pair of protein names occurring together in a sentence whether the two proteins interact or not. Xiao et al. used Maximum Entropy models to combine diverse lexical, syntactic and semantic features for PPI extraction (Xiao et al., 2005). Zhou et al. employed a semantic parser using the Hidden Vector State (HVS) model for protein-protein interactions which can be trained using only lightly annotated data whilst simultaneously retaining sufficient ability to capture the hierarchical structure (Zhou et al., 2006). Yang et al. used Support vector machines to combine rich feature sets including word features, Keyword feature, protein names distance feature, Link path feature and Link Grammar extraction result feature to identify protein interactions (Yang et al., 2010).

A wide range of results have been reported for the PPI extraction systems, but differences in evaluation resources, metrics and strategies make direct comparison of the numbers presented problematic (Airola et al., 2008). Further, PPI extraction methods generate poorer results compared with other domains such as newswire. In general, biomedical IE methods are scored with F-measure, with the best methods scoring about 0.85 without considering the limitation of test corpus, which is still far from users' satisfaction.

This chapter introduces three different protein-protein interactions extraction approaches which represent the state-of-the-art research in this area.

2. Methods

2.1 Multiple kernels learning mehtod

Among machine learning approaches, kernel-based methods (Cristianini & Taylor, 2000) have been proposed for PPI information extraction. Kernel-based methods retain the original representation of objects and use the object only via computing a kernel function between a pair of objects. Formally, a kernel function is a mapping K: X ×X $\rightarrow [0,\infty)$ from input space X to a similarity score $K(x,y)=\phi(x)\cdot\phi(y)=\Sigma_i\phi_i(x)\phi_i(y)$, where $\phi_i(x)$ is a function that maps X to a higher dimensional space without the need to know its explicit representation. Such a kernel function makes it possible to compute the similarity between objects without enumerating all the features.

Several kernels have been proposed, including subsequence kernels (Bunescu & Mooney, 2006), tree kernels (Moschitti, 2006), shortest path kernels (Bunescu & Mooney, 2005a), and graph kernels (Airola et al., 2008). Each kernel utilizes a portion of the structures to calculate useful similarity. The kernel cannot retrieve the other important information that may be retrieved by other kernels.

In recent years researches have proposed the use of multiple kernels to retrieve the widest range of important information in a given sentence. Kim et al. suggested four kernels: predicate kernel, walk kernel, dependency kernel and hybrid kernel to adequately encapsulate information required for a relation prediction based on the sentential structures involved in two entities (Kim et al., 2008). Miwa et al. proposed a method to combine BOW kernel, subset tree kernel and graph kernel based on several syntactic parsers, in order to retrieve the widest possible range of important information from a given sentence (Miwa et al., 2009).

However, these methods assign the same weight to each individual kernel and their combined kernels fail to achieve the best performance: in Kim's method, the performance of the hybrid kernel is worse than that of one of the individual kernels - the walk kernel. In Miwa's method, graph kernels outperform the other individual kernels. When combined with the subset tree kernels, it achieves better performance. However, when further

combined with BOW kernels, the performance deteriorates. In fact, the performance of BOW kernel and graph kernels combination is worse than that of graph kernels alone.
In this chapter, we propose a weighted multiple kernels learning based approach to extracting protein-protein interactions from biomedical literature. The approach combines feature-based kernel, tree kernel, and graph kernel with different weights: the kernel with better performance is assigned higher weight. Experimental results show the introduction of each individual kernel contributes to the performance improvement. The other novelties of our approach include: a) in addition to the commonly used word feature, our feature-based kernel includes the protein name distance feature as well as the Keyword feature. Especially, the introduction of Keyword feature is a way of employing domain knowledge and proves to be able to improve the performance effectively. b) with our tree kernel, we extend Shortest Path-enclosed Tree and dependency path tree to capture richer contextual information.

2.1.1 Methods

A kernel can be thought of as a similarity function for pairs of objects. Different kernels calculate the similarity with different aspects between two sentences. Combining the similarities can reduce the danger of missing important features and produce a new useful similarity measure. In this work, we combine several distinctive types of kernels to extract PPI: feature-based kernel, tree kernel, graph kernel.

2.1.1.1 Feature-based kernel

The following features are used in our feature-based kernel:

Word feature

A bag-of-words kernel takes two unordered sets of words as feature vectors, and calculates their similarity, which is simple and efficient There are two sets of word features used in our method.
Words between two protein names: These features include all words that are located between two protein names.
Words surrounding two protein names: These features include N words to the left of the first protein name and N words to the right of the second protein name. N is the number of surrounding words considered which is set to be three in our experiment.

Protein name distance feature

The shorter the distance (the number of words) between two protein names is, the more likely the two proteins have interaction relation. Therefore the distance is chosen as a feature. If there are less than three words between two proteins, the feature value is set to "DISLessThanThree"; if there are more than or equal to three words but less than six words between two proteins, the feature value is set to "DISBetweenThreeSix". The other feature values include "DISBetweenSixNine", "DISBetweenNineTwelve" and "DISMoreThanTwelve".

Keyword feature

The existence of an interaction keyword (the verb expressing protein interaction relation such as "bind", "interact", "inhibit", etc) between two protein names or among the surrounding words of two protein names often implies the existence of the protein-protein interaction. Therefore, the existence of the keyword is chosen as a binary feature. To identify the keywords in texts, we built an interaction keyword list of about 500 entries manually, which includes the interaction verbs and their variants (for example, interaction verb "bind" has variants "binding" and "bound", etc. The list can be provided upon request).

2.1.1.2 Tree kernel

A convolution kernel aims to capture structured information in terms of substructures. As a specialized convolution kernel, convolution tree kernel K_C (T_1, T_2) counts the number of common sub-trees (sub-structures) as the syntactic structure similarity between two parse trees T_1 and T_2 (Collins & Duffy, 2001):

$$K_C(T_1, T_2) = \sum_{n_1 \in N_1, n_2 \in N_2} \Delta(n_1, n_2) \quad (1)$$

where N_j is the set of nodes in tree T_j, and $\Delta(n_1,n_2)$ evaluates the common sub-trees rooted at n_1 and n_2.

Parse tree kernel

A relation instance between two entities is encapsulated by a parse tree. Thus, it is critical to understand which portion of a parse tree is important in the tree kernel calculation.
Zhang et al. explored five tree spans in relation extraction and found that the Shortest Path-enclosed Tree (SPT, an example is shown in Figure 1) performed best (Zhang et al., 2006). SPT is the smallest common sub-tree including the two entities. In other words, the sub-tree is enclosed by the shortest path linking the two entities in the parse tree. But in some cases, the information contained in SPT is not enough to determine two entities' relationship. For example, "interact" is critical to determine the relationship between "ENTITY1" and "ENTITY2" in the sentence "ENTITY1 and ENTITY2 interact with each other." as shown in Figure 1. However, it is not contained in the SPT (dotted circle in Figure 1) to determine their relationship. By analyzing the experimental data, we found in these cases the number of leaf nodes in a SPT is usually less than four, following the pattern like "ENTITY1 and ENTITY2" and including little information except the two entity names.
Here we employ a simple heuristic rule to expand the SPT span. By default, we adopt SPT as our tree span. When the number of leaf nodes in a SPT is less than four, the SPT is expanded to a higher level, i.e. the parent node of the root node of the original SPT is used as the new root node. Thus the new SPT (solid circle in Figure 1) will include richer context information comprising the original SPT. In the above example, the flat SPT string is extended from "(NP (NN PROTEIN1) (CC and) (NN PROTEIN2))" to "(S (NP (NN PROTEIN1) (CC and) (NN PROTEIN2)) (VP (VBP interact) (PP ((IN with) (NP (DT each) (JJ other)))))" and includes richer context information.

Dependency path tree kernel

The other type of tree structure information included in our tree kernel is from parser dependency analysis output. For dependency based parse representations, a dependency path is encoded as a flat tree as depicted as follows: (DEPENDENCY (NSUBJ (interacts ENTITY1)) (PREP (interacts with)) (POBJ (with ENTITY2))) corresponding to the sentence "ENTITY1 interacts with ENTITY2". Because a tree kernel measures the similarity of trees by counting common subtrees, it is expected that the system finds effective subsequences of dependency paths.
Similar to SPT parse tree, in some cases, dependency path tree also needs extension. Taking the sentence "The expression of rsfA is under the control of both ENTITY1 and ENTITY2." as an example (its dependency parse is shown in Figure 2), the path tree between ENTITY1 and ENTITY2 is "(DEPENDENCY (CONJ (ENTITY1, ENTITY2))." Obviously, the information in this path tree is insufficient to determine the relationship between the two entitles. Our solution is to extend the length of dependency path between two proteins to

three when it is less than three. In such case, if there exist two edges in the left of the first protein in the whole dependency parse path, they will be included into the dependency path. Otherwise, the right two edges of the second protein will be included into the dependency path. In the above example, the path tree between ENTITY1 and ENTITY2 is extended from "(DEPENDENCY (CONJ (ENTITY1, ENTITY2))" to "(DEPENDENCY (PREP(control, of)) POBJ((of, ENTITY1)) (CONJ(ENTITY1, ENTITY2)))". The example is shown in Figure 2. The optimal extension threshold three is determined through experiments to achieve the best performance.

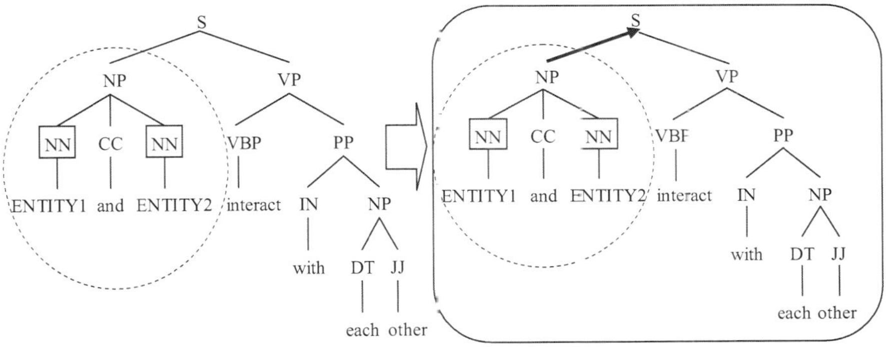

Fig. 1. An example of the extension of Shortest Path-enclosed Tree (the original SPT is in dotted circle and extended SPT in solid circle.)

2.1.1.3 Graph kernel

A graph kernel calculates the similarity between two input graphs by comparing the relations between common vertices (nodes). The graph kernel used in our method is the all-paths graph kernel proposed by Airola et al. (Airola et al., 2008). The kernel represents the target pair using graph matrices based on two subgraphs, and the graph features are all the non-zero elements in the graph matrices. The two subgraphs are a parse structure subgraph (PSS) and a linear order subgraph (LOS). More complete detail about the all-paths graph kernel is presented in (Airola et al., 2008).

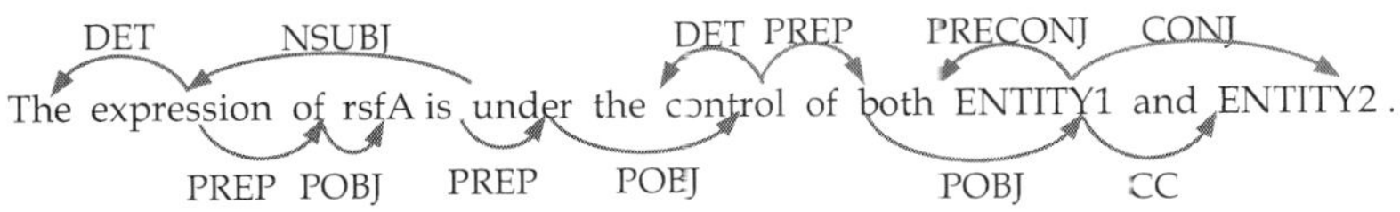

Fig. 2. An example of dependency path tree extension. The edge marked with red color is the original dependency path and the edge marked with blue color is included into the new dependency path.

2.1.1.4 Combination of kernels

Each kernel has its own advantages and disadvantages. The dependency path kernel ignores some deep information, and conversely, the parse tree kernel does not output certain shallow relations. All of them ignore the words. The feature-based kernel is simple and efficient, but can not capture the sentence structure. The graph kernels can treat the parser's

output and word features at the same time. However, they cannot treat them properly without tuning the kernel parameters. They may also miss some distant words, and similarities of paths among more than three elements (Airola et al., 2008).
The kernels calculate the similarity with different aspects between the two sentences. Combining the similarities can reduce the danger of missing important features and produce a new useful similarity measure. To realize the combination of the different types of kernels based on different parse structures, we sum up the normalized output of several kernels K_m as:

$$K(x,x') = \sum_{m=1}^{M} \sigma_m K_m(x,x') \tag{2}$$

$$\sum_{m=1}^{M} \sigma_m = 1,\ \sigma_m \geq 0,\ \forall m \tag{3}$$

where M represents the number of types of kernels, σ_m is the weight of each K_m which is determined through experiments: we tune the weight for each kernel until the overall best results are achieved. We found that each kernel has different performance and only when the kernel with better performance is assigned higher weight can the combination of each individual kernel produce the best result. In our experiments, the weights for feature-based kernel, tree kernel, and graph kernel are set to 0.6, 0.2 and 0.2 respectively in the order of performance rank (the weights of each individual kernel in combined kernels are shown in Table 5). This is a very simple combination, but the resulting kernel function contains all of the kernels' information. Comparatively, the methods in (Kim et al., 2008; Miwa et al., 2009) assign the same weight to each individual kernel and their combined kernels fail to achieve the best performance.

2.1.2 Experiments

2.1.2.1 Experimental setting

We evaluate method using a publicly available corpora AImed (Bunescu et al., 2005b) which is sufficiently large for training and reliably testing machine learning methods. It has recently been applied in numerous evaluations (Airola et al., 2008) and can be seen as an emerging de facto standard for PPI extraction method evaluation. Further, like in (Airola et al., 2008), we do not consider self-interactions as candidates and remove them from the corpora prior to evaluation. In our implementation, we use the SVMLight package (http://svmlight.joachims.org/) developed by Joachims for our feature-based kernel. The polynomial kernel is chosen with parameter d = 4. Tree Kernel Toolkits developed by Moschitti is used for our tree kernel (http://dit.unitn.it/~moschitt/Tree-Kernel.htm) and the default parameters are used. All-paths graph kernel proposed by Airola et al. (http://mars.cs.utu.fi/PPICorpora/GraphKernel.html) is used for our graph kernel.
In the test we evaluate our method with 10-fold document-level cross-validation so that no two examples from the same document end up in different cross-validation folds.

2.1.2.2 Experimental results and discussion

In this section, we firstly discuss the effectiveness of different features used in the feature-based kernel, SPT and dependency tree and their extensions, and different kernels on

AImed corpus. Here AImed is used since it is sufficiently large for training and reliably testing machine learning methods. It has recently been applied in numerous evaluations (Moschitti, 2006) and can be seen as an emerging de facto standard for PPI extraction method evaluation. Then we provide a comprehensive evaluation of our method across five PPI corpora, and compare our results with earlier work.

Effectiveness of different features in the feature-based kernel

In our method, no feature selection is performed. We tried stemming, but found little decline in performance. The classification performances of different features in the feature-based kernel tested on AImed are shown in Table 1 (the precision, recall, F-score values are achieved with the optimal threshold values obtained from the 10-fold cross-validations).
With the feature-based kernel, an F-score of 50.82% and an AUC of 77.69% are achieved using only word features. With the introduction of protein names distance and Keyword feature the F-score and AUC are improved to 52.69% and 80.71% respectively. Compared with protein names distance feature, the Keyword feature contributes more to the performance improvement (1.39 percentage units' increase in F-score and 2.48 percentage units' increase in AUC). The reason is that the Keyword feature employs domain knowledge, which proves to be able to improve the performance effectively. Exploiting domain knowledge may be a promising method to further improve PPI extraction performance. Similar works have been reported recently. Danger et al. defined a PPI ontology, PPIO, and showed some preliminary results guided by the ontology (Danger et al., 2008). He et al. proposed a novel framework of incorporating protein-protein interactions ontology knowledge into PPI extraction from biomedical literature in order to address the emerging challenges of deep natural language understanding (He et al., 2008).

Effectiveness of SPT parse tree, dependency tree and their extensions

The performances of SPT parse tree, dependency path tree and their extensions tested on AImed are shown in Table 2. Using only SPT achieves an F-score of 50.13% and an AUC of 76.32% while, after the introduction of SPT extension, dependency tree and its extension, the F-score and AUC are improved to 52.24% and 79.19% respectively (2.11 percentage units' increase in F-score and 2.87 percentage units' increase in AUC). Though the performance of dependency tree kernel itself is poor (an F-score of 30.03% and an AUC of 56.11% after extension), when combined with SPT parse tree kernel, it can help improve the total performance (0.68 percentage units' increase in F-score (52.24-51.56) and 1.14 percentage units' increase in AUC (79.19-78.05)).

	P	R	F	σ_F	AUC	σ_{AUC}
Words	42.58	62.9	50.82	2.9	77.69	3.4
Words + Protein names distance	43.65	62.3	51.3	5.4	78.23	3.6
Words + Protein names distance + Keyword	46.32	61.1	52.69	4.9	80.71	4.1

Table 1. Effectiveness of different features in the feature-based kernel and their combinations on AImed

In addition, as discussed in Section 2.1.1.2, SPT and dependency path tree extensions can improve the performance by including richer context information outside SPT and dependency path. They together contribute to the improvement of performance by almost 0.7 percentage units in F-score (52.24-51.52) and 2 percentage units in AUC (79.19-77.24).

	P	R	F	σ_F	AUC	σ_{AUC}
SPT	40.09	66.74	50.13	3.2	76.32	2.7
SPT Extension	42.37	65.8	51.56	3.3	78.05	2.2
Dependency	18.76	58.33	29.17	3.2	54.37	2.3
Dependency Extension	20.49	56.18	30.03	3.6	56.11	2.1
SPT + Dependency	42.29	65.65	51.52	5.1	77.24	2.8
SPT Extension +Dependency Extension	43.71	64.65	52.24	4.8	79.19	2.6

Table 2. Effectiveness of SPT, dependency tree and their extensions on AImed

Effectiveness of different kernels

The performances of different kernels tested on AImed are shown in Table 3. Among the four individual kernels, the performance of the graph kernel is the best. As discussed in Section 2.1.1.4, the reason is that the graph kernels can treat the parser's output and word features at the same time. The performance of the feature-based kernel ranks second since it uses protein names distance and Keyword feature besides words features (otherwise, with only words features, its performance (an F-score of 50.82% and an AUC of 77.69%) is worse than that of the tree kernel). The performance of the tree kernel is almost the same with that of the feature-based kernel.

	P	R	F	σ_F	AUC	σ_{AUC}
Feature-based kernel	46.32	61.1	52.69	3.6	80.71	2.7
BOW(Miwa)			52.8		82.1	
Tree kernel	43.71	64.65	52.24	3.1	79.19	2.6
Tree kernel(Miwa)			58.2		82.5	
Graph kernel	52.66	64.56	57.20	5.6	83.27	2.8
Graph kernel(Miwa)			59.5		85.9	
Tree kernel(0.5)+ Feature-based kernel(0.5)	50.44	68.49	58.05	3.3	84.19	2.3
Tree kernel + BOW (Miwa)			60.5		85.9	
Graph kernel(0.7) +Feature-based kernel(0.3)	51.33	69.58	59.02	4.1	84.68	3.1
Graph kernel + BOW (Miwa)			57.8		85.2	
Graph kernel(0.7)+ Tree kernel(0.3)	53.43	68.57	59.66	5.8	85.51	3.4
Tree kernel+ Graph kernel (Miwa)			61.9		87.6	
Feature-based kernel(0.2) + Tree kernel(0.2)+ Graph kernel(0.6)	57.4	70.75	63.9	4.5	87. 83	2.9
Tree kernel+ Graph kernel + BOW (Miwa)			60.8		86.8	

Table 3. Effectiveness of different kernels and performance comparison with those of Miwa's method on AImed. The weights of each individual kernel in combined kernels are in the parentheses after the kernel name.

The experimental results show that, when two or more individual kernels are combined, better performances are achieved. When the graph kernel is combined with the feature-based kernel, the performance is improved by 1.82 percentage units in F-score and 1.41

percentage units in AUC. When further combined with the tree kernel, the performance is improved by 4.88 percentage units in F-score and 3.15 percentage units in AUC. The results show that the combined kernel can achieve much better performance than each individual kernel. As discussed in Section 2.1.1.4, the different kernels calculate the similarity with different aspects between the two sentences and the combination of kernels covers more knowledge by introducing more kernels and is effective for PPI extraction.
The performance comparison between our kernels and those in (Miwa et al., 2009) is also made in Table 3. Our feature-based kernel, tree kernel, graph kernel corresponds to the BOW, tree kernel, graph kernel in Miwa's method respectively. The performance of the BOW kernel Miwa's method is almost the same as our feature-based kernel in F-score (52.69% to 52.8%). The performance of the tree kernel in Miwa's method is better than our tree kernel (58.2% to 52.4% in F-score and 82.5% to 79.19% in AUC) the reason is that it uses the predicate type information to represent the dependency types (Miwa et al., 2009). The performance of the graph kernel in Miwa's method is also better than our graph kernel (59.5% to 57.2% in F-score and 85.9% to 83.27% in AUC). The reasons are: First, each word in the shortest path has two labels, and the relations in the shortest path are not replaced, but duplicated in the first subgraph. Second, the shortest path is calculated by using the constituents in the PAS structure. The words in the constituents in the shortest path are distinguishably marked as being "in the shortest path" (IP). Finally, the POS information for protein name is not attached (Miwa et al., 2009).
However, different from our results, the combination of kernels in (Miwa et al., 2009) doesn't always contribute to performance improvement. Among their kernels, the graph kernel performs best. When it is combined with the tree kernel, the performance is improved by 2.4 percentage units in F-score and 1.7 percentage units in AUC. However, when further combined with the BOW kernel, the performance drops by 1.1 percentage units in F-score and 0.8 percentage units in AUC. In fact, the performance drops when the graph kernel itself is combined with the BOW kernel. That shows the introduction of the BOW kernel into the graph kernel leads to the deterioration of the performance. Similarly, the performance of the hybrid kernel in (Kim et al., 2008) is worse than that of one of the individual kernels - the walk kernel. The reason may be that in their methods each kernel is assigned the same weight when combined. As discussed in Section 2.1.1.4, we found that only when the kernel with better performance is assigned higher weight can the combined kernel produce the best result. In our experiments the weights for feature-based kernel, tree kernel, and graph kernel are set to 0.6, 0.2, and 0.2 respectively in the order of performance rank.

Performance compared to other methods

Method	P	R	F	AUC
Our: Combined Kernel	57.4	70.75	63.9	87. 83
Miwa et al., 2008			63.5	87.9
Miwa et al., 2009	58.7	66.1	61.9	87.6
Miyao et al., 2009	54.9	65.5	59.5	
Airola et al., 2008	52.9	61.8	56.4	84.8

Table 4. Comparison on AImed. Precision, recall, F-score and AUC results for methods evaluated on AImed.

The comparison with relevant results reported in related research is summarized in Table 4. The best performing system combines multiple layers of syntactic information by using a combination of multiple kernels based on several different parsers and achieves an F-score of 63.5% and an AUC of 87.9% (Miwa et al., 2008). Our method uses only the Stanford parser output to achieve parse tree, dependency structure (path and graph) information and the performance is comparable to the former. This is due to the following three key reasons: 1) with feature-based kernel, besides the commonly used word feature, protein names distance and Keyword feature are introduced to improve the performance. Especially, the introduction of Keyword feature is a way of employing domain knowledge and proves to be able to improve the performance effectively. With the appropriate features, feature-based kernel performs best among three individual kernels. 2) the tree kernel can capture the structured syntactic connection information between the two entities. Our tree kernel combines the information of parse tree and dependency path tree and introduces their extensions to capture richer context information outside SPT and dependency path when necessary. 3) different kernels calculate the similarity with different aspects between the two sentences. Our combined kernel can reduce the danger of missing important features and, therefore, produce a new useful similarity measure. Especially, we use a weighted linear combination of individual kernel instead of assigning the same weight to each individual kernel and experimental result show the introduction of each kernel contributes to the performance improvement.

2.2 Uncertainty sampling based active learning method

One problem of applying machine learning approaches to PPI extraction is that large amounts of data are available but the cost of correctly labeling it prohibits its use. For example, MEDLINE is the most authoritative bibliographic database which has covered over 17 million references to articles from over 4800 journals, newspapers and magazines and updates weekly in the Web of knowledge. On the other hand, though the amount of unlabeled data is increasing fast, the existing labeled data can not meet research needs, for which people have to tag a lot of samples manually. However, corpus annotation tends to be costly and time consuming. People would like to minimize human annotation effort while still maintaining desired accuracy.

To accomplish this, we turned to the uncertainty sampling method of active learning. Active learning is a research area in machine learning that features systems that automatically select the most informative examples for annotation and training (Angluin, 1988).

The primary goal of active learning is to reduce the number of examples for annotation that the system is trained on, while maintaining the accuracy of the acquired information. It may construct their own examples, request certain types of examples, or determine which of a set of unsupervised examples are most usefully labeled (Cohn et al., 1994). The last approach is particularly attractive in text mining since there is an abundance of data and we would like to tag the samples as few as possible (i.e. selecting only the most informative ones for tagging). The basic idea is to combine obtaining samples and model, not like passive learning which considers each part separately. The method has been applied to text classification (McCallum & Nigam, 1998), natural language parsing (Thompson et al., 1999), name entity recognition (Shen et al., 2004) and information extraction (Thompson et al., 1999).

To reduce annotation effort in PPIs from biomedical text, we present an uncertainty sampling based method of active learning in a lexical feature-based SVM model. To verify the effectiveness the AImed corpus and the CB corpus (Krallinger et al., 2007) are used and a 10-fold cross validation is applied.

2.2.1 Methods

The process flow of uncertainty sampling based active learning (USAL) method includes two stages. Firstly, the corpus is divided into three parts: the initial training set, the unlabeled the training set and the test set. Secondly, USAL method is introduced to select the most informative samples and add them into training set. The details are described in the following sections.

2.2.1.1 Lexical feature and preprocessing

The words surrounding the tagged protein names are used as lexical features. We divide lexical features into three types: left words, middle words and right words. Left words are the words to the left of the first protein name, middle words are the words between the first protein name and the second protein name, and right words are the words to the right of the second protein name.

A few preprocessing steps are performed before the lexical feature extraction including stopword elimination and stemming. Stopword elimination can reduce the noise, and stemming can relieve the sparse problem.

2.2.1.2 Uncertainty sampling

Uncertainty sampling (Lewis & Catlett, 1994) is an active learning method. It iteratively requests informative examples to label from unlabeled samples. Comparing to random sampling which randomly selects samples to label and train, the idea of USAL is that people only find the most informative unlabeled samples to tag.

In our method the "most informative" unlabeled samples are defined as those with the lowest absolute value of the predict scores outputted by our lexical feature-based SVM model (the lexical features used are discussed in Section 2.2.1.1). We think the smaller a sample's absolute value of the predict score is, the more uncertainty the sample has and, therefore, is more informative. Learning begins with a small pool of annotated samples and a large pool of unannotated samples. The USAL attempts to choose the most uncertain additional samples. The iterative process will not stop until the pool of unlabeled samples is empty or any other indicator reaches a threshold.

2.2.2 Experiment and discussion

2.2.2.1 Datasets

One problem in current PPI extraction research is the lack of defined criteria for evaluating the PPI systems: researchers develop and test on their own corpus and, therefore, their results are not comparable. In our experiments we used two standard datasets: AImed corpus and CB corpus. CB corpus is provided by as BioCreAtIvE II (Krallinger et al., 2007) challenge evaluation.

In our experiments, each corpus is divided into three parts The first part is initial training set composed of 400 randomly selected samples, the second is unlabeled training set and the third is the test set composed of 400 samples which are also randomly selected.

We use Precision, Recall, F-score and Accuracy as metrics to evaluate the performance. Three group experiments are designed to verify the effectiveness and efficiency of USAL method. In the first group USAL is evaluated on using how much of the training set can achieve the best performance; In the second group how much the learning process could be accelerated is tested by only considering one of the same uncertainty samples while keeping the PPI performance; In the third group a threshold is used to restrict the uncertainty so as to further speed up learning process, i.e. samples whose uncertainties are within the threshold are picked up to label, and the other samples are ignored.

During every round in uncertainty sampling, samples selected by the classifier from the unlabeled train dataset are added into the initial dataset. In the last round the final actual training set is formed. Assuming that e denotes the proportion between the sizes of the actual and total training set, the values of Precision, Recall, F-score and Accuracy are observed on the test set with increasing e. A 10-fold cross-validation is applied to verify the effectiveness of USAL method.

2.2.2.2 Results and discussion

First, on AImed dataset, USAL is put up as N=10 and N=100 (N denotes the number of samples which are picked up in each round). In each round a prediction is done on the test set. As shown in the Fig. 3 and Fig. 4, the performance is steadily improved by increasing the amount of training data, and when e=0.6 almost each evaluation metric (Precision, Recall, F-score and Accuracy) reaches its optimal value. It shows that labeling cost can be reduced by 40% using USAL while the performance doesn't decline.

USAL selects the unlabeled samples with most uncertainty to label (i.e. the samples with the lowest absolute value of predict scores outputted by our lexical feature-based SVM model), adds them into training set and re-trains the SVM model to pick up another N informative samples. It is an iterative process that gradually makes the training model rich and perfect. As shown in Fig. 3 and Fig. 4, on AImed dataset, no matter how many samples are selected in each round, almost each evaluation metric reaches its optimal values as e=0.6. However, sometimes the result may decline a little when e is increasing. It is a self-improvement process in which the model improves itself constantly.

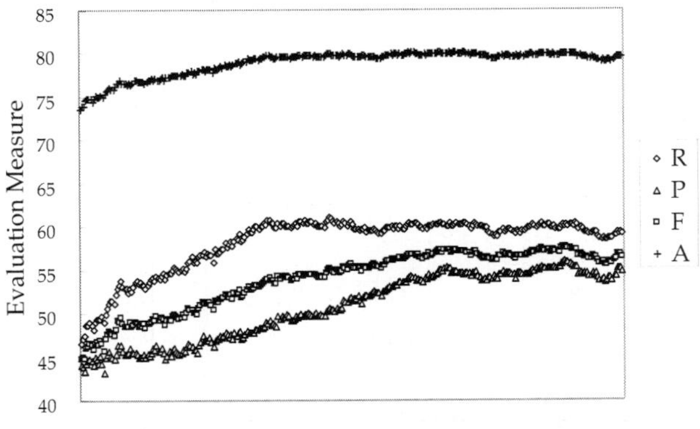

Fig. 3. Performance on AImed dataset when N is set to 10

From the above discussion, we can draw a conclusion that USAL could reduce the labeling cost without sacrificing the PPI performance. Besides, as shown in Fig. 3 and Fig. 4, Accuracy is much higher than F-score. By analyzing the result we found that as the number of positive instances is much less than that of negative instances, F-score (which is calculated in allusion to the number of positive instances) can not be as high as Accuracy(which is calculated in allusion to the number of instances classified correctly including positive and negative instances).

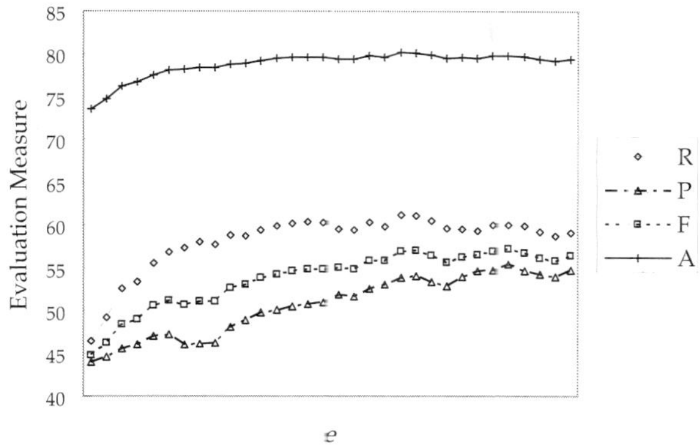

Fig. 4. Performance on AImed dataset when N is set to 100

The experiment results on CB dataset are similar to those on AImed dataset: the performance is steadily improved by increasing the amount of training data, and when e=0.8 almost each evaluation metric reaches its optimal value. It shows that annotation effort can be reduced by 20% using USAL. In addition, Accuracy is almost the same as F-score since the positive instances are almost as many as the negative instances.

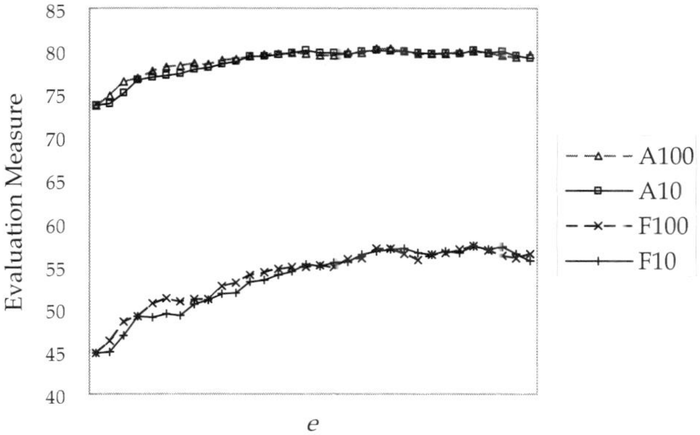

Fig. 5. F-score and accuracy comparison when N=100 and N=10 on AImed dataset

The experiment results on both AImed and CB datasets verify the effectiveness of USAL method. In addition, some experiments are designed to verify the effect of accelerating the learning process by only considering one of the same uncertainty samples. F100 and A100 denote F-score and Accuracy when N is set to 100; F10 and A10 denote F-score and Accuracy of when N is set to 10. They are compared on AImed and CB datasets respectively.

As shown in Fig. 5, the results on AImed dataset show that there is no obvious difference between N=10 and N=100 which means that N can be set to a large value to speed up learning process with less training time while keeping the performance. The similar result is found on CB dataset.

During the process of USAL, many unlabeled samples have the same uncertainty in each round. We only consider one of these samples and the others are ignored. In this way a faster learning process could be achieved while still maintaining desired performance. In order to further speed up, a threshold is used to restrict the uncertainty. Samples whose uncertainties are within the threshold are picked up to tag, and the others are ignored.

Assuming that the method used in the phase is denoted by f (T, IU) where T is the threshold and IU denotes to whether the same uncertainty samples are combined as one. RT (rounds of training) is used to measure the speed of learning process. FTS is the number of samples in final training set after USAL. The achieved F-score and accuracy of different strategies are shown in Table 5.

f (T, IU)	AImed				CB			
	RT	FTS	F	A	RT	FTS	F	A
f (∞, *False*)	32	3626	56.43	79.47	31	3656	84.34	84.23
f (∞, *True*)	28	3066	56.22	79.18	28	3042	84.5	84.39
f (3, *True*)	21	2411	56.96	79.83	27	2934	84.25	84.12
f (2, *True*)	14	1769	55.49	79.34	23	2552	83.44	83.38
f (1, *True*)	9	1087	51.4	79.05	12	1456	77.8	77.94

Table 5. Comparison of different strategies based on four indicators: RT, FTS, F and A.

In Table 5 f (∞, False) is used as the baseline in which all the training samples are used to predict the test set and the samples with same uncertainty are not combined as one. There are four group experiments with varying T and IU. Compared with f (∞, False), f (∞, True), in which all the training samples are used and the samples with same uncertainty are combined as one, reduces 3 RT and more than 600 FTS while maintaining the performance. Further, when the threshold T is introduced, f (3, True) reduces 7 RT and more than 600 FTS in AImed dataset while it reduces 1 RT and more than 100 FTS in CB dataset. While when T is set to smaller values, the performance begins to decline, and when T is set to 1 the performance degrades sharply. If T is set to an optimal threshold value (e.g. 2) keeping only one sample with the same uncertainty and using a threshold could help to reduce much training time with slight loss of performance.

2.3 Feature coupling generalization method

Many recent works (Airola et al., 2008; Bunescu et al., 2005a; Miwa et al., 2008; Miyao et al., 2009) focus on the syntactic-based methods where examples are represented by features or kernels derived from the outputs of syntactic parsers.These methods are capable of capturing syntactic relationships between entities, and show over 10% better performance than lexical features (Miwa et al., 2008; Miyao et al., 2009).

One could wonder whether methods without using syntactic information can also achieve state-of the-art performance or not. In this work, we present a novel feature representation method for the PPIE task, which is an application of our recently proposed semi-supervised learning strategy – feature coupling generalization (FCG) (Li et al., 2009). The general idea of

FCG is to learn a novel feature representation from the co-occurrences of two special types of raw features: example-distinguishing features (EDFs) and class-distinguishing features (CDFs). EDFs and CDFs refer to strong indictors for examples and for classes respectively. Intuitively, their co-occurrences in huge unlabeled data will capture indicative information that could not be obtained from labeled training data due to data sparseness. We used this method to learn an enriched representation of entity names from 17GB unlabeled biomedical texts for a gene named entity classification (NEC) task (Li et al., 2009) and found that the new features outperformed elaborately designed lexical features.
It is natural to think of applying FCG to PPIE as well as the NEC task, since there are huge amount of biomedical literatures available online which provide rich unlabeled resources. Our primary work here is to design proper EDFs, CDFs and other settings of FCG framework for the PPIE task. We also compare the performance of our methods with other syntactic-based methods proposed in previous researches on AImed corpus.

2.3.1 Feature coupling generalization

2.3.1.1 The general framework

In short, feature coupling generalization is a framework for creating new features from old features (referred to as "prior features" (Li et al., 2009)). We introduced two types of prior features: example-distinguishing features (EDFs) and class-distinguishing features (CDFs). EDFs are intuitively defined as "strong indicators" for the current examples, and CDFs are "strong indicators" for the target classes. The relatedness degree of an EDF fe and a CDF fc estimated from the unlabeled data U is defined as feature coupling degree (FCD), denoted by FCD (U, fe, fc). The FCG algorithm describes how to convert FCDs into new features. The assumptions behind this idea are: 1) the relatedness of an EDF and a CDF provides indicative information for classifying the current examples that contains the EDF. 2) Given more unlabeled data, more FCDs that cannot be obtained from labeled data can be estimated from unlabeled data.
Assuming that $F = \{f_1, \ldots, f_n\}$ is the feature vocabulary of "raw data" that contains every Boolean feature one could enumerate to describe an example, and $\mathbf{X} \subseteq \mathbf{R}^n$ is the vector space of the raw data, where each example is represented by a n-dimensional vector $\mathbf{x} = (x_1, \ldots, x_n) \in \mathbf{X}$. The algorithm process of FCG can be summarized as follows:

1. Select the "example-distinguishing" part of F as EDFs, denoted by $E \subseteq F$.
2. Map each element in E to a unique higher-level concept (EDF root) in the set H, denoted by root (e): $E \rightarrow H$.
3. Select the "class-distinguishing" part of F as CDFs, denoted by $C \subseteq F$.
4. Define the set of FCD types T to measure the relatedness of EDFs and CDFs.
5. Let the vocabulary of FCD features be $H \times C \times T$ so that each FCD feature maps a tuple (h, c, t), where $h \in H$, $c \in C$, and $t \in T$.
6. Calculate FCDs from unlabeled data and convert each example from the old representation x to a new feature vector $\tilde{\mathbf{x}}$ by the equation:

$$\tilde{x}_i = \tilde{x}_{(h,c,t)} = \sum_{root(e)=h} band(e,\mathbf{x}) * FCD\,(U,e,c) \qquad (4)$$

where $e \in E$, $\tilde{x}_i \in \tilde{\mathbf{x}}$, i indexes each triple (h, c, t) in $H \times C \times T$. The operator band(e, x) equals 1 if the feature e appears in the example x, and 0 otherwise.
For simplicity, here we assume that EDFs and CDFs are all extracted from F. In a broader sense, we can use the transformed feature set of original data to generate EDFs or CDFs. For

example, the "CDF II" used in the NEC task is the combination of local context words by a classifier. In the above algorithm, we assume F contains all the "feasible" combinations of original features derived from the data, and all the EDFs and CDFs are limited to be generated from this set.

2.3.1.2 Why it works

In supervised learning, usually only a subset of elements in F can be utilized. This means features that don't lead to performance improvement are regarded as irrelevant ones which are either removed before training or assigned very small weights during training to degrade their impact. In FCG framework, we also need to select a subset of F as EDFs or CDFs, but the criterion for feature selection is rather different. Here "good" EDFs or CDFs mean the performance of FCD features generated by them is good, although the single performances of them might be poor in a supervised setting. In other words, irrelevant features in supervised learning may be good EDFs or CDFs that produce indicative FCD features, so that FCG could utilize the features discarded by supervised learning.

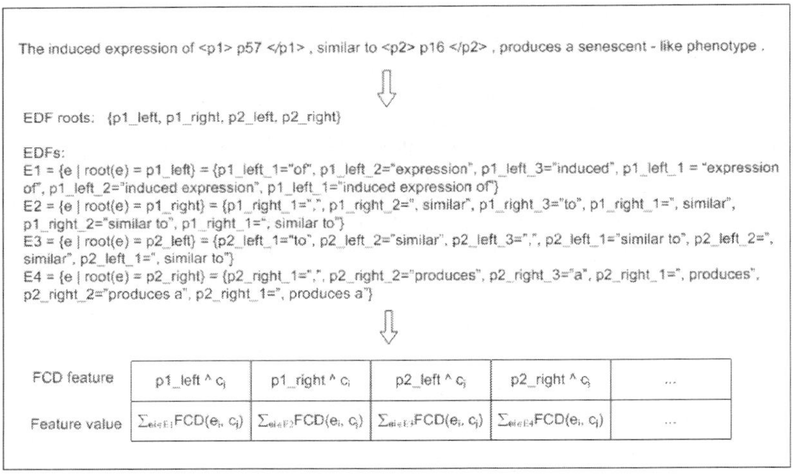

Fig. 6. An example that shows how FCG generates new feature for the PPIE task. Here only SP-EDFs are considered, and they are divided into four groups according to different EDF roots. A CDF is denoted by cj. Since only one FCD type is used here, the FCD features are indexed by the conjunction of EDF roots and CDFs.

The selection of EDFs and CDFs plays a central part in this framework. We suggested that when selecting these features, a trade-off between "indicative" and "informative" should be considered (Li et al., 2009). In the NEC task (Li et al., 2009) for determining whether an entity is a gene or protein name, the EDFs were selected as the whole entities and boundary word-level n-grams, and the CDFs were context patterns (such as "X gene" and "the expression of X") and the discretized scores of a SVM trained by local contexts. The experiments show that good results can be achieved when various types of EDFs together with hundreds of CDFs are used. We also found that these FCD features performed better in non-linear classifiers than linear ones.

2.3.2 Methods for protein-protein interaction extraction

Similar to the research methodology in our previous work (Li et al., 2009), we first designed an enhanced lexical feature set considering words and n-grams in specific positions of sentences, and then proposed several types of EDFs and CDFs for the PPIE task. We also combined lexical features and FCD features to get a higher performance

2.3.2.1 Corpus and preprocessing

We used AImed corpus to examine our methods. We converted each sentence to lowercase, replaced XML tags like """ by their standard ASCII characters, and then tokenized a sentence by splitting tokens from non-letter or digit characters, e.g., "wild-type (d)" -> "wild - type (d)". We replaced the two focus proteins in the current example by "prot1" and "prot2", and the other proteins in the same sentence by "prot0". We also replaced all the examples with overlapping "prot1" and "prot2" (self-interactions) by the same sentence "prot1 prot2 ."

Before introducing lexical features and FCD features, we give some notions that describe words, n-grams, areas or positions in sentences with regard to interacting proteins.

Vocabularies of words: LW = {words in labeled data}, and UW = {words in unlabeled data}.

Vocabularies of n-grams: LN = {1-3 grams in labeled data}, and UN = {1-3 grams in unlabeled data}.

General areas: *GA* = *{left_area, inner_area, right_area}* -text snippets split by *"prot1"* and *"prot2"* in each sentence denoted by *"left_area prot1 inner_area prot2 right_area"*.

Surrounding areas: *SA* = *{p1_left, p1_right, p2_left, p2_right}* - texts surrounding *"prot1"* or *"prot2"* within a 3-word window.

Specific positions: *SP* = *SA* × *{1, 2, 3}* = *{p1_left_1, p1_left_2, ...}* - words or n-grams that appear in certain positions of *SA*. See also the example in Figure 6.

Cross patterns: CP = {p1_dirction_offset ^ p2_direction_offset ^ distance | direction ∈ {left, right}, offset ∈ {1}, distance ∈ {0, 1, 2, 3, 4, 5, (6~7), (8~10), (11~15), (16~20), (21~30), (31~40), (40~) } } - "cross-entity" conjunctions of partial elements in SP and the discretized word count between the two proteins.

2.3.2.2 Lexical features

Note that the lexical features used in the recent works (Miwa et al., 2008; Miyao et al., 2009) based on AImed corpus only involved bag-of-words or simple variants. Here we attempt to enhance lexical-level representation by incorporating n-gram and position information and give a detailed evaluation of the contribution of each feature type. Four types of features are investigated in our work:

Bag-of-words (GA-BOW): features derived from *LW*×*GA*, e.g., *word_in_left_area* =*"expression"*. These features ignore word positions in the current area, which are almost the same as features of the baselines used in the works (Miwa et al., 2008; Miyao et al., 2009).

Bag-of-n-grams (GA-Lex): features from *LN*×*GA*. It simply enriches the bag-of-words representation by bigrams and trigrams.

Surrounding n-grams (SA-Lex): features from *LN*×*SA*, e.g., *p1_right="interacts with"*. They are used to highlight n-grams in the "indicating areas" since intuitively features surrounding candidate protein pairs are more indicative.

Specific n-grams (SP-Lex): features from *LN*×*SP*, which gives the information of the specific distances from protein candidates to n-grams in *SA*, e.g., *p1_right_1="interacts"*, and *p1_right_2="with"*. It provides more specific information than the "surrounding n-grams".

Our classifier for all the lexical features is SVM light (http://svmlight.joachims.org/) with linear kernel and default parameters.

2.3.2.3 FCD features

FCD measure and unlabeled data

In this work, we consider one type of FCD measure:

$$FCD1 = \frac{\log_{10}(co(x,y)+b)}{\log_{10}(count(x)+b) * \log_{10}(count(y)+b)} \tag{5}$$

where x is an EDF, y is a CDF, and co(x, y) is the co-occurrence count of x and y. The smoothing factor b is assigned 1. We log the term count to avoid highly biased values in very large corpus. This measure can be viewed as a variant of pointwise mutual information (PMI). We discussed its advantage in our previous work (Li et al., 2009).
The experimental results in our previous work (Li et al., 2009) show that the performance of FCD features increases when more unlabeled data are added. So in this work, we downloaded more data, which include all the PubMed abstracts (up to 2009) and data collection of TREC genomics track 2006 (Hersh et al., 2006; Li et al., 2009), with the total size of 20GB. We tokenized the texts in the same way as the method in Section 2.3.2.1 and tagged the protein names using the gene/protein mention tagger developed in our previous work (Li et al., 2009). We used the "dictionary-based" method because it is very fast. The method for the dictionary construction was also based on FCG and it achieved an F-score of 86.2 on BioCreative 2 Gene Mention test corpus (Wilbur et al., 2007). Note that in the PPIE task, "unlabeled" means no need to label the protein-protein interactions, but the protein names should be recognized first.

EDF selection

We examine the performances of two types of EDFs which are also derived from the lexical information introduced in Section 2.3.2.1:
SP-EDF: EDFs derived from UN×SP. It can be viewed as the extension of SP-Lex features to the vocabulary of UN. Obviously it has stronger discriminating ability than features derived from GA or SA. But the set of EDF roots was selected as SA not SP because SP resulted in higher feature dimension and space cost but the performance varied little (not reported in this work due to page limitation).
CP-EDF: text patterns derived from the set UN×CP. The set of EDF roots is CP′ = {p1_direction ^ p2_direction ^ distance | direction ∈ {left, right}, distance ∈ {0, 1, 2, 3, 4, 5, (6~7), (8~10), (11~15), (16~20), (21~30), (31~40), (40~)}}. One SP-EDF only considers a text snippet surrounding one protein, which may limit its discriminating ability, while a CP-EDF incorporates information from both sides across "prot1" and "prot2".

CDF selection

The method for generating CDFs is very simple. We used information gain - a popular feature selection technique - to rank lexical features introduced in Section 2.3.2.2 and selected top 400 ones as CDFs. This idea is similar to our prior wok on named entity classification (Li et al., 2009).
Note that rather different from lexical features, these EDFs and CDFs are not elements of the input vectors of the target classifiers. They are used only for generating FCD features which

belong to part of the final feature vectors. Figure 6 shows an example of the generation of FCD features for the PPIE task, where only SP-EDFs and one type of FCD measure are considered, so the FCD features are indexed by the conjunction of EDF roots and CDFs. It can be seen clearly that the "sparse" EDFs are "generalized" to a "higher-level" representation.

Classification model

In the work (Li et al., 2009), we found the density of FCD features was much higher than lexical features widely used in NLP and was somewhat like the feature spaces for image recognition, which inspired us to make use of non-linear classifiers. We used SVD plus RBF kernel and achieved better results than linear kernel. Similarly, for the PPIE task we also investigated the two models: linear SVM and RBF kernel based SVM. For the RBF model, we first used SVD to get a sub-space of FCD features and then used the new features as the inputs of SVM with RBF kernel. In our experiments, SVD was done on the entire AImed corpus and top 300 most significant features in left-singular matrix were selected. The parameter "-c" and "-g" of SVM light were set at 3.0 and 20.0 respectively. Then we combined the prediction scores of lexical features and FCD features given by SVMs using a simple weighted linear function, where their weights were set at 0.5 and 0.5 respectively.

2.3.3 Results and discussion

2.3.3.1 Evaluation metrics

We attempt to keep our evaluation metrics as the same as most recent works (Airola et al., 2008; Miwa et al., 2008; Miyao et al., 2009). We used F-score as the primary evaluation measure and also reported AUC. They suggested that for this task, abstract-level cross validation should be done to avoid sentences in the same abstract are both used for training and testing. We also performed abstract-wise 10-cross validation, where abstracts were divided into 10 groups, and one was used for testing and the others for training in each turn. We also extracted CDFs from each training data separately to avoid the use of answers in testing data at training time.

2.3.3.2 Lexical features

Features	P	R	F	AUC
F1	41.9	62.8	50.0	78.7
F1+F2	46.5	61.6	52.1 (+2.1)	80.5
F1+F2+F3	54.3	61.5	57.2 (+7.2)	83.6
F1+F2+F3+F4	56.8	63.1	59.0 (+9.0)	84.9

Table 6. Performance of lexical features. F1: GA-BOW, F2: GA-Lex, F3: SA-Lex, F4: SP-Lex.

Table 6 shows the performances of various combinations of lexical features. We can see the F-score of GA-BOW features is 50.0, which is similar to the results reported in the recent work (Miyao et al., 2009), where the F-score of a similar feature set is 51.1. The discrepancy may be caused by lemmatization they used, or the detailed methods in data preprocessing and splitting stages. It can be seen that features derived from n-grams, surrounding areas and specific position information improve the performance significantly and produce a surprisingly good result – 59.0 F-score and 84.9 AUC, which is competitive to most of the recent works based on syntactic parsing (Airola et al., 2008; Miwa et al., 2008; Miyao et al.,

2009) (see also Table 8). Note that this run only used simple Boolean lexical features, so it is much faster and easier to implement than syntactic based methods, which will make it of great value in practice. To our best knowledge, the features (F2, F3, and F4) are not explicitly used as Boolean lexical features in the PPIE task and their contribution is not examined well on the AImed corpus. The simple idea of creating these lexical features is similar to our work on entity classification (Li et al., 2009), just following the cue: "word -> n-grams -> n-grams in specific positions".

2.3.3.3 FCD features

Table 7 shows the performances of runs with FCD features. It can be seen that the F-score of SP-EDFs is lower than CP-EDFs, possibly because features derived from SP only consider specific n-grams surrounding one protein, so they have lower example-discriminating ability than CP, thus produce weaker FCD features. However, SP-EDFs yield higher recall and seem benefit more from non-linear classifier than CP-EDFs. From Run 2 to Run 5, we cannot see the significant advantage of non-linear classifiers, but Run 7 outperforms Run 6 by near 3 points in F-score, since in our experiments we fixed the parameters of SVD and RBF kernels for all the runs, which were tuned to optimize the performance of FCD features with both EDFs. So the results also support the fact that RBF kernel performs better for these FCD features. In Table 7, we also find that the runs with both the two EDFs (Run 6 and 7) produce a further improvement over each single feature (Run 2-5). Note that Run 7 doesn't use any classical features, while its performance is competitive to any single type of features proposed by previous researchers.

ID	Features (Models)	P	R	F	AUC
1	lexical (linear)	56.8	63.1	59.0	84.9
2	SP-EDF (linear)	43.2	58.1	49.9	76.7
3	SP-EDF (SVD + RBF)	47.9	58.5	51.4	79.8
4	CP-EDF (linear SVM)	49.5	55.9	52.2	80.3
5	CP-EDF (SVD + RBF)	50.1	54.4	52.3	78.6
6	SP+CP EDF (linear)	49.7	62.9	54.2	81.3
7	SP+CP EDF (SVD + RBF)	59.9	57.8	58.1	83.1
8	lexical +FCD (1 + 7)	59.3	68.2	62.9	87.3

Table 7. Performance of FCD features

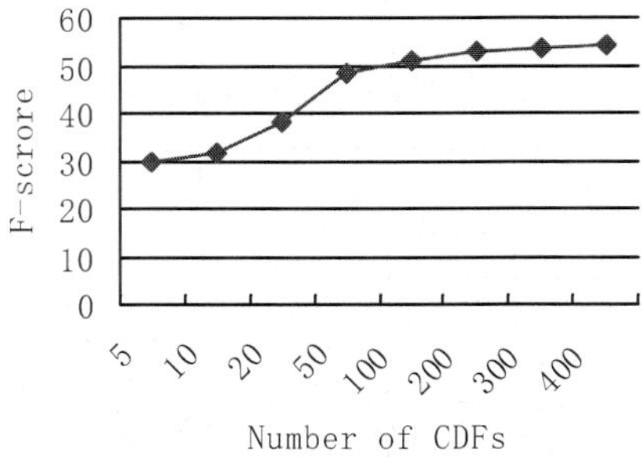

Fig. 7. Relationship between the number of CDFs and the performance of FCD features.

It is promising to see that Run 8 (Table 7) that combines the results of lexical and FCD features by simple average produces a significant improvement over the lexical features on both F-score and AUC, although the baseline is rather strong. The results in Table II have proved the success of applying FCG to the PPIE task. However, the improvement of FCD features is not as huge as the entity classification task (Li et al., 2009), where the improvement is over 6 points in F-score. We think it is mainly because the EDFs and CDFs investigated here are relatively simple. For example, only information of words surrounding the interacting proteins within a 3-word window is considered in EDFs. Also the EDFs in the PPIE task are not so "obvious" as that in the NEC task, since it is more difficult to select the "example-distinguishing" part of a sentence concerned with two interacting proteins. In addition, the introduction of more types of CDFs would also enhance the performances, since in Figure 7, the performance of PPI extraction increases when more CDFs are incorporated.

2.3.3.4 Comparison with other systems

Methods	F	AUC
Our method (Combined)	62.9	87.3
(Miwa et al., 2008)	62.7 (64.3)	83.2 (87.9)
(Miyao et al., 2009)	59.5	
Our method (Lex)	59.0	84.9
Our method (FCD)	58.1	83.1
(Airola et al., 2008)	56.4	84.8
Bag-of-words	50.0	78.7

Table 8. Comparison with other systems

For the work in (Miwa et al., 2008), the scores in brackets are their reported results obtained by removing all the examples with self-interaction protein pairs in AImed corpus.

In Table 8, we compare the performances of our methods with other results reported in previous researches evaluated on AImed corpus. Although it is difficult to make strict comparison due to different methods for data splitting and pre-processing, it can be seen that our combined method is among the state-of-the-art systems. It is an important finding for both biomedical text mining and NLP community, because unlike other methods, not any syntactic information is used in this run. Another interesting finding is that our simple lexical features create a strong baseline for other methods to challenge, since it not only achieves good results but is much more efficient than syntactic based methods.

In our previous work (Li et al., 2009), we discussed the efficiency of FCG in real world applications. In summary, for real-time application, it needs the support of "feature-level" search engine. Alternatively if the task can be divided into non-real-time sub-tasks, we can run FCG on each sub-task in an offline manner. For example, in this task, we can generate a huge number of lexical patterns indicating for PPI and used FCG to remove noisy patterns. Then the refined patterns are used as features integrated into the lexical feature-based method (Section 2.3.2.2). The idea is similar to the dictionary construction for the NER task (Li et al., 2009). In this way, we can both utilize the information from unlabeled data and make the system efficient.

3. Conclusions

In this chapter, three different protein-protein interactions extraction approaches representing the state-of-the-art research in this area are introduced.

Firstly, we present a multiple kernels learning based approach to extracting protein-protein interactions from biomedical literature. The approach combines feature-based kernel, tree kernel, and graph kernel with different weights and achieves much better performance than each individual kernel. This indicates that the features in individual kernels are complementary and the combined kernel can well integrate them: 1) the flat entity information captured by the feature-based kernel; 2) the structured syntactic connection information between the two entities captured by the tree kernel, graph kernel and POS path kernel.

Secondly, we present a lexical feature-based SVM model to extract PPI information from biomedical literature. During the supervised learning process, to reduce annotation effort while maintaining the PPI extraction performance, we employ an uncertainty sampling based method of active learning to tag the most informative unlabeled samples. The experiment results show that our method can reduce the labeling cost by 40% and 20% on the two corpora respectively without degrading the performance. In addition, the number of samples picked up in each round can be set to a large value to speed up learning process. Besides, to further accelerate USAL process, our method only reserves one of the same uncertainty samples. To further speed up learning process, a threshold is used to restrict the uncertainty. The samples whose uncertainties are within the threshold are picked up to tag, and the other samples are ignored. The experiment results show these methods reduce much annotation effort and training time with slight loss of performance.

Finally, we present the application of FCG semi-supervised learning strategy to the PPI extraction task and show that FCD features derived from simple lexical information can achieve good results and produce further improvement over a high baseline.

Currently, PPI extraction methods generate poorer results compared with other domains such as newswire and there is still much room for performance improvement. In the future work, we will focus on designing EDFs and CDFs that cover more lexical or linguistic information (e.g., from shallow or syntactic parsing) of the whole sentences. Since many experiments show that FCD features perform well in non-linear classifiers, we will examine other popular learning techniques in pattern recognition. It is encouraging to see that FCG can perform well in the two different NLP tasks: entity classification and relation extraction, so we will continuously examine this method in more tasks on natural language processing and machine learning. In addition, as discussed in Section 2.1.2.2, introducing more domain knowledge such as protein-protein interactions ontology into PPI extraction from biomedical literature may help address the emerging challenges of deep natural language understanding.

4. References

Airola, A., Pyysalo, S.; Björne, J.; Pahikkala, T.; Ginter, F. & Salakoski, T. (2008). All-paths graph kernel for protein-protein interaction extraction with evaluation of cross-corpus learning. *BMC Bioinformatics*, no.9(Suppl 11):S2.

Angluin, D. (1988). Queries and concept learning. *Mach Learn*, vol. 2, no. 4, pp., 319-342.

Bader, G.D.; Betel, D. & Hogue, C.W. (2003). BIND: the biomolecular interaction network database, *Nucl. Acids Res*, vol. 31, no. 1, pp. 248-250.

Blaschke, C. & Valencia, A. (2002). The frame-based module of the Suiseki information extraction system. *IEEE Intelligent Systems*, vol. 17, no. 2, pp.14-20.

Bunescu, R.C. & Mooney, R.J. (2005a). A shortest path dependency kernel for relation extraction. In: *Proceedings of Human Language Technology and Empirical Methods in Natural Language Processing*, pp. 724-731, British Columbia, Canada.

Bunescu, R.C.; Ge, R.; Kate, R.J.; Marcotte, E.M.; Mooney, R.J.; Ramani, A.K. & Wong, Y. (2005b). Comparative Experiments on Learning Information Extractors for Proteins and their Interactions. *Artif Intell Med*, vol. 33, no. 2, pp. 139-155.

Bunescu, R.C. & Mooney, R.J. (2006). Subsequence kernels for relation extraction. In: *Advances in Neural Information Processing Systems 18*, Weiss Y, Schölkopf B, Platt J, (Ed.), pp. 171-178. MIT Press, Cambridge, MA.

Cohn, D., Atlas, L., & Ladner, R. (1994). Improving generalization with active learning. *Machine Learning*, vol. 15, no. 2, pp. 201-221.

Collins, M. & Duffy, N. (2001). Convolution Kernels for Natural Language", In: *Proceedings of 14th Conference on Neural Information Processing Systems*, pp. 625-632, Cambridge, MA.

Corney, D.P.; Buxton, B.F.; Langdon, W.B. & Jones D.T. (2004). BioRAT: extracting biological information from full-length papers. *Bioinformatics*, vol. 20, no. 17,pp.3206-3213.

Cristianini, N. & Taylor, J.S. (2000). *An introduction to support vector machines and other kernel-based learning methods*. Cambridge University Press, 0521780195, New York.

Danger, R.; Rosso, P.; Pla, F. & Molina, A. (2008). PPIEs: Protein-protein interaction information extraction system. *Journal of Procesam ento del lenguaje natural*, no. 40, pp. 137-143.

Fundel, K.; Küffner, R. & Zimmer, R. (2007). RelEx-Relation extraction using dependency parse trees. *Bioinformatics*, vol. 23, no. 3, pp.365-371.

He, Y.L.; Nakata, K. & Zhou, D. (2008). Ontology-Based Protein-Protein Interactions Extraction from Literature Using the Hidden Vector State Model. In: *Proceedings of 2008 IEEE International Conference on Data Mining Workshops*, pp.736-743,Pisa, Italy.

Hersh, W.; Cohen, A.; Roberts P. & Rekapalli, H.K. (2006). TREC 2006 genomics track overview, In: *Proceedings of 15th Text REtrieval Conference (TREC)*, Gaithersburg, Maryland.

Kim, S.; Yoon, J. & Yang, J. (2008). Kernel approaches for genic interaction extraction, *Bioinformatics*, vol. 24, no. 1, pp. 118-126.

Krallinger, M.; Leitner, F. & Valencia, A. (2007). Assessment of the second BioCreative PPI task: automatic extraction of protein-protein interactions. In: *Proceedings of the 2nd BioCreAtIvE Workshop*, pp. 41-54,Madrid, Spain: CNIO.

Lewis, D., & Catlett, J. (1994). Heterogeneous uncertainty sampling for supervised learning. In: *Proceedings of the Eleventh International Conference on Machine Learning*, pp.148-156. New Brunswick, USA.

Li, Y. P.; Lin, H.F. & Yang.Z.H. (2009). Incorporating Rich Background Knowledge for Gene Named Entity Classification and Recognition, *BMC Bioinformatics*, no. 10:223.

McCallum, A. & Nigam, K. (1998). Employing EM and Pool-Based Active Learning for Text Classification. In: *Proceedings of the Fifteenth International Conference on Machine Learning*, pp.350-358. Madison, USA.

Miwa, M.; Sætre, R.; Miyao, Y.; Ohta, T. & Tsujii, J. (2008). Combining Multiple Layers of Syntactic Information for Protein-Protein Interaction Extraction. In: *Proceedings of the Third International Symposium on Semantic Mining in Biomedicine*, pp.101-108, Turku, Finland: Centre for Computer Science.

Miwa, M.; Soetre, R.; Miyao, Y. & Tsujii, J. (2009). Protein-protein interaction extraction by leveraging multiple kernels and parsers, *Int. J. Med. Inform.* vol. 78, no. 12, pp. e39-46.

Miyao, Y.; Sætre, R.; Sagae, K.; Matsuzaki; T. & Tsujii J. (2009). Evaluating contributions of natural language parsers to protein-protein interaction extraction. *Bioinformatics*, vol. 25, no. 3, pp. 394-400.

Moschitti, A. (2006). Making tree kernels practical for natural language processing. In: *Proceedings of the 11th Conference of the European Chapter of the Association for Computational Linguistics*, Trento, Italy.

Ono, T.; Hishigaki, H.; Tanigam, A. & Takagi, T. (2001). Automated extraction of information on protein-protein interactions from the biological literature. *Bioinformatics*, vol. 17, no. 2, pp.155-161.

Sekimizu, T.; Park, H.S. & Tsujii, J. (1998). Identifying the interaction between genes and gene products based on frequently seen verbs in MEDLINE abstracts. *Genome Inform*, vol. 9,pp. 62-71.

Shen, D.; Zhang, J.; Su, J.; Zhou, G. D. & Tan, C. L. (2004). Multi-Criteria-based Active Learning for Named Entity Recognition. In: *Proceedings of the 42nd Association of Computational Linguistic*, pp.589-596. Barcelona, Spain.

Thompson, C. A.; Cali, M. E. & Mooney, R. J. (1999). Active learning for natural language parsing and information extraction. In: *Proceedings of the 16th International Conference on Machine Learning*, pp.406-414. Bled, Slovenia.

Wilbur, J.; Smith, L. & Tanabe, L. (2007). BioCreative 2. gene mention task, In: *Proceedings of the Second BioCreative Challenge Evaluation Workshop*, pp. 7–16, Madrid, Spain: CNIO.

Xenarios, I.; Rice, D.W.; Salwinski, L.; Baron, M.K.; Marcotte, E.M.; Eisenberg, D. (2000). DIP: the Database of Interacting Proteins, *Nucleic Acids Res*, vol. 28, no. 1, pp. 289-291.

Xiao, J.; Su, J.; Zhou, G.D. & Tan, C.L. (2005). Protein-Protein Interaction Extraction: A Supervised Learning Approach. In: *Proceedings of the First International Symposium on Semantic Mining in Biomedicine*, pp. 10-13, Hinxton, Cambridge, UK.

Yang, Z.H.; Lin, H.F. & Li, Y.P. (2010). BioPPISVMExtractor: A protein-protein interaction extractor for biomedical literature using SVM and rich feature sets. *J Biomed Inform*, vol. 43, no. 1, pp.88-96.

Zanzoni, A.; Montecchi-Palazzi, L.; Quondam, M.; Ausiello, G.; Helmer-Citterich, M. & Cesareni, G. (2002). Mint: A molecular interaction database, *FEBS Lett.* vol. 513, no. 1, pp. 135-140.

Zhang, M.; Zhang, J.; Su, J. & Zhou, G.D. (2006). A Composite Kernel to Extract Relations between Entities with both Flat and Structured Feature. In: *Proceedings of the 21st International Conference on Computational Linguistics and 44th Annual Meeting of the ACL*, pp. 825-832, Sydney, Australia.

Zhou, D.; He, Y. & Kwoh, C.K. (2006). Extracting Protein-Protein Interactions from the Literature Using the Hidden Vector State Model. In: *Proceedings of the International Workshop on Bioinformatics Research and Applications*, pp. 718-725, Reading, UK. LNCS 3992, Springer-Verlag.

Part 8

Technology and Instrumentation

27

Recent Research and Development of Open and Endo Biomedical Instrument in Surgical Applications

Zheng (Jeremy) Li
University of Bridgeport
United States of America

1. Introduction

The biomedical surgical instruments are mainly designed to perform specific functions during the surgical procedures including modifying biological tissue, open and close the organs and tissues, and providing access to view it. The surgical instruments are designed for general or specific procedures in surgery, and specialized professionals and engineers can provide assistance to surgeon with proper handling of surgical instruments in surgical operation. The important difference in surgical instruments is the amount of bodily disruption and tissue trauma that instruments might cause the patients. The development of minimally invasive surgical instruments is in the positive and future directions for surgical product industry. Surgical instruments were designed and developed since ancient times. The following real breakthrough in surgical instrument development comes with advanced biomedical technologies, better materials, and improved manufacturing techniques (Lin et al., 2007). Later more new surgical instruments were again invented and designed with the new biomedical engineering technologies to allow surgeon performing more complicated surgical procedures to patients. Some precision medical instruments were developed for microsurgery and endoscopic surgery in the late 20th century (Cheng et al., 2004). In order to prevent the instruments from corrosion due to blood contamination and sterilization, the nontoxic, durable and anti-corrosion materials were developed for surgical instruments. The modern manufacturing techniques help to produce the cost effective biomedical surgical instruments. The advanced biomedical researches over the past centuries significantly improve human's life quality. Biomedical instrument design and development is to apply engineering principles and techniques to the biomedical fields to reduce the gap between engineering and surgery and combine the engineering design knowledge and problem solving with biomedical and surgery science to improve surgical procedures, diagnosis and treatment. Biomedical surgical instrument design and development is an interdisciplinary field that affected by other technological and biomedical fields including mechanical, electrical and chemical engineering. The surgical instrument design should be collaborated regarding prospective design improvements based on clinical experiences. The development progression of the state-of-the-art instruments must be traced to reconstruct procurement patterns and influence the trajectory of surgical instrument innovation accordingly. Biomedical Surgical instruments are developed to facilitate many different procedures and operations. The good understanding of fundamental engineering knowledge, different engineering disciplines, human anatomy and physiology is required in surgical instrument design and development.

The surgical instruments include the devices performing clamping, occluding, probing, suturing, and ligating. Improper use of surgical instruments will lead alignment problems (Piatt et al., 2006). While using surgical instruments, the institutional and professional protocols must be strictly followed, and necessary medical trainings will be required. In surgical procedure, the previously sterilized instruments must be maintained clean to keep blood and tissues from hardening, otherwise the blood and hardened tissues will be trapped between organ surface and surgical instruments. The minimally invasive surgery, aided by improved surgical instruments, can minimize the trauma to patients, reduce health care costs, and shorten the recovery time after surgery. Similar to ligatures, suture might cause the suppuration surround the wound edges (Evans et al., 2006). The process is slow and patients feel pain when remove the sutures. Our new surgical instruments including open and endo clip instruments can speed up the suture process and improve surgical procedure. This chapter introduces the new surgical open and endo clip instruments with improved mechanism to apply the metal clips to patient's vessel / tissues in the surgical operations. The new surgical instrument design aids in better ergonomic design, reliable functionality, continuous cost reduction, and minimally invasive therapy procedure. The improved clip delivery systems have been designed and developed in these two types of surgical instruments to improve the clip distal move from clip channel into jaw guide track and resolve the problems of clip accidental shooting out when surgical clips are being loaded into jaw pair by compression spring that has been normally used in some current surgical clip instruments. With this improvement, the new surgical open and endo clip instruments can prevent patient's vessels and tissues from being damaging because the distal move of clips are well controlled without clip drop-off incident. Plus the operational forces to form the open or endo surgical clips are lower than regular surgical instruments due to new mechanism design. Moreover, the manufacturing and product costs of these two surgical instruments can be decreased because the dimensional tolerance of components, such as clip channel and jaw guide track, can be wider due to the new instrument design. The prototype of these new open and endo surgical instruments are analyzed and optimized through computer aided modeling and simulation to prove its feasible function, reliable performance, and mechanical advantage. All these improved features have also been tested and verified through the prototype.

2. Open surgical instrument:

In the surgical operations, surgeons and doctors need to apply the hemostasis instrument to the severed organs or tissues to stop the bleeding. The instrument jaw pair is placed at the organ or vessel structures. When instrument handles are being brought together, the clip can close and secure the tissue or vessel to prevent them from bleeding. The next surgical clip is automatically loaded into the instrument jaw when instrument handles are released. Surgical procedures need ligation of blood vessels, severed tissues and organs to stop bleeding. Surgical clip instruments for quickly applying a surgical clip onto tissue or vessel include single clip and multiple clip applications (Sun et al., 2005). A new clip is loaded into the apparatus after applying each clip in single clip applications and the multiple clip applications include a series of clips that can be sequentially applied to tissue during the course of a surgical procedure. Open surgical clip instruments normally have a trigger handle mechanism, a major body portion, a clip crimping assembly and some other functioning components including a pair of jaws. Although the current surgical instruments for continuously advancing individual clip have been proposed, the continuing improvements for better surgical clip delivery with cost-effective apparatus is required to provide efficient occlusion of a blood vessel.

Currently some feedbacks from clinic fields indicated the incidents of clip dropping off from clip channel while being delivered to the jaw pair in the existing open surgical clip instruments. In these cases, the closed jaw pair will sever or damage the tissue if there is no surgical clip in the jaw pair. The clip drop-off problem is mainly caused by improper dimensional tolerance control in clip channel, clip guide track in jaw pair, and transition area between these components during production process. In order to smoothly load the clips through compression spring, the high cost manufacturing process is required to precisely maintain the high surface quality and accurate dimension controls on these components, otherwise the clips will be dropping off if the dimensional tolerance is too wider or clips will not be moving by spring force if the dimensional tolerance is too tight. The clip delivery mechanism of new surgical clip instrument is different from current clip instrument. In this new design, clips are advanced to jaw pair through distal movement of clip pusher which is driven by instrument handles. When surgeons and doctors bring the instrument handles together, the clip will be fully formed after clip pusher distally delivers clip into the jaw guide track. When surgeons release instrument handles, the clip pusher returns proximally to original home position and then picks up next clip. Because the clip advancing process can be easily and well controlled in this new design, the high dimensional tolerance control is not required to these components in manufacturing process. This can ease the machining process, increase the productivity, and save the production cost.

The prototype tests have been carried out on dogs including vascular occlusion, ligating for tubular ducts, and applying the surgical clip to the tissue. The preliminary testing results indicated no clip drop-off incident in this new surgical instrument design and the closure force to fully form the clip is between 3.38 lbf that is lower than 4 lbf in current surgical clip instrument.

2.1 Analysis on new open surgical instrument

The surgical clip instrument, shown in Figures 1, 2 and 3, is first placed around patient's body tissue or vessel, and then clip is distally moving to jaw pair through clip pusher and secured onto the tissue or vessel when surgeons close the trigger handles. When surgeons release the trigger handles, jaw pair is open, clip pusher and driving bar return to their original positions. Compared with the current clip delivery apparatus in which the clip is advancing to jaw pair through compression spring that sometime causes accidental clip shooting out from instrument, the clip delivered into jaw pair in this new instrument design is well guided and controlled. The driving bar that linked to the pivot pin in handles moves distally to advancing clip into jaw pair when surgeons gradually close the instrument handles. Such clip linear motion can be easily and well controlled by surgeons to prevent the clip from accidentally shooting out from instrument. The preliminary prototype testing of this new design has proved its proper and reliable performances since there is no clip shoot out and operational force is lower than usual.

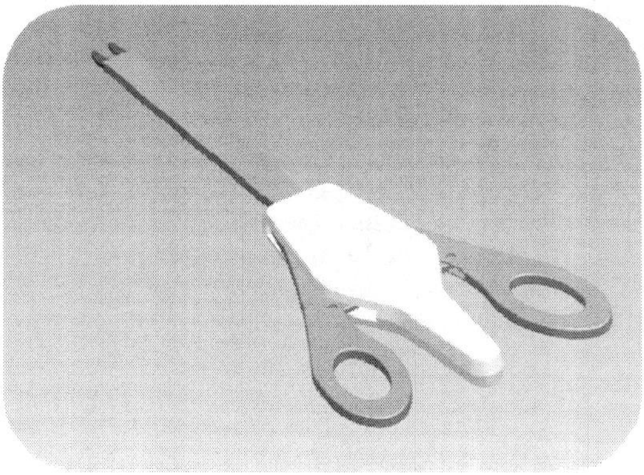

Fig. 1. Prototype of new open surgical instrument

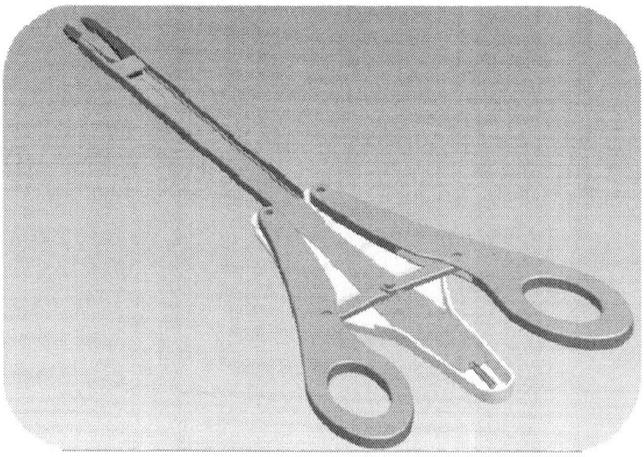

Fig. 2. New mechanisms including handle, linkages, driving bar and clip pusher

2.2 Computer aided modeling and analysis on new design

The velocity ratio of ($V_{angular}$ / V_{linear}) can be determined through computational simulation targeting the optimized instrument performance, and simulation results are indicated in Figures 4 and 5.

The mechanical advantage of this new instrument can be determined when surgical clip has been fully formed:

$$\text{Mechanical advantage} = (VR) * 2.148$$

$$= (.04866 / .03533) * 2.148 = 2.958 \quad (1)$$

The above result shows that if 20 lbf forces are required to fully form or close the surgical clip, the force loaded on surgeon's finger will be 3.380 lbf which are lower than the normal spec of 4 lbf in surgical operation procedure and this meets the surgeons' requirement. Also, the results of this computational simulation and prototype testing are very close to each other which verify the credibility of this new instrument design and research methodology.

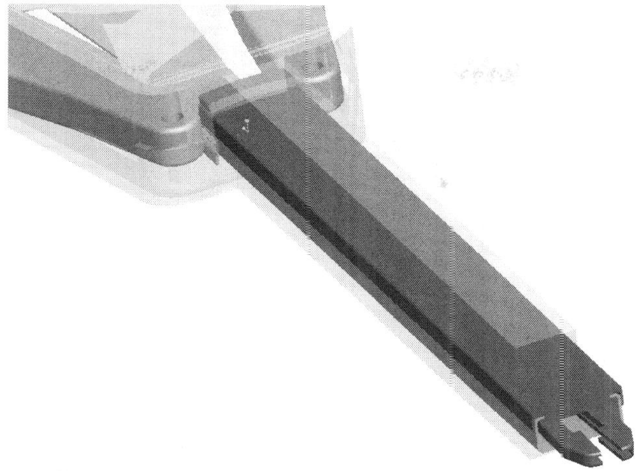

Fig. 3. Front view of new open surgical instrument

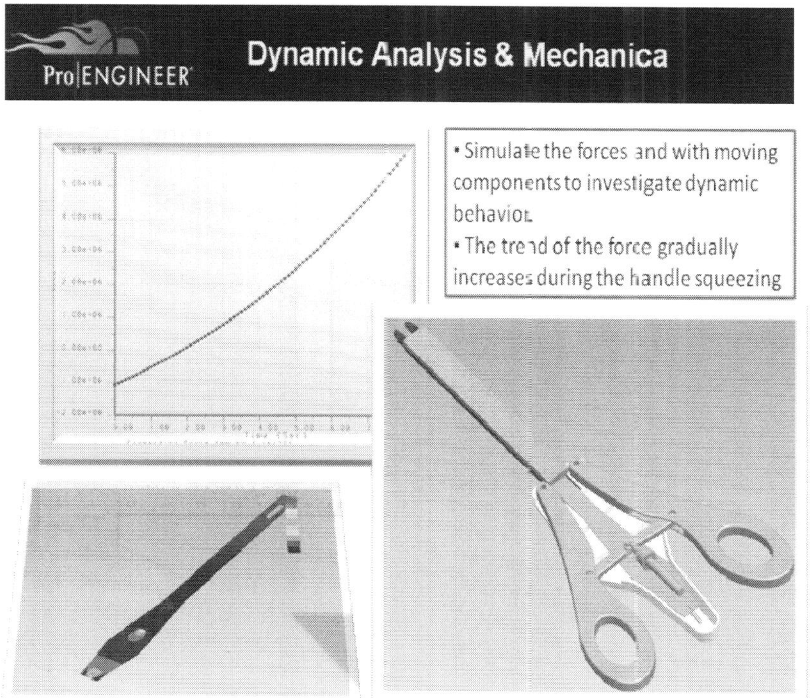

Fig. 4. FEA and dynamic analysis of mechanism in this surgical instrument

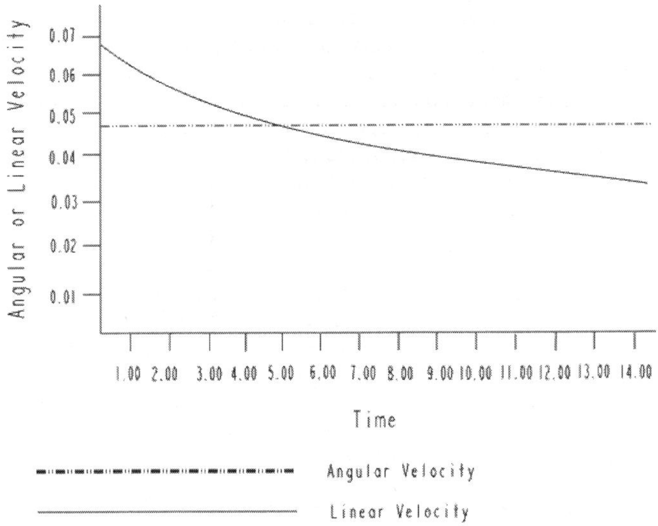

Fig. 5. Linear and angular velocity vs. time phase in operating the instrument

2.3 Discussion

The feasible functioning and reliable performance of this new open surgical instrument has been preliminarily proved based on the instrumental functional study, computerized simulation and prototype testing. The major advantages of this new surgical instrument include that the clip distal advancing can be well guided and controlled to prevent patient's vessel and tissue from damage due to accidental clip shooting out during surgical procedure, operational force to fully form clip is lower than usual, manufacturing and product cost will be decreased because of this new instrument design. The prototype of this new surgical instrument has been tested and the preliminary results show the potential improvement. While this new instrument is being sent to fields for clinical evaluation, the further improvement will be considered including enhancing the structure of jaw pair to prevent jaw pair from twisting in case the instrument is not being used properly in the field, adding supporting feature to prevent jaw pair from accidental close when unanticipated side load exerted to the jaw pair, and simplifying the instrument design to further reduce the product cost.

3. Endo surgical instrument.

The biomedical/surgical instrument market is very competitive and has been measured and controlled for its performance, feasibility, safety, and production cost (Chu et al., 2005). This market is price sensitive and dominated by different advanced technologies. Biomedical/surgical instrument is technology based product which requires the special techniques to compete today's challenging market. The endo surgical instruments can be applied to close tissue defects, perforations, and anastomotic leakage in the esophagus and stomach (Starly et al., 2005). The recent studies indicate the versatility of endo surgical clips in therapeutic and endoscopic applications (Laufer et al., 2007). Endo surgical instruments have been normally applied in hemostasis using endoscopy to the upper and lower gastrointestinal tract in which the bleeding lesions can be effectively clipped. The methods other than endoscopic clipping of peptic ulcers are thermal therapy or injection of epinephrine to constrict the blood vessel (Kassam et al., 2007). Comparative studies between endo surgical clips and thermal therapy verify that endo surgical clips cause fewer traumas to the mucosa around the ulcer than electrocautery.

3.1 Analysis of endo surgical instrument

The operation of this endoclip instrument is illustrated as follows. An endo surgical clip is loaded and retracted into a protective sheath in this endo surgical instrument. The instrument is inserted through the open channel of an endoscope and the sheath is forced backwards by the instrument handle which can drive the clip from the sheath. The clip can be pulled back to open its prongs. The distance between the clip prongs reaches the maximum when instrument jaw tips fully open. Turning the instrument handle clockwise can adjust and control the orientation of endo surgical clip prongs and pulling the clip proximally can fully close the surgical clip.

The figure 6 shows this new endo surgical instrument, figure 7 indicates the cross-section view of endo surgical instrument.

3.2 Computer modeling and simulation

Referring figure 8, the energy balance and force equations in this new endo surgical instrument design can be derived as follows.

AB represents the pushing bar and EF is the trigger handle. Considering the ergonomic factor, the length of EF should properly fit most surgeons' hand size. When calculating the geometry factor of this mechanism, the length of BC, CD, DE and angle should be first determined. Assume the squeeze force is F, angle EDC is θ, angle ABC is α.

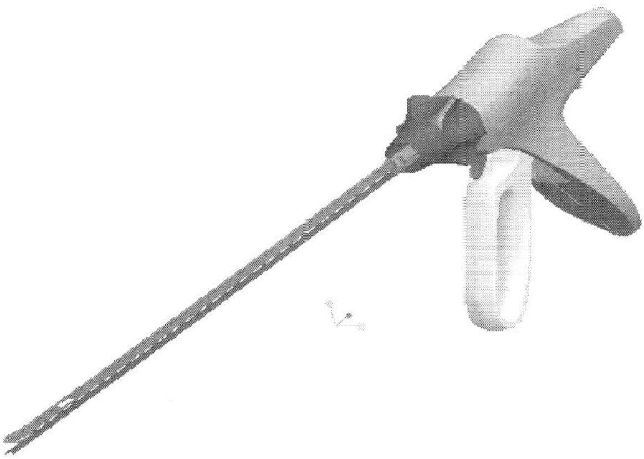

Fig. 6. Endo surgical instrument

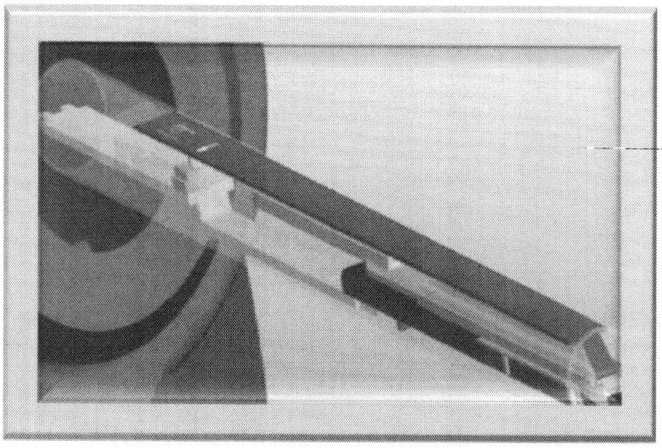

Fig. 7. Cross section view of endo surgical instrument

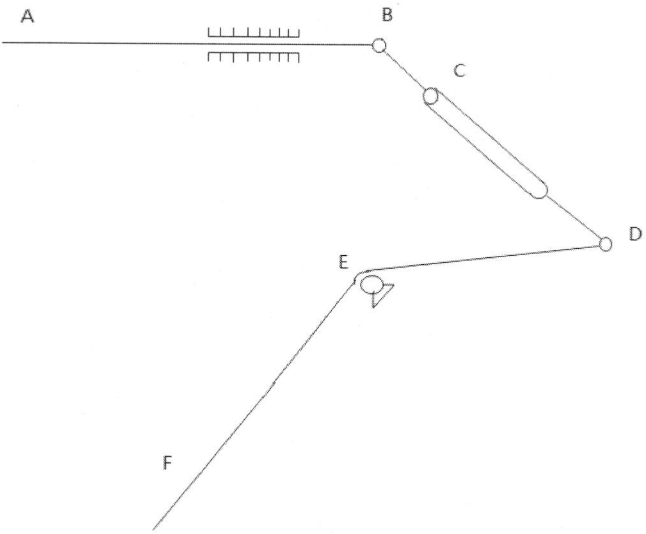

Fig. 8. Mechanism diagram

$$F * 0.5\ EF = F_1 * DE \tag{2}$$

$$F_1 * \cos(\theta) = N * \cos(180-\alpha) \tag{3}$$

N is the force exerted onto pushing bar.

The velocity ratio of ($V_{angular}$ / V_{linear}) can be determined by computer aided simulation targeting optimized instrument performance, and simulation results are shown in Figure 9.

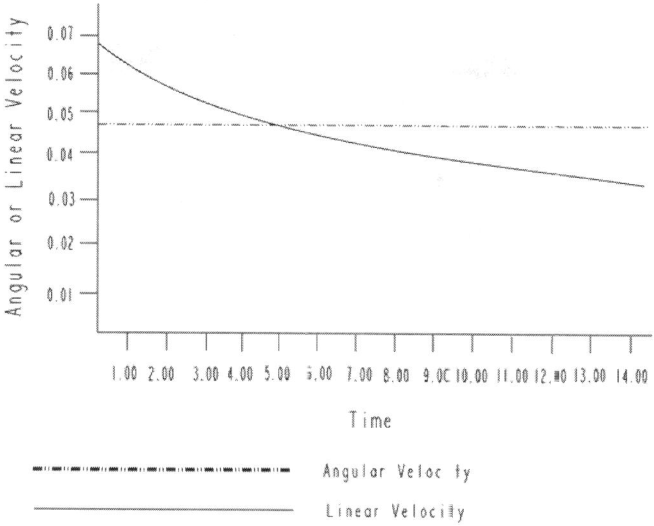

Fig. 9. Linear and angular velocity vs. time phase of instrument operation

The mechanical advantage of this new instrument can be found when surgical clip is fully formed:

$$\text{Mechanical advantage} = (VR) * (3.75 / 1.70)$$

$$= (.04840 / .03125) * (3.75 / 1.70) = 3.415 \quad (4)$$

This result shows that, if 20 lbf forces are required to fully form the surgical clip, the operational force that surgeon needed is 2.928 lbf that is lower than normal spec of 4 lbf and this will benefit surgeons in their surgical procedure. Also, both computational simulation and prototype testing results are very close which verify and prove the credibility of this new instrument design and research methodology.

3.3 Discussion

This section presents the results of a new endo surgical/biomedical instrument design using 3D modeling simulations with CAD modeling software and structure/stress analysis by FEA simulation software. 3D modeling and computer aided simulation can benefit geometrical and dynamical analysis in conceptual and feasible design of biomedical surgical instruments. The geometric, dynamical and visual limitations of the surgical instruments are analyzed to assist the surgeon in surgical procedures. 3-D CAD modeling simulation is applied to the endo surgical equipment based on its feasible geometry and weeping boundary. The kinematics of precision mechanism design can be simulated and modeled as either an open or closed-loop joint chain with some rigid bodies connected to each other in a series format, driven by actuated mechanism. The analysis of kinematical structure in mechanism can provide a systematic and general approach to determine and calculate mechanism motion functionality. This new endo surgical instrument shows its feasible and reliable functionality, better mechanical advantage, cost effective in manufacturing process, and safe in use. This new biomedical/surgical instrument design has been analyzed and verified through the computational simulation and prototype testing. In addition to the preliminary lab testing, this new instrument has been sent for further hospital and field evaluations to continuously improve this instrument including enhancement of jaw section to keep instrument jaw tip portion from extra deformation when instrument is not being operated correctly in surgical processes, adding wedge plate between jaw area to keep jaw from unanticipated closure while additional side load exerted to the jaw tips, and modifying the instrument mechanism to further reduce the manufacturing cost.

4. References

Lin HJ, Lo WC, Cheng YC, Peng, CL (2007), "Endoscopic Hemoclip Versus Triclip Placement in Patients with High Risk Peptic Ulcer Bleeding", *Journal of Gastroenterol*, Vol. (102), pp 539-543.

Cheng AW, Chiu PW, Chan PC, Lam SH (2004), "Endoscopic Hemostasis for Bleeding Gastric Strormal Tumors by Application of Hemoclip", *Journal of Laparoendoscopic & Advanced Surgical techniques*, Vol. (14), pp 169-171.

Piatt, J., Starly, B., Faerber, E. and Sun, W. (2006), "Application of Computer-Aided Design Methods in Craniofacial Reconstructive Surgery Using a Commercial Image-Guidance System", *Journal of Neurosurgery*, Vol. (104), pp. 64-67.

Evans, P., Starly, B. and Sun, W. (2006), "Computer-Aided Tissue Engineering for Design and Evaluation of Lumbar-Spine Arthroplasty", *Journal of Computer-Aided Design and Application*, Vol. 3(6), pp. 771-778.

Sun, W., Starly, B., Nam, J. and Darling, A. (2005), "Bio-CAD Modeling and Its Application in Computer-Aided Tissue Engineering", *Journal of Computer- Aided Design*, Vol. 37(11), pp. 1097-1114.

Chu, Fang-Cheng and Chang, B. C. (2005), "Automatic Visual Tracking Control System Using Embedded Computers", *Proceeding of the 2005 IEEE International Conference on Mechatronics*, July 10-12.

Starly, B., Fang, Z., Sun, W. and Regli, W. (2005), "Three-Dimensional Reconstruction for Medical-CAD Modeling", *Journal of Computer-Aided Design and Application*, Vol. (2), pp. 431-438.

Laufer, Llya, Anand, Vijay and Schwartz, Theodore H. (2007), " Endoscopic, endonasal extended transsphenoidal, transplanum transtuberculum approach for resection of suprasellar lesions", *Journal of Neurosurgery, Vol. (*106). pp. 400-406.

Kassam, Amin, Thomas, Ajith, Snyderman, Carl, Carrau, Ricardo, Gaedner, Paul, Mintz, Arlan, and Kanaan, Hilal (2007), "Fully endoscopic expanded endonasal approach treating skull base lesions in pediatric patients". *Journal of Neurosurgery*, Vol. (106), pp. 75-86.

28

Critical Issues in Reprocessing Single-Use Medical Devices for Interventional Cardiology

Francesco Tessarolo[1], Iole Caola[2] and Giandomenico Nollo[1,3]
[1]BIOtech, Interdepartmental Center on Biomedical Technologies. University of Trento,
[2]Department of Microbiology and Virology, Azienda Provinciale per i Servizi Sanitari,
[3]Department of Physics. University of Trento,
Italy

1. Introduction

1.1 Single-use vs. multiple use medical devices

During the 1960s and the early 1970s, most medical devices made of glass, rubber, or metal were generally considered to be reusable. This concept did not change until the late 1970s, when medical devices started to enter the market labelled "single-use only".

During the same decades, clinical medicine has undergone substantial changes, with traditional open surgical procedures giving way to new minimally invasive techniques such as endovascular and laparoscopic intervention. Such procedures required new instruments allowing delicate and complex manipulations through small incisions, with the effector portion of the device located some distance from the operator's hand, demanding stable and predictable performance. During this same period, patients and clinicians have become increasingly concerned about the risk of infectious disease transmission, particularly human immunodeficiency virus and hepatitis B and C viruses.

One solution to both demands was found in single-use devices (SUDs), shaped from newly developed fabrication materials, firstly polymers, and intended to be discarded after use on a given patient. Consequently, the past three decades have seen an explosion in the production and use of single-use medical devices, stemming from a desire to improve product performance and minimize the potential for disease transmission, and enabled by advances in manufacturing techniques.

1.2 SUDs reprocessing

Although a number of advantages are related to the use of disposable goods in medicine, single-use devices are typically more costly on a per-use basis. SUDs are relatively expensive to purchase and their one-patient/one-product nature made necessary enlargement of hospital inventories and the resulting stream of medical waste.

These aspects have led to the interest in reprocessing and reuse of these devices. Many hospitals began to explore the reprocessing and a limited reuse of products intended for single use, initially using on-site facilities as they have traditionally done with multiple-use metallic surgical instruments. As single-use products became more complex, hospitals began to turn to third-party reprocessors to handle reprocessing needs.

Differently from the simple re-sterilization, the reprocessing practice is generally perceived to mean the cleaning, disinfection and sterilization of a medical device, including related procedures, as well as the functional testing and repackaging, carried out on a medical device after it has been put into service (EU Public Consultation, 2007).

Reprocessing and reuse of SUDs have gained wide popularity in the last years as a result of the escalating cost of health care. A survey conducted in 2000 revealed that approximately 20%−30% of hospitals in the United States reprocess SUDs (GAO, 2000). Data are likely underestimated because hospitals tend not to report their use of reprocessed SUDs. According to the United States General Accounting Office, substantial cost savings can be achieved by reprocessing SUDs because the cost of in-house reprocessing can be less than 10% of the cost of a new device and the cost of third-party reprocessing is approximately 50% of the cost of a new device (GAO, 2000). A national survey in Canada, investigating the current practices of reprocessing and reusing SUDs in Canadian acute-care hospitals indicates that 28% of hospitals participating in the survey reprocessed single-use devices (Polisena et al., 2008), and gave an overview on the types of SUDs most frequently reprocessed at acute-care hospitals in Canada.

The basic and legitimate questions before starting a reprocessing policy are: i) Are reprocessed SUDs as good as the original devices in terms of chemical and physical characteristics? ii) Is it safe and economically convenient to use reprocessed SUDs? iii) How should reprocessing be regulated to ensure public health?

In a commentary on reusing SUDs it is agreed that the answer to these questions depend on to whom they are addressed (Quian & Castaneda, 2002). Most of the opposition against reprocessing of SUDs comes from the original equipment manufacturers (EUCOMED, 2002), whereas the medical community is generally supportive of reprocessing (Lindsay et al., 2001). In general, legislation advocates the precautionary approach till scientific evidences are sufficient to guarantee safeness and efficiency. Anyhow, commentary in the scientific literature on this subject is relatively sparse.

1.3 The current status about reprocessing SUDs

Nowadays, the practice of reusing SUDs prevails in almost all developing countries of Africa, Asia, Eastern Europe, Central America, and South America, where there are shortages of medical supplies and financial resources (Quian & Castaneda, 2002). The rationale behind the reuse of disposable devices in these countries is simple and forceful. The overwhelming public demand for minimally invasive procedures made the single-use of devices financially and ethically unsustainable: otherwise, only those patients with sufficient resources would avail themselves of these new procedures because public institutions could not afford the use of disposable devices for the indigent population (Ruffy, 1995).

The evidence for the safety and effectiveness of reusing SUDs is indirect with the majority of studies set in laboratory contexts evaluating surrogate outcomes such as medical device integrity and contamination after reprocessing. Few studies involved outcomes directly related to patients. It is difficult to define adequately a direct causal link between patient exposures to contaminated or faulty medical devices and adverse patient outcomes due to a lack of data on cross-infection and loss of device functionality.

Conflicting results comes from the available studies. Some studies concluded that the reuse of SUDs is potentially safe and effective with strict reprocessing protocols and standards.

Others do not recommend reprocessing and reuse because the evaluated devices were not clean or sterile and changes in device integrity were evident. These conflicting results were apparent for anaesthesia devices (Daggan et al., 1999; Lipp et al., 2000), airways devices (Vezina et al., 2001), and disposable plastic trocars (Chan et al., 2000; Roth et al., 2002). The reprocessing and reuse of sphincterotome devices was considered safe and effective with proper reprocessing standards (Kozarek at al., 1999). Studies investigating biopsy forceps consistently showed that reprocessing standards were not met as the devices were not clean nor sterile (Hambric 2001, Kinney et al., 2002). In general there are ethical constraints in using patients in studies designed to determine the 'risk' associated with reusing SUDs, thereby limiting the overall evidence base. However, despite the existence of some recommendations and protocols governing the reuse of SUDs many items are still being reprocessed and reused without definitive evidences on the safety of these practices. Reports of cases where the use of reprocessed medical devices intended for single-use have caused harm to patients are scarce. It is thus difficult to estimate the incidents frequency as, in general, the personnel involved is likely to be reluctant to report the incidents for insurance or other reasons. In most European countries, the reporting of incidents is not mandatory. In the United States, reporting of incidents involving medical devices is mandatory and all reported incidents are integrated into a searchable database. However, when analysing the reported incidents, the Government Accounting Office did not find any evidence that reprocessed SUDs caused more incidents than other devices (GAO, 2008).

2. Reusing SUDs in interventional cardiology

Nowadays, one of the few areas where reprocessing and reuse of SUDs seems suitable both for safeness and cost effectiveness is interventional cardiology (Lindsay et al., 2001; Bourassa, 1996, CETSQ, 1994; Krause et al., 2000; Day, 2004). Radiofrequency catheter ablation and percutaneous transluminal coronary angioplasty have emerged as important therapeutic options for patients suffering respectively from a variety of arrhythmias and coronary diseases. A significant portion of the cost for the procedure is represented by the cost of the multielectrode diagnostic and ablation electrophysiology catheters (EP) or the coronary angioplasty balloon catheter (PTCA). Both catheter types are nowadays labelled and marketed as single use only.

Similarly to other SUDs, in the past, as the demand for disposable equipment rose, hospital administrators and physicians began to notice that some products labelled "single use only" were similar to devices that had been formerly distributed as "reusable". It was reported about a letter by one of the major cardiac catheter manufacturer that stated, "our manufacturing processes of Woven Dacron Intracardiac Electrodes have not changed. These electrodes are made with the same materials and in the same manner they have been in the past" (CCHR, 2000). In response to what many physicians and hospital administrators perceived as an arbitrary labelling policy, the practice of reprocessing SUDs evolved to reduce costs and the amount of medical waste. As this practice encompassed critical devices such as electrophysiology and PTCA catheters the complexity of decontamination and sterilization procedure increased. The role of hospital committees (physicians, nurses, infection control specialists, risk managers, hospital lawyers, and professional reprocessors) evolved to monitor the safety of repeocessing methods. Many hospital administration believed this practice was safe, some made use of third party reprocessors, and others abandoned the practice altogether.

In the present context, material and technological advancements brought to produce and place on the market high-quality and technologically advanced devices for interventional cardiology with higher therapeutic efficiency but considerably more expensive interventions. Considering the worldwide shortening of economic resources in healthcare systems, the issue of reuse and reprocessing feasibility in a field like interventional cardiology, reveal a great interest and represent a very topical problem.

2.1 The clinical knowledge on reprocessing SUDs in interventional cardiology

The issue of reprocessing single use devices in interventional cardiology has been debated from many years and literature presents some investigations which have been conducted to explore technical feasibility, safety, and efficacy of introducing a reprocessing policy in hospital and health care institutions (Bloom et al., 1997; Blomstrom-Lundqvist, 1998; Azyman et al., 2002; Brown et al., 2001; Browne et al., 1997; Chaufour et al., 1999; Granados et al., 2001; Luijt et al., 2001; Ma et al., 2003). Available scientific evidences are of utmost importance for in deep addressing this topic and pointed out the need for new experimental data on technical feasibility, and clinical effectiveness since new materials, manufacturing advancements and substantial technological improvements are frequently introduced in the production of new medical device generations.

Some clinical studies tried to convey clinical data on safety and efficiency by introducing reprocessing and reuse practices in the interventional context and retrospectively or prospectively evaluating patients' outcome. Moreover, some case studies highlighted important benefits and limitations of the reprocessed instrumentation that arose during clinical reuse. All these evidences will constitute the starting point for approaching the reprocessing issue and formulating recommendations and guidelines even more efficient and precise.

The issues pertaining to the safety and efficacy of reusing catheters focus on the risk of transmitting an infection from one patient to an other and the structural and functional integrity of a catheter that is used more than once on different patients. Differently from resterilization procedures that are quite well established, protocols for SUDs disinfection and cleaning are often lacking or improperly designed. Moreover, objective procedure for the measurement of catheter integrity and functionality are not as well documented since they are highly related to materials and design. Some catheters are subjected to very little stress during a procedure, while the deflectability or manoeuvrability of others may change considerably. Lumen cleaning, disinfection and patency are critical due to the peculiarity of catheter design and, sometimes, rapid and effective procedures are to be implemented. Moreover, reprocessing may affect catheter materials and could have a significant impact on functionality.

2.2 Electrophysiology and ablation (EP) catheters

A few published studies have evaluated the safety of reusing catheters for electrophysiological studies and have addressed some of these issues. O'Donoghue and Platia surveyed 12 medical centres to determine the safety of reusing EP catheters (O'Donogue & Platia, 1988). The incidence of infection related to a total of 14640 electrophysiological studies, involving 48075 catheter uses, was reported. At three centres, catheters were automatically discarded after a single use. These centres carried out 1245 electrophysiological studies using 3125 catheters. At the other nine centres, the catheters were sterilized for reuse. There were 13395 interventions using 44950 catheters in the reuse group. The incidence of bacteraemia (blood borne infection) and superficial skin infection at the site of catheter insertion were respectively 0.03% and 0.03% for the single use group and 0.018% and 0.002% for the reuse group. The authors concluded that sterilization and reuse of the catheters used in this study did not result in an increase in the risk of infection. They felt the catheters were sufficiently durable to be reused well in excess of five times, and that one-time use of such catheters appeared to be an unnecessary and expensive policy.

Dunnigan et al. obtained similar results in a prospective study that evaluated catheter reuse over a 5-year period during which 178 catheters were used 1576 times for 847 electrophysiological studies (Dunnigan et al., 1987). No complications were encountered during the study period. All reused catheters were effective for cardiac pacing and recording of cardiac electrical signals. Surveillance cultures and biological indicators revealed that adequate sterilization procedures were used. The authors concluded that electrophysiological catheter may be safely reused provided a thorough cleaning, testing, and record keeping system is instituted. They also concluded that the practice of reusing catheters would result in substantial cost savings to hospitals.

The clinical trials presented above were conducted in patients undergoing diagnostic electrophysiological studies before the advent of deflectable catheters and arrhythmia ablation procedures.

Avital et al. prospectively investigated the time course of electrical, physical, and mechanical changes in ablation catheters to determine the effect of reuse on safety and efficacy (Avital et al., 1993). They studied 69 ablation catheters made by a single manufacturer that were used in 336 procedures. Testing of physical integrity consisted of visual and stereoscopic examination of handle function, catheter shaft, and the deflectable tip. Specific attention was paid to the ablation electrode attachment to the catheter shaft, and the ablation tip electrode was scrutinized for pitting. The electrical integrity of the catheters was checked by measuring the electrical resistance from the handle connector to the recording rings and to the tip electrode. Deflection and torque measurements were made to assess mechanical integrity. During the course of this study 36 catheters (52%) were rejected at some point because of mechanical or electrical failure. Eighteen catheters were repeatedly sterilized and 11 of the catheters were used 10 times. The most common reasons for catheter rejection were tip electrode glue separation after 4.3±4.3 uses and loss of deflection after 5.0 ± 3.3 uses. The glue that covers the most proximal portion of the distal electrode was shiny and uniform before any use. The application of radiofrequency energy causes a rise in tissue temperature and the electrode tip is heated secondarily. Small fractions of glue were missing and may have been released into the bloodstream. Catheters with blood that collected in this space could not be properly cleaned. There was no evidence that the tip to shaft attachment was affected by the outer glue separation; however, the possibility that the attachment of the tip electrode was weakened by the glue separation was not excluded by the authors. Electrical discontinuity was observed after 10.0±3.7 uses. There was no significant decrease in the catheter torquing ability that determines the steering responsiveness of the catheter. The medical records of 140 patients who had arrhythmia ablation procedures in this study revealed only one case (0.7%) of local infection at the insertion site that was treated effectively by antibiotics. There were no other complications.

Avital and co-workers concluded that the catheter model used in this study could be reused an average of five times. They recommended that, after each use, catheters be carefully examined under magnification with special attention to the tip electrode. They also recommended that the catheters be tested for deflection and electrical integrity after each use.

As part of an internal quality review process Aton et al. determined the effects of reprocessing on mechanical integrity, sterility, and chemical residuals to establish and validate an institutional policy for reuse (Aton et al., 1994). A total of 12 commercially available catheters from two manufacturers were analysed. Eleven of the catheters were randomly selected from the catheter inventory of the clinical electrophysiological laboratory after being used one to four times. They were manually cleaned, repackaged, and gas sterilized with ethylene oxide. To assess the sterility of reused catheters, three were cut into 2-inch segments, placed in bacterial culture media, and incubated for 5 days. Six of the catheters were analysed for chemical residuals after gas sterilization. Two catheters were examined for evidence of component failure. Visual inspection and microscopy were used to determine the mechanical integrity of the catheter surface, and x-ray inspection was performed to assess interior structures.

The study results of Aton et al. showed no bacterial growth detected on any of the cultures, which indicated that reprocessed electrode catheters are effectively sterilized. The chemical analysis demonstrated that the concentrations of ethylene oxide detected in extraction liquid exceeded standards established by the FDA. Microscopic examination of reprocessed catheters demonstrated inconsequential metal and fibre particulates on the catheter surface and at some electrode to catheter interfaces. Fluid entrapment around the distal pole may occur in catheters with tip electrodes. The shaft of the catheters and the electrodes remained intact. No evidence of electrical discontinuity was found and the integrity of the internal structures was confirmed by x-ray inspection. The authors concluded that, with the sterilization techniques frequently used at that time by hospitals, the potential for chemical residual contamination might exist after sterilization with ethylene oxide.

2.3 Percutaneous coronary angioplasty (PTCA) catheters

Similarly to EP catheters, a few clinical trials were performed to assess safety and efficiency of PTCA reprocessed catheters and only a single randomised, double blind, clinical trial was found in the English literature.

In 1994 a first relevant and debated study by Plante et al. was designed to determine the effectiveness, safety and costs associated with reuse of angioplasty catheters and to compare these results with those of a contemporary centre that employed a single-use strategy in Canada (Plante et al., 1994). In a prospective observational study, data forms were completed after each angioplasty procedure and before patient discharge over a 10-month period. A total of 693 patients were enrolled in the two centres. Clinical and lesion characteristics were similar except for a higher incidence of unstable angina at the reuse centre. The angiographic success rate was identical (88%) at both centres, but the reuse strategy was associated with a higher rate of adverse events, prolonged procedure time and increased use of contrast medium, especially in lesions that were not crossed by the initial balloon and in patients with unstable angina. Whether these differences are related to the reuse strategy or to differences in patient groups cannot be ascertained by this observational study as pointed out by Rozeman and colleagues (Rozemann et al., 1995).

Mak et al. re-evaluated clinical data from Plante's study using a multivariate statistical model with the purpose to control for the differences in the baseline clinical characteristics of the patients at the two centres and to determine if catheters reuse was associated with an increase in complication rate (Mak et al., 1996). The reanalysis showed that the reuse of balloon catheters was not associated with an increased in-hospital event.

A study conducted in the United States by Browne and co-workers aimed at evaluating the performance of angioplasty catheters, restored under a strict remanufacturing process (Browne et al., 1997). Used PTCA balloon catheters were shipped to a central facility and were decontaminated, cleaned and tested for endotoxins. Physical testing and quality assurance were performed before the products were packaged and sterilized with ethylene oxide. Catheter performance was assessed in a pilot study powered to detect a 5% difference in the angiographic failure rates of new and reused balloons. Under specific indication for PTCA procedure, 107 patients were enrolled, 106 had a successful laboratory outcome, and 1 required coronary artery bypass graft surgery after failed rescue stenting. Over 122 lesions attempted, the angiographic failure rate was 7% (10 of 108) comparable to the 10% rate seen with new balloons in other studies. Authors concluded that restoration of disposable coronary angioplasty catheters using a highly controlled process appears to be safe and effective, with success rates similar to those of new products and no detectable loss of performance. Moreover the reported cost analysis suggested that implementation of reuse technology for expensive disposable equipment may offer cost savings for U.S. hospitals, without sacrifice of quality.

Shaw et al. examined the effects of catheter reuse on duration of PTCA procedures and clinical outcomes by retrospectively analysing clinical data of two patients group isolated before and after July 1996 in Canada (Shaw et al., 1999). In July 1996, because of concern regarding the possible transmission of Creutzfeldt-Jakob disease, the province of Quebec stopped the reuse of PTCA catheters. Prior to this time, PTCA balloon catheters were commonly used a maximum of four times in the enrolled health centre. After this time, only new catheters were used. Fifty-three consecutive patients undergoing PTCA prior to 21 July 1996 were compared with 54 consecutive patients undergoing PTCA after that time. It was concluded that there were no significant differences between the single-use and reuse groups with respect to baseline characteristics, no significant differences in the numbers of PTCA catheters used (97 vs. 103) or angiographic success rates (88% vs. 83%). Authors stated that, if catheter reuse is not found to be associated with infectious disease transmission, its widespread use should be considered.

The first randomised, double-blind, controlled, single centre, clinical trial has been performed by Zubaid and colleagues (Zubaid et al., 2001). The study compared the safety (clinical success) and efficacy (angiographic success) of reused versus new coronary angioplasty balloon catheters on a total of 377 procedures, 178 performed by reused catheters and 199 by new catheters. No significant differences in clinical or lesion characteristics between the two approaches were found. The incidence of first balloon failure in reused catheter was similar to that of the new catheter (7% vs. 5%) and the angiographic success rate was also similar with 176 cases (98.9%) in reused catheters and 196 cases (98.5%) in new catheters. The number of balloon catheters used per lesion, amount of contrast, and procedural and fluoroscopy time were similar in the two arms. At 30 days, the incidence of major adverse cardiac events was similar in both cases (4.5% vs. 5%). The study concluded that, in a wide variety of patients, the clinical results of reused balloon catheters are similar to those of new catheters and reused catheters are as effective and safe as new catheters.

A prospective randomised trial comparing new and reprocessed balloons, including stented and stand-alone balloons, has been more recently proposed by Unverdorben and colleagues

(Unverdorben et al., 2005). Percutaneous coronary interventions were performed randomly in 238 consecutive patients with either new or 1 to 3 times reused balloon catheters. Crossing of the stenosis decreased from 96% with new balloon catheters to 93.2%, with 1 time reused balloon catheters to 81.8% with 2 times reused catheters and to 80.8%with 3 times reused catheters. In all primary failures using resterilized balloon catheters, new ones of the same nominal diameter were successful. The angiographic follow-up rates were 77.4 % for new balloon catheter, 79.5% for 1 time reused balloon catheters, 75.0 % for 2 times reused balloon catheters, and 80.8% for 3 times reused balloon catheters. The percent stenosis was higher in reused versus new balloon catheters, as was the restenosis rate. There was one death in reused balloon catheter category but no event of myocardial infarction. Rates of target lesion revascularizations were similar in stent recipients and more frequent after stand-alone balloon angioplasty with reused versus new balloon catheters. According to clinical data, authors concluded that the use of two or three times resterilized balloon catheters does not seem to be justified in stand-alone balloon angioplasty of *de novo* coronary stenoses and should be limited to stent procedures until data will be available for other indications.

2.4 Limitations of available clinical data

Some criticisms could be made of the above reported studies. Retrospective surveys might depend on the memory of those who responded. Isolated events could escape the attention of the participants in the survey or they may have forgotten complicating events. Some of the prospective studies involved small numbers of patients. In general the methodology of these studies varied and is unlikely to meet recognized standards. Specifically, reprocessing procedures are not harmonized and sometimes not clearly reported. It is also unclear if the protocols used to reprocess the devices were insufficient or if the devices could indeed not be properly reprocessed. Studies claiming safety of reprocessed device do not cover any form of long-term observation of patients regarding the development of infectious diseases and/or immunological complications following exposure. Moreover, the catheters used in the majority of these studies are old designs. Because changes in materials or/and functions might have a significant impact on the durability of electrophysiology and angioplasty catheters, it should not be assumed that prior safety data is applicable to new catheter designs that are nowadays used in the clinical practice.
This chapter aims at eliciting, discussing and integrating recent experimental findings for the assessment of a reprocessing policy on interventional cardiac catheters labelled as "single use only". The experimental techniques here reviewed supply new parameters for the assessment of quality and safety of reprocessed devices before starting a clinical trial on patients. To this end, technical data and legal, ethical, and economic issues are integrated in order to define the applicability and suitability of SUDs reprocessing.

3. Technical issues

3.1 Chemical and physical analysis of new and reprocessed devices

The reprocessing protocol should be conceived and designed according to the peculiar characteristics of the device to reuse (Fig. 1). Manufacturers of reusable devices are required to specify in details the proper cleaning, disinfection and (whenever required) sterilization methodologies for guaranteeing a safe and effective reuse on patient. Differently, disposable devices, labelled as "single-use only" do not provide any information addressing for reprocessing procedures. Moreover there is a diffused scarcity of materials and designs details on the accompanying documentation. This lack of technical data demands for a complete and exhaustive characterization of the device, posing a particular attention to materials, coatings, and design.

Tessarolo et al. applied a wide number of experimental analytical technique to address essential information about polymer composition and fillers, metals and coatings, surface and bulk parameters, mechanical and thermodynamic materials properties, micro and macro design of PTCA and EP catheters The preliminary characterization of device, allowed to define detergents, procedures, and sterilization methods according to procedural standards, materials composition, and design. Long and narrow lumens of PTCA catheters demanded for ethylene oxide sterilization, while gas-plasma sterilization was applicable for non irrigated EP catheters (Tessarolo et al., 2004a).

The reprocessing feasibility from a technical point of view has been evaluated on non-irrigated electrophysiology and non-stented coronary angioplasty devices produced by the major worldwide manufacturers. Chemical-physical properties have been assessed on both new and reprocessed devices by using advanced analytical techniques for surface and bulk material characterization such as optical microscopy (OM), electron microscopy (EM), atomic force microscopy (AFM), and infrared spectroscopy (IR).

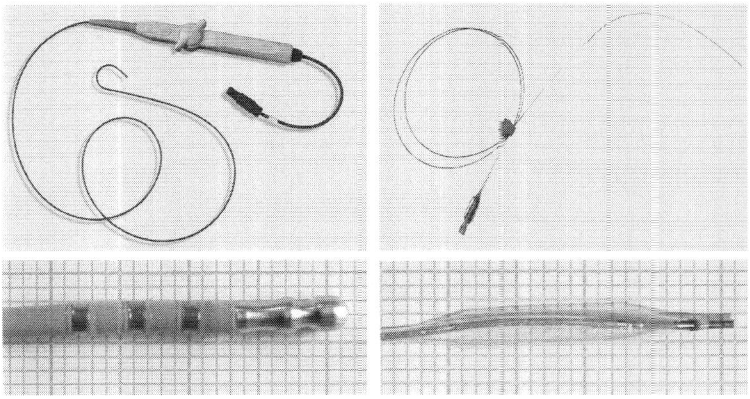

Fig. 1. Representative electrophysiology (upper left) and angioplasty (upper right) catheter for interventional cardiology marketed as single-use only. Images in the bottom show distal portions of the catheters including the functional units: electrodes for recording endocardiac ECG signal and ablation of myocardial tissue (lower left) and an inflated ballon for coronary reprocessing, chemical and physical characterization was carried out at different number of arthery dilation in case of stenosis (lower right). The grid is 1x1mm squared. Adapted from Tessarolo et al., 2004a.

To identify device alterations induced by clinical use and/or reprocessing cycles catheters were characterized after clinical use, simulated reuse, and repeated reprocessing (from 0 to 14 cycles for EP and from 0 to 6 cycles for PTCA) (Fedel et al., 2006; Tessarolo et al., 2004b; Tessarolo et al., 2005; Tessarolo et al., 2006a). OM on EP catheters revealed reprocessing-dependent scratches on the polyurethane shaft's surface (Fig. 2) (Tessarolo et al., 2004b). EM and AFM documented a physical-chemical etching on polymers, due to plasma sterilization, and a significant increasing in nano-roughness after 7±4 cycles of reprocessing (Fig.3) (Tessarolo et al., 2004b).

Residuals of iodate contrast medium in PTCA underlined the need for a timely and efficient cleaning of balloon lumen to avoid crystallization and loss of functionality. Infra-red spectrum suggests that ethylene oxide did not significantly modify polymer's bulk characteristics (Fedel et al., 2006). These studies elicited that materials are highly model dependent and should be verified after each reprocessing cycles. Critical steps for materials modifications were identified in cleaning and sterilization phases.

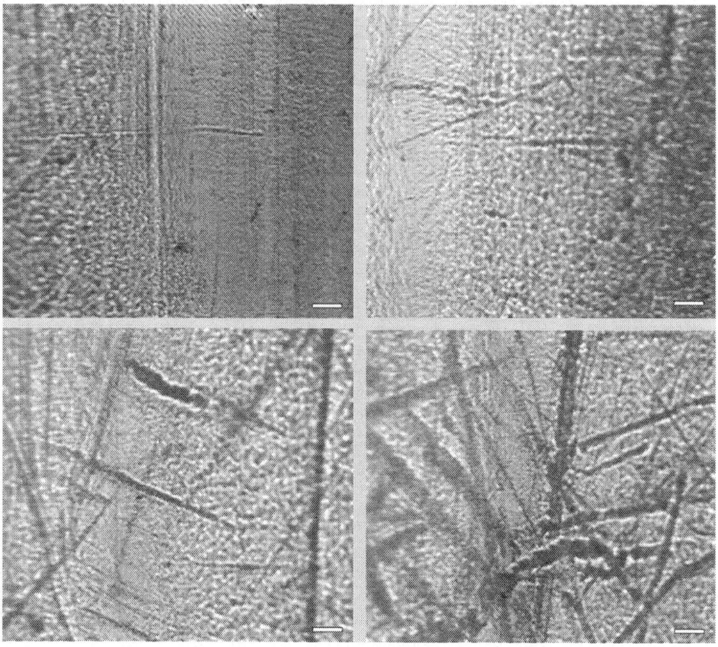

Fig. 2. Optical microscopy on EP catheter shafts. Scratches and indentations were caused by both clinical use and mechanical and/or manual brushing during cleaning procedures. The amount of scratches was related to the number of reprocessing cycles. From left to right and from top to bottom: new device, 1, 4, 8 times regenerated devices. Bar is 20 μm.

3.2 Functional testing of reprocessed devices

To estimate the maximum number of reuses sustainable by the device in an effective status, functionality was assessed by realizing specific experimental set-ups for both EP and PTCA catheters. Tissue- and organ-synthetic phantoms were realized for simulating clinical use and obtaining quantitative an reproducible functional measurements. Radiofrequency ablation efficiency, electrical characteristics, and catheter slipperiness were quantified in EP devices until 10 cycles of reprocessing (Tessarolo et al., 2004a). Compliance curve, crossing profile, burst pressure, and slipperiness were checked at different steps of the protocol on new and reprocessed PTCA catheters up to three uses (Fedel et al., 2006).

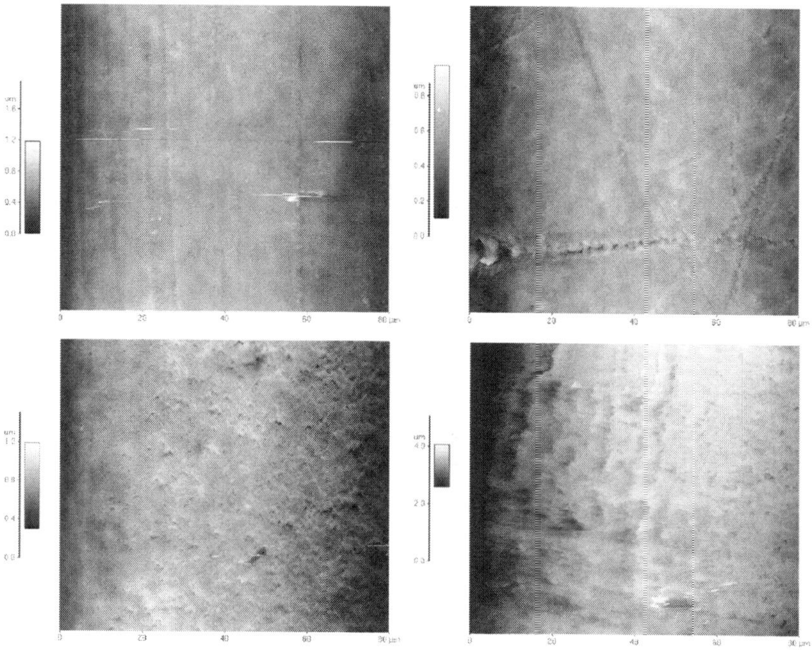

Fig. 3. AFM on EP catheter shaft. Polyurethane underwent progressive nanometric roughening with repetitive gas plasma sterilization. Alterations were induced by the chemical and physical etching of the sterilization technique. From left to right and form top to bottom: new device, 1, 4, 8 cycles regenerated devices. Adapted from Tessarolo et al., 2004b.

Functionality tests on EP catheters elicited no variations in ablation efficiency, electrodes conductivity, thermometric sensor's precision and accuracy (Tessarolo et al., 2005). Differently, slipperiness tests showed a worsening of lubricious properties in regenerated EP devices after 4 cycles in accordance to the increase of surface roughness. Conversely, functional properties of PTCA catheters were affected by both clinical use and reprocessing procedures (Fig. 4) (Fedel et al., 2006). As a consequence of the mechanical stress in clinical use, balloon diameter at nominal pressure tended to increase. Differently thermo-chemical stress due to cleaning and sterilization induced balloon shrinkage after the first reprocessing cycle. Subsequent cleaning and sterilization did not induce further dimensional alterations. However these modifications did not affect the performance of the device because compliance tests showed the conformity of reprocessed balloons within the 10% limit of acceptance of manufacturers' original specifications. Anyway, the authors suggested that in case of PTCA catheter reprocessing, it would be profitable to introduce a new calibration curve, with new nominal diameter values. Slipperiness and friction patterns were strictly dependent on PTCA device manufacturer and model but the magnitude of modifications did not compromise in-vitro catheters functionality up to three uses (Fedel et al., 2006).

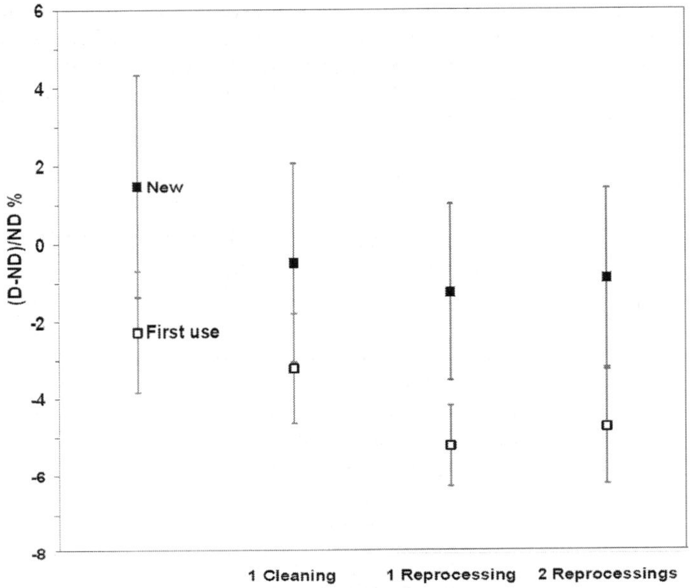

Fig. 4. Effects of cleaning and reprocessing on balloon working diameter (D) normalized to nominal specifications (ND). Data refer to new PTCA devices (full squares), and to products used once on patients (empty squares). The gap between new and used catheters could be caused by exceeding the nominal pressure during in vivo inflation. Both new and used catheters underwent a progressive shrinking after cleaning and first complete reprocessing. Adapted from Fedel et al., 2006.

4. Hygienic issues

Hygienic issue should consider a wide spectrum of microbiological tests at different steps of the reprocessing procedure. The bioburden after clinical use and decontamination should be quantified and decontamination-cleaning efficacy, pyrogenic load and device sterility have to be guaranteed. Pathogenic agents/substances include: bacteria in vegetative or sporulated form, fungi, viruses, microscopic parasites, and prions which are agents responsible for transmissible spongiform encephalopathies. Furthermore, endotoxins (which are part of the bacterial cell wall of Gram-negative bacteria and can be responsible for septic shock) may remain on a SUD even after sterilization as they have a very high resistance to disinfection or sterilization processes. A specific hazard is the possible contamination with agents causing transmissible spongiform encephalopathies as they are particularly resistant to commonly used physical and chemical methods of cleaning, disinfection and/or sterilization. The causative agent of these diseases consists of the pathogenic isoform of the prion protein, which is misfolded into an infectious agent. It is known that iatrogenic infection of Creutzfeldt-Jakob disease can occur in specific situations associated with medical interventions (Armitage et al. 2009). To date, processes ensuring a total inactivation of the transmissible spongiform encephalopathy agents are relatively aggressive precluding their application to materials used for the production of single-use medical devices (Fichet et al., 2004). Anyway, new association of chemical disinfection and low temperature gas plasma sterilization seemed are promising for prion inactivation from thermo-sensitive materials (Rogez-Kreutz et al., 2009).

4.1 Collection, cleaning and disinfection of used devices

Tessarolo et al. conducted cultural tests on patient-used catheters to determine and quantify the possible microbial species which could contaminate devices surfaces in clinical procedures (Tessarolo et al., 2004a). Cultural quantitative test on PTCA devices showed that 50% of the samples were contaminated after use with a microbial bioburden lower than 6 CFU per device (Table 1). Isolated genera were typical of the skin resident microbial flora. Equivalent test on clinically used catheters subjected to decontamination confirmed that inappropriate or untimely procedures might generate bacterial contamination and microbial dissemination in formerly sterile device's surfaces (Table 2). Moreover the use of low quality water might induce contaminations by environmental microorganisms.

Catheter	Bacterial Load/catheter	Isolated species	Notes
A	6 CFU	*Staphylococcus spp.* *Corynebacterium spp.* Aerobial sporigenes	-
B	5 CFU	*Staphylococcus spp.* Aerobial sporigenes	-
C	2 CFU	*Staphylococcus aureus*	-
D	5 CFU	*Staphylococcus spp.* *Corynebacterium spp.*	-
E	4 CFU	*Staphylococcus spp.* *Corynebacterium spp.*	Positive culture of the distal tip *Corynebacterium jeikeium*
F	1 UFC	*Staphylococcus. auricolaris*	Positive culture of the lumen eluate
G	sterile	-	-
H	sterile	-	-
I	sterile	-	-
L	sterile	-	-
M	sterile	-	-
N	sterile	-	-
Mean device	2 CFU		

Table 1. Bioburden on PTCA catheters immediately after use on patients. In 50% of the examined catheters showed the growth of typical resident microbial flora of the skin. A very low number of CFU per devices was revealed as outlined in the "mean devices" bacterial load.

Catheter	Bacterial Load/catheter	Isolated species	Notes
O	2 CFU	*Staphylococcus spp.* (CoNS)	
P	109 CFU	*Staphylococcus spp.*	Distal tip: *S. warneri* Lumen eluate: *S. auricolaris*
Q	2 CFU	*Staphylococcus warneri* *Staphylococcus hominis hominis*	-
R	11 CFU	*Staphylococcus warneri* *Staphylococcus spp.* (CoNS)	-
S	sterile	-	-
Mean device	**25 CFU**		

Table 2. Bioburden on PTCA catheters used on patients and decontaminated. A significantly higher number of CFU per device was revealed in respect to used but untreated devices (See Table 1). CoNS: Coagulase negative staphylococci

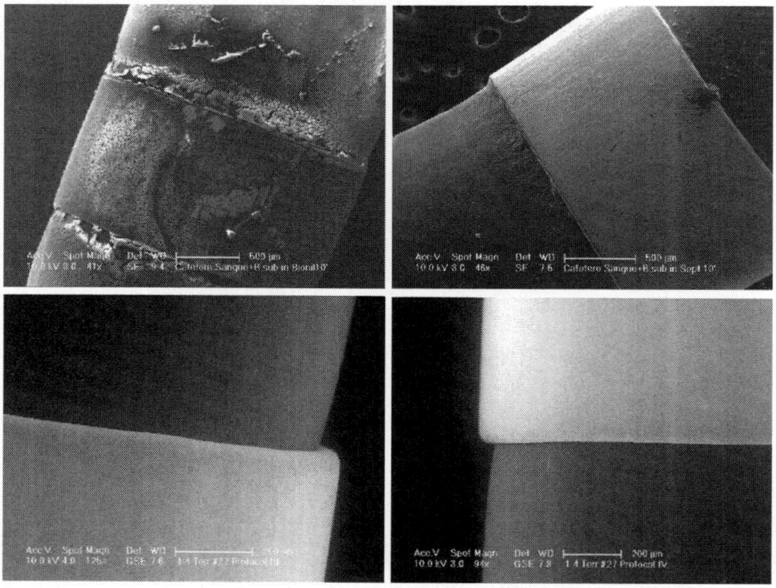

Fig. 5. Scanning Electron Microscopy on decontaminated and cleaned EP catheter by four different protocol: 1) chlorine-enzymatic solutions 2) enzymatic-chlorine solutions; 3) polyphenolic emulsion 4) polyphenolic plus enzymatic treatment. From top to bottom and from left to right is reported the electrode-shaft interface of catheter after protocol 1, 2, 3, and 4. Adapted from Tessarolo et al., 2004c and Tessarolo et al., 2007a.

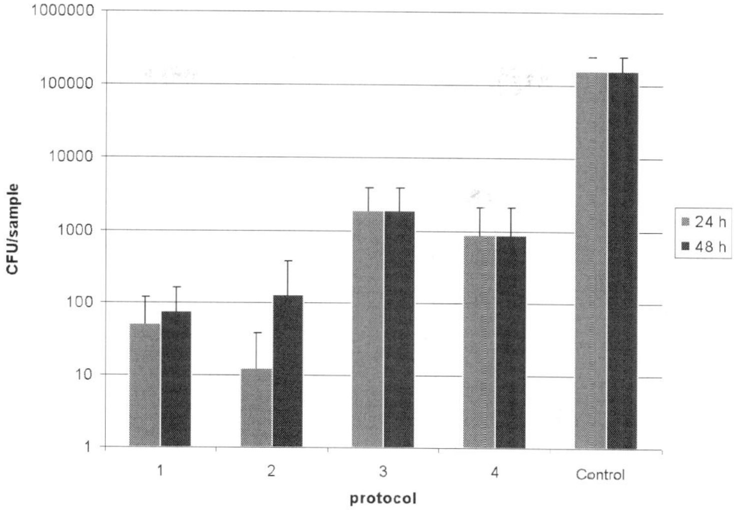

Fig. 6. Survival of *P. aeruginosa* after the exposure of the contaminated catheter shaft to the same four different protocol for decontamination and clearing described in Fig 5. Colony count was performed at 24 and 48 hours to evidence any eventual bacteriostatic effect. Initial bacterial load (conrol) was 1.6×10^5 CFU per catheter.

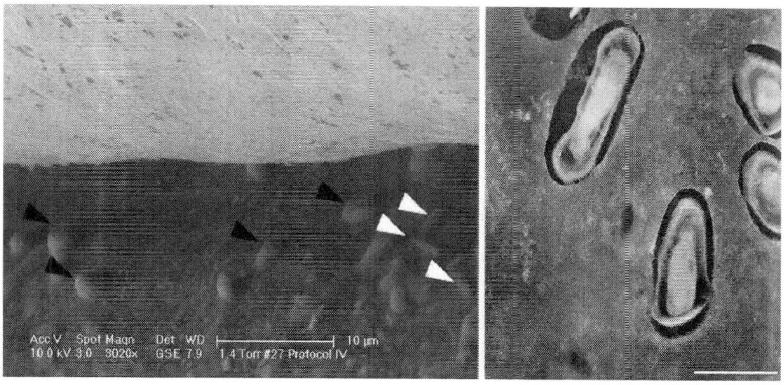

Fig. 7. Electron microscoscopy images of biologic residuals including *Bacillus subtilis* in catheters processed for resterilization. Left: Low-vacuum SEM at electrode-polymer interface showing bacterial shaped corpuscles embedded in the organic coating residual. Sporulated (black arrowheads) and vegetative (white arrowheads) forms of *B. subtilis* might be associated to this debris according to morphology and size. Right: TEM on a ultrathin section (bar is 1µm) of blood clot scraped from the catheter surface after treatment by polyphenolic solution and enzymatic detergent. The inclusion of B. subtilis in vegetative and sporulated forms are shown. TEM image was negative filtered. Adapted from Tessarolo et al. 2007a.

Since the efficacy of pre-sterilization device treatments is fundamental for sterilization success, different decontamination, disinfection and cleaning protocols were tested to identify biocide properties and cleaning effectiveness. Tessarolo and co-workers reported about 80 catheters samples, contaminated with bacteria-spiked human blood and subjected to different pre-sterilization protocols including chlorine releasing agent, polyphenolic emulsion, and enzymatic detergent (Tessarolo et al., 2004c; Tessarolo et al., 2007a). Treated samples were analysed by electron microscopy for biologic and inorganic residuals characterization, while cultural quantitative methods assessed chemicals' bactericidal effectiveness. Significant differences by using different chemicals were found. The use of chlorine solution as first treatment left relevant blood residuals on the exposed device surfaces while protocols including the polyphenolic emulsion, realized a deep cleaning of the surfaces with a very limited lasting bioburden (Fig. 5). Interaction and absorption of polyphenols on polymers has to be also considered for potential toxicity in re-use. Cultural quantitative methods showed the highest biocide properties of hypochlorous-acid based protocols while a lower bactericidal activity was documented for polyphenolic based solutions (Fig 6). Authors elicited the need to optimize both the disinfection efficiency and the biologic burden removal. It is also mandatory to provide for protecting the personnel from infectious agents. This threefold aim ask for defining structured protocols based on the synergic integration of mechanical and chemical agents.

Finally, the problem of pyrogenic risk related to reuse of single use devices, got in contact with blood, was specifically addressed (Tessarolo et al., 2006b). With this purpose the pyrogenic status of 61 catheters was monitored in three fundamental steps of the reprocessing protocol: untreated, after decontamination-cleaning procedure and after complete reprocessing. Endotoxin content was assayed by LAL test both after standard clinical use conditions and worst-case contamination by in-vitro high inocula endotoxins spiking. Experimental results demonstrated that standard clinical use did not represent a critical source of endotoxins contamination. Differently, the use of tap water and manual cleaning processing increased the pyrogenic load by introducing gram-negative microorganisms and by favouring bacterial growth on residual moisture. Microbiologically high quality water for limiting gram-negative contamination and overgrowth, is mandatory to avoid pyrogenic risk in reusing single use devices. Microbiological data suggested that the use of automated cleaning system instead of or in addition to manual device processing is more suitable for guaranteeing a reliable and standardized cleaning of complicated designs and sensitive materials.

4.2 Sterilization of processed SUDs

High-sensitive and reproducible sterility testing methodologies were developed by Tessarolo and co-workers to evaluate performances and limitations of a regeneration protocol for EP catheters (Tessarolo et al., 2006c). Devices were collected after clinical use on patient, underwent repeated cycles of simulated-use (bacteria spiked blood) and regeneration (decontamination, cleaning and sterilization), and were cultured for 28 days in trypticase soy broth. Sterility tests provided experimental evidences on 208 samples, six cycles of regeneration, and four inoculating bacteria species. Sterility investigations showed no positive sample to the inoculated strain until the fourth cycle of reprocessing (Table 3). The inoculated Bacillus subtilis strain was recovered in samples reprocessed five and six times. These results were in accordance with surface analysis which pointed out alterations on materials' properties that might favour bacterial persistence and limit reprocessing effectiveness after repeated reprocessing cycles. Hence, over-reuse of the devices could affect both safeness and efficacy as documented by sterility data and surface worsening after five reuses (Tessarolo et al., 2004b, Tessarolo et al., 2006c). Coming from experimental conditions conducted in worst case scenarios, this estimation of the maximum number of reprocessing cycles was precautionary.

Lot	Tested devices	Positive devices to inoculated strain	Positive devices to inoculated strain %
I regeneration	54	N.A.	N.A.
II regeneration	36	0	0%
III regeneration	24	0	0%
IV regeneration	28	0	0%
V regeneration	35	1	2.9%
VI regeneration	22	1	4.5%

Table 3. Sterility tests on EP catheters. Regeneration procedures were ineffective in restoring sterility of devices reused more than five times. Data are reported for 2nd to 6th regeneration after simulated in-vitro contamination by using bacterial spiked human blood (10^7 CFU/mL.). Due to first patient clinical use, data on possible contaminating species in I regeneration lot are not available (N.A.). Adapted from Tessarolo et al., 2006c.

5. The ethical and legal context

5.1 Juridical issues about reprocessing SUDs

There is no uniform policy governing the reuse of SUDs in the European Community. Finland, France, Germany, UK, Portugal, Spain and Sweden have all introduced various degrees of regulation (including a total ban) on refurbishing and reuse of SUDs. Despite this, the practice remains present in EU countries.

Directive 93/42/EEC on medical devices (MDD), adopted on 14 June 1993, stated that medical devices intended for single-use must bear on their label an indication that the device is for single-use. Directive 2007/47/EC, adopted on 5 September 2007, amending Directive 93/42/EEC, provided further clarification defining a "single-use" medical device as "a device intended to be used once only for a single patient". The Directive also introduced the requirement that if the device is for single-use, information on characteristics and technical factors known to the manufacturer that could pose a risk if the device were to be re-used must be provided in the instructions for use. According to the Directive and to national legislations of European countries, producers of medical devices are held to guarantee the number of times the product can be reused, assuming the complete liability during the whole life cycle. A disposable device ends its intended life after the first use so losing any manufacturer's responsibility for subsequent reuse. On the other hand, in most of European countries, no bans are clearly provided by the law for a reprocessor who intends to enter in the market proving a safe reuse of this kind of devices. The freedom of enterprise and the free competition, submitted to strict market regulation, could in fact promote competition and products improvement. Consequently, many European countries assumed that the certificate of conformity system should be extended to the reprocessor's activity, since CE mark is a guarantee for product compliance with all of the essential requirements for medical devices.

In the United Kingdom, France, Spain, and Switzerland, recommendations, legislation, or notes have been published forbidding or warning on the reuse of SUDs. Conversely, in Germany, the Medical Device Act does not ban the reprocessing of medical devices labelled for single use and advises users and institutions to use their own discretion. Therefore, catheters are processed for reuse in many hospitals in Germany. The regulative answer provided by the German legal system to reprocessing represents a possible balance between the need to maximize the efficiency of the health care system and the safeguard of patient health and safety. German legislation on matter of reprocessing comes from specific definitions in the MDD European directive transposition. In the German case, manufacturer's indication for "single usage" is not considerable in the notion of "intended purpose". This eliminates any implicit ban of reprocessing practice and avoids the assimilation of reprocessor to manufacturer, so considering the reprocessing activity differently from "fully refurbishing". Moreover reprocessing does not entail a placing of the device in the market since after process it is still delivered to the first purchaser who represents the effective owner. This fact allowed to not re-marking the devices with a new CE label. The third party reprocessor provides the possibility of unique identification and the re-delivering to the sole owner. However, according to German regulation, the reprocessor is not exempted from carrying on complex procedures for process control and validation.

The United States Food and Drug Administration increased its oversight of SUDs reprocessing gradually. On August 14, 2000, a new FDA policy entitled, "Enforcement Priorities for Single-Use Devices Reprocessed by Third Parties and Hospitals," was released to regulate third-party and hospital reprocessors of SUDs. Under the new guidelines, these reprocessors are considered device manufacturers. Therefore, third-party firms and reprocessing hospitals have to obtain pre-market approval (PMA) from the FDA for their products and are obligated to follow the same adverse-event reporting requirements (Medical Device Reporting) as OEMs.

The reprocessors, whether third-party firms or hospitals, are also required to register their establishment with the FDA, provide a list of devices they reprocess, establish a medical-device tracking system, conform to good manufacturing practice requirements, and follow general labelling requirements regarding the name and site of reprocessing and inclusion of adequate directions for use.

The Australian Government does not endorse the reuse of SUDs and requires informed consent from patients if a reprocessed device is to be used.

Reuse of SUDs was common practice in Canada before august 1996. At that time the government advised to discontinue the practice of reusing SUDs primarily because of concern about the potential risk of blood borne Creutzfeldt-Jakob disease. However, in Canada, there are no Federal or Provincial regulations governing the reuse of single-use medical devices. Currently, Health Canada does not regulate the reuse of medical devices by health care facilities or reprocessing of these devices by third-party reprocessors. The use or reuse of medical devices falls outside the governance of the Food and Drugs Act and the Medical Devices regulations. These acts have authority over the manufacture and sale of medical devices and were never intended as regulations over the use (including reuse) of such medical devices.

5.2 The ethical issue

From an ethical standpoint, two main aspects have to be considered: patients safety and distributive justice in allocating available resources. The focus of the concern should be upon the ethical obligation of all health care professionals/institutions to cause no harm or injury to their patients, but the issue is complicated by important considerations involving the appropriate allocation of increasingly scarce health resources. In an era of enormous restriction of resources in the health care system, the incentive to save money is a legitimate claim. From an ethical perspective, any wastefulness in unjustifiable in a health care system where a patient may be denied a service because a lack of resources, (CETSQ, 1994). As such, reuse may not be unethical so long as it is established that the quality of care is maintained and there is no significant loss of device effectiveness and no unreasonable increased risk of harm to the patient. Anyway, economic saving should not be at the expense of patient safety and the focus of any consideration of the practice of reuse must be the patient (NHMRC, 1997).

At the same time it is included in the ethical debate the importance to spread goods and technologies in less privileged countries. It was reported that in different health systems the risk/efficacy ratio could be substantially different and the most of the clinical work can be done with less technological support than that typically available in more affluent countries (Ruffy, 1995). On a secondary level, hospitals which reuse SUDs may be fulfilling their societal obligations to protect the environment through decreased landfill disposal, providing that the substituted cleaning and sterilization procedures are not of increased harm to the environment (CHA, 1996).

5.3 Patient's informed consent

Patients have the right to know and physician should not be reluctant to disclose information about reuse and reprocessing of single use devices to the patient. Both individual patients and public trust requires that openness is exercised and that the practice of reuse is not concealed in any way. A hospital's policy in this regard must therefore be public knowledge and clearly disclosed (CETSQ, 1994). However there are different opinions regarding the need for obtaining patient's consent about reusing SUDs. Usual ethical perspectives on informed consent could be grouped in two different positions.

The first concludes that patients should be always advised when reusing SUDs because the risk of this practice has not been adequately studied. Some ethicists believe, moreover, that the informed consent of a patient is ethically necessary, since there is an obligation on medical staff not to lie, deceive or otherwise interfere with a patient's free choice (Hall, 1991). This opinion is, in some points also reflected in the original equipment manufacturers (OEMs) position about SUDs reuse. Producer remarks that it is a basic principle of medical treatment that the patient should consciously agree to the form of treatment. It is OEMs' opinion that patient should be clearly told of all relevant factors, including the fact that he is to be treated with a reused single-use device contrary to the manufacturer's instructions, and that this may expose the patient to possible additional risks (EUCOMED, 2002).

The second ethicists' perspective concluded that the need to obtain informed consent for reused SUDs depends on if the physician believes there is an appreciable and significant risk for the patient. In this approach it is supposed that no substantial differences in safety and efficiency are imputable to reprocessed devices in respect to new ones. This perspective considers that the risk of a life-threatening or fatal complication during the clinical intervention is always present. As an example, in the case of electrophysiological studies, such a risk is in the range of 1:1000 (Horowitz, 1986). Conversely, the risk of reusing electrophysiological catheters appears to be so low that no reasonable estimate has been

identified yet. Relative to the overall risk of the procedure, the risk of reusing the devices might become insignificant.
It is in the opinion of the North America Society of Pacing and Electrophysiology (Lindsay et al., 2001) that, if the use of reprocessed EP devices is not associated with material and functional risk, then there is no ethical reason why this issue must be added to the long list of risks known to be associated with the procedure. Patients should be informed if they ask about the hospital's policy and they have the right to request that reprocessed catheter not be used. The decision to include this discussion when informed consent is obtained should be determined by the attending physician. If a patients objects to the use o a reused catheters it is up to the hospital to decide whether a new catheter will be provided or whether the patient will have to assume the risk of a delay in treatment until a new catheter became available in the course of routine (CETSQ, 1994).
A study on the patient acceptance of reused angioplasty equipment showed that a sufficient number (68%) of patients would be willing to permit reused PTCA devices (Vaitkus & Burlington, 1997). The same study pointed out that the disapproval by one third of patient raises the possibility of adverse publicity and litigation for institution implementing a reuse policy. However the perception of duplicity in medical care when informed consent is obtained is of particular concern.

6. Economic issues

6.1 Cost-minimization model

To estimate the potential saving for budgets of cardiology departments, a cost-minimization model was developed by Capri and colleagues (Capri et al. 2005) and applied to data pertaining to the Italian health system (Tessarolo et al., 2007b; Tessarolo et al., 2009). The model was developed in the hypothesis that reprocessing and reuse of SUDs is performed by guaranteeing safety and efficiency of the reconditioned device as high as the new one.
The model was used to describe the costs associated to catheters for interventional cardiology at departmental level in two different scenarios: single-use policy and re-use policy. Device reprocessing in case of reuse policy was designed by considering a third party professional reprocessor. Accordingly to the model, the single-use catheter's cost (c_K) was computed by the following expression:

$$c_K = P_K + S + \frac{G_K}{3N} \tag{1}$$

Where P_k is the new catheter price, S is the cost related to special waste disposal per single device, N is the total number of used catheters per year in the modelled cardiology department, and G_K is the cost for a competitive triennial contracts allocation of new devices. Differently, in case of reprocessing and reuse of cardiac catheters, the expression was modified as follows:

$$c_R = i\frac{P_K + (n-1)P_R}{n} + (1-i)P_K + \frac{S}{n} + C + \frac{G_K}{3N} + \frac{G_R}{3N} \tag{2}$$

Where c_R is the cost for n-times used device, i is the reprocessing rate, P_R is the reprocessing cost per catheter, n is the maximal number of uses sustainable by the catheter. Additional parameters were considered, as costs related to collection and handling of used catheter after each use (C), and costs for competitive triennial contracts allocation of reprocessing service (G_R). Potential saving, related to the introduction of a reprocessing SUDs policy, were eventually calculated by the following expression:

$$\text{Saving\%} = \frac{c_K - c_R}{c_K} \cdot 100 \tag{3}$$

6.2 Potential saving from SUDs reprocessing in interventional cardiology

Accordingly to previous finding on safety and effectiveness, the maximum number of uses (n) to enter in the cost-minimization model was set at 6 and 3 for EP and PTCA catheters respectively.

For a cardiology department with a median number of intervention (600 angioplasties and 200 electrophysiological studies per year) the model forecasted a potential saving of about 12% in the expenditure for PTCA catheter if reprocessing and reuse policy is adopted (Tessarolo et al., 2009). A markedly higher saving of about 41% and 33 % was computed for EP diagnostic and ablation procedures respectively. The sensitivity analysis on the three main variables, those are regeneration rate, number of uses, and catheter consumption per year, showed that significant differences in savings between EP and PTCA catheters reprocessing are mostly related to the annual catheter consumption that is proportional to cardiac department activity (Fig. 8). Major variations in savings occurred in the range between 1 and 200 catheters per year.

Percent savings generally grew as a function of regeneration rate (i) and maximum number of uses (n), but for high number of catheter usage per year (i.e. greater than 300) there was a tendency to a linear relation between percent savings and regeneration rate, while a plateau in percent saving was reached by increasing the maximum number of uses.

The economic analysis indicated that reuse of SUDs might be a source of savings for the cardiology department. However, the scaling to a specific working unit should be done cautiously. Since the cost saving depends on the number of devices used per year, regeneration might be economically unfavourable if a small number of clinical interventions is performed. The number of catheter used per year is therefore the most immediate parameter for establishing the cut off between benefits and charges in reprocessing SUDs. An additional critical point is the price of new device. Namely, decrease in the cost of new devices could sensibly modify potential saving and, in case of limited percents of benefits as PTCA catheters, a decrease in new device price could nullify the benefit of reprocessing (Capri et al., 2005). Moreover innovations in devices or reprocessing technology could affect the final savings by altering the maximum number of regenerations and the regeneration rate. Anyway, market dynamics forces to make stable the ratio between new catheter prices and regenerated device's cost, usually placed in the range of 0.4-0.5 by third party reprocessor.

Finally, quotes for patient's insurance and risk management should be introduced in the model, and more complex cost-effective analyses and decisional processes have to be applied in case reprocessed device is not as safe and effective as the new one (Sloan, 2007).

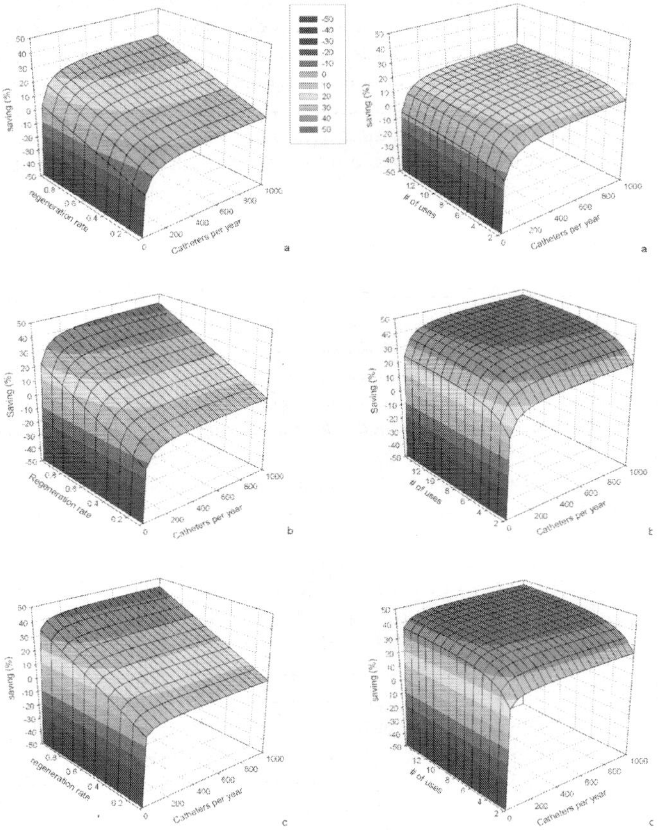

Fig. 8. Sensitivity analysis surface plots for potential percents saving of a reprocessing policy calculated according to the economic model. Left column: variation of the regeneration rate. The number of uses per catheter type has been set to 3, 6, and 6 for (a) PTCA, (b) EP diagnostic, and (c) EP ablation catheters respectively. Right column: variation of the number of uses. The regeneration rate per catheter type has been set to 0.48, 0.95, and 0.95 for (a) PTCA, (b) EP diagnostic, and (c) EP ablation catheters respectively. Adapted from Tessarolo et al., 2009.

7. Conclusions

From a technical and hygienic perspective the most efficient and safe reprocessing protocol should contemplate a unique and continuative solution, which provide for all the treatments starting from collection of used devices in cardiology departments to sterilization. This approach to regeneration, while assuring the best hygienic performances, requires devoted infrastructures, trained staff and specific knowledge. These technical considerations added to organizational, economic, and legal requirements connected to the need to qualify and certify all reprocessing procedures, suggest the introduction of this practice only in hospitals and health care structures with a significant workload. Anyway the more and more stringent criteria required by legislation and regulative policies underline the need for guaranteeing a certified reprocessing procedure, with the same quality issues supplied by the original manufacturers. These requirements may be unlikely achieved by small or medium hospitals, but could be affordable by relevant health care institutions or by third party industry reprocessors.

8. References

Armitage, WJ.; Tullo, AB. & Ironside JW. (2009). Risk of Creutzfeldt-Jakob disease transmission by ocular surgery and tissue transplantation. *Eye.* 23, 1926-1930.

Aton, EA.; Murray, P.; Fraser, V.; Conaway, L. & Cain ME. (1994). Safety of reusing cardiac electrophysiology catheters. *American Journal of Cardiology*, 74, 1173-1175.

Avitall, B.; Khan, M.; Krum, D.; Jazayeri, M. & Hare, J. (1993). Repeated use of ablation catheters: a prospective study. *Journal of the American College of Cardiology*, 22, 367-372.

Ayzman, I.; Dibs, SR.; Goldberger, J.; Passman, R. & Kadish, A. (2002). In vitro performance characteristics of reused ablation catheters. *Journal of Interventional Cardiac Electrophysiology*, 7, 53-59.

Bloom, DF.; Cornhill, JF.; Malchesky, PS.; Richardson, DM.; Bolsen, KA.; Haire, DM. et al. (1997). Technical and economic feasibility of reusing disposable perfusion cannulas. *Journal of Thoracic & Cardiovascular Surgery*, 114, 448-460.

Blomstrom-Lundqvist, C. (1998). The safety of reusing ablation catheters with temperature control and the need for a validation protocol and guidelines for reprocessing. *Pacing & Clinical Electrophysiology*, 21, 2563-2570.

Bourassa, MG. (1996). The reuse of single use balloon angioplasty catheters:it is now legitimate? *The American Journal of Cardiology*, 78, 673-674.

Brown, SA.; Merritt, K.; Woods, TO. & Hitchins, VM. (2001). The effects of use and simulated reuse on percutaneous transluminal coronary angioplasty balloons and catheters. *Biomedical Instrumentation and Technology*, 35, 312-322.

Browne, KF.; Maldonado, R.; Telatnik, M.; Vlietstra, RE & Brenner AS. (1997). Initial experience with reuse of coronary angioplasty catheters in the United States. *Journal of the American College of Cardiology*, 30, 1735-1740.

Capri, S.; Ferrari, P.; Tessarolo, F.; Guarrera, GM.; Fontana, F. & G Nollo. (2005). Modello di calcolo della convenienza economica per l'ospedale: il caso dei cateteri cardiaci rigenerabili vs. i cateteri monouso. *Politiche Sanitarie*, 6, 188-196.

CCHR. (2000). Reuse of single use devices. Hearing before the Subcommittee on Oversight and Investigations of the Committee on Commerce House of Representative. Serial n°106-89. Attacchmnent C, 138. February 10, 2000. US Government Printing Office Washington, 2000.

CETSQ. (1994). Conseil d'Evaluation des Technologies de la Santé du Quebec. The reuse of single use cardiac catheters: safety, economical, ethical and legal issues. *Canadian Journal of Cardioloy*, 10, 413-421.

CHA. (1996). Canadian Hospital Association. The reuse of single-use medical devices. Available at: http://sprojects.mmi.mcgill.ca/heart/carecha2ca.html.

Chan, AC.; Ip, M.; Koehler, A.; Crisp, B.; Tam, JS. & Chung, SC. (2000). Is it safe to reuse disposable laparoscopic trocars? An in vitro testing. *Surgical Endoscopy*, 14, 1042-1044.

Chaufour, X.; Deva, AK.; Vickery, K.; Zou, J.; Kumaradeva, P.; White, GH. & Cossart, YE. (1999). Evaluation of disinfection and sterilization of reusable angioscopes with the duck hepatitis B model. *Journal of Vascular Surgery*, 30, 277-282.

Daggan, R.; Zefeiridis, A.; Steinberg, D.; Larijani, G.; Gratz, I. & Goldberg, ME. (1999). High-quality filtration allows reuse of anesthesia breathing circuits resulting in cost savings and reduced medical waste. *Journal of Clinical Anesthesia*, 11, 536-539.

Day, P. (2004). What is the evidence on the safety and effectiveness of the reuse of medical devices labelled as single-use only? *New Zeland Health Technology Assessment, Technical Brief Series*, 3.

Dunnigan, A.; Roberts, C.; McNamara, M.; Benson, DW. & Benditt, DG. (1987). Success of re-use of cardiac electrode catheters. *American Journal of Cardiology*, 60, 807-810.

EUCOMED. (2002). Patients in danger: the reuse of single use medical devices in Europe. June 2002.

Fedel, M.; Tessarolo, F.; Ferrari, P.; Lösche, C.; Ghassemieh, N.; Guarrera, GM. & Nollo G. (2006). Functional Properties and Performance of New and Reprocessed Coronary Angioplasty Balloon Catheters. *Journalof Biomedical Materiasl Research B Applied Biomaterials*, 78, 364-372.

Fichet, G.; Comoy, E.; Duval, C.; Antloga, K.; Dehen, C.; Charbonnier, A. et al. (2004). Novel methods for disinfection of prion-contaminated medical devices. *Lancet*, 364, 521-526.

GAO. (2000). US General Accounting Office. GAO Report: single-use medical devices: little available evidence of harm from reuse, but oversight warranted. June 20, 2000.

GAO. (2008). US General Accounting Office. GAO Report: Reprocessed single-use medical devices. FDA oversight has increased, and available information does not indicate that use presents an elevated health risk. January 31, 2008.

Granados, DL.; Jimenez, A. & Cuadrado, TR. (2001). Assessment of parameters associated to the risk of PVC catheter reuse. *Journal of Biomedical Materials Research*, 58, 505-510.

Hall, W. (1991). Ethical issues in the reuse of single-use medical products. In *"Reuse of single-use medical devices: reviewing the issues"*. Chatswood, NSW: Medical Industry Association of Australia Inc., pp. 45-49.

Hambrick, D. (2001). Reprocessing of single-use endoscopic biopsy forceps and snares. One hospital's study. *Gastroenterology Nursing*, 24, 112-115.

Horowitz, LN. (1986). Safety of electrophysiology studies. *Circulation*, 73, 28-31.

Kinney, TP.; Kozarek, RA.; Raltz, S. & Attia, F. (2002). Contamination of single-use biopsy forceps: a prospective in vitro analysis. *Gastrointestinal Endoscopy*, 56, 209-212.

Kozarek, RA.; Raltz, SL.; Ball, TJ.; Patterson, DJ. & Brandabur, JJ. (1999). Reuse of disposable sphincterotomes for diagnostic and therapeutic ERCP: a one-year prospective study. *Gastrointestinal Endoscopy*, 49, 39-42.

Lindsay, BD.; Kutalek, SP.; Cannom, DS.; Hammill, SC. & Naccarelli, GV. (2001). NASPE policy statement. Reprocessing of electrophysiology catheters: clinical studies, regulations, and recommendations. A report of the NASPE Task Force on Reprocessing of Electrophysiological Catheters. *Pacing & Clinical Electrophysiology*, 24, 1297-1305.

Lipp, MD.; Jaehnichen, G.; Golecki, N.; Fecht, G.; Reichl, R. & Heeg, P. (2000). Microbiological, microstructure, and material science examinations of reprocessed combitubes after multiple reuse. *Anesthesia & Analgesia*, 91, 693-697.

Luijt, DS.; Schirm, J.; Savelkoul, PHM. & Hoekstra, A. (2001). Risk of infection by reprocessed and resterilized virus-contaminated catheters: an in-vitro study. *European Heart Journal*, 22, 378-384.

Ma, N.; Petit, A.; Huk, OL.; Yahia, L. & Tabrizian, M. (2003). Safety issue of re-sterilization of polyurethane electrophysiology catheters: a cytotoxicity study. *Journal of Biomaterials Science, Polymer Edition*, 14, 213-226.

Mak, KH.; Eisenberg, MJ.; Plante, S.; Strauss, BH.; Arheart, KL. & Topol, EJ. (1996). Absence of increased in-hospital complications with reused balloon catheters. *American Journal of Cardiology*, 78, 717-719.

NHMRC. (1997). National Health and Medical Research Council. Report of the NHMRC expert panel on re-use of medical devices labelled as single use. Canberra: Commonwealth of Australia, 1997.

O'Donoghue, S. & Platia, EV. (1988). Reuse of pacing catheters: a survey of safety and efficacy. *Pacing & Clinical Electrophysiology*, 11, 1279-1280.

Plante, S.; Strauss, BH.; Goulet, G.; Watson, RK. & Chisholm RJ. (1994). Reuse of balloon catheters for coronary angioplasty: a potential cost-saving strategy? *Journal of the American College of Cardiology*, 24, 1475-1481.

Polisena, J.; Hailey, D.; Moulton, K.; Noorani HZ.; Jacobs, P.; Ries, N. et al. (2008). Reprocessing and reuse of single-use medical devices: a national survey of Canadian acute-care hospitals. *Infection Control and Hospital Epidemiology*, 29, 437-439.

Quian, Z. & Castaneda WR. (2002). Can labelled single use devices be reused? An old question in the new era. *Journal of the Vascular Interventional Radiology*, 13, 1183-1186.

Roth, K.; Heeg, P. & Reichl, R. (2002). Specific hygiene issues relating to reprocessing and reuse of single-use devices for laparoscopic surgery. *Surgical Endoscopy*, 16, 1091-1097.

Rozenman, Y. & Gotsman, MS. (1995). Reuse of balloon catheters for coronary angioplasty *Journal of the American College of Cardiology*, 26, 840-841.

Ruffy, R. (1995). Catheter ablation in a less privileged country: the importance of spreading the goods. *Pacing & Clinical Electrophysiology*, 18, 1463-1464

Rogez-Kreuz, C.; Yousfi, R.; Soufflet, C.; Quadrio, I.; Yan, ZX.; Huyot, V. et al. (2009). Inactivation of animal and human prions by hydrogen peroxide gas plasma sterilization. *Infection Control and Hospital Epidemiology*, 30, 769-777.

Shaw, JP.; Eisenberg, MJ.; Azoulay, A. & Nguyen N. (1999). Reuse of catheters for percutaneous transluminal coronary angioplasty effects on procedure time and clinical outcomes. *Catheterization &Cardiovascular Interventions*. 48, 54-60.

Sloan, TW. (2007). Safety-cost trade-offs in medical device reuse: a Markov decision process model. *Health Care Manage Science*, 10:81–93.

Tessarolo, F.; Fedel, M.; Ferrari, P.; Caola, I ; Guarrera, GM.; Favaretti, C.; Migliaresi, C. & Nollo, G. (2004a). Reuse of single use devices for interventional cardiology: a HCTA approach. *IFMBE Proceedings*, 6.

Tessarolo, F.; Ferrari, P.; Nollo, G.; Motta, A.; Migliaresi, C.; Zennaro, L. et al. (2004b). Evaluation and quantification of reprocessing modification in single use devices in interventional cardiology. *Applied Surface Science*, 238, 341-346.

Tessarolo, F.; Caola, I.; Fedel, M.; Caciagli, P.; Guarrera, GM.; Nollo, G. (2004c). Effects of chlorine-releasing compounds on medical devices decontamination. *Journal of Applied Biomaterials and Biomechanics*, 2, 219.

Tessarolo, F.; Ferrari, P.; Antolini, R. & Nollo, G. (2005). Radiofrequency ablation on heart-equivalent phantom. Functionality testing of percutaneous single-use catheter. In: *Recent Advances in Multidisciplinary Applied Physics*, Mendez-Vilas A. ed., Elsevier; pp. 229-234.

Tessarolo, F.; Fedel, M.; Nollo, G. & Motta, A. (2006a). A novel phantom for the in-vitro quantification of electrophysiology catheter slipperiness: implementation and testing. *Journal of Applied Biomaterials and Biomechanics*, 4, 70.

Tessarolo, F.; Caola, I.; Nollo, G.; Antolini R.; Guarrera, GM. & Caciagli, P. (2006b). Efficiency in endotoxins removal by a reprocessing protocol for electrophysiology catheters based on hydrogen peroxide sterilization. *Journal of Hygiene and Environmental Health*, 209, 557-565.

Tessarolo, F.; Caola, I.; Caciagli, P.; Guarrera, GM. & Nollo, G. (2006c). Sterility and microbiological assessment in reusing single-use cardiac electrophysiology catheters. *Infection Control and Hospital Epidemiology*, 27, 1385-1392.

Tessarolo, F.; Caola, I.; Fedel, M.; Caciagli, P.; Guarrera, GM.; Motta, A. & Nollo, G. (2007a). Different protocols for decontamination affect cleaning of medical devices. A preliminary electron microscopy analysis. *Journal of Hospital Infection*, 65, 326-333.

Tessarolo, F.; Disertori, M.; Caola, I.; Guarrera, GM.; Favaretti, C. & Nollo, G. (2007b). Health technology assessment on reprocessing single-use catheters for cardiac electrophysiology: results of a three-years study. *Conference Proceeding IEEE Engineering in Medicine and Biology Society*, 2007, 1758-1761.

Tessarolo, F.; Disertori, M.; Guarrera, GM.; Capri, S. & Nollo, G. (2009). Reprocessing single use cardiac catheters for interventional cardiology. Potential savings at the laboratory scale and at national level. *International Journal of Public Health*, 6, 38-47.

Unverdorben, M.; Degenhardt, R.; Erny, D.; Scholz, M.; Wagner, E.; Kohler, et al. (2005). Clinical and angiographic procedural and mid-term outcome with new versus reused balloon catheters in percutaneous coronary interventions. *Indian Heart Journal*, 57, 114-120.

Vaiktus, P. & Burlington, VT. (1997). Patients acceptance of reused angioplasty equipment. *American Heart Journal* 134, 127-130.

Vezina, DP.; Trepanier, CA.; Lessard, MR.; Gourdeau, M. & Tremblay C. (2001). Anaesthesia breathing circuits protected by the DAR Barrierbac S breathing filter have a low bacterial contamination rate. *Canadian Journal of Anaesthesia*, 48, 748-754.

Zubaid, M.; Thomas, CS.; Salman, H.; Al-Rashdan, I.; Hayat, N.; Habashi, A. et al. (2001). A randomized study of the safety and efficacy of reused angioplasty balloon catheters. *Indian Heart Journal*, 53, 167-171.

Krause, G.; Dziekan, G. & Daschner, FD. (2000). Reuse of coronary angioplasty balloon catheters: yes or no? *European Heart Journal*, 21, 185-189.